The Specialty Practice of
Rehabilitation Nursing

A Core Curriculum
Fourth Edition

Editor

Patricia A. Edwards, EdD RN CNAA
Nurse Educator, Graduate Nursing
Regents College
Albany, NY

Rehabilitation Nursing Consultant, Private Practice
Greenfield Center, NY

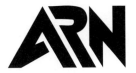

Association of Rehabilitation Nurses
4700 W. Lake Avenue • Glenview, IL 60025-1485
800/229-7530, 847/375-4710 • Fax 847/375-6310
E-mail info@rehabnurse.org • Web site http://www.rehabnurse.org

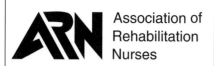

Association of Rehabilitation Nurses

STAFF

Executive Director
Anne Cordes

Director of Communications
Dot Vartan

Managing Editor
Nancy Poore

Copy Editor
Phoebe King

Graphic Designer
Eric Trisilla

Editorial Assistant
Heather Forkos

Cover Design
Jodi Cook

Library of Congress Catalog Card Number: 00-190797
ISBN 1-884278-11-6

Note. As new scientific information becomes available through basic and clinical research, recommended treatments and drug therapies undergo changes. The authors, editors, and publisher have done everything possible to make this book accurate, up-to-date, and in accord with standards accepted at the time of publication. The authors, editors, and publisher are not responsible for errors or omissions or for consequences from application of the book and make no warranty, expressed or implied, in regard to the contents of the book. Any practice described in this book should be applied by the healthcare practitioner in accordance with professional standards of care used in regard to the unique circumstances that may apply in each situation. The reader is advised always to check product information (package inserts) for changes and new information regarding dose and contraindications before administering any drug. Caution is especially urged when using new or infrequently ordered drugs or treatments.

This volume contains many references and resources utilizing Internet addresses. Although these sites were current at the time of research, writing, and/or publication, many Internet postings are volatile and subject to expiration or deletion over time. Therefore, ARN cannot guarantee currency of electronic references. (Readers who wish to pursue the latest information on a cited topic are likely to find new or updated postings via online search engines.)

Last digit is the print number: 9 8 7 6 5 4 3

Foreword

It is an honor to write a foreword for this vital and influential publication. In the past 20 years, the Association of Rehabilitation Nurses has published four editions of this core curriculum. The evolution of rehabilitation nursing as a specialty practice can clearly be seen from edition to edition. The first edition, *Rehabilitation Nursing: Concepts and Practice: A Core Curriculum,* was the result of a 1977 directive by a very young ARN to identify and commit to paper the central body of rehabilitation nursing knowledge. Editor Shannon Sayles, MSN RN, and a group of regional editors took on the daunting task of writing the first edition in 1981. From the beginning, a conceptual focus, rather than a disease-oriented model, was used as a guiding framework. The first edition was dedicated to "individuals with a disability and to their families—it is hoped that their care will be enhanced as a result of this effort."

In 1987, the second edition of *Rehabilitation Nursing: Concepts and Practice* was developed and edited by Christina M. Mumma, PhD RN CS CRRN, and her associate editors. This ambitious work expanded on the work of the original core, using nursing process and nursing diagnoses as its conceptual framework. This edition also incorporated the newly developed Rehabilitation Nursing Standards of Practice. Chapters covered legislative involvement, quality assurance, research, healthcare economics, and educational preparation, and continued learning for rehabilitation nurses. This second edition was dedicated to "rehabilitation nurses, in recognition of their commitment to individuals with disability, the families of those individuals, their colleagues, and their profession." The first stanza of Robert Frost's poem *"Stopping by Woods on a Snowy Evening"* served as a metaphorical description of the commitment of those who contributed to this body of work and as a reflection of the dedication of rehabilitation nurses everywhere. The continuing evolution of future editions of the core curriculum was predicted "as rehabilitation nursing knowledge develops and expands."

That evolution was reflected in the 1993 publication, *The Specialty Practice of Rehabilitation Nursing: A Core Curriculum(3rd ed.).* This edition was dedicated to "those who have made rehabilitation nursing a specialty practice." Under the leadership of Ann E. McCourt, RN, MS, this third edition emphasized the use of functional health patterns as an organizing framework for clinical practice issues. Chapters on functional health patterns promoted in-depth discussion of relevant theory and identified common nursing diagnoses, interventions and outcomes. A section on common neuromuscular disorders whose sequelae produce health problems treated by rehabilitation nurses was added. Additional content on ethics, economics, healthcare legislation, and the role of the rehabilitation nurse case manager reflected the expansion of rehabilitation nursing practice. Research works were highlighted in the reference lists, in keeping with the specialty's growing emphasis on research.

Those responsible for this fourth edition of ARN's core curriculum carry the torch of rehabilitation nursing knowledge into a new millennium. Edited by Patricia A. Edwards, EdD RN CNAA, *The Specialty Practice of Rehabilitation Nursing: A Core Curriculum (4th ed.)* has a strong focus on community, family, and rehabilitation across the life continuum. It includes content on ethical, legal, and moral considerations, and supplies much-needed information about cardiovascular and pulmonary rehabilitation, acute and chronic pain, economics and health policy, the delivery and evaluation of rehabilitation services, and the impact of information technology and computer applications. A growing emphasis on nursing research is reflected in this edition in the form of research perspectives. These sidebars summarize a research work and suggest implications for rehabilitation nursing practice.

Although the content of successive editions has changed to reflect research findings, practice changes, and new roles for rehabilitation nurses, the commitment of rehabilitation nurses to share knowledge that will improve the lives of people with disabilities is an enduring constant. Hundreds of ARN members have made contributions to this effort. Each edition is a tribute to the vision and courage of ARN's founding leaders, to the leadership of editors Shannon Sayles, Christina M. Mumma, Ann E. McCourt, and Patricia A. Edwards, and to the work of the associate editors, authors, and reviewers who have devoted countless hours to help each edition become a reality. The pioneers responsible for the first core curriculum charted new territory, commenting that " a commencement has been made and a future exists." That future is contained within the pages of this book.

—*Maureen Habel, MA RN CRRN*
July 2000

Preface

As we begin the 21st century, we face numerous daily challenges as professional nurses. It is imperative that we maintain current knowledge about all facets of rehabilitation and use our abilities to the fullest in creating a healthy environment for our clients.

This newest edition of the Association of Rehabilitation Nurses (ARN) core curriculum is a comprehensive guide, designed to assist both new and experienced nurses who practice rehabilitation in any setting. It is an authoritative resource for the rehabilitation component of nursing practice, a text for individuals learning or teaching rehabilitation nursing, and a resource for preparing for the Certified Rehabilitation Registered Nurse (CRRN) examination. The fourth edition was conceived and designed as a Year 2000 epitome of what rehabilitation nursing is and where it is going in the new millennium.

In 1998, the ARN Board of Directors recognized the need for a review of the core curriculum and appointed a task force to do an in-depth examination of the third edition. That group, chaired by Shirley Hoeman, was composed of rehabilitation nurses with a variety of backgrounds. The task force members, Lisa Cyr Buchanan, Nancy Dayhoff, Deirdre Jackson, Suzanne MacAvoy, Jeanne Mervine, Judy Salter, and Nancy Sislow, reviewed sections of the basic core based on their areas of expertise and interest. They also reviewed the entire core curriculum to assess timeliness, scope, and breadth of the publication regarding format, conceptual framework, organization, and content.

The task force recommended that the third edition be revised and that additional content be added to reflect the advances and changes in rehabilitation nursing practice. As a result of their extensive review, they suggested that the core curriculum required more content about pediatrics, family, home health care, and community re-entry. They also recommended expanding or providing content in areas such as gerontology, common disorders encountered by rehabilitation nurses in practice, and outcome measures. They felt that this publication should focus on current practice with an eye to the future, while keeping in mind the purpose of the core curriculum, which is to provide the basic information a nurse needs to know to practice rehabilitation in any setting. Additionally, the task force identified the importance of reformatting and reorganizing the topics to provide a more futuristic look.

My first task as editor was to develop a content outline for the new edition based on these recommendations and input from other rehabilitation nurse colleagues. With this edition, a number of new features have been added, including research perspectives within six of the chapters, special teaching boxes, online references and resources, and an appendix that contains case studies with accompanying thought-provoking questions. Logistically, the book is divided into six sections that employ both narrative and outline formats. The narrative format is used to enhance the readability of broad general topics as well as introduce each chapter. The outline format is used extensively to present scientific data and to show the hierarchy of information under each topic, and to aid in teaching and learning. Throughout the book, the terms *patient* and *client* are used interchangeably and the term *family* includes significant others.

To introduce the reader to the specialty, **Section I** provides a broad overview of the philosophy, goals, and process of rehabilitation and examines the roles, educational preparation, and competencies for the practice of rehabilitation nursing. This section includes a focus on the shift in care delivery to the community and the importance of family-centered nursing. An overview of ethical and moral issues and legal considerations frequently encountered in rehabilitation nursing practice is included, as well as a review of the important issues related to the economics of healthcare delivery and policy development.

Section II focuses on the clinical practice of rehabilitation nursing and begins with an overview of neuroanatomy that provides the foundation for discussing specific nursing interventions. Functional health patterns are a unifying framework, with chapters on health maintenance and management of the therapeutic regimen, physical healthcare patterns and psychosocial healthcare patterns. The concepts of health promotion and disease prevention are included, and emphasis is placed on identifying problems that result from the disruption of physical, and psychosocial healthcare patterns and promoting health over the life span.

Section III contains new material that will improve and update knowledge relating to stroke, traumatic brain injury, spinal cord injury and musculoskeletal disorders. Three new chapters provide information about cardiovascular and pulmonary rehabilitation, acute and chronic pain, and a number of specific disease processes, including diabetes mellitus, Parkinson's disease, multiple sclerosis, HIV/AIDS, burns, and cancer.

Section IV provides an overview of individual human development, family development, and functioning across the life span. Issues specific to children with rehabilitation needs and their families, as well as the special knowledge and training rehabilitation nurses need to meet the demands of an aging society, are described in two specialized chapters.

The changing environment in which rehabilitation nursing is practiced and the changing role of rehabilitation nurses in all healthcare settings led to the inclusion of **Section V**, which addresses the delivery and evaluation of rehabilitation services. Models of care and service delivery are described, and rehabilitation environments throughout the continuum of care are contrasted. Outcomes of care in rehabilitation are examined and data collection tools are described. The impact of information technology and the range of computer applications used in health care are reviewed, and the reader is introduced to computer technology and resources.

The concluding chapters in **Section VI** detail the changes in health care and their implications for rehabilitation so that nurses are more prepared to move across settings and meet the needs of individuals of any age with a disability or chronic illness. The last chapter chronicles the history of rehabilitation and includes a glimpse into the future through the eyes of a group of prominent rehabilitation nurses. Historical information may not be seen as essential for entering the specialty, but it does provide a very helpful perspective on past accomplishments and goals to be set for the future. This book concludes with appendixes that contain case studies that cover a variety of ages, problems, and issues, and lists of community resources and health-related organizations.

—Patricia A. Edwards, EdD RN CNAA, Editor
July 2000

Acknowledgments

The development of the fourth edition of this core curriculum was a complete team effort, accomplished through the combined knowledge and total commitment of 29 chapter authors and 37 reviewers. It has been a pleasure to work with these dedicated rehabilitation nurses who have expended their energy to produce timely, comprehensive chapters and provide thoughtful critiques to enhance each chapter's content. I have also been very fortunate to work with Carol Dikelsky, an extremely competent project coordinator, who was my guide through the whole process and made my job so much easier.

Dedication

To the spirit and energy of rehabilitation nurses everywhere who have created a body of knowledge and who will chart the course of our practice in the new millennium.

Authors

Chapters and Case Studies

Penny A. Adsit, MHSA BSN RN CRRN
Specialist, Research/Protocol
Shriners Hospitals
Greenville, SC

Maria J. Amador, BSN RN CRRN
Nurse Specialist
The Miami Project to Cure Paralysis
University of Miami School of Medicine
Miama, FL

Terrie Black, MBA BSN RN BC CRRN
Rehabilitation Consultant
Hospital for Special Care
New Britain, CT
and FIM Trainer–Uniform Data System for Medical
  Rehabilitation
Buffalo, NY

Barbara Brillhart, PhD RN CRRN FNP-C
Associate Professor
Arizona State University, College of Nursing
Tempe, AZ

Teresa A. Bryan, BSN RN CRRN
Nurse Manager
Craig Hospital
Englewood, CO

Lynn M. Carbone, BSN RN CRRN
Clinical Supervisor, Level III
St. Joseph's Regional Medical Center
South Bend, IN

Karen Cervizzi, MSN RN CRRN CAN
Nurse Educator/Infection Control Coordinator
HealthSouth Saint Joseph's Healthcare Center
Lowell, MA

Kelly Coleman, RN CRRN
Unit Manager
Shepherd Center
Atlanta, GA

Marjorie J. Culbertson, MSE MSN RN CS
Instructor of Nursing
Medical College of Ohio, School of Nursing
Toledo, OH

Anne Deutsch, MS RN CRRN
Research Associate
Uniform Data System for Medical Rehabilitation
  and Adjunct Instructor
State University of New York at Buffalo,
School of Nursing
Buffalo, NY

Kristen L. Mauk, PhD RN CRRN-A APRN
Assistant Professor of Nursing
Valparaiso University
and Community Health Education Director
Porter Memorial Hospital
Valparaiso, IN

Patricia A. Edwards, EdD RN CNAA
Nurse Educator
Regents College
Albany, NY

Jenecia Fairfax, PhD RN
Instructor, Community Health Nursing
Medical College of Ohio, School of Nursing
Toledo, OH

Cynthia Kraft Fine, MSN RN CRRN
Program Director
Magee Rehabilitation Hospital
Philadelphia, PA

Patricia Ann Haldi, MN RN CRRN CDE
Certified Diabetes Educator
Saint Luke's Rehabilitation Institute
Spokane, WA

Judy A. Harris, MS BSN RN CRRN CRC CCM LHCRM
Nurse, Case Manager
Florida State University, School of Nursing,
Graduate Program
Tallahassee, FL

Dalice Hertzberg, MSN RN CRRN
Instructor
JFK Partners and the School of Nursing
University of Colorado Health Sciences Center
Denver, CO

Carla J. Howard, MS RN CRRN
Clinical Nurse Manager
Parkview Center for Rehabilitation–Parkview Medical
Center
Pueblo, CO

Barbara A. Naden, MSN RN CRRN GNP
Clinical Nurse II
Kernan Hospital
Baltimore, MD

Carol Ann Ottey, MSN RNC CRRN
Nurse Practitioner
The Reading Hospital School of Nursing
Reading, PA

Bonnie J. Parker, MSN RN CRRN
Medical/Legal Nurse Consultant
Waterford, VA

Linda L. Pierce, PhD RNC CRRN CNS
Associate Professor
Medical College of Ohio, School of Nursing
Toledo, OH

Patricia A. Quigley, PhD CRRN ARNP
Rehabilitation Clinical Nurse Specialist
Associate Director, Clinical Division, Patient Safety
    Center–VISN 8
James A. Haley Veterans Hospital
Tampa, FL
and Faculty Member
University of Phoenix, College of Nursing
Phoenix, AZ

Rhonda J. Reed, MSN RN CRRN
Instructor and Learning Resources Center
    Technology Coordinator
Indiana State University, School of Nursing
and PRN Staff Nurse
Union Hospital, Medical Rehabilitation
Terre Haute, IN

Suzanne T. Rogers, MA RN CRRN
Clinical Nurse Specialist
HealthSouth New England Rehabilitation Hospital
Woburn, MA

Lyn R. Sapp, BSN RN CRRN
Rehabilitation Department
Children's Hospital and Regional Medical Center
Seattle, WA

Mary Ann Sawalski, MSEd BSN RN CRRN
Consultant/Educator
Lexington Health Care
Lombard, IL

Janet A. Secrest, PhD RN
Assistant Professor
University of Tennessee–Chattanooga
Chattanooga, TN

Linda Dufour, MSN RN CRRN
Clinical Nurse Specialist
Shepherd Center
Atlanta, GA

Teresa L. Thompson, PhD RN CRRN-A
Assistant Professor
Oakland University, School of Nursing
Rochester, MI

Kay Viggiani, MS RN CS
Associate Professor of Nursing
Keuka College
Keuka Park, NY

Joan Williams, MSN RN CRRN ARNP-C
Nurse Practitioner
Jackson Memorial Medical Center
Miami, FL

Reviewers

Chapter 1: Rehabilitation and Rehabilitation Nursing

Rose Butler, MS RNC CRRN CCM
Education Coordinator
Brooks Health System
Jacksonville, FL

Sue Sheridan, BSN RN CRRN
Director of Education
Kethley House at Benjamin Rose Place
Cleveland, OH

Chapter 2: Community and Family-Centered Rehabilitation Nursing

Leslie J. Neal, PhD RNC CRRN CS
Assistant Professor
Marymount University
Arlington, VA

Lois Schaetzle, MS RN CRRN
Rehabilitation Manager
Centura Porter Adventist Hospital
Denver, CO

April Struck, BSN RN
Regis University Case Manager
Boulder Manor's Progressive Care Center
Boulder, CO

Chapter 3: Ethical, Moral, and Legal Considerations

Judy Harris, MS BSN RN CRRN CRC CCM LHCRM
Healthy Start/ FSU
Tallahassee, FL

Sherry Liske, MS RN CRRN
Senior Clinical Nurse
Rush Presbyterian–St. Luke's Medical Center
Chicago, IL

Chapter 4: Economics and Health Policy in Rehabilitation

Carol Gleason, MM RN CRRN CCM LRC
Regional Director of Marketing and Census Development
Mariner Post Acute Network
Marblehead, MA

Nancy Lynn Whitehead, MS RNC CSN
Clinical Examiner
Midwestern Performance Assessment Center, Inc.
Regents' College
Madison, WI

Chapter 5: Neuroanatomy

Patricia S. Palmer, RN CRRN
Staff Nurse
Piedmont Hospital, Center for Rehabilitation Medicine
Atlanta, GA

Nancy Lynn Whitehead, MS RNC CSN

Chapter 6: Health Maintenance and Management of Therapeutic Regimen

Aleisa E. Kyper, BSN RN CRRN CNRN
Nurse Clinician
Hurley Rehabilitation Center
Flint, MI

Nancy Youngblood, PhD CRNP
Director, Adult and Family Nurse Practitioner Programs
La Salle University, School of Nursing
Philadelphia, PA

Chapter 7: Physical Healthcare Patterns and Nursing Interventions

Tonnie Glick, MEd RN CRRN CCRN
Acute Care Coordinator
Kessler Institute for Rehabilitation
West Orange, NJ

Patricia Ann Haldi, MN RN CRRN CDE
Certified Diabetes Educator
Saint Luke's Rehabilitation Institute
Spokane, WA

Sandra A. Huntington, MBA BSN RN CRRN
Rehabilitation Nurse Manager
Columbus Regional Hospital
Columbus, IN

Chapter 8: Psychosocial Healthcare Patterns and Nursing Interventions

Pamala D. Larsen, PhD CRRN
Associate Dean for Academic Affairs
University of North Carolina at Charlotte, College of Nursing and Health Professions
Charlotte, NC

Penelope (Penny) A. Taylor, BA RNC CRRN
Nurse Education Clinician
UNC Rehabilitation Unit
Chapel Hill, NC

Chapter 9: Stroke

Kathleen Gresser Fritzman BSN RN
Staff Nurse
Board of Education, City of New York, P.S. 144
Forest Hills, NY

Nancy Youngblood, PhD CRNP

Chapter 10: Traumatic Injuries: TBI and SCI

Teresa A. Bryan, BSN RN CRRN

Tonnie Glick, MEd RN CCRN CRRN

Bonnie J. Parker, MSN RN CRRN
Medical Lagal Nurse Consultant
Waterford, VA

Chapter 11: Musculoskeletal and Orthopedic Disorders

Kathy G. Dale, MS-HSA RN CRRN
Nurse Educator/Coordinator
Learning to Live
Arthritis and Osteoporosis Care Center–Baptist
  Hospital
Nashville, TN

June Webber BSL CRRN
Staff Nurse–Orthopedic, Cardiac, and TBL
Burke Rehabilitation Center
White Plains, NY

Chapter 12: Cardiovascular and Pulmonary Rehabilitation: Acute and Long-Term Management

Aleisa E. Kyper, BSN RN CRRN CNRN

June Webber, BSL CRRN

Chapter 13: Understanding Acute and Chronic Pain

Kathy G. Dale, MS-HSA RN CRRN

Cynthia Kraft Fine, MSN RN CRRN

Renee Steele Rosomoff, MBA RN CRRN CRC
Adjunct Associate Professor
University of Miami, School of Medicine and School
  of Nursing
and Programs Director
University of Miami Comprehensive Pain and
  Rehabilitation Center
Miami Beach, FL

Chapter 14: Specific Disease Processes Requiring Rehabilitation Interventions

Patricia S. Palmer, RN CRRN

Penelope (Penny) A. Taylor, BA RNC CRRN

Chapter 15: Developmental Theories and Tasks Across the Life Span: Individuals and Families

Cindy Gatens, MN RN CRRN-A
Clinical Nurse Specialist
The Ohio State University
Columbus, OH

Nancy Youngblood, PhD CRNP

Chapter 16: Pediatric Rehabilitation Nursing

Kathleen Gresser Fritzman, BSN RN

Dalice Hertzberg, MSN RN CRRN
Instructor
JFK Partners and the School of Nursing
University of Colorado Health Sciences Center
Denver, CO

Deirdre Jackson, MSN CRRN CPN
Nursing Education Director/Clinical Nurse Specialist
Children's Specialized Hospital
Mountainside, NJ

Chapter 17: Gerontological Rehabilitation Nursing

Sue Sheridan, BSN RN CRRN

Margaret (Peg) L. Toth, RNC CRRN
Manager, Clinical Services
HCR ManorCare
Toledo, OH

Chapter 18: Environment of Care and Service Delivery

Carol Gleason, MM RN CRRN CCM LRC

April Struck, BSN RN

Chapter 19: Program Evaluation and Outcome Measurement

Rose Butler, MS RNC CRRN CCM

Chapter 20: Impact of Information Technology and Computer Applications on Rehabilitation Nursing

Dalice Hertzberg, MSN RN CRRN

Chapter 21: Changes in American Healthcare and Its Implication for Rehabilitation Nurses

Dalice Hertzberg, MSN RN CRRN

Leslie J. Neal, PhD RNC CRRN CS

Chapter 22: Rehabilitation Nursing: Past, Present, and Future

Terrie Black, MBA BSN RNC CRRN
Rehabilitation Consultant
Hospital for Special Care
New Britain, CT
and FIM Trainer–Uniform Data System for Medical
    Rehabilitation
Buffalo, NY

Susan Dean-Baar, PhD RN CRRN FAAN
Associate Professor
University of Wisconsin–Milwaukee, School of
Nursing
Milwaukee, WI

Cynthia S. Jacelon, MS RN CRRN-A
Clinical Assistant Professor
University of Massachusetts, School of Nursing
Amherst, MA

Kelly Johnson, MSN RN CFNP CRRN
Vice President, Patient Care
Craig Hospital
Englewood, CO

Ann E. McCourt MS RN
Consultant, formerly Editor of
*The Specialty Practice of Rehabilitation Nursing:
    A Core Curriculum, Third Edition*
Ormand Beach, FL

Lois Schaetzle, MS RN CRRN

Marilyn Ter Maat, MSN RNC CRRN-A CNAA
Rehabilitation/Restorative Nurse Consultant
The Evangelical Lutheran Good Samaritan Society
Sioux Falls, SD

Teresa L. Thompson, PhD RN CRRN-A

Catherine A. Tracey, MS RN CRRN
Project Manager, Disease Management
Tufts Health Plan
Waltham, MA

Barbara H. Warner, MS RN
Director of Nursing
Ohio State University Hospitals
Columbus, OH

Appendix A: Case Studies and Questions for Thought

Jill Derstine, EdD RN
Chair–Nursing Department
Temple University, College of Allied Health
Philadelphia, PA

Dalice Hertzberg, MSN RN CRRN

The Specialty Practice of Rehabilitation Nursing

A Core Curriculum
Fourth Edition

Table of Contents

SECTION V: The Delivery and Evaluation of Rehabilitation Services

SECTION VI: Rehabilitation Nursing in the 21st Century

APPENDIXES

INDEX

Section 1

General Principles and Concepts of Rehabilitation Nursing as a Specialty

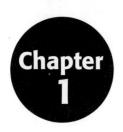

Chapter 1

Rehabilitation and Rehabilitation Nursing

Janet A. Secrest, PhD RN

Advances in health care have enabled people to survive injuries and illnesses and to live longer than in the past. Over the next few decades, the numbers of people with chronic illness and disability are expected to rise, increasing the need for rehabilitation. Rehabilitation is a philosophy of and an attitude toward caring for people with disabilities. The overall goal of rehabilitation is to improve quality of life and to help a person "reach the fullest physical, psychological, social, vocational, avocational, and educational potential consistent with his or her physiologic or anatomic impairment, environmental limitations, and desires and life plans" (DeLisa, Currie, & Martin, 1998, p. 3). Rehabilitation is contingent upon a team approach; an integral discipline on the team is nursing. Rehabilitation nursing is a specialty practice that offers a unique perspective to the care of clients with disabilities.

This chapter reviews rehabilitation philosophy, goals, and process and examines the nursing role, including nurses' values and philosophical perspectives. Nursing science—the relationship among theory, research, and practice—provides a basis for professional rehabilitation nursing practice. This chapter also describes role responsibilities, educational preparation, competencies, certification, professional associations, and resources for the specialty practice of rehabilitation nursing.

The Evolution of Rehabilitation
Historical Trends

Advances in health care over the past century have enabled people to live longer lives and to recover from injuries and illnesses that were previously lethal. With these advances, however, have come disabilities and chronic illnesses that profoundly and forever change the way a person lives in the world. The field of rehabilitation arose to help individuals and families integrate the changes associated with disability and chronic illness into their lives. Rehabilitation is a philosophy, an attitude, and an approach to caring for people with disabilities that improves the quality of their lives and provides a meaningful context in which to live.

The concept of rehabilitation as a philosophy and attitude is important. Attitudes toward people with disability, which arise from a philosophy, determine societal responsibilities and approaches. For example, in ancient Western civilization, disease and disability were often thought to be the result of evil spirits. Consequently, those so "possessed" were feared and shunned. Parents in ancient Rome could legally drown infants with congenital anomalies, and in Sparta, such infants were left to die of exposure. This situation did not improve in the Middle Ages. Some people with disabilities were burned as witches, others were used as court jesters, and all who had disabilities were shunned from everyday societal functions (World Book, 1997). Fortunately, philosophical approaches and attitudes have changed radically since that time. *[Refer to Chapter 22 for a historical overview of rehabilitation.]*

Rehabilitation, as an interdisciplinary healthcare specialty, grew out of the wars that occurred in the 20th century: World War I, World War II, the Korean Conflict, and the Vietnam War. Large numbers of soldiers—young men for the most part—survived their injuries, but often faced serious disability. As a result, military hospitals established rehabilitation units that focused extensive efforts on returning these young men to society. Dr. Howard Rusk, head of the American Air Force Convalescent Training Program, was a strong leader in organizing rehabilitation programs (Lyons & Petrucelli, 1978). Soon, rehabilitation units and hospitals sprang up around the country and the interdisciplinary specialty of rehabilitation gained importance. By 1974, the Association of Rehabilitation Nurses

(ARN) was formed, and nursing, which had always been involved in rehabilitation, formally became recognized as a rehabilitation specialty.

Legislative Initiatives

Legislation in the United States has played a significant role in rehabilitation. The Rehabilitation Act of 1973 encouraged efforts to hire people with disabilities and prohibited unfair treatment of individuals with disabilities in activities supported in any way by federal funds. In 1975, the Education for All Handicapped Children Act required states to provide education free of cost to any school-age child. The Americans with Disabilities Act (ADA) of 1990 has required that public buildings and transportation be made accessible to all (World Book, 1997). This act also prohibits discrimination against people with disabilities in the workplace. The result of these legislative acts has been to increase societal acceptance of individuals with disabilities and provide opportunities for them to maximize their potential. *[Refer to Chapter 4 for more on legislation.]*

Rehabilitation is a vital component of health care. Today, it is not so much war that creates disabilities, but modern life—high speeds, athletics, and longer lives. The need for rehabilitation today is greater than ever before.

Rehabilitation Across Disciplines
Philosophy and Goals

Regardless of discipline, rehabilitation assumes a common philosophical base. It has been defined as "a process of helping a person to reach the fullest physical, psychological, social, vocational, avocational and educational potential consistent with his or her physiologic or anatomic impairment, environmental limitations, and desires and life plans" (DeLisa et al., 1998, p. 3). It is an inherently collaborative endeavor, and it places the client and family in the center of the healthcare team. Rehabilitation is contingent upon a team approach. Indeed, most rehabilitation professionals would agree that the healthcare system would flourish if the ideals of rehabilitation permeated all aspects of health care.

In 1980, the World Health Organization (WHO) developed the International Classification of Impairment, Disability, and Handicap (cited in Kirby, 1998, pp. 55-57). This classification system has been translated into 13 languages and distinguishes among the following terms:
- **Impairment:** A loss or abnormality of a psychological, physiological, or anatomical structure and function

- **Disability:** A restriction or lack (resulting from an impairment) of ability to perform an activity in the manner or within the range considered normal for a human being
- **Handicap:** A disadvantage for a given individual resulting from impairment or disability that limits or prevents fulfillment of a role that is normal for that individual

Thus, impairment occurs at the organ level, disability at the level of the person, and handicap at the societal level. These definitions provide a framework and a language that is not just for rehabilitation, but for society as well.

While many goals of rehabilitation have been articulated, improvement in quality of life is the ultimate goal (e.g., DeLisa et al., 1998). This goal can be accomplished through many avenues, and each member of the rehabilitation team contributes to this goal.

Process
Rehabilitation Team Models

The rehabilitation team consists of, first and foremost, the individual and his or her family. DeLisa et al. (1998) defined the team as "a group of healthcare professionals from different disciplines, who share common values and objectives" (p. 3). Team members contributing to a person's rehabilitation are varied and cross many disciplines (see Figure 1-1). Four models for team functioning have been described: medical, multidisciplinary, interdisciplinary (DeLisa et al., 1998), and transdisciplinary (Mumma & Nelson, 1996). In all models, nursing is an integral part of the rehabilitation team.

Medical model: The medical model is the traditional way of providing healthcare services, in which the physician directs care. This model is not consistent with rehabilitation philosophy or goals, and it is uncommon in rehabilitation practice.

Multidisciplinary model: The multidisciplinary team, which may be seen in rehabilitation, is one that takes on a pyramid-like shape. The medical literature places the physician at the top; however, Lydia Hall's model, implemented at the Loeb Center, placed nursing at the top (Alfano, 1988). Communication is more vertical than lateral, with the leader controlling team conferences. This model is effective when the team is not stable (e.g., when there are different team members for different clients).

Interdisciplinary model: The interdisciplinary model is a matrix-like model in which communication is primarily lateral. This is an effective model when team members are stable (e.g., in an inpatient rehabilitation unit). Decisions are determined by the group, which means that mutual trust among team members must be established, and conflict resolution is an important skill used by team members.

Transdisciplinary model: A newer team model is the transdisciplinary model, in which the client has a primary therapist from the team, who then is guided by the team in caring for the client. For example, the primary therapist may be a nurse, who then provides physical, speech, and occupational therapy based on the advice and counsel he or she receives from team members in those disciplines. Similarly, the primary therapist could be a physical therapist. Mumma and Nelson (1996) noted that this model requires flexibility and receptiveness on the part of team members, because individual roles become less distinct. This model also raises many issues regarding licensure and accountability. It may be best suited for situations in which the client is stable and in need of long-term services.

Regardless of the rehabilitation team model, all team members can increase their effectiveness by understanding collaborative practice, group dynamics, conflict resolution, and team functioning. Youngblood (1999) stated the two goals of a rehabilitation team are to provide care to the individual and family and to ensure "self-maintenance" (p. 114). Components necessary for self-maintenance of a team include trust, knowledge, shared responsibility, mutual respect, communication, cooperation and coordination, and optimism. Effective teams require a commitment from each member.

Figure 1-1. Members of the Rehabilitation Team

Client and family
Nurses
Physiatrists
Other physicians
Physical therapists
Occupational therapists
Speech/language pathologists
Psychologists
Recreational therapists
Vocational therapists
Orthotists
Chaplains
Insurance case managers or representatives
Employers
Teachers
Audiologists
Nutritionists
Home health professionals

Provision of Services

The rehabilitation philosophy can infuse any healthcare setting. Collaboration between team members (through any of the team models), the individual, family, and community is a vital aspect of rehabilitation. Mumma and Nelson (1996) offered a useful categorization of models for provision of services: client-centered, setting-centered, provider-centered, and collaborative. For the purposes of this chapter, a collaborative model (i.e., a team concept) is assumed in all rehabilitation models.

Client-centered care: Client-centered models are those serving specialized populations. The focus may be on a specific developmental stage, such as pediatric or elderly clients, or on a type of impairment, such as spinal cord or head injury. With a population-specific focus, providers can focus their resources and gain extensive expertise through experience.

Setting-centered care: Acute, long-term, outpatient, home care, and community are the traditional models focusing on settings. Each describes where rehabilitation takes place. The trend away from inpatient care has accelerated in recent years, as a result of changing funding practices. A newer category of setting-focused rehabilitation is subacute care. Subacute care settings provide rehabilitation to individuals who continue to require substantial medical care and who are slower to progress. For adults, subacute care units are usually inpatient settings and are often housed within an acute care, traditional rehabilitation unit or long-term care facility. However, in the pediatric population, subacute rehabilitation is seen more often in day treatment programs, whereby the children return to home or residential settings at night (Hertzberg & Edwards, 1999).

Provider-centered care: Provider-centered models reflect how healthcare providers have decided to organize the provision of care. Many models have been used over the years with the goal of maximizing the use of human resources. Within nursing, functional, team, and primary nursing, and more recently, case management have been the models. In functional nursing, the tasks are divided (e.g., one nurse delivers all the medications). In team nursing, a nurse oversees the care of a group of clients by providers of various skill levels. Primary nursing (not to be confused with primary care) became popular in the 1980s as a means of providing client-centered care. One nurse provides direct total care to a group of clients and is responsible for planning and coordinating that care when he or she is not on duty. This model spawned several variations. Primary nursing has coordinated, client-centered care as its goal, not unlike case management.

Case management, though not a new concept in nursing and health care, is currently a common provider-centered model within rehabilitation. With this model, the goal is to provide quality, individualized, cost-effective care through an ongoing process of assessment, planning, implementing, coordinating, and evaluating care and services (Youngblood, 1999). Because of nursing's holistic focus, nurses are ideal case managers; however, this is not always the case. While theoretically the case manager is the client advocate, it is important to recognize to whom the case manager is accountable (e.g., the insurance company, the hospital).

In the rehabilitation field, no single model dominates, and several models coexist. For example, a case management system may be operating within a subacute pediatric day treatment program. As health care continues to evolve, new models of providing services will undoubtedly emerge, and nurses are in an important position to lead the way.

Rehabilitation Nursing Perspectives
Nursing's Focus and Core Values

Nursing brings a unique, holistic focus to rehabilitation. While members of other disciplines treat particular aspects of a person, nurses focus on the person as a whole, thus providing continuity and integrity to the client's rehabilitation experience.

Fawcett (1984) defined the central foci (or metaparadigm) of nursing as person, health, environment, and nursing. The individual's philosophical view of these concepts lays the foundation for how he or she will approach nursing care. The philosophy of rehabilitation nursing involves a statement of beliefs and values, or what is assumed to be true, regarding the focus of this specialty practice (Fawcett, 1995). The core values of rehabilitation as an interdisciplinary practice are congruent with those of nursing.

As a profession, nursing has stated its ethical foundation in the *Code for Nurses* (American Nurses' Association [ANA], 1985). In 1991, more than 70 nursing organizations endorsed *Nursing's Agenda for Health Care Reform* (ANA, 1991), a public policy agenda that further explicated disciplinary values with respect to provision of services. This was an important document developed as a public proclamation of nursing's values and desire to influence health care on a national scale. Some of the values purported that all U.S. residents and citizens must have equitable access to essential healthcare services and that consumers must be the central focus of the healthcare system (see Figure 1-2). ARN was among the organizations that endorsed this document.

Rehabilitation nursing arises as a specialty practice from the nursing discipline. Values and assumptions for the discipline are explicated in *Nursing's Social Policy Statement* (ANA, 1995, pp. 3-4), which states the following:

- Humans manifest an essential unity of mind/body/spirit.
- Human experience is contextually and culturally defined.
- Health and illness are human experiences.
- The presence of illness does not preclude health nor does optimal health preclude illness.

Rehabilitation nursing, as a specialty of the nursing discipline at large, embraces these values and further explicates its core values, which include the following (ARN, 1994, p. 3):

Figure 1-2. Nursing's Agenda for Healthcare Reform: An Explication of Nursing Values

1. All citizens and residents of the United States must have equitable access to essential healthcare services.
2. Primary healthcare services must play a very basic and prominent role in service delivery.
3. Consumers must be the central focus of the healthcare system.
4. Consumers must be guaranteed direct access to a full range of qualified healthcare providers who offer their services in a variety of delivery arrangements at sites that are accessible, convenient, and familiar to the consumer.
5. Consumers must assume more responsibility for their own care and become better informed about the range of providers and potential options for services.
6. Healthcare services must be restructured to create a better balance between the prevailing orientation toward illness and cure and a new commitment to wellness and care.
7. The healthcare system must assure that appropriate, effective care is delivered through efficient use of resources.
8. A standardized package of essential healthcare services must be provided and financed through an integration of public and private sources.
9. Mechanisms must be implemented to protect against catastrophic costs and impoverishment.

Reprinted with permission of the American Nurses Association from American Nurses Association. (1991). *Nursing's agenda for health care reform.* Kansas City, MO: Author.

- Individuals with functional limitations have intrinsic worth that transcends their disability and/or chronic illness.
- Individuals are complex yet unified, whole persons who have the right and the responsibility to make informed decisions about their future.

Goals of Rehabilitation Nursing

Rehabilitation nursing is defined as "the diagnosis and treatment of human responses of individuals and groups to actual or potential health problems relative to altered functional ability and lifestyle" (ARN, 1994). This is congruent with the ANA (1980) definition of nursing: "the diagnosis and treatment of human responses to actual or potential health threats." The overall goal of rehabilitation has consistently been cited as the promotion of a higher quality of life (DeLisa et al., 1998; Kottke, 1982; McCollom, 1988; Secrest & Thomas, 1999) (see Research Perspective in this chapter). The goal of rehabilitation nursing, according to ARN (1994), is "assisting the individual with a disability or a chronic disease toward maximal health through health restoration, maintenance, and promotion" (p. 3). Nursing interventions, in promoting maximal health, promote the client's quality of life. Explicitly essential and inherent in achieving this goal is collaboration with the client, his or her significant others, and other health-care providers. Rehabilitation nursing is client-centered, goal-oriented, and outcome-based.

Nursing Science as a Basis for Rehabilitation Nursing Practice
Philosophical Worldviews

Nursing's body of knowledge—its science—derives from the relationship among practice, theory, and research with respect to the focus of the discipline (i.e., the metaparadigm). The metaparadigm concepts provide the focus of nursing, and the nursing models provide the context. These models or frameworks provide a lens through which nursing phenomena are viewed, and thus, reveal how nursing care is approached. An example of how different lenses determine approaches in another discipline would be (a) a behavioral psychologist, who sees the person in terms of behavior that can be manipulated through environmental changes and (b) a cognitive psychologist, who sees a person's behavior as changeable through talk therapy. Similarly, nursing models provide differing ways of practicing nursing. What is common to all nursing models, however, is the holistic view of human beings (see Table 1-1).

Whereas core values undergird all nursing models, philosophical worldviews shape the development of metaparadigm concepts in the models. They provide a broad understanding of the models in which the metaparadigm concepts are explicated. Although many categorizations of worldviews exist, Fawcett (1995) offered a synthesis of three categories:

- **Reaction:** The person is seen as the sum of parts (e.g., biological, psychological, sociological, spiritual) and responds to external stimuli in a linear, causal way. Change is predictable and necessary for survival. Nursing models do not mirror this view; however, it can be seen, for example, in B.F. Skinner's behaviorism model and in the germ theory model.

- **Reciprocal interaction:** Human beings are holistic, not reducible to parts, and in reciprocal interaction with the environment. Although the "parts" are not reducible, they are recognized and seen only in context of the whole. Change is the result of multiple factors in the person and the environment, and is probabilistic, though not entirely predictable. Examples of this view in nursing theory include King's (1981, 1995) Systems Framework, Orem's (1995) Self-Care Framework, and Hall's (1964, 1969) Core, Cure, and Care Model.

- **Simultaneous action:** Human beings are more than and different from the sum of their parts. They are seen as unitary, irreducible, and known by patterns of behavior. Change is continuous, moving into an ever-complex organization, and is unpredictable. A nursing example of this worldview is Rogers' (1970, 1992) Science of Unitary Human Beings.

Nursing Models that Guide Practice

Nursing models are frameworks that guide practice and research. Within the models are theories, which propose relationships among concepts. The nurses who developed the models and theories are referred to as nursing theorists. These theorists drew from existing knowledge in nursing as well as from other disciplines. For example, nursing theorists have drawn from general system theory (e.g., King), adaptation theory (e.g., Roy), learning and motivational theories (e.g., Hall), various developmental theories, and even physics (e.g., Rogers). Theorists incorporate their knowledge of existing theories with their nursing knowledge and perspectives to create models and theories that are unique to nursing. So, whereas nursing is a discipline within the larger community of scientific disciplines in which knowledge is shared, this knowledge is applied in nursing situations with a nursing perspective.

One discipline with which nursing is intimately involved is medicine, and, at times, nurses may confuse nursing knowledge with medical knowledge. Of course, it is important for nurses to understand disease processes, but their goal is different from medical specialists. The question nurses must ask is "Why do nurses need to know this?" The answer differs from that of the originating discipline. By using nursing models to guide practice, nurses can gain a clear understanding of their discipline and its unique contribution to health care in general and rehabilitation in particular. When nurses have a clear understanding of their discipline, its role, and the differences from other disciplines, they can confidently assume leadership roles in rehabilitation. Practicing nursing from a nursing model perspective provides that clear understanding.

All of the nursing models have a holistic focus, and thus all are appropriate to guide rehabilitation nursing practice. Nurses can make individual choices regarding their preferred nursing model, depending on their own philosophy of nursing. Rehabilitation nurses are encouraged to first consult an overview of nursing models and theories (e.g., Tomey & Alligood, 1998) to find one that resonates with their own philosophy and then consult the primary sources of the theory. Selected theorists have been included in this chapter as examples for nursing practice (see Table 1-1), although many others exist. These models were chosen because of their emphasis on interaction with clients and on the importance of setting goals from the client's perspective, both of which are of paramount importance in rehabilitation.

Lydia Hall

Lydia Hall is best known for her work at the Loeb Center at Montefiore Hospital in New York. This was a rehabilitation unit with a primary focus on nursing care. It was a nurse-run center; members of other disciplines, including medicine, served in a consultant role to nursing (Alfano, 1988). Hall's theory of nursing provided the framework for the care. Research demonstrated that clients' length of stay was shortened and life satisfaction improved (Pearson, Durand, & Punton, 1988).

Three interlocking circles represent Hall's theory: the person ("core"), the body ("care"), and the disease ("cure"). She asserted that nurses provide different types of care in each circle and different types of care

Principle	Hall	King	Orem	Rogers
Person	A unity of 3 interrelated parts: the person (core), disease/treatment (cure), and body (care); people strive for their own goals, and behavior is more directed by feelings than by knowledge	An open system; a social, rational, and sentient being; major concepts include perception, self, growth and development, body image, time, and space	A unity, functioning biologically, symbolically, and socially, who values self-care	Unitary human beings who cannot separate from environment knowledge
Health	A behavior; achieves maximum potential through learning, particularly about oneself	Dynamic life experiences, adjusting to stressors; ability to function in social roles	A wholeness of body and mind; integrated	Individually defined; an expression of the life process
Nursing	A teacher and nurturer: By understanding the three aspects of a person, the nurse helps the client understand goals and motivation. Nursing should be provided by professional nurses.	An interactive endeavor in which the nurse and client share perceptions and mutually identify goals and means to reach those goals	A helping profession in which nurses help others meet therapeutic self-care demands	A learned profession; a science and art of promoting health

Table 1-1. Comparison of Selected Nursing Models

over the course of a person's illness (see Figure 1-3.). She further asserted that "wholly professional" nursing care would hasten recovery.

Hall believed that nursing care should only be provided by professional nurses. While the person is in the first stage of illness, medical specialists direct the care, with nurses in a supportive role. Nurses assume dominance in the second stage of illness, when the body and person assume greater importance. Her view of health can be inferred from her belief that people achieve their maximum potential through learning; however, because people behave according to their feelings, inattention to the person while teaching will not change their behavior. She specified that rehabilitation is a process of learning to live within limitations (Tomey & Alligood, 1998). Therefore, nursing intervenes to facilitate learning about not only physical and mental skills, but also about self and one's feelings, behavior, and motivations. Hall was one of the first to assert that setting goals for clients that do not reflect the client's own goals is counter therapeutic.

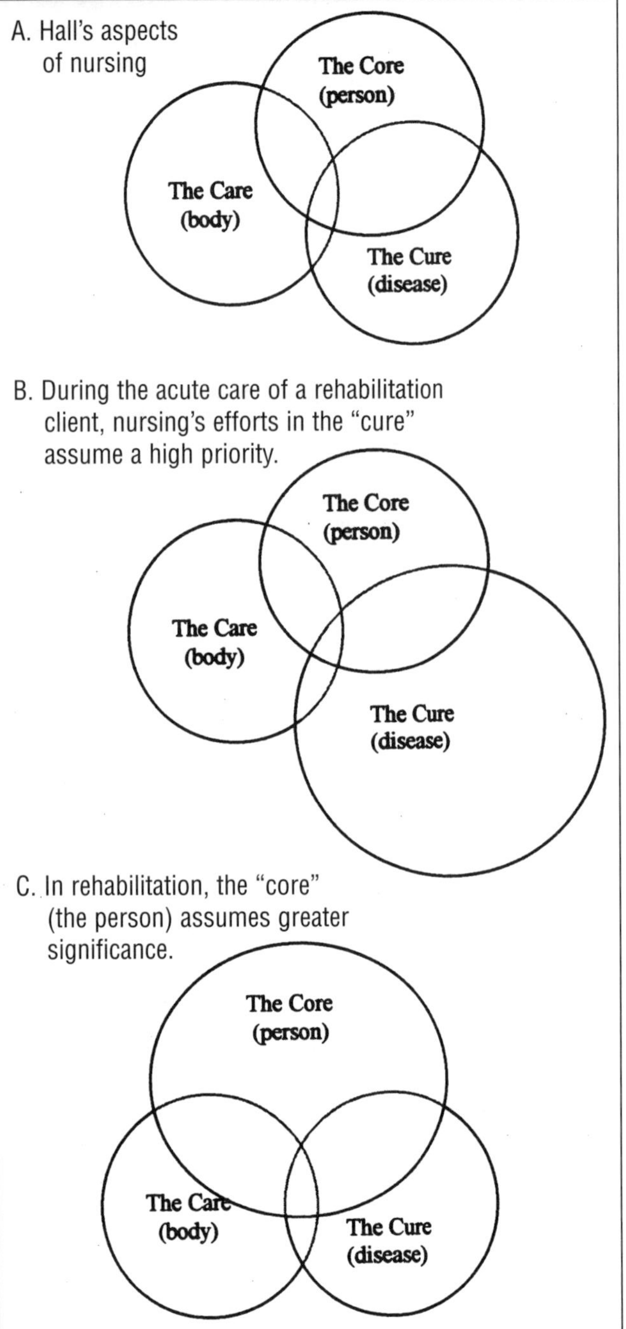

Clinical application: When a stroke survivor, for example, enters the healthcare system, the cure circle assumes dominance. Nurses assist during the biological crisis, still attending to the person and body. During rehabilitation, the nurse attends to intimate body functions. Through communication, the nurse becomes the therapeutic modality in treating the person. By helping the person explore his or her feelings, behavior, and motivation, the nurse can work with the client to establish goals for rehabilitation. As rehabilitation progresses, the client assumes more responsibility for the body; in the diagrammatic representation of Hall's theory, the circles expand and contract relative to nursing's role.

The nurse's approach to assessment is organized into three areas: the disease (cure), the body (care), and the person (core). The intervention approach, similarly, would be organized around the three aspects of the model. In the disease realm, interventions are primarily medically directed (e.g., administering medications, monitoring biological functions). In the body realm, nurses assist with the bodily functions the person is unable to manage (e.g., elimination). Finally, and most importantly in nursing, is the person. Nurses employ the therapeutic use of self to guide clients into a greater understanding of themselves and to help them achieve their maximal potential through learning. The nurse would focus teaching and learning on the client. For example, the nurse would help the stroke survivor set and continually evaluate goals.

Nurses who are developing a multi-, inter-, or transdisciplinary team could use Hall's model as a structure and a process. This, in fact, was how the Loeb Center functioned.

Imogene King

Imogene King (1981) developed a framework for nursing based on systems theory, and within this framework, a theory of nursing. Her framework consists of three interacting systems: personal system (an individual), interpersonal system (two or more personal systems), and social systems (social forces) (see Figure

Figure 1-3. Hall's Aspects of Nursing

A. Hall's aspects of nursing

The Core (person)

The Care (body)

The Cure (disease)

B. During the acute care of a rehabilitation client, nursing's efforts in the "cure" assume a high priority.

The Core (person)

The Care (body)

The Cure (disease)

C. In rehabilitation, the "core" (the person) assumes greater significance.

The Core (person)

The Care (body)

The Cure (disease)

1-4). People, including nurses, function in all three systems. From the interpersonal system, she developed a theory of goal attainment. Mutual goal attainment results from transactions between nurse and client. Both must communicate and have clarity of each other's role to understand each other's perspective of a situation (perceptual congruence). With this understanding, goals can be mutually set, and transactions can occur, resulting in mutual goal attainment (see Figure 1-5). Thus, mutuality achieved through perceptual congruence is the keystone. King's (1981) theory "focuses on goals to be attained in specific nursing situations through participative decision making by nurses and patients" (p. 155).

King (1981) views the person as an open system in interaction with the environment, who is unique, holistic, and has intrinsic worth. Individuals are capable of making decisions in most situations, and they differ in their needs, wants, and goals. Health is defined as a dynamic life cycle that has different meanings for people and "implies continuous adjustment to stress in the internal and external environment through optimum use of one's resources to achieve maximum potential for daily living" (p. 5).

King (1981) sees nursing as an inherently interactive endeavor, in which "nurse and client share information in the nursing situation" (p. 2). Nurses have special knowledge of nursing, and the client has special knowledge of himself or herself. By sharing this knowledge with each other, goals and the means to achieve goals can be mutually developed. The goal of nursing is "to help individuals maintain their health so they can function in their roles" (p. 4).

Clinical application: When a stroke survivor enters the healthcare system, the nursing assessment focuses on concepts in the personal, interpersonal, and social systems (see Table 1-2). Perceptual congruence in the assessment is crucial (e.g., Does the nurse understand the client and does the client understand the nurse?). Unless there is communication, perceptual congruence will not occur, and goals will not be met. Communication occurs in many ways, and goal setting is not necessarily a formalized procedure. For example, the stroke survivor may communicate his fear of this bewildering event entirely nonver-

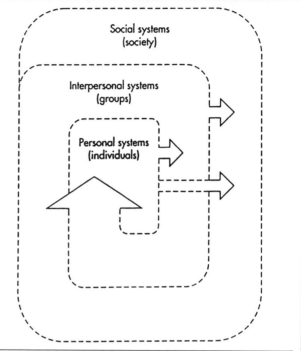

Figure 1-4. King's Conceptual Framework for Nursing, Demonstrating the Relationship Among Each System

Reprinted with permission of Sage Publications, from Frey, M.A., & Sieloff, C.L. (Eds.). (1995). *Advancing King's systems framework and theory of nursing* (p. 19). Thousand Oaks, CA: Sage.

bally. The nurse validates his or her perception of the client's experience and uses "special knowledge" (of nursing) to reassure and comfort the client. The goal for the client is perhaps reassurance, comfort, and information, whereas the nurse's goal is to provide that reassurance, comfort, and information. Because the client

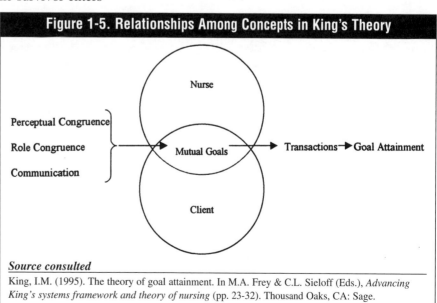

Figure 1-5. Relationships Among Concepts in King's Theory

Source consulted

King, I.M. (1995). The theory of goal attainment. In M.A. Frey & C.L. Sieloff (Eds.), *Advancing King's systems framework and theory of nursing* (pp. 23-32). Thousand Oaks, CA: Sage.

Table 1-2. Concepts in King's Framework

Personal System	Interpersonal System	Social System
Perception	Interaction	Organization
Self	Communication	Authority
Body image	Transaction	Power
Space	Role	Status
Time	Stress	Decision making
Growth and development		

Sources consulted

Frey, M.A., & Sieloff, C.L. (Eds.). (1995). *Advancing King's systems framework and theory of nursing*. Thousand Oaks, CA: Sage.

King, I.M. (1981). *A theory for nursing: Systems, concepts and process*. New York: John Wiley.

is a personal system embedded within interpersonal and social systems, the context of the client's life is vital. For many stroke survivors, explicit goals that extend beyond moment-to-moment care are often difficult to negotiate. In these cases, the nurse may set goals with the client's significant others, using the best data available. As the client progresses, he or she is more able to be an active participant in setting goals. It is important to note that goal setting is not a one-time event, but rather an ongoing process.

Goal attainment based upon mutuality of all participants is process-oriented. King's theory of goal attainment, while originally meant for nurse-client interactions, also provides a firm foundation upon which nurses can build an effective interdisciplinary team.

Dorothea E. Orem

Dorothea Orem (1995) sees self-care as essential for health, well-being, and life itself. Orem's model focuses on individuals' self-care needs or demands (self-care requisites) and the ability of the person to meet those needs (self-care agency). The three groups of self-care requisites (universal, developmental, health deviation) are influenced by conditioning factors (see Figure 1-6). Self-care agency is the ability of an individual to meet these self-care requisites. When self-care requisites exceed self-care agency, nursing may intervene (see Figure 1-7).

Orem views health as a state of wholeness or integrity, and nurses design systems to facilitate this state. Nursing systems are action systems in which nurses design their care. These include wholly compensatory, partly compensatory, and supportive-educative systems (see Figure 1-8). Orem's theory specifically recognizes that clients may be dependent on others outside the healthcare system to meet self-care demands. Those who fulfill the responsibility to assist with the self-care agency of another are called dependent care agents.

Clinical application: When a stroke survivor enters the healthcare system, the nurse assesses the person's self-care requisites and self-care agency. The stroke increases the person's self-care requisites and, at the same time, diminishes the person's self-care agency. In the acute care setting, a wholly compensatory nursing system may be most appropriate. As the person begins rehabilitation, the nurse employs a partially compensatory system and begins to form a supportive-educative system. As rehabilitation progresses, a supportive-educative system assumes primacy. During rehabilitation, the focus of the supportive-educative system may be a dependent care agent, such as a spouse.

Figure 1-6. Orem's (1995) Self-Care Requisites

Universal self-care requisites	Developmental self-care requisites	Health-deviation self-care requisites	Basic conditioning factors
"Common to all human beings during all stages of the life cycle, adjusted to age, developmental state, and environmental and other factors. They are associated with life processes, with the maintenance of the integrity of human structure and functioning, and with general well-being" (pp. 108-109)	"Associated with human developmental processes and with conditions and events occurring during various stages of the life cycle (e.g., prematurity, pregnancy) and events that can adversely affect development" (p. 109)	"Associated with genetic and constitutional defects and human structural and functional deviations and with their effects and with medical diagnostic and treatment measures" (p. 110)	Age Gender Developmental state Health state Sociocultural orientation Healthcare system factors Family system factors Pattern of living, including routine activities Environmental factors Resource availability and adequacy

Source consulted

Orem, D.E. (1995). *Nursing concepts of practice* (5th ed.). St. Louis: Mosby.

The Specialty Practice of Rehabilitation Nursing: A Core Curriculum, 4th Ed.

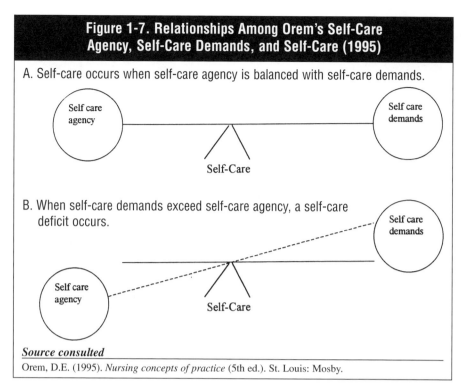

Figure 1-7. Relationships Among Orem's Self-Care Agency, Self-Care Demands, and Self-Care (1995)

A. Self-care occurs when self-care agency is balanced with self-care demands.

Self care agency — Self-Care — Self care demands

B. When self-care demands exceed self-care agency, a self-care deficit occurs.

Self care agency — Self-Care — Self care demands

Source consulted

Orem, D.E. (1995). *Nursing concepts of practice* (5th ed.). St. Louis: Mosby.

is an expression of the life process. Rogers' view of nursing is that of "knowing" rather than "doing"; in other words, nursing is an abstract body of knowledge. She describes nursing as a learned profession, with the goal of promoting health and well-being. Human beings have the capacity to knowingly participate in change, which is creative and innovative—and nurses help people knowingly participate in change.

Clinical application: The nurse assesses the stroke survivor entering the healthcare system through a pattern appraisal. Gordon's (1987) functional health patterns (see Figure 1-9) as a means of client assessment is particularly well suited to Rogers' model

Martha Rogers

Martha Rogers' Science of Unitary Human Beings theory focuses on "people and their worlds in a pandimensional universe" (Rogers, 1992, p. 29). Human beings are viewed as unified wholes, not parts. In this model, the human and the environment are energy fields that are inextricably intertwined and are irreducible—essentially, a unitary field. Rogers calls this concept integrality. People, therefore, are always viewed in the context of the environment, never separate from it. People are known by patterns, which are manifestations of the whole.

Change is fundamental to life—it is unidirectional, increasingly complex, and creative. This means that one never repeats patterns, but rather, continues to grow. "Each repatterning is a revision of the immediately preceding pattern" (Rogers, 1970, p. 98). For example, if a person vacations at the same location each year, and if all of the elements of the vacation remain the same, it is still a different experience that has built on previous experience. In this model, the notion of an individual returning to (as near as is possible) his previous existence is rejected because change is unidirectional and increasingly complex. After rehabilitation, the person has grown or developed into a more complex person than his or her previous existence.

Rogers' theory does not specifically define health but views health as a value-laden term imposed by society. It is not the opposite of illness, but as with illness, health

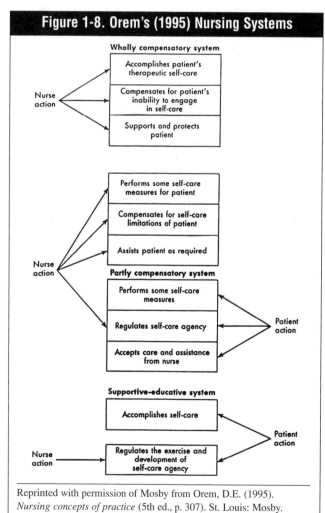

Figure 1-8. Orem's (1995) Nursing Systems

Wholly compensatory system

Nurse action →
- Accomplishes patient's therapeutic self-care
- Compensates for patient's inability to engage in self-care
- Supports and protects patient

Nurse action →
- Performs some self-care measures for patient
- Compensates for self-care limitations of patient
- Assists patient as required

Partly compensatory system
- Performs some self-care measures
- Regulates self-care agency
- Accepts care and assistance from nurse
← Patient action

Supportive-educative system
- Accomplishes self-care
← Patient action

Nurse action →
- Regulates the exercise and development of self-care agency

Reprinted with permission of Mosby from Orem, D.E. (1995). *Nursing concepts of practice* (5th ed., p. 307). St. Louis: Mosby.

Figure 1-9. Gordon's (1987) Functional Health Patterns

Health perception–health management: The client's perceived pattern of health and well-being, and how health is managed

Nutritional–metabolic: The client's pattern of food and fluid consumption relative to metabolic and pattern indicators of local nutrient supply

Elimination: The client's patterns of excretory function (e.g., bowel, bladder, skin)

Activity–exercise: The client's patterns of exercise, activity, leisure, and recreation

Sleep–rest: The client's patterns of sleep, rest, and relaxation

Cognitive–perceptual: The client's sensory-perceptual and cognitive patterns

Self-perception: The client's self-concept pattern and perceptions of self

Role–relationship: The client's patterns of satisfaction and dissatisfaction with sexuality

Sexuality–reproductive: The client's patterns of satisfaction and dissatisfaction with sexuality and reproductive patterns

Coping–stress tolerance: The client's general coping pattern and the effectiveness of the pattern in terms of stress tolerance

Value–belief: The client's patterns of values, beliefs, and goals that guide the client's choices or decisions

Source consulted

Gordon, M. (1987). *Nursing diagnosis: Process and application* (2nd ed.). St. Louis: McGraw-Hill.

because it offers a holistic assessment of a person's interrelated patterns, and therefore, manifestations of the whole. Gordon's functional health patterns are useful for nursing assessments in most nursing models, and, in fact, all nursing diagnoses can be grouped under the various patterns (Carpenito, 1997). In Rogers' model, dissonance in patterns is identified. Nursing interventions focusing on the dissonance aim to help the person with patterning to achieve resonance. For example, if the pattern appraisal reveals a dissonance in urinary and bowel elimination, the nurse facilitates harmonious patterning in establishing new toileting routines, using data regarding past patterns.

Many nursing models and theories are useful in nursing practice. What distinguishes nursing models from those in other disciplines is their holistic focus. All of the models "see" clinical situations from a different perspective. It can be argued that if a clinical situation cannot be framed in a nursing model, then perhaps it is not a situation that is suited for nursing. Rehabilitation nurses are urged to explore nursing models (using primary

sources) to find one that is congruent with their philosophy of nursing. Practicing from a conceptual or theoretical base is an important aspect of professional practice and it reinforces nursing's unique contributions to health care.

In all nursing endeavors, the client is at the center. Nursing models and theories can be used not only in the direct provision of care, but also in designing nursing care delivery systems (e.g., Hall's model). Rehabilitation is inherently a team concept, and any model for care delivery systems must begin with this premise.

Nursing Research to Guide Practice

Research is necessary to provide a scientific foundation and to establish accountability for professional nursing practice. Health care in general, and nursing in particular, is becoming increasingly complex and costly; these trends place increasing demands on nursing care to be validated through systematic study.

The word *research* means simply "to search again." Scientific nursing research is the systematic study of phenomena that are of interest to nursing for the purposes of validating existing knowledge and/or developing new knowledge. Research allows nurses to understand phenomena (through qualitative research), and to describe, explain, predict, and ultimately control events (through quantitative research).

Nurses in all areas and levels of practice have an important role in research. The ANA (1989) delineated the levels of nurses' involvement in research. Nurses with associate degrees can help identify research problems, assist with data collection, and utilize findings in practice with supervision. Nurses who have baccalaureates must be able to access and evaluate research for utilization in practice. Master's-level nurses create the environment in which research and its utilization are fostered, collaborate with experienced investigators, and provide the clinical expertise required for research. Doctoral and postdoctoral nurses develop nursing knowledge through research and theory with funded research.

ARN's *Standards and Scope of Rehabilitation Nursing Practice* (in press) reinforce ANA's recommendations for professional rehabilitation nurses. These standards state that a research attitude (i.e., one of systematic searching) is important in all aspects of care. Whether by identifying particular problems in rehabilitation, using the research literature to determine practice approaches, or systematically evaluating nursing practices, nurses can use research to play an important role. Research should be considered an integral aspect of professional decision making.

The Specialty Practice of Rehabilitation Nursing

Rehabilitation nursing is viewed as a specialty practice by both ARN and ANA. ARN's standards (in press) outline the scope of practice, standards of care, and standards of professional performance. The Rehabilitation Nursing Foundation (RNF, 1994) outlined specific competencies in a separate manual.

Professional rehabilitation practice is guided by philosophy, theory, and research, and thus can be practiced in any setting. When the client is at the center of care, and the goals are to optimize health (however it is defined) and to improve the quality of life for those with disability or chronic disease, the boundaries of the healthcare system become less important. Instead, what assumes importance are the client's and his or her significant others' goals to reintegrate their lives. Practice settings for rehabilitation nursing may include the home, work settings, insurance companies, community centers, residential centers, day care centers, clinics, skilled care facilities, inpatient rehabilitation centers, subacute units, and acute care facilities.

Role Responsibilities

The American Association of Colleges of Nursing (AACN, 1998) described the following role responsibilities for generalist nursing practice:

- **Provider of care:** The nurse "uses theory and research-based knowledge in the direct and indirect delivery of care...in the formation of partnerships with clients and the interdisciplinary health care team" (p. 16). Particular roles in rehabilitation with these responsibilities include caregiver, client advocate, client educator, counselor, nurse practitioner, expert witness, and researcher.

- **Designer, manager, and coordinator of care:** The nurse requires skills such as communication, collaboration, negotiation, delegation, coordination, and evaluation of interdisciplinary work. These are particularly important skills for rehabilitation nurses, who are team members and/or leaders. Rehabilitation roles fulfilling these responsibilities include care manager, case manager, consultant, administrator or manager, and clinical nurse specialist. Designing and coordinating care becomes increasingly important in nursing as healthcare systems use various skilled and semiskilled workers in direct care. Additionally, nurses are in a key position to assume leadership in the coordination of care across disciplines.

- **Member of a profession:** Professionals have a responsibility to value lifelong learning, identify with the profession's values, and incorporate professionalism into practice. Client advocacy is an important aspect of professional rehabilitation practice, and although this is an integral aspect of everyday practice, advocacy assumes a particularly important aspect in a larger societal sense. Rehabilitation nurses have a responsibility for helping shape public policy in such endeavors as advocating for dismantling societal barriers to people with disabilities and educating the public to prevent disease and trauma. Although many of these role opportunities already exist, many more roles could be developed by creative and entrepreneurial nurses. In today's dynamic healthcare system, nurses have the opportunity to develop unique nursing roles that will meet the goals of rehabilitation.

Educational Preparation

ARN's standards (in press) do not mandate which type of basic nursing preparation is necessary for generalist practice or certification. The ANA has long since recommended a bachelor's degree for entry into practice. A baccalaureate better prepares practitioners for the high level of flexibility necessary as health care becomes increasingly sophisticated and provides a basis for practitioners to participate in, evaluate, and utilize research findings as greater evidence is required to support practice. A baccalaureate, thus, is important for specialty practice.

Competencies

The specialty practice of rehabilitation nursing has a defined area of competence within nursing. RNF (1994) has described these competencies, which provide a foundation of content and behaviors that can be evaluated in nurses' cognitive, affective, and psychomotor domains. Competencies provide accountability and standards of practice for the specialty.

Certification

Certification in rehabilitation nursing is a means of validating specialized knowledge and skills and displays a sense of accountability to the public. The Rehabilitation Nursing Certification Board (RNCB) offered its first certification examination in 1984. Those who meet the criteria and pass the exam earn the Certified Rehabilitation Registered Nurse (CRRN) credential. Since 1984, more than 12,500 candidates have earned their certification in rehabilitation nursing.

Professional Associations

Associations have played a crucial role in the development of nursing as a profession. They establish standards of practice and control policies and activities of nursing practice. To regulate its own practice is a hallmark of a profession; and professional nursing associations ensure that nurses control nursing practice. Incumbent upon being a member of a profession is belonging to professional organizations. Associations provide nurses with a voice as well as information in the form of newsletters, books, journals, educational conferences, and other resources.

The ANA is the primary voice for professional nurses. Professional rehabilitation nurses should also belong to ARN, the specialty organization for rehabilitation nurses. ARN's purpose is "to promote and advance professional rehabilitation nursing practice through education, advocacy, collaboration, and research to enhance the quality of life for those affected by disability and chronic illness." Other professional associations that may be of interest to rehabilitation nurses include the American Association of Spinal Cord Injury Nurses, the American Society for Long Term Care Nurses, the American Society of Pain Management Nurses, the Association of Nurses in AIDS Care, the Developmental Disabilities Nurses Association, and the National Association of Orthopedic Nurses.

Research Perspective

Secrest, J., & Thomas, S.P. (1999). Continuity and discontinuity: The quality of life following stroke. *Rehabilitation Nursing, 24*(6), 240-246.

The ultimate goal of rehabilitation is to improve quality of life, yet the meaning of this concept varies among clients, families, and providers of care. Many instruments that measure quality of life exist. None of the instruments, however, address the meaning that life has following stroke. The purpose of this existential-phenomenological study, therefore, was to investigate the experience of life following stroke rehabilitation to provide understanding of quality of life from the stroke survivor's perspective.

In-depth phenomenological interviews were conducted with 14 stroke survivors (7 men, 7 women). The median length of time since stroke was 2 years. Participants exhibited many disabilities; three of them had nonfluent aphasia. The opening interview question asked participants to describe specific experiences since the stroke that stood out for them. Subsequent questions were designed to validate and clarify information. Pollio's (Pollio, Henley, & Thompson, 1977) approach, which involved a part-to-whole dialectic—some of which occurred within an interdisciplinary interpretive research group, was used for analysis.

Prior to the interviews, the researcher underwent a "bracketing" interview to uncover any biases related to the phenomenon. The results revealed that the world of the stroke survivor is grounded in a life of loss and effort. From this background of loss and effort emerged themes that were inextricably related:

* independence/dependence
* in control/out of control
* connection/disconnection with others

Fundamental to these themes was the essence of the experience, which was a sense of continuity while at the same time discontinuity in the experience of self.

Implications for practice

The themes revealed in this study provide a foundation from which nurses can assess stroke survivors. Rather than focusing on neurological impairments or levels of functioning, nurses can explore what these mean to the person with respect to control, independence, connection with others, and a sense of continuity. Goal setting, then, can be individualized to help clients progress toward the positive poles of the themes, rather than toward standardized goals of functioning.

An unexpected finding was that the three participants with nonfluent aphasia seemed to become more fluent as the interview progressed. This was attributed to the fact that they were not asked for specific information; rather, they could talk about what they chose, in the detail they chose, and at the pace they chose to an interested, attentive listener who made no demands. Participants thanked the researcher for listening and said that they had not heretofore had this opportunity. Perhaps if nurses were less inclined to seek specific information from clients with aphasia and were more able to let the client choose what to share, the client's level of effort may decrease while the sense of connection and continuity will increase. This is an area for further study.

Resources

In this information age, resources are readily available to all nurses. The Cumulative Index of Nursing and Allied Health Literature (CINAHL) can be accessed electronically through libraries that subscribe to the service. Interlibrary loans provide articles that are not locally available. Also, MedLine is available, free of charge, through the Internet. Other electronic databases of interest to nurses are PsychLit and ERIC. Nearly all professional associations have Web sites, and most have links to many other relevant sites. The ability to access information in a timely manner is a skill that all nurses must master in order to provide competent, evidence-based care to rehabilitation clients. *[Refer to Chapter 20 for more on information technology and computer applications. See Appendix C, "Community Resources and Health-Related Organizations" for resource listings.]*

References

Alfano, G. (1988). A different kind of nursing. *Nursing Outlook, 36,* 34–37.

American Association of Colleges of Nursing (AACN). (1998). *The essentials of baccalaureate education for professional nursing practice.* Washington, DC: Author.

American Nurses' Association (ANA). (1980). *Nursing's social policy statement.* Kansas City, MO: Author.

American Nurses' Association (ANA). (1985). *Code for nurses with interpretive statements.* Kansas City, MO: Author.

American Nurses' Association (ANA). (1989). *Education for participation in nursing research.* Kansas City, MO: Author.

American Nurses' Association (ANA). (1991). *Nursing's agenda for health care reform.* Kansas City, MO: Author.

American Nurses Association (ANA). (1995). *Nursing's social policy statement.* Washington, DC: Author.

Association of Rehabilitation Nurses (ARN) (in press). *Standards and scope of rehabilitation nursing practice* (4th ed.). Skokie, IL: Author.

Carpenito, L.J. (1997). *Nursing diagnosis. Application to clinical practice* (7th ed.). Philadelphia: Lippincott.

DeLisa, J.A., Currie, D.M., & Martin, G.M. (1998). Rehabilitation medicine: Past, present, and future. In J.A. DeLisa & B.M. Gans (Eds.), *Rehabilitation medicine: Principles and practice* (pp. 3-32). Philadelphia: Lippincott-Raven.

Fawcett, J. (1984). The metaparadigm of nursing: Current status and future refinements. *Image: The Journal of Nursing Scholarship, 16,* 84-87.

Fawcett, J. (1995). *Analysis and evaluation of conceptual models of nursing* (3rd ed.). Philadelphia: F.A. Davis.

Frey, M.A., & Sieloff, C.L. (Eds.). (1995). *Advancing King's systems framework and theory of nursing.* Thousand Oaks, CA: Sage.

Gordon, M. (1987). *Nursing diagnosis: Process and application* (2nd ed.). St. Louis: McGraw-Hill.

Hall, L.E. (1964). Nursing: What is it? *Canadian Nurse, 60,* 150–154.

Hall, L.E. (1969). The Loeb Center for Nursing Rehabilitation. *International Journal Nursing Studies, 6,* 81-95.

Hertzberg, D., & Edwards, P.A. (1999). Introduction to pediatric rehabilitation nursing. In P.A. Edwards, D.L. Hertzberg, S.R. Hays, & N.M. Youngblood (Eds.), *Pediatric rehabilitation nursing* (pp. 3–19). Philadelphia: W.B. Saunders.

King, I.M. (1981). *A theory for nursing: Systems, concepts, process.* Albany, NY: Delmar Publishers.

King, I.M. (1995). The theory of goal attainment. In M.A. Frey & C.L. Sieloff (Eds.), *Advancing King's systems framework and theory of nursing* (pp. 23–32). Thousand Oaks, CA: Sage.

Kirby, R.L. (1998). Impairment, disability and handicap. In J.A. DeLisa & B.M. Gans (Eds.), *Rehabilitation medicine: Principles and practice* (pp. 55–60). Philadelphia: Lippincott-Raven.

Kottke, J.J. (1982). Philosophic considerations of quality of life for the disabled. *Archives Physical Medicine & Rehabilitation, 63,* 60-62.

Lyons, A.S., & Petrucelli, R.J. (1978). *Medicine: An illustrated history.* New York: Harry N. Abrams, Inc.

McCollom, P. (1988). Quality of life versus cost of life. *Rehabilitation Nursing, 13,* 116.

Mumma, C.M., & Nelson, A. (1996). Models for theory-based practice of rehabilitation nursing. In S.P. Hoeman (Ed.), *Rehabilitation nursing. Process and application* (2nd ed.), (pp. 21–31). St. Louis: Mosby.

Orem, D.E. (1995). *Nursing concepts of practice* (5th ed.). St. Louis: Mosby.

Pearson, A., Durand, I., & Punton, S. (1988). The feasibility and effectiveness of nursing beds. *Nursing Times, 84*(47), 48–50.

Pollio, H.R., Henley, T., & Thompson, C. (1977). *The phenomenology of everyday life.* Cambridge, UK: Cambridge University Press.

Rehabilitation Nursing Foundation (RNF). (1994). *Basic competencies for rehabilitation nursing practice.* Skokie, IL: Author.

Rogers, M.E. (1970). *An introduction to the theoretical basis of nursing.* Philadelphia: F.A. Davis.

Rogers, M.E. (1992). Nursing science and the space age. *Nursing Science Quarterly, 5,* 27–34.

Secrest, J., & Thomas, S.P. (1999). Continuity and discontinuity: The quality of life following stroke. *Rehabilitation Nursing, 24*(6), 240-246.

Tomey, A.M., & Alligood, M.R. (1998). *Nursing theorists and their work* (4th ed.). St. Louis: Mosby.

World Book. (1997). *World Book encyclopedia.* Chicago: Author.

Youngblood, N.M. (1999). Models for practice and service. In P.A. Edwards, D.L. Hertzberg, S. R. Hays, & N.M. Youngblood (Eds.), *Pediatric rehabilitation nursing* (pp. 113–126). Philadelphia: W.B. Saunders.

Suggested resources

Alligood, M.R., & Marriner-Tomey, A. (Eds.). (1997). *Nursing theory: Utilization and application*. St. Louis: Mosby.

Davidson, A.W., & Young, C. (1985). Repatterning of stroke rehabilitation clients following return to life in the community. *Journal Neurosurgical Nursing, 17*, 123–128.

Edwards, P.A., Hertzberg, D.L., Hays, S.R., & Youngblood, N.M. (Eds.). (1999). *Pediatric rehabilitation nursing*. Philadelphia: W.B. Saunders.

Folden, S.L. (1993). Effects of a supportive educative nursing intervention on older adults' perceptions of self-care after stroke. *Rehabilitation Nursing, 18*, 162–167.

Hoeman, S.P. (Ed.). (1996). *Rehabilitation nursing. Process and application* (2nd ed.). St. Louis: Mosby.

Smith, D.W. (1995). Power and spirituality in polio survivors: A study based on Rogers' science. *Nursing Science Quarterly, 8*, 133–139.

Taylor, S.G. (1990). Nursing practice applications of self-care deficit nursing theory. In M. Parker (Ed.), *Nursing theories in practice* (pp. 61-70). New York: National League for Nursing.

Temple, A., & Fawdry, K. (1992). King's theory of goal attainment: Resolving filial caregiving role strain. *Journal of Gerontological Nursing, 18*, 11–15.

Woods, E.C. (1994). King's theory in practice with elders. *Nursing Science Quarterly, 7*, 65–69.

Chapter 2

Community and Family-Centered Rehabilitation Nursing

Bonnie J. Parker, MSN RN CRRN

As the healthcare profession continues to strive for a balance between quality of care and fiscal responsibility, the emphasis of care delivery will continue to move toward a community focus. Healthcare professionals are accepting this shift and recognizing that communities support and nurture the health of individuals. With this recognition comes the realization that structures must be in place to support these relationships. The family provides the nucleus of the community support structure. As a result, rehabilitation nurses must focus on defining family and the relationships that exist for rehabilitation clients. Providing education and training to facilitate weaknesses and maximize strengths is an integral part of the rehabilitation process. The rehabilitation team process draws upon the expertise of many individuals to provide a plan to meet the needs of clients and families and to promote health within the community.

I. Overview

A. Definitions of Community

1. A community is a group of people who reside in a specific locality, share government, and often have a common cultural and historical heritage (*Webster's American Family Dictionary*, 1998).

2. Community is a complex concept that refers to individuals in the context of an environment and the relationships that exist between them.

   a. A community is an ever-changing system that responds to input and output, which can occur at any time.

   b. The reciprocal nature of the relationships between individuals and their community greatly affects health. For example, just as family members function in specific roles to serve its members, a community functions in roles such as caregiving agent, nurturer, and sustainer (Klainberg, Holzemer, Leonard, & Arnold, 1998) to serve the individuals who reside within it.

   c. The needs of a healthy community can be viewed in terms of Maslow's hierarchy of individuals' needs (Table 2-1).

3. A community involves "people, location, and social systems" (Hunt & Zurek, 1997, p. 9).

B. Theory of Community Nursing

1. Margaret Newman's theory (1994) focuses on community- and family-centered rehabilitation nursing.

2. Newman (1994) views the meaning of life and health in terms of "an evolving process of expanding consciousness" (p. xxiv).

3. "The pattern of the whole contains the individual as an open system interacting with the family as an open system interacting with the community as an open system. The previous assumptions apply also when focusing on the community. Health of the community is con-

Table 2-1. Maslow's Hierarchy of Individuals' Needs as Compared to Community Needs

Individual needs	Community needs
Self-actualization	Community-actualization
Esteem	Community pride
Belongingness	Educational preparation
Safety	Security
Physiological needs	Life-sustaining activities

Source consulted

Klainberg, M., Holzemer, S., Leonard, M., & Arnold, J. (1998). *Community health nursing: An alliance for health.* St. Louis: McGraw-Hill Nursing Core Series.

ceptualized in terms of changing patterns of energy in the evolution of the system. A pattern of disease endemic to a community can be considered a manifestation of the pattern of the community health.... The diversity and quality of interaction within the community and between the community and its larger environment are indicators of the level of consciousness and thus of the health of the community" (Newman, 1994, pp. 28-29).

   a. Health and illness are viewed as being different patterns in the life of the individual as opposed to being considered a dichotomy or a continuum.

   b. Disease or chronic illness are manifestations of health.

   c. Changes in the health status of an individual or family result in changes in the pattern as related to the whole community.

   d. The problem with trying to separate the views of health and illness is that it becomes more than just a useful way of thinking—it becomes reality. For example, our language promotes the thought process that one object can act on another (e.g., "the person had a stroke" or "the person sustained a spinal cord injury").

   e. By viewing health as encompassing disease and nondisease states, health can be considered just one of the underlying patterns of the person-environment.

4. Rehabilitation nursing as a specialty practice meshes with Newman's concept of community-based nursing practice.

C. Principles of Community-Based Rehabilitation Care

   1. Self-care (client and family responsibility)

      a. The client and family retain primary responsibility for healthcare decisions.

      b. Empowering the client through education allows him or her to make informed healthcare choices about issues such as advance directives and living wills.

   2. Emphasis on the client achieving goals to improve quality of life

      a. Goal development may be short-term, long-term, or lifelong.

      b. Importance is placed on goals being

mutually developed by the client, the family, and the nurse.

      c. Goals are developed in the context of the client's community.

   3. Preventive care

      a. "Treatment efficacy rather than technologic imperative promotes nursing care that emphasizes prevention" (Hunt & Zurek, 1997, p. 18).

      b. Community-based rehabilitation primarily involves tertiary prevention (e.g., teaching a client with spinal cord injury [SCI] about skin care to prevent pressure ulcers).

   4. Care within the context of the community

      a. The nurse recognizes that the health of the client and family is linked to the health of the community.

      b. Nursing care considers culture, values, and available resources.

      c. The community's location and social systems influence care: Location often determines eligibility for healthcare resources; therefore, access to and availability of services can affect the health of the community (Hunt & Zurek, 1997). For example, a client with a stroke may require outpatient rehabilitation services that he or she cannot continue to receive after discharge because the rehabilitation facility is located 150 miles from the client's home.

   5. Continuity of care

      a. Acute care nursing services typically are episodic (i.e., treatment is rendered for a specific disease or condition for a short period of time).

      b. Community-based rehabilitation is marked by the continuity of care that the individual experiences as he or she moves from one healthcare setting to another.

      c. "Continuity is the glue that holds community-based nursing care together" (Hunt & Zurek, 1997, p. 20).

   6. Collaborative care

      a. Collaborative care, which is a hallmark of rehabilitation nursing, is a basic tenet of community-based care.

b. All members of the healthcare team should work with the client and family to achieve goals.

c. The team may use an interdisciplinary model, a transdisciplinary model, or an interagency model. *[Refer to Chapter 1 for more on rehabilitation team models.]*

d. The nurse is often designated as the coordinator of communication.

7. Communication

a. Principles of interpersonal communication are applied in all interactions with clients, families, and healthcare professionals.

b. Interpersonal communication skills are essential to establish, maintain, and terminate therapeutic relationships (Hunt & Zurek, 1997).

D. Levels of Community-Based Services

1. Health

a. The focus of community-based rehabilitation nursing

b. A pattern of wholeness that encompasses the individual (as opposed to the opposite of illness)

c. Maximization of the client's potential in terms of independence and quality of life in the client's own environment

2. Preventive health care (Neal, 1998)

a. Primary prevention: Interventions that promote optimal health and provide special protection to prevent illness, disabilities, or injuries

b. Secondary prevention: Interventions that limit disabilities and are done primarily by early identification and prompt treatment

c. Tertiary prevention: Interventions that decrease disabilities and impairments caused by illness or injury

3. Health maintenance

a. Maintaining the current status of one's health

b. Interventions directed at the client's level that facilitate sequential learning of health activities (e.g., teaching a client with SCI to perform active range-of-motion exercises to maintain flexibility)

c. Activities directed to achieving goals that are part of the client's community regardless of the setting

4. Health restoration

a. Interventions aimed at maximizing the client's and family's level of health

b. Interventions incorporate the client's values and culture (e.g., the nurse recognizes the client's Jewish faith and schedules visits accordingly), and goal setting takes place in active participatory fashion.

E. The Continuum of Community-Based Care

1. Care is delivered in many practice settings (Hoeman, 1996) (see Table 2-2).

a. Acute care (e.g., hospitals, freestanding rehabilitation facilities)

b. Long-term care (e.g., nursing homes, extended care facilities, subacute rehabilitation units or facilities)

c. Community-based settings (e.g., outpatient clinics, day treatment programs, independent living centers, community reentry programs, rural outreach programs)

d. Home care (i.e., continuing rehabilitation services that have been initiated in other settings)

2. The practice area or setting provides the impetus for the primary focus of the role of the nurse across the spectrum of health care (see Table 2-3).

II. Rehabilitation Nurses in Community-Based Care

A. Skills and Competencies That Healthcare Professionals Need to Practice in the Community (Pew Health Professions Commission, 1995)

1. Have an interest in community health

2. Expand access to effective care

3. Provide contemporary clinical care

4. Emphasize primary care

5. Participate in coordinated care

6. Ensure cost-effective, appropriate care

7. Practice prevention

8. Involve clients and families in decision-making process

Table 2-2. Settings, Models, and Programs Where Community-Based Rehabilitation Is Used

Setting	Purpose	Types of Clients	Delivery System	Nursing Roles
Home health care	To provide health care to individuals and families in their place of residence for the purpose of prompting or restoring health, maximizing independence, and minimizing the effects of disability (Hankwitz, 1993)	All age levels Common conditions: • Fractures • Degenerative joint disease • Multiple sclerosis • Parkinson's disease • Cancer • Alterations in function secondary to neuropathy or myopathy • Amputations • Burns	Primary care Case management	Partner Teacher Resource manager Clinician (Neal, 1998)
Subacute care	To serve clients whose medical treatment does not allow for participation in acute rehabilitation programs or who are classified as slow to progress or who cannot qualify for a standard rehabilitation program (Mumma & Nelson, 1996)	Typically older than age 16, although specialty pediatric facilities are available Common conditions: • Closed head injury with quadriparesis • Anoxic encephalopathy secondary to cardiac arrest • Strokes • Aneurysms	Team nursing Primary care delivered by licensed vocational nurses (LVNs) and nursing assistants with RNs serving in the case coordination and management role	Planner Coordinator Evaluator of client outcomes Client advocate
Long-term care	To serve clients who are unable to live independently and meet their self-care needs	Primarily the geriatric population, as well as an unknown number of younger people with chronic disabilities Common conditions: • Joint fractures • Strokes • Closed head injury • Anoxia • Rheumatoid arthritis	Team nursing Primary care delivered by nursing assistants; LVNs provide unit supervision and treatments; RNs serve in the case management and coordination role	Planner Coordinator Evaluator of client outcomes Client advocate
Independent living	To serve individuals who want to take control of their lives, participate in decision making, and achieve the highest level of independence possible	Primarily adults Common conditions • SCI • Closed head injury	Care provided by personal care attendants RN serves as care manager	Partner Educator Client advocate

9. Promote healthy lifestyles

10. Assess and use technology appropriately

11. Improve the healthcare system

12. Manage information

13. Understand the role of the physical environment

14. Provide counseling on ethical issues

15. Accommodate expanded accountability

16. Participate in a racially and culturally diverse society

17. Continue to learn (Hunt & Zurek, 1997, pp. 21–22)

B. Primary Nursing Roles in the Community

1. Partner or physical caregiver (Neal, 1998)

    a. As clients and families become more educated consumers and take responsibility for making healthcare choices, the relationship between the nurse and client will naturally shift toward a partnership.

    b. The client takes primary responsibility for setting goals; the nurse's role varies depending on the client's degree of independence.

2. Teacher

    a. The most important goal of teaching in community-based rehabilitation is to help the client and family achieve the highest level of independence possible.

    b. Quality teaching results in positive outcomes.

        1) Improvements in care

        2) Facilitation of health promotion

        3) Reduction of complications

        4) Resumption of functional activities

    c. Sharing knowledge concerning health care improves client and family satisfaction (Hunt & Zurek, 1997).

    d. Education increases the client's and family's sense of control by encouraging mutual participation in the planning of care (see Figure 2-1).

3. Resource and/or care manager

    a. The nurse maintains responsibility for tracking and directing the client's care and progress throughout the healthcare system.

    b. The nurse oversees the client's primary needs.

        1) Assesses the client appropriately

        2) Establishes the plan of care

        3) Delegates specific nursing care tasks to other qualified personnel

        4) Initiates interventions

        5) Coordinates and collaborates with the healthcare team

        6) Evaluates outcomes

    c. Collaboration and coordination is vital to the implementation of this role, because rehabilitation clients and families interact with many healthcare professionals who have different areas of expertise and training.

    d. The care manager facilitates the client's treatment plan to ensure that it is consistent with the client's needs and is achieved in a timely manner.

    e. Culture is an important part of the

Table 2-3. Role Differentiation of Nurses Based on Practice Setting

Roles	Percentage of time on each role spent by hospital-based nurses	Percentage of time on each role spent by home care nurses	Percentage of time on each role spent by community-based health nurses
Physical caregiver	84%	61%	63%
Manager, administrator	2%	10%	10%
Manager, supervisor	6%	12%	9%
Communicator, teacher, consultant	5%	14%	15%

Sources consulted

Hughes, K., Kostbade, K., & Marcantoinio, R. (1992). Practice patterns among home health, public health and hospital nurses. *Nursing and Health Care, 13*(10), 532–536.

Hunt, R., & Zurek, E. (1997). *Introduction to community based nursing*. Philadelphia: Lippincott.

client's environment.

1) Cultural norms are often implied and influence the client's behavior.
2) Culture provides the foundation for the client's social behavior.
3) It is imperative that the nurse use knowledge of cultural diversity to positively affect the client's health (see Figure 2-2).

4. Advocate
   a. An advocate defends the cause of another individual.
   b. In nursing, advocacy involves empowering clients, families, and client populations through knowledge.
   c. Advocacy involves changing the system, collaborating with other professionals, role modeling, and maximizing the use of community resources (see Figure 2-3).

C. Types of Community-Based Nurses
   1. Nurses in outpatient rehabilitation clinics: Focus on integrating rehabilitation principles into the individual's community
   2. Nurses in assisted living environments: Focus on promoting health in a structured community living setting that is accessible for people with disabilities
   3. Home healthcare nurses: Provide hands-on nursing care in the client's home
   4. School nurses: Provide education, counseling, and referral services for health promotion and health prevention and in meeting the needs of children with disabilities
   5. Parish nurses: Act as health counselors, educators, and referral sources for meeting the needs of individuals; use a holistic focus with a foundation based on spiritual health; usually provide care within the realm of a faith community
   6. Case managers: Act as liaisons, health educators, health promoters, and referral sources
      a. To facilitate return to work for workers with injuries
      b. To integrate workers with catastrophic injuries into the community

III. **Community Reentry and Reintegration**
   A. Overview
      1. Focuses on transition from an acute care environment to the community through a gradual acquisition of community skills and training with active participation by the family
      2. Focuses on self-care, leisure, and vocational activities, as well as psychosocial integration into the client's environment
      3. Focuses nursing services on education, resource management, and advocacy
      4. Threads structure and consistency

Figure 2-1. Benefits of Quality Client Education

Better Outcomes for Client and Family
- Improved care
- Reduction of complications
- Development of self-care skills
- Achievement of highest possible level of independence
- Provision for personal needs
- Resumption of functional activities

Improved Client and Family Satisfaction
- Acquisition of knowledge
- Acquisition of confidence
- Sense of control through participation
- Allows individual decision making

Improved Staff Satisfaction
- Satisfaction regarding safety to move through different types of healthcare services
- Positive results from discharge
- Client successfully manages care

Continuity of Care
- Identical plans and actions by all professionals
- Movement through different types of healthcare services that does not disrupt treatment

Cost Containment While Maintaining Quality Care
- Efficient use of resources
- Prevention strategies incorporated into care

Source consulted

Hunt, R., & Zurek, E. (1997). *Introduction to community based nursing.* Philadelphia: Lippincott.

Figure 2-2. Cultural Interventions for Community-Based Rehabilitation Nurses

Be aware of differences and similarities among cultures
Possess and model a high commitment to culturally competent care
Promote culture-specific care
Demonstrate knowledge of diverse cultures when developing interventions

Source consulted

Hunt, R., & Zurek, E. (1997). *Introduction to community based nursing.* Philadelphia: Lippincott.

throughout the interventions

5. Focuses on acquiring skills through training and education, resulting in behavioral changes

6. Involves addressing or overcoming community-based barriers and handicaps (*handicap* is defined as the result of an impairment or disability—a disadvantage that limits or prevents normal role performance [World Health Organization, 1980] and measured by the interaction and adaptation the client has to his or her surroundings).

   a. Personal barriers: Barriers that are controlled by the individual

---

Figure 2-3. Keys to Developing Advocacy Skills

Understanding and Knowledge of Self Personally and Professionally
- Knowledge of oneself: Awareness of personal goals and how these goals affect relationships with clients
- Realistic self-concept: Awareness of own limitations and abilities that will affect client care
- Values clarification: Awareness of personal bias and prejudices, moral and ethical values; knowledge of personal perceptions concerning what is fair and acceptable and how these perceptions may affect relationships with clients

Knowledge of Treatment and Intervention Options
- Development of a strong knowledge base concerning interventions and outcomes
- Awareness of rationale for interventions

Knowledge of the Healthcare System
- Awareness of how the healthcare system relates to clients, families, and the community
- Awareness of specific aspects of community (e.g., politics, economy) and how these factors affect the healthcare system

Knowledge of How To Put Advocacy into Action
- Assessment
  - What does the client identify as the problem?
  - What support or resources does the client already have?
  - What knowledge does the client have concerning health services and treatment options?
  - In what areas does the client feel a need for more personal control?
- Planning: Mobilizing resources, consulting, collaborating with the healthcare team
- Implementation: Educating and empowering the client (the nurse helps the client assert control over variables affecting the client's life)

---

1) Negative attitude
2) Poor self-esteem
3) Lack of motivation
4) Poor self-image
5) Feelings of dependence
6) Insecurity
7) An inability to plan and meet goals
8) Unrealistic expectations (Frieden, 1992)

b. Transportation issues, which greatly affect a client's environment and community reintegration efforts and can make the difference between community reintegration and reinstitutionalization

   1) Accessibility of healthcare services
   2) Ability to pursue vocational interests
   3) Accessibility to public facilities
   4) Participation in social and recreational activities
   5) Ability to pursue education
   6) Ability to achieve independence in high-level self-care skills

c. Issues related to quality attendant care

   1) Attendant care is often linked with eligibility requirements and income.
   2) Waiting lists for programs can be lengthy.
   3) The types of services provided by attendants and homemaker services are often deemed custodial by third-party payers and may not be reimbursable.
   4) Responsibility for hiring, firing, and training is placed on the client and family.
   5) Training can be very costly and can involve limited staff retention.
   6) If an attendant is sick or unable to attend work for personal reasons, the client must have alternative resources to meet his or her needs.

d. Housing barriers

   1) Accessible housing in many communities is not adequate to meet the needs of the population.
   2) There are several causes for inadequate housing (Buchanan, 1996).
      a) Insufficient supply
      b) Inaccessibility
      c) Architectural barriers

d) Long waiting lists

e) Poor location and high cost

3) "Independent living has been associated with promoting general well-being and self-esteem of persons with disabilities; however, discrimination continues even when housing is erected to accommodate them under federal mandates" (Buchanan, 1996, p. 117).

e. Barriers to financial independence, identity, and life satisfaction through employment opportunities

1) Budget restraints in federal and state agencies limit the access to vocational rehabilitation programs for individuals with disabilities.

2) A limited number of job coaches are available to help train and supervise individuals with disabilities (Grossi, Test, & Keul, 1991).

3) Return to work is affected by the client's level of disability, level of education, gender, age, and preinjury wages (Tate, 1992).

4) New opportunities may exist for individuals with disabilities as the trends continue toward more home-based businesses and the use of computer technology.

f. The tremendous cost of health care and the client's inability to meet financial needs

1) Individuals with chronic illness or disability are often faced with incredible financial burdens.

2) Lost or reduced employment can lead to a loss of insurance benefits, which places further burdens on the client and family.

3) Often, the client's spouse or caregiver must face additional stress in trying to meet the needs of the client in the home setting while balancing work and home obligations.

g. Issues related to appropriate caregiving at home

1) Caregiver and family needs must be assessed to identify potential handicaps for the client.

2) When an individual with a chronic illness or disability returns home, the entire family system is affected.

3) Research has demonstrated that the lack of preparation and training, information, skills, support resources, respite care, and financial concerns can cause tremendous burdens for the family (DeGraff, 1992; Frieden, 1992).

4) Community-based rehabilitation nurses use their skills and training to identify needs regardless of the setting to help the client and family reduce their burdens as much as possible.

B. Life Skills and Independent Living

1. Overview

a. Whether they express it or not, individuals with chronic illness or disability begin to wonder almost from the point of diagnosis about their future outcomes (Frieden, 1992).

b. Early in the rehabilitation process, their expectations may be unrealistic and extreme.

c. As the client and family gather more information and training and synthesize this knowledge into their personal environment, they can begin to adjust and readapt to the community.

2. History: The concept of independent living began with a focus on quality-of-life issues during the late 1960s and early 1970s.

3. The essence of independent living: The ability for individuals to have control over their lives based on choice

a. Minimizing dependence on other individuals for daily living needs

b. Managing personal affairs

c. Participating in community life

d. Fulfilling social roles

e. Having options

4. Grassroots efforts: Lobby groups (including policy makers, politicians, healthcare professionals, community members, family members) were formed to promote independent living programs.

a. Developed new laws that protect the rights of people with disabilities

b. Required the new construction of or adaptations to public buildings, housing, transportation, schools, and places of employment to ensure accessibility

c. Initiated changing public attitudes about and toward people with disabilities

d. Provided new opportunities for individuals with disabilities to enjoy opportunities that enhance quality of life

C. A Conceptual Model for Nurses Working in Community Reentry and Independent Living Programs

1. The client serves as manager of his or her life and care in a community-based or independent living setting.

   a. Based on the knowledge and skills that the client acquires during the acute phase of rehabilitation, options are considered and decisions are made.

   b. The nurse's role is one of an active participant to help the client through education, coordination of resources, and understanding how the community's needs and resources will affect his or her health as well as the health of the family (see Figure 2-4).

2. The client's lifestyle and needs are considered in terms of his or her environment and community.

   a. Health is promoted by determining accessibility for meeting self-care needs and by facilitating opportunities for community reintegration.

   b. The nurse's role is to facilitate communication and collaborate with other healthcare professionals so that the client's energy can be optimized during the transition period.

3. Client and family education is an ongoing process.

   a. Initially, education is focused and goal-directed to help the client and family meet the client's basic self-care needs.

   b. As the client reintegrates into the community, the focus of education changes to enhance the client's problem-solving skills and to learn strategies to maximize health by identifying resources.

c. Preventive care is always emphasized— from the time of initial education through the rehabilitation process. Preventing complications is the simplest way to diminish handicaps and barriers that can increase the stress and burden on the client and family.

4. The management of attendant care training and services facilitates independent living and helps the client maintain a community-based living environment.

5. Equipment and supplies should be evaluated prior to discharge from the acute rehabilitation setting.

   a. The nurse communicates with the family during acute care and the transition to the community to ensure that equipment and supplies meet the client's needs.

   b. The nurse establishes a partnership with the client and family and maintaining the lines of communication.

   c. The nurse coordinates the equipment and monitors its effectiveness in meeting the client's needs while monitoring cost.

6. The client and family's financial resources must be assessed in terms of current availability but also in terms of future projections.

   a. As part of the educational process, the nurse helps the client and family identify

---

Figure 2-4. Rehabilitation Nursing Competencies for Helping Clients in Community Reintegration and Independent Living

- Identify the family's role in the rehabilitation process
- Involve the client's family in the rehabilitation process
- Discuss factors that influence community reentry of a person with a disability
- Provide family with appropriate strategies to use and options to seek in the community to cope with the client's and/or the family's dysfunctional behavior
- Collaborate with the team to develop a resource bank of supportive services for clients
- Collaborate with the rehabilitation team to develop an appropriate home program that includes interventions to manage severe cognitive or physical deficits
- Provide a resource list to help clients with community reintegration

Source consulted

Rehabilitation Nursing Foundation (RNF). (1994). *Basic competencies for rehabilitation nursing practice*. Skokie, IL: Author.

---

options and make choices that will meet their future needs.

b. Identifying barriers early in the community living process gives the client and family time to make calm, informed choices rather than having to make decisions during times of crisis.

c. By helping the client and family realistically appraise their financial needs and available resources, the nurse helps the client maintain ongoing success and health in the community setting.

7. Identifying barriers and options in the community helps the client and family make good healthcare and personal choices.

a. In the management role, the nurse can help educate the client and family about housing alternatives and architectural designs that maximize independence in the community.

b. Through collaboration with other healthcare professionals and coordination of efforts within the healthcare system, the nurse can use community resources to help the client and family make the transition to independent living.

8. Independent living is fostered in environments where cooperation exists among healthcare providers.

a. Collaboration and coordination of services between agencies and healthcare systems maximizes clients' resources in terms of financial and self-care needs.

b. Identification of resources and plans of action that incorporate healthcare emergencies facilitate clients' transition to independent living as well as their overall health.

D. Housing Issues
1. Components of an in-depth assessment of housing alternatives and the client's needs

a. Awareness of the client's functional ability

b. Family needs and support

c. The client's goals

d. Availability of resources

2. Considerations for the client's transition to the community

a. Necessary modifications to the home

environment (e.g., building ramps, widening doorways, making bathroom and kitchen modifications, and ensuring accessibility to the community)

b. Independent living environments that allow the individual to maintain his or her own residence while providing support services in specific areas

1) Communication techniques
2) Homemaking skills
3) Transportation skills
4) Recreational opportunities
5) Emergency procedures
6) Management of attendants
7) Advocacy services
8) Peer counseling
9) Personal business management

3. Residential living arrangements: Housing in which a group of individuals with disabilities live in the same geographic area or building and share support services

4. Extended care facilities (e.g., subacute rehabilitation, neurobehavioral programs, skilled care facilities)

5. Laws that affect housing availability and accessibility

a. Housing Act (1959): Provided funds for mortgage loans to developers to build housing for people who are disabled or elderly

b. Architectural Barriers Act (1968): Mandated that all federally funded buildings being constructed must be made accessible for people with disabilities

c. Rehabilitation Act (1973): Prohibited discrimination against people with disabilities when they purchase or rent federally subsidized housing

d. Housing and Community Development Act (1974): Allowed families with low incomes to receive subsidized rent payments

e. Rehabilitation, Comprehensive Services, and Developmental Disabilities Amendment (1978): Issued grants for housing

f. Americans with Disabilities Act (1990): Established new laws concerning physical access to the community; the laws are evaluated in relation to access to services and ways to implement them in communities to ensure access for all individuals

6. Components of a home assessment

   a. Safety of the client in the home environment and the ability to maximize function while meeting healthcare needs

   b. Availability of healthcare services to continue to meet the client's needs

   c. Architectural design of the building and accessibility

   d. Assistive devices to promote community living skills

   e. Availability of support services, transportation, and recreational and leisure opportunities in the community

   f. Furniture, floor surfaces, and clutter that can lead to client safety issues

   g. Adequacy of lighting, ventilation, and toileting facilities

   h. Accessibility of parking to residence entrance

   i. Availability of emergency services (e.g., telephone, fire alarms, emergency exits)

E. Financial Issues

   1. Individuals often have limited life skills or financial resources to deal with catastrophic illness.

   2. Stress from financial burdens can result in a diminished ability to continue the rehabilitation process and ultimately prevent reaching the maximum health potential.

   3. Rehabilitation nurses can help perform a realistic assessment of the client's financial resources and potential future burden to the client and family as a result of disability or chronic illness.

   4. Rehabilitation nurses can enlist a representative from the client's payer or reimbursement source as part of the treatment team to facilitate communication and provide prompt justification of resources. *[Refer to Chapter 4 for more information on economics and health plans.]*

      a. Group health

      b. Self-insurance

   c. Health maintenance organization (HMO) or preferred provider organization (PPO) plans

   d. Third-party payers

   e. Workers' compensation

   f. Medicare

   g. Medicaid

F. Transportation Issues

   1. Legislation that guarantees basic rights for all people

      a. Equal access to public transportation

      b. Equal access to airplanes, terminals, buses, subways, and public railway systems

   2. Roles of the rehabilitation nurse in facilitating transportation for rehabilitation clients

      a. Provide education concerning the availability of community resources and how to problem solve when moving to other communities

      b. Advocate to ensure that the transportation needs of clients are met in the community

      c. Collaborate with other healthcare professionals to expand knowledge of available resources and support services

   3. Considerations for assessing clients' transportation needs

      a. Hand controls, lifts, transfer mechanisms, and seating in existing vehicles

      b. Adaptive training with modified vehicles

      c. Financial considerations for vehicle modifications

      d. Travel programs or clubs for people with disabilities

G. Issues Concerning Care Providers

   1. Making the choice to use care providers

      a. Facilitation of the client and family's transition to the community must include in-depth consideration of the client's self-care needs.

      b. The burden of care for the family attempting to meet the client's needs and the implications for home management and finances must be assessed.

      c. Sometimes the client's quest for independence is completed at the risk of self-harm, which may be demonstrated by various problems (e.g., shoulder joint damage, stress-related illnesses, psychological alterations).

    d. When the rehabilitation nurse helps maintain the lines of communication, provides education, and helps the client evaluate options, the client and family may decide that using care providers is a valid option.

2. Steps in using care providers

    a. Determine hiring strategy

    b. Determine need for training (e.g., should care providers be competent upon hiring or is training on the job an option?)

    c. Determine what support services are available to the client and care providers

    d. Solidify the role of the family and consider the implications of having nonfamily members in the home setting

    e. Address financial implications

    f. Consider the philosophies and definitions of care providers, which vary from state to state (e.g., what can a care provider do in this client's community?)

    g. Address safety issues

    h. Determine ways to terminate the relationship with a care provider

    i. Establish emergency measures to meet personal needs in case a care provider is unable to meet work obligations

3. Freedoms of clients who use care providers (DeGraff, 1992)

    a. Freedom from having to use parents or relatives as attendants

    b. Freedom from having to use a spouse or lover as an attendant or sole attendant

    c. Freedom to directly control the type, quality, and schedule of attendants and to change attendants whenever necessary

    d. Freedom from being dependent on referral agencies or pools of aides and from being forced to relocate wherever and whenever necessary

    e. Freedom from having to use agency or college campus attendant training services

    f. Freedom from having to pay high hourly administrative rates to professional home

health aide agencies if the individual is not eligible for third-party funding

4. A three-pronged model for nurses who training clients and care providers to work together (DeGraff, 1992)

    a. Instruct the client

        1) Teach which skills qualify as self-care skills and which skills require attendant services

        2) Teach safe and efficient methods to instruct others to provide self-care

        3) Encourage self-advocacy when needs are not being met or the quality of care is unacceptable

        4) Teach the client how to be assertive

    b. Offer support services: Provide education about safe and efficient personal care methods and how to find, manage, and cope with care attendants (see Figure 2-5)

    c. Provide practical opportunities: Behavioral changes and integration of knowledge cannot occur without the ability to practice new skills.

        1) Allow practice time that addresses specific skill training and that follows instruction

        2) Encourage or require practice sessions with the healthcare professional acting as the attendant in the client's room.

        3 Allow for mistakes without instilling a fear of punishment

        4) Schedule additional practice opportunities with support when necessary (DeGraff, 1992)

H. Finding Natural Supports in the Client's Community

1. Definition: Natural supports are defined as "...resources and strategies that promote [the] interests and causes of an individual with or without disabilities that enable him or her to access resources, information, and relationships inherent within integrated work and living environments, and that result in [the] person's enhanced independence, productivity, community integration, and satisfaction (Karan & Greenspan, 1995, p. 210).

    a. This term is borrowed from vocational literature; it refers to the use of community resources from everyday life to help people with disabilities find employment in the community (Edwards, Hertzberg, Hays, Youngblood, 1999).

   b. All attempts to return clients in the community should include an assessment of the natural supports present in the community.

2. Importance of natural supports: The foundation of community-based rehabilitation care involves using the options available in the community that support and facilitate the health of the client. Natural supports are the community's internal mechanisms that are unrelated to disability services but that facilitate and enhance the client's options and opportunities for maintaining a gainful and healthy lifestyle within the environment.

Figure 2-5. Topics with Which Clients and Families Who Will Be Using Care Providers Should Be Familiar

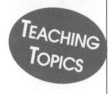

Management skills
Management situations
Qualities of a good manager
Styles of management
Training and ongoing management
Predicting and recognizing problems
Ways to maintain independent living
Rights of people with disabilities and care attendants
Settings in which people with disabilities may use help
Types of help and services that providers can perform
Job expectations
Work environments
Abusing help or taking advantage of assistance (e.g., not completing tasks that could be done independently because it is easier to have someone else do it)
Activities that qualify for attendant services
Making a master list of needs
Residence locations for attendants
Reasons why attendants quit and are fired
Paying salaries and taxes
Recruiting, interviewing, training, and parting with help
Creating a job description
Sources of recruiting
Methods of recruiting
Interviewing and screening
Parting ways with a care attendant

Source consulted

DeGraff, D. (1992). Teaching attendant management skills. In C.P. Zedjlik (Ed.), *Management of spinal cord injury* (2nd ed., pp. 661–671). Boston: Jones and Bartlett.

---

3. Examples of natural supports
   a. Churches
   b. Neighbors
   c. Friends
   d. Public or private services

4. Parish nursing: An evolution of natural supports in the community

   a. Parish nursing provides an alternative means for health care for those who might otherwise not be served.

   b. Parish nursing focuses on holistic health care and integrates spiritual health. It is practiced within the context of the values, beliefs, and practices of a faith community.

   c. Parish nursing began in the 1970s in the Chicago area through the efforts of Reverend Granger Westburg.

      1) In his work as a hospital chaplain, Westburg found that nurses frequently took on responsibility of decoding medical terminology for clients, making it more understandable and, often, basing it in the context of faith and healing.

      2) Westburg was impressed with the work of a nurse educator at the University of Arizona who served in the position of "minister of health." As a health promoter in the local Lutheran church, this nurse spread her message through programs that were focused on health promotion and disease prevention. Westburg took these principles and started the first parish nursing program in the Chicago area.

   d. The primary roles of parish nurses include health education, health counseling and referral, and health screening. Hands-on nursing is not a component of this role.

   e. Parish nurses believe that all human beings are sacred and deserve to be treated with respect and dignity and empower individuals to become active partners in their health by managing their healthcare resources.

   f. Parish nurses recognize that spiritual health is fundamental to well-being and

---

that health and illness can occur simultaneously. Therefore, using illness to evaluate life goals can mobilize untapped strengths. Healing may take place in the absence of cure, because physical well-being is only one dimension of an individual's health.

I. Research Validating the Need for Rehabilitation Nursing Skills in Community Settings
    1. Neal (1999) evaluated the congruence between rehabilitation nursing principles and home health nursing practice.
    2. Neal's findings determined that rehabilitation principles are congruent with home health nursing principles and that educating and training home health nurses about rehabilitation principles may result in better health outcomes for clients.

IV. **Employment Opportunities for People with Disabilities in the Community**
    A. Vocational Rehabilitation
        1. Each state is mandated by federal law to have an office of vocational rehabilitation that provides vocational services for people with disabilities.
        2. Funding is available to help individuals seek gainful or supported employment.
            a. To make home or vehicle modifications
            b. To participate in work hardening programs or functional work capacity examinations: Work hardening programs are custom-designed programs that are formulated to address a client's specific needs based on his or her ability to perform activities of daily living. The goal is for the client to achieve the highest level of function, which will prepare him or her for returning to work.
            c. To determine the client's vocational strengths or weaknesses
            d. To identify abilities, previous work experiences, or vocational interests
            e. To assess the job market
            f. To educate and train employers
            g. To match the client's functional and cognitive abilities with job options
        3. Supported employment allows people with disabilities to integrate into employment settings.

            a. In 1986, the amendments to the Rehabilitation Act described how supported employment programs would be implemented. Prior to this act, vocational rehabilitation programs met the needs of people with disabilities through sheltered workshops.
            b. Key aspects of supported employment
                1) Meet the employment needs of people with severe disabilities
                2) Pay all workers
                3) Integrate the work environment by placing able-bodied workers with workers with disabilities
                4) Provide support and job supervision
                5) Provide training that includes job adaptations, money management, personal care, and social skills
                6) Provide transportation
    B. Rehabilitation Nurses' Role in Disability Management in the Workplace
        1. Rehabilitation nurses are uniquely qualified to provide disability management in the workplace.
            a. By identifying potential sources of work-related injury
            b. By providing education and training on preventive techniques as well as health maintenance
        2. When injuries occur, rehabilitation nurses serve as care managers and emphasize prompt assessment and intervention by using the healthcare team to facilitate return to work as soon as possible for the injured employee.
        3. Rehabilitation nurses perform other case management tasks such as job analysis, job modification and training, and education for employers concerning job placement.
        4. Rehabilitation nurses can provide training for employers regarding work-hardening programs
        5. Rehabilitation nurses facilitate positive outcomes by being involved in disability management.
            a. Lower workers' compensation costs
            b. Decreased absenteeism
            c. Decreased cost of rehabilitation services for injured employees
            d. Increased employee satisfaction
            e. Increased employee retention

References

Buchanan, L.C. (1996). Community-based rehabilitation nursing. In S.P. Hoeman (Ed.), *Rehabilitation nursing: Process and application* (2nd ed., pp. 114-129). St. Louis: Mosby.

DeGraff, D. (1992). Teaching attendant management skills. In C.P. Zedjlik (Ed.), *Management of spinal cord injury* (2nd ed., pp. 661-671). Boston: Jones and Bartlett.

Edwards, P., Hertzberg, D., Hays, S., & Youngblood, N. (Eds.). (1999). *Pediatric rehabilitation nursing.* Philadelphia: W.B. Saunders.

Frieden, L. (1992). Is there life after rehabilitation? In C.P. Zedjlik (Ed.), *Management of spinal cord injury* (2nd ed., pp. 631-641). Boston: Jones and Bartlett.

Grossi, T.A., Test, D.W., & Keul, P.K. (1991). Strategies for hiring, training and supervising job coaches. *Journal of Rehabilitation, 57,* 37-42.

Hankwitz, P.E. (1993). Role of physician in home care. In B.J. May (Ed.), *Home health and rehabilitation concepts of care* (pp. 1-23). Philadelphia: F.A. Davis.

Hocman, S. (Ed.). *Rehabilitation nursing: Process and application* (2nd ed.). St. Louis: Mosby.

Hughes, K., Kostbade, K., & Marcantoinio, R. (1992). Practice patterns among home health, public health and hospital nurses. *Nursing and Health Care, 13*(10), 532-536.

Hunt, R., & Zurek, E. (1997). *Introduction to community based nursing.* Philadelphia: Lippincott.

Karan, O., & Greenspan, S. (Eds.). (1995). *Community rehabilitation services for people with disabilities.* Boston: Butterworth-Heinemann.

Klainberg, M., Holzemer, S., Leonard, M., & Arnold, J. (1998). *Community health nursing: An alliance for health.* St. Louis: McGraw-Hill Nursing Core Series.

Mumma, C., & Nelson, A. (1996). Models for theory-based practice of rehabilitation nursing. In S.P. Hoeman (Ed.), *Rehabilitation nursing: Process and application* (2nd ed., pp. 21-33). St. Louis: Mosby.

Neal, L. (Ed.). (1998). *Rehabilitation nursing in the home health setting.* Glenview, IL: Association of Rehabilitation Nurses.

Neal, L. (1999). Research supporting the congruence between rehabilitation principles and home health nursing practice. *Rehabilitation Nursing, 24*(3), 115-121.

Newman, M.A. (1994). *Health as expanding consciousness* (2nd ed.). New York: National League for Nursing.

Pew Health Professions Commission. (1995). *Health America: Practitioners for 2005.* Durham, NC: Author.

Rehabilitation Nursing Foundation (RNF). (1994). *Basic competencies for rehabilitation nursing practice.* Skokie, IL: Author.

Tate, D.G. (1992). Workers' disability and return to work. *American Journal of Physical Medicine and Rehabilitation, 71,* 92-96.

Webster's American family dictionary. (1998). Springfield, MA: Merriam-Webster, Inc.

World Health Organization (WHO). (1980). *International classification of impairments, disabilities, and handicaps.* Geneva: Author.

Suggested resources

McCourt, A.E. (Ed.). (1993). *The specialty practice of rehabilitation nursing: A core curriculum* (3rd ed.). Skokie, IL: Rehabilitation Nursing Foundation of the Association of Rehabilitation Nurses.

Zedjlik, C.P. (Ed.). (1992). *Management of spinal cord injury* (2nd ed.). Boston: Jones and Bartlett.

Chapter 3

Ethical, Moral, and Legal Considerations

Patricia A. Edwards, EdD RN CNAA

Rhonda J. Reed, MSN RN CRRN

Rehabilitation nurses are confronted with a variety of ethical and moral dilemmas in their varied practice settings. They often face the problem of working with clients and families whose decisions may not reflect their own values and beliefs about health, self-care, and independence and whose quality of life has been significantly affected by technological advances in medicine and health care.

To help clients and families make informed decisions about care and treatment options, rehabilitation nurses should be careful to adhere to established parameters and to seek ethical and legal consultation when necessary to determine the most appropriate course of action. Rehabilitation nurses' participation in collaborative decision making with clients, families, and other health professionals should reflect the understanding that care should be ethical, legal, compassionate, and culturally sensitive, and that those affected by the care should be well informed.

Rehabilitation services have a significant effect on clients' future abilities and the continued need for costly services. "Understanding how ethical conflicts affect the delivery of rehabilitation services is necessary to improve the delivery of these services into the next century" (Redman & Fry, 1998, p. 184). This chapter provides an overview of the ethical and moral issues and legal considerations that are frequently encountered in rehabilitation nursing practice.

I. Ethical and Moral Considerations
A. Definitions
1. "Ethics: Study of the nature and justification of general ethical principles that can apply to special areas where there are moral problems
2. Morality: Traditions of belief about right and wrong moral conduct
3. Bioethics: Ethics applied to health care including moral rules, principles, and values that guide healthcare professionals in relationships with clients and families" (McCourt, 1993, p. 230)
4. Rehabilitation nursing ethics: "Judgments about decisions to act and subsequent actions based on the rules of conduct or precepts of rehabilitation nursing practice" (Graham-Eason, 1996, p. 35)

B. Ethical Theories and Principles
1. Models
   a. Deontologic: Assumes the "rightness or wrongness of an act does not depend on the consequence; the rightness or wrongness is inherent in the act" (Graham-Eason, 1996, p. 35)
   b. Theologic or utilitarian: Is based on the assumption that actions lead to maximizing the overall good
   c. Intuitionist: Assumes that practitioners consider all points and use their own moral intuition to determine what is good or bad
   d. Personalized: Contains no universal laws and allows nurses to choose when to make compromises
2. Factors for choosing a model that fits the individual nurse (Graham-Eason, 1996)

a. Choices are based on the individual's philosophy of life, religious practice, secular habits, practice setting, political beliefs, and other factors.

b. Intuitionist and personalized theories offer options based on current reality.

c. By choosing one model, the individual can discern moral answers where many values exist.

d. There are few simple, final solutions to ethical dilemmas.

e. Choosing a model can help the individual build a compendium of potential solutions and consequences from previous situations.

f. Each situation must be assessed and acted upon individually.

C. Moral Principles
   1. Defining attributes of a dilemma (Sletteboe, 1997)
      a. Engagement
      b. Equally unattractive alternatives
      c. Awareness of alternatives
      d. Need for a choice
      e. Uncertainty of action
   2. Recognition of a dilemma: Integrating an initial assessment with information about specific needs and resources and data from other team members' analyses
   3. Types of moral conflict (Redman & Fry, 1998)
      a. Moral dilemma: Occurs when two or more clear moral principles apply but they support mutually inconsistent courses of action
      b. Moral distress: Occurs when a person knows the right thing to do but institutional constraints make it nearly impossible to pursue the right course of action
      c. Moral uncertainty: Occurs when a person is unsure about which moral principles or values apply or even about what the moral problem is
   4. Assessment and moral principles (see Table 3-1) and the specific dilemmas and concerns that may arise in rehabilitation (Graham-Eason, 1996)

a. Autonomy
b. Nonmaleficence
c. Beneficence
d. Advocacy
e. Veracity
f. Client fiduciary responsibility
g. Ethic of care
h. Reciprocity
i. Protection of dignity
j. Respect that acknowledges the interdependence of individuals

D. Professional Ethics Codes, Standards, and Statements
   1. American Nurses Association's (ANA) *Code for Nurses with Interpretive Statements* (1985)
   2. Association of Rehabilitation Nurses (ARN) standards of ethical rehabilitation nursing practice (1994) (see Figure 3-1)
   3. ANA (1996) position statements regarding ethics
      a. Active euthanasia
      b. Assisted suicide
      c. Ethics and human rights
      d. Foregoing medical provision of nutrition and hydration
      e. Nonnegotiable nature of ANA's *Code for Nurses with Interpretive Statements*
      f. Nursing and the Patient Self-Determination Act
      g. Nursing care and do-not-resuscitate (DNR) decisions
      h. Risk versus responsibility in providing nursing care
   4. The influence of codes as the cornerstone of nursing practice in specific areas (Esterhuizen, 1996)
      a. Moral decision making
      b. Administration and management
      c. Education

E. Models of Ethical and Moral Decision Making
   1. Nursing process
   2. Three-step ACT model (Graham-Eason, 1996)
      a. A: Anticipate obstacles to action

Table 3-1. Assessment and Moral Principles*

Principle	Descriptor	Dilemma or Concern
Autonomy	Patient has right to choose; self-determination	1. Informed consent—related to research 2. Ventilator-dependent client feels he has no quality of life; lives in a nursing home, has no resources—financial or family. Wants to die. Questions to ask relate to whether the client has been informed of all resources.
Nonmaleficence	Do no harm	Should a client be sent home with family member if it appears as though the family member is not interested or just cannot follow through? Should a head-injured client be restrained? Is this protection?
Beneficence	Doing good	When dealing with adolescents or children who are comatose: Are parents always in the best position to make decisions? What is the nurse's role in the situation where the family or caregiver's decision is not consistent with philosophy of rehabilitation?
Advocacy (loyalty)	Standing for client	
Veracity	Truth telling: Client needs information before he or she can consent	When a client is admitted to rehabilitation, how "honest is honest" when giving prognosis while "still offering hope"?
Client fiduciary responsibility	Recognize costs to client when provided or do not provide treatments	1. Is length of stay determined by insurance? 2. Who determines level of care?
Ethic of care	Gives rise to compassion, equity, fairness, envisions problem in context—framework of relationships, dignity	Dilemma is that nurses work in situations and institutions where policies and practices may be based on paternalistic views of what is right. Nurses in rehabilitation also work with other team members who are involved with client. Nurse-client relationship here is one that takes into consideration other relationships and available resources. Does not act on what is understood common right but looks at the unique rights of the client now.
Reciprocity	Develop one's talents, integrity—be true to one's self, impartial, consistent, having respect for client's goals and values	Setting contracts with clients. They need to behave in manner consistent with plan of care. Staff members need to be fair, impartial in contract setting, and be able to keep their end of the deal. Involves having relationship. Are staff members open to compromises with clients who want to tailor a trust contract?
Fidelity	Always keep promises	Promise to keep child from ever hurting again—find out client to be returned to family that caused injury. Need to consider promises in ethical dilemma, especially in light of legal consequences or long-term outcomes.
Concern for community as a whole	Costs to the community; values of the community	1. Who will take care of indigent rehabilitation clients? 2. Client has placement problem—will end up in nursing home. Do costs that allow independence in the nursing home balance with benefits? 3. Is rehabilitation necessary when many in community do not even have access to basic healthcare needs? Is rehabilitation a basic healthcare need?
Sanction for life	Maintaining life rather than intent to end life	Persons with Parkinson's disease and others may benefit from fetal transplant neuron tissue. Is it ethically responsible to end one life to benefit another? What if fetus will be aborted anyway? Who benefits from abortion?

*Note. *Moral principles form bases for nursing practice. Dilemmas or concerns may arise for one or more principles, as with these examples from rehabilitation practice.*

Reprinted with permission of Mosby from Graham-Eason, C. (1996). Ethical considerations for rehabilitation nursing. In S. Hoeman (Ed.), *Rehabilitation nursing: Process and application* (2nd ed., p. 37). St. Louis: Mosby.

      b. C: Clarify position related to planning action

      c. T: Test choice

  3. Savage model (Savage & Michalak, 1999) for facilitating ethical decision making (see Figure 3-2)

  4. Josephson Institute of Ethics (1999) decision-making model

      a. All decisions must take into account and reflect a concern for the interest and well-being of stakeholders.

      b. Ethical values and principles always take precedence over nonethical ones.

      c. It is proper to violate an ethical principle only when it is clearly necessary to advance another true ethical principle, which, according to the decision maker's conscience, will produce the greatest balance of good in the long run.

  5. Other ethical decision-making models (see Figure 3-3)

F. Ethical Principles Associated with a Family-Centered Approach to Decision Making

  1. Autonomy: Moral obligation to respect self-determination

  2. Beneficence: Moral obligation to do good for others

  3. Justice: Fair distribution of benefits and burdens

  4. Nonmaleficence: Moral obligation not to inflict harm

G. Ethics Committee

  1. Definition: A multidisciplinary group of healthcare professionals established specifically to address ethical dilemmas that occur within a particular setting (McCourt, 1993)

  2. Pros (Savage & Michalak, 1999)

      a. Allows multidisciplinary perspectives to be considered

      b. Provides a forum for communication

      c. Allows anticipatory discussion of potential conflicts

      d. Has a clinical focus

      e. Allows for objective, detached deliberation

      f. Fosters policy development

      g. Promotes awareness of ethical issues

  3. Cons (Savage & Michalak, 1999)

      a. Can involve dominant members' opinions to prevail

      b. Can be intrusive in a physician-patient relationship

      c. Has the potential for bureaucratic inefficiency

      d. Can become a "rubber-stamp" for physician opinion

      e. Has the potential for disenfranchising interested parties who are not included on the committee

  4. Responsibilities of an ethics committee (McCourt, 1993)

      a. Address issues of informed consent

      b. Render decisions for incompetent or

Figure 3-1. ARN Standards Regarding Ethics

Standard V. Ethics: The rehabilitation nurse's decisions and actions on behalf of clients are determined in an ethical manner.

- The rehabilitation nurse's practice is guided by *Code for Nurses with Interpretive Statements* (ANA, 1985) and ARN's position statement on ethical issues.
- The rehabilitation nurse maintains a client's confidentiality.
- The rehabilitation nurse acts as a client advocate.
- The rehabilitation nurse delivers care in a nonjudgmental and nondiscriminatory manner that is sensitive to clients' diversity.
- The rehabilitation nurse delivers care in a manner that preserves and protects the client's autonomy, dignity, and rights.
- The rehabilitation nurse maintains an awareness of his or her beliefs and value systems and what effect they may have on care he or she provides to the client and client's significant others.
- The rehabilitation nurse supports the client's right to make decisions that may not be congruent with the values of the rehabilitation team.
- The rehabilitation nurse seeks available resources to help formulate ethical decisions.
- The rehabilitation nurse promotes the provision of information and discussion that allows the client to participate fully in decision making.
- The rehabilitation nurse participates in decision making regarding allocation of resources.

Reprinted with permission of the Association of Rehabilitation Nurses (ARN) from ARN. (1994). *Standards and scope of rehabilitation nursing practice* (3rd ed.). Skokie, IL: Author.

incapacitated patients when an emergency exists or an immediate decision is needed

    c. Rule on difficult decisions that present a compelling case

    d. Attempt resolution of treatment differences

    e. Serve as a forum for discussion of such concerns and act in an advisory capacity prior to judicial review

    f. Educate staff

  5. Special responsibilities of a nursing ethics committee (Habel, 1999)

    a. Address unique concerns of nursing

    b. Help nurses identify, explore, and resolve ethical issues in practice

    c. Provide education and staff development

    d. Develop and follow a defined model of critical thinking

    e. Review department policies related to ethics

II. Legal Issues and Considerations

  A. Patient Self-Determination Act: Requires that individuals receiving medical care must be given written information about their right to make decisions

  B. Patients' Bill of Rights

    1. Adopted in 1973 by the American Hospital Association and revised in 1992

    2. Includes the following rights for patients:

      a. The right to receive considerate and respectful care

      b. The right to obtain relevant, current, and understandable information regarding diagnosis, treatment, and prognosis

      c. The right to make decisions regarding the plan of care

      d. The right to have advance directives regarding treatment

      e. The right to privacy in all aspects of care

      f. The right to expect that all communication and records will be treated confidentially

      g. The right to review records pertaining to care

Figure 3-2. Savage Model for Facilitating Ethical Decision Making

1. Gather facts of the case and understandings of those parties involved
2. Identify the questions and goals
3. Organize a meeting with key players—parents, physicians, nurses, social workers, therapists, and others who might assist in the decision making
  a. Pose questions, clarify information, set goals
  b. Explore options and their consequences and ethical ramifications
  c. Make plan for future management of case
4. Provide information, referrals, education, and emotional support to family
5. Participate in implementation of decision, if appropriate
6. Review the process, evaluate your role, and revise process as needed

Reprinted with permission of W.B. Saunders from Savage, T., & Michalak, D. (1999). Ethical, legal, and moral issues in pediatric rehabilitation. In P.A. Edwards, D.L., Hertzberg, S.R. Hays, & N.M. Youngblood (Eds.), *Pediatric rehabilitation nursing* (p. 67). Philadelphia: W.B. Saunders.

Figure 3-3. Two Models of Ethical Decision Making

Model 1 (Aiken & Catalano, 1994)	Model 2 (Blanchard & Peale, 1988)
1. Collect, analyze, and interpret data	1. Ask "Is it legal?" If the answer is yes, then stop. If no, go on to Items 2 and 3.
2. State dilemma clearly	
3. Consider choices for action	2. Ask "Is it balanced?" This will help answer issues of fairness vs. giving advantages to one or more parties.
4. Consider and weigh choices	
5. Analyze advantages and disadvantages of each choice	3. Ask "How will the decision make me feel?" This will help answer issues of personal standards of morality.
6. Make decision from choices	

Primary Sources: Model 1: Adapted with permission of F.A. Davis Company from Aiken, T., & Catalano, J. (1994). *Legal, ethical, and political issues in nursing* (pp. 31–35). Philadelphia: F.A. Davis. Copyright 1994 by F.A. Davis Company. Model 2: Adapted with permission of William Morrow & Company, Inc., from Blanchard, K., & Peale, N. (1988). *The power of ethical management* (pp. 20–27). New York: William Morrow & Company. Copyright 1988 by Blanchard Family Partnership and Norman Vincent Peale by William Morrow & Company, Inc.

Secondary Source: Armstrong, M. (Ed.). (1998). *Telecommunications for health professionals: Providing successful distance education and telehealth* (p. 247). New York: Springer Publishing Company.

---

h. The right to expect reasonable responses to requests for appropriate and medically indicated care and services

i. The right to be informed about business relationships that may influence treatment and care

j. The right to consent to or decline participation in proposed research studies

k. The right to expect reasonable continuity of care

l. The right to be informed about hospital policies and practices that relate to patient care, treatment, and responsibility

C. Living Wills and Life-Prolonging Declarations: Allows individuals to make their wishes known prior to hospitalization regarding medical care, illness, or conditions resulting in incompetency (McCourt, 1993)

D. Durable Power of Attorney: Enables a competent individual to appoint a surrogate decision maker who is empowered to act legally for the patient (Romano, 1998)

E. Guardianship: A position of responsibility granted to an individual by the court to make decisions for the incapacitated individual's life

F. Incompetence: A court decision based upon clinical opinion of the individual's mental fitness

G. Natural Death Acts: State legislation that allows for the creation of documents to provide a way to express desires related to medical decisions (McCourt, 1993)

H. Informed Consent: Full description about the risks and consequences of agreeing or refusing to have an operation or procedure

I. Estate Planning: Long-term planning for future care and expenses

J. Legal Death or Brain Death: Legal parameter of when life ceases

K. Withholding or Withdrawing Treatment
   1. Withholding is often termed *omission*
   2. Withdrawal is often termed *commission*
   3. The patient must consider whether either one achieves the expected benefit (McCourt, 1993)

L. Do-Not-Resuscitate (DNR) Order

M. Research on Human Subjects
   1. Basic rules and requirements for research studies can be found in various codes and regulations

   2. Participants should understand the purpose of the research and what is expected of them

   3. Participants should be competent to make the decision to participate

   4. Policies regarding compensation for individuals who become injured by research procedures should be in place (McCourt, 1993)

III. **Ethical, Legal, and Moral Issues in Practice**
   A. Diagnosis and Prognosis
      1. Involves withholding or withdrawing treatment
      2. Requires consideration of the presence of chronic illness
      3. Involves patients' participation in treatment decisions

   B. Collaborative Decision Making and Effective Communication
      1. Involves discussing the intensity of medical care with the individual and family
      2. Encourages a dialogue to determine cultural and socioeconomic attitudes related to defining an appropriate level of care
      3. Identifies components of life support systems, policies of the healthcare setting, and resources for support
      4. Involves the entire rehabilitation team in communicating with the family and discussing their concerns regarding treatment

   C. Acute Care vs. Long-Term Care: Involves making decisions in the best interest of the patient

   D. Allocation of Resources
      1. Involves microallocation, or deciding what to spend on a specific patient's care
      2. Involves macroallocation, or deciding how to distribute spending across a patient population, including rationing health care

   E. Ethical Rehabilitation (Graham-Eason, 1996)
      1. Client participates in the plan of care as fully as possible
      2. Client values independence and wellness
      3. Client regains self-worth as well as makes other physical gains
      4. Nurse collaborates with other team members
      5. Nurse demonstrates caring, good judgment, and advocacy
      6. Rehabilitation helps an individual regain his or her lost capabilities and self-worth

7. Rehabilitation happens in the shortest possible time and is cost-effective

F. Team Issues
   1. Team members should be aware of the roles and core values of all team members
   2. Team members should show respect for relationships and functions
   3. Team members should place self-care, independence, and client well-being as the ultimate goals

G. Ethical Conflicts Reported by Certified Rehabilitation Registered Nurses (CRRNs) (Redman & Fry, 1998) [*See "Research Perspective" on page 40*]
   1. Disagreements about medical or institutional practice (e.g., overtreatment, undertreatment, treatment that does not meet standards)
   2. Patients' rights (e.g., confidentiality, family issues, code status, advance directives, treatment refusal)
   3. Payment issues (e.g., managed care, insurance)
   4. Other issues (e.g., institutional downsizing, reorganization)

H. Ethical Issues Related to Alternative and Complementary Medicine and Therapies
   1. The patient's right to choose alternative and complementary medicine and therapies
      a. Acupuncture
      b. Chiropractic therapy
      c. Herbal medicine
      d. Naturopathic medicine
      e. Homeopathic medicine
   2. Possible interactions between alternative or complementary medicine and traditional Western medicine

I. Ethical Implications of Caring
   1. Maintain the status of special relationships within a healthcare organization
   2. Maintain personal and professional standards in a managed care environment
   3. Maintain an administrative perspective on pursuing the good of the patient and the organization

J. Ethical Foundations of Healthcare Reform (as cited in Graham-Eason, 1996, p. 46)
   1. Universal access: Every American citizen and legal resident should have access to health care without financial or other barriers.
   2. Comprehensive benefits: Guaranteed benefits should meet the full range of health needs, including primary, preventive, and specialized care.
   3. Choice: Each consumer should have the opportunity to exercise effective choice about providers, plans, and treatments. Each consumer should be informed about what is known and not known about the risks and benefits of available treatments and be free to choose among them according to his or her preferences.
   4. Equity of care: The system should avoid the creation of a tiered system providing care based only on differences of need, not individual or group characteristics.
   5. Fair distribution of costs: The healthcare system should spread the costs and burdens of care across the entire community, basing the level of contribution required of consumers on ability to pay.
   6. Personal responsibility: Under health reform, each individual and family should assume responsibility for protecting and promoting health and contributing to the cost of care.
   7. Intergenerational justice: The healthcare system should respond to the unique needs of each stage of life, sharing benefits and burdens fairly across generations.
   8. Wise allocation of resources: The nation should balance prudently what it spends on healthcare against other important national priorities.
   9. Effectiveness: The new system should deliver care and innovation that works and that patients want. It should encourage the discovery of better treatments. It should make it possible for the academic community and healthcare providers to exercise effectively their responsibility to evaluate and improve health care by providing resources for the systematic study of healthcare outcomes.
   10. Quality: The system should deliver high-quality care and provide individuals with the information necessary to make informed healthcare choices.
   11. Effective management: By encouraging

simplification and continuous improvement, as well as making the system easier to use for patients and providers, the healthcare system should focus on care, rather than administration.

12. Professional integrity and responsibility: The healthcare system should treat the clinical judgments of professionals with respect and protect the integrity of the provider-patient relationship while ensuring that health providers have the resources to fulfill their responsibilities for the effective delivery of quality care.

13. Fair procedures: To protect these values and principles, fair and open democratic procedures should underlie decisions concerning the operation of the healthcare system and the resolution of disputes that arise within it.

14. Local responsibility: Working within the framework of national reform, the new healthcare system should allow states and local communities to design effective, high-quality systems of care that serve each of their citizens.

IV. Future Considerations and Directions
A. End-of-Life Issues
  1. Making "no code" decisions
  2. Dying at home
  3. Limiting treatment for dementia
  4. Withholding nutrition and fluids
  5. Using euthanasia, including assisted suicide

B. Genetic Research
  1. Decoding genes that are responsible for specific diseases
  2. Gene therapy
  3. Genetic engineering
  4. Use of genetic information

C. Beginning-of-Life Issues
  1. Abortion
  2. Newborns with severe defects
  3. Fetal tissue experimentation
  4. Genetic counseling
  5. Genetic manipulation
  6. Surrogacy

D. Resource Allocation
  1. Microallocation
  2. Macroallocation
  3. Cost containment
  4. Individual access to services
  5. Clinical decisions made by for-profit managed care organizations (Habel, 1999)

E. Issues That Rehabilitation Professionals Must Address
  1. Balancing medical and rehabilitative needs that present moral quandaries
  2. Team contributions to decision making with regard to services for clients, as well as clients' progress and outcomes
  3. Definitions of quality-of-life issues
  4. Access to rehabilitative services regardless of the client's disability or funding level
  5. Legal requirements for providing rehabilitation services
  6. Meeting standards and regulations imposed by various entities
  7. Client decisions to adhere or not to adhere to recommended regimens as defined by the rehabilitation team

Research Perspective

Redman, B., & Fry, S. (1998). Ethical conflicts reported by certified registered rehabilitation nurses. *Rehabilitation Nursing, 23*(4), 179-184.

This research, which represented an initial step in studying ethical conflicts in rehabilitation care, identified the types of ethical conflict certified rehabilitation registered nurses (CRRNs) reported in practice. The study was guided by a conceptual framework of ethical decision making and was structured around utilitarian and deontologic theory and the principles of beneficence, autonomy, nonmaleficence, and justice. The sample was drawn from CRRNs who were actively practicing in Maryland, Virginia, and the District of Columbia. Two instruments were used for data collection: the Demographic Data Form (designed to collect vital statistics and information on educational preparation and clinical practice) and the Moral Conflict Questionnaire (designed to elicit descriptions of ethical conflicts in practice).

A descriptive analysis was done on the demographic data, and four content analysis schemes were created to analyze the described ethical conflicts. These encompassed the practice context of the conflict, the ethical principles and values used when describing the conflict, how the conflict was experienced, and how it was resolved. The clinical context conflicts involved payment policies, patients' rights issues, and disagreement with medical and/or institutional practice. The ethical principles and moral values conflicts related to fair allocation of resources and disagreement between beneficence and nonmaleficence. Most participants experienced the conflicts as moral dilemmas or moral distress. Nurses took action to resolve conflicts through discussions, patient and family education, and initial activities to protect the patient. One-third of the conflicts were not resolved, and it was noted that ethics committees or consultants were infrequently used.

Implications for practice

Understanding how ethical conflicts affect rehabilitation nurses' ability to serve clients who are experiencing major health alterations is essential to enhancing the quality of care in all practice settings. Further study is necessary to verify the situations reported and to develop assessment strategies and educational interventions to help rehabilitation nurses resolve ethical and moral conflicts. As healthcare and payment systems continue to shift, rehabilitation professionals should advocate for policies that support appropriate services and participate in activities that quantify cost-effective, nurse-sensitive outcomes.

References

Aiken, T., & Catalano, J. (1994). *Legal, ethical, and political issues in nursing*. Philadelphia: F.A. Davis.

American Nurses' Association (ANA). (1985). *Code for nurses with interpretive statements*. Kansas City, MO: Author.

American Nurses Association (ANA). (1996). *Compendium of American Nurses Association position statements*. Washington, DC: American Nurses Publishing.

Armstrong, M. (Ed.). (1998). *Telecommunications for health professionals: Providing successful distance education and telehealth* (p. 247). New York: Springer Publishing Company.

Association of Rehabilitation Nurses (ARN). (1994). *Standards and scope of rehabilitation nursing practice*. Skokie, IL: Author.

Blanchard, K., & Peale, N. (1988). *The power of ethical management*. New York: William Morrow & Company.

Esterhuizen, P. (1996). Is the professional code still the cornerstone of clinical nursing practice? *Journal of Advanced Nursing, 23*(1), 25–31.

Graham-Eason, C. (1996). Ethical considerations for rehabilitation nursing. In S. Hoeman (Ed.), *Rehabilitation nursing: Process and application* (2nd ed., pp. 34–46). St. Louis: Mosby.

Habel, M. (1999). Bioethics: Strengthening nursing's role. *Nurse Week* [On-line]. Available: http://www.nurseweek.com/ce/ce420a

Josephson Institute of Ethics. (1999). [On-line]. Available: http://www.josephsoninstitute.org

McCourt, A. (Ed.). (1993). *The specialty practice of rehabilitation nursing: A core curriculum* (3rd ed.). Skokie, IL: Rehabilitation Nursing Foundation of the Association of Rehabilitation Nurses.

Redman, B., & Fry, S. (1998). Ethical conflicts reported by certified registered rehabilitation nurses. *Rehabilitation Nursing, 23*(4), 179–184.

Romano, J. (1998). *Legal rights of the catastrophically ill and injured: A family guide* (2nd ed.). Norristown, PA: Joseph L. Romano.

Savage, T., & Michalak, D.R. (1999). Ethical, legal and moral issues in pediatric rehabilitation. In P.A. Edwards, D.L. Hertzberg, S.R. Hays, & N.M. Youngblood (Eds.), *Pediatric rehabilitation nursing* (pp. 62–83). Philadelphia: W.B. Saunders.

Sletteboe, A. (1997). Dilemma: A concept analysis. *Journal of Advanced Nursing, 26*(3), 449–454.

Suggested resources

Andrews, M., Goldberg, K., & Kaplan, H. (1996). *Nurses' legal handbook* (3rd ed.). Springhouse, PA: Springhouse.

Guidelines on reporting incompetent, unethical or illegal practices. (1994). Washington, DC: ANA Publishing.

Hall, J. (1996). *Nursing ethics and the law*. Philadelphia: W.B. Saunders.

Jamison, S. (1997). *Assisted suicide*. San Francisco: Jossey-Bass.

Lucke, K. (1998). Ethical implications of caring in rehabilitation. *Nursing Clinics of North America, 33*(2), 253-264.

Nursing Ethics Network (NEN). [On-line]. Available: http://www.bc.edu/bc_org/avp/son/ethics/purposes

Petrozella, O. (1999). *Development of a nursing ethics elective course* [On-line]. Available: http://www.nln.org/abstracts

Rumbald, G. (1999). *Ethics in nursing practice* (3rd ed.). Philadelphia: W.B. Saunders.

Salladay, S. (1996). Rehabilitation ethics and managed care. *Rehab Management, 9*(6), 38-42.

Scanlon, C., & Fibison, W. (1995). *Managing genetic information: Implications for nursing practice*. Washington, DC: ANA Publishing.

Silva, M. (1995). *Ethical guidelines in the conduct, dissemination, and implementation of nursing research*. Washington, DC: ANA Publishing.

Trandel-Korenchuk, D., & Trandel, K. (1997). *Nursing and the law*. Gaithersburg, MD: Aspen.

White, G. (Ed.). (1993). *Ethical dilemmas in contemporary practice*. Washington, DC: ANA Publishing.

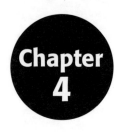

Chapter 4

Economics and Health Policy in Rehabilitation

Anne Deutsch, MS RN CRRN

The American healthcare system, including the delivery of rehabilitation services, is largely financed through federal and state programs and private sector health insurance. Rising healthcare costs, due in part to an aging population and the high cost of new technology, have resulted in shifting the reimbursement of healthcare services by insurance and government agencies from a fee-for-service model to managed care and prospective payment models with shared financial risks. In addition to medical care coverage, various income support programs (e.g., workers' compensation) are available for people with disabilities.

The rising cost of providing health care is only one of the many important themes in the development and modification of healthcare policy. Two other important health policy issues are access to health care and the quality of health services. The process of developing and modifying health policy provides opportunities for rehabilitation nurses to share their expertise with local, state, and federal government agencies and legislators. Rehabilitation nurses' unique knowledge and understanding of the needs of people with disabilities position them to advocate for health policy reform. A rehabilitation nurse's involvement may include a range of activities including educating the public about health issues (i.e., at schools or senior centers) or promoting letter-writing campaigns to garner support for a proposed bill.

The Association of Rehabilitation Nurses (ARN) Health Policy Committee represents ARN members and monitors pending legislation. In addition, the committee serves as a resource for individual members and ARN chapters to actively participate in local and state issues.

This chapter reviews the important issues related to the economics of healthcare delivery, including financing of health care, reimbursement (payment) models, and income support programs. It also describes how health policy is developed and modified and how rehabilitation nurses can influence policy.

Economics

I. Financing the Delivery of Healthcare Services (see Table 4-1)

A. Federal Programs
 1. Medicare: A federal health insurance program for people who are elderly or disabled under the authority of the U.S. Department of Health and Human Services (DHHS); began with the enactment of Title XVIII of the Social Security Act of 1965

 a. Administration: Managed by the Health Care Financing Administration (HCFA), which designates intermediaries on a regional basis to process claims (e.g., Blue Cross plans)

 b. Services

 1) Medicare Part A: Hospital insurance plan that covers services provided by hospitals, skilled nursing facilities (SNFs), home health programs (skilled care only), hospice, and nursing homes; financed by employees and employers through the Social Security system

 2) Medicare Part B: Insurance plan that covers physicians' services; paid for by federal taxes and monthly premiums from beneficiaries

 c. Program options

 1) Traditional fee-for-service

 a) This plan offers the beneficiary a choice of hospital and provider, but requires the payment of a fee each time a service is used and the payment of the difference between the bill amount and the Medicare payment

    b) The healthcare provider bills for every service rendered, based on previously established rates

  2) Medicare managed care

    a) Prepaid coordinated health plans contract with the Medicare program to provide services to Medicare beneficiaries

    b) Most plans charge a copayment each time a service is used.

    c) Benefits vary greatly by plan, but they usually include preventive care services and optional prescription drug coverage for an additional premium

    d) Under the Medicare+Choice program, groups of physicians and hospitals (i.e., preferred provider organizations [PPOs]) contract with insurers to serve a group of enrollees on a fee-for-service basis, but the rates charged are supposed to be lower than those charged to nonenrollees

  d. Eligibility

    1) Upon reaching age 65, people who are eligible for Social Security are automatically enrolled in Medicare Part A whether or not they are retired.

    2) People younger than age 65 who are totally and permanently disabled may enroll in Medicare Part A after they have been receiving Social Security disability benefits for 24 months. People with chronic renal disease requiring dialysis or a transplant are eligible for Medicare Part A without the 2-year waiting period

2. Medicaid: Federal grants provided to states for medical assistance programs; enacted under Title XIX of the Social Security Act of 1965 (see details in the following section on state programs)

B. State Programs

  1. Medicaid: Medical assistance program for certain individuals and families with low incomes and resources

    a. Administration: Managed by each state; funded by federal, state, and (sometimes) local taxes

    b. Services: Required by the federal government to provide hospital, physician, laboratory, X-ray, prenatal, and preventive care services; nursing home and home health care; and medically necessary transportation. States can add services to this list and can place certain limitations on the federally mandated services

Table 4-1. Funding Resources for Healthcare and Rehabilitation Programs

	Programs			
	Medicare (Federal)	**Medicaid** (State)	**Workers' compensation**	**Private health insurance**
Eligibility Requirements	Must be over the age of 65 or have been disabled for 2 years	Categories include the medically needy (e.g., AFDC recipients, blind people)	Workers injured in the course of employment	Policyholders
Benefits	Part A—hospital Part B—supplemental medical insurance (individual must enroll) Part C—miscellaneous (e.g., for those with end-stage renal disease)	Hospital costs and visits to a physician Care in a skilled nursing facility	Medical care related to a compensable injury Income support during period of disability	Hospital costs and outpatient treatment, as specified in policy Physicians' visits, as specified in policy May or may not cover rehabilitation therapies

Sources consulted

Health Care Financing Administration (HCFA). (1997). *Your Medicare desk reference* [HCFA Publication No. 10937]. Baltimore, MD: Author. Reprinted with permission by ARN from McCourt, A.E. (Ed.). (1993). *The specialty practice of rehabilitation nursing: A core curriculum* (3rd ed., p. 227). Skokie, IL: Rehabilitation Nursing Foundation of the Association of Rehabilitation Nurses.

c. Eligibility
   1) The federal government requires state Medicaid programs to cover specific groups of people:
      a) Recipients of Aid to Families with Dependent Children (AFDC), a federal-state cash assistance (welfare) program for which states set eligibility standards
      b) Recipients of Supplemental Social Security Income (SSI)
      c) Infants born to Medicaid-eligible women
      d) Pregnant women (for pregnancy-related services) and children younger than age 6 whose family incomes are up to 133% of the federal poverty line
      e) Recipients of adoption assistance and foster care
      f) Special protected groups who lose cash assistance because of the cash program's rules but who may keep Medicaid for a period of time
   2) States have the option to cover "medically needy" people, that is, those who are poor but earn too much money to qualify for AFDC or SSI, but who would otherwise be eligible for one of these programs by virtue of being in a family with dependent children, older than age 65, blind, or totally and permanently disabled.
d. Program options: Traditional or managed care plans
2. Child Health Insurance Plan: Health insurance plan for children and working families who do not earn enough to afford coverage for their children
   a. Administration
      1) States are given broad flexibility in tailoring programs to meet their own circumstances.
      2) States can create or expand their own separate insurance programs, expand Medicaid, or combine both approaches.

b. Eligibility: States have the opportunity to set eligibility criteria regarding age, income, resources, and residency within broad federal guidelines.
3. Workers' compensation: Government-sponsored and employee-financed systems for compensating employees who incur an injury or illness in connection with their employment. Benefits provided include medical care, disability payments, rehabilitation services, survivor benefits, and funeral expenses.
   a. Administration: Each state, as well as the District of Columbia, Puerto Rico, and the U.S. Virgin Islands, designates an agency that will administer the program (e.g., state department of labor, independent workers' compensation agency, court administration).
   b. Eligibility: Workers who are disabled by injury or families of a worker whose death "arose out of and in the course of employment"
   c. Coverage: Provides both medical care related to the compensable injury and income benefits through the following sources:
      1) Private commercial insurance companies
      2) Self-insurance (corporations that are able to carry the risk)
      3) State funds
      4) State's second injury fund
   d. Medical care provisions
      1) Treatment and rehabilitative programs for work-related injury
      2) Reimbursement in full or, in certain states, according to a medical fee guide
   e. Vocational rehabilitation benefits: Most states provide job retraining, education, and job placement.
C. Private Health Insurance
   1. Purchasing private health insurance plans
      a. An individual may purchase private health insurance and pay the full premium.
      b. Entities (e.g., an employer) may purchase private health insurance on behalf

of a group of individuals. Purchasing groups often negotiate coverage, thus benefits often vary by group. Group members (e.g., employees) contribute to the insurance premium.

2. Types of health insurance and service plans

   a. Indemnity plans: Provide comprehensive coverage for medical and hospital services

     1) The employer and/or subscriber pays a premium, and the subscriber agrees to pay any required deductible, copayments, and amounts over the insurer's usual and customary rate for specific services

     2) The subscriber may receive services from physicians, hospitals, or other qualified providers of his or her choice for services that are medically necessary and meet accepted standards of medical practice

     3) Preapproval for coverage may be required

     4) Experimental and other noncovered services may be negotiable under certain circumstances

   b. Managed care plans (Kongstvedt, 1997)

     1) Overview

       a) Managed care plans provide an identified set of medical and/or hospital care services for a fixed, predetermined premium

       b) The managed care organization (MCO) may restrict the subscriber's choice of providers and control subscriber access through utilization management

       c) Subscribers often choose or are assigned a primary care physician (PCP) who is employed or under contract with the MCO. In many cases, the PCP acts as a gatekeeper for all other medical and hospital services.

       d) The different types of insurance plans were reasonably distinct until the late 1980s. Since that time, the differences between traditional forms of health insurance (e.g., indemnity plans) and managed care plans have reduced substantially.

       e) MCOs vary greatly in terms of their focus on controlling costs and quality (see Figure 4-1).

         (1) Less controlled: Managed indemnity plans that may include precertification of elective admissions and case management of catastrophic cases

         (2) More controlled: Group and staff model health maintenance organizations (HMOs)

     2) Types of managed care plans

       a) HMOs: Organized healthcare systems that are responsible for both the financing and the delivery of a broad range of healthcare services to an enrolled population. The original definition of HMO also included financing health care for a prepaid fixed fee. HMOs must ensure that their members have access to

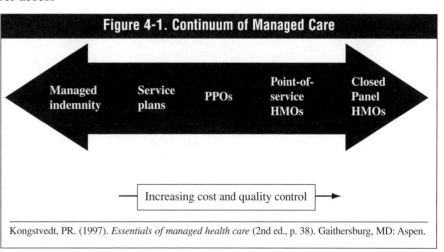

Figure 4-1. Continuum of Managed Care

Managed indemnity — Service plans — PPOs — Point-of-service HMOs — Closed Panel HMOs

Increasing cost and quality control →

Kongstvedt, PR. (1997). *Essentials of managed health care* (2nd ed., p. 38). Gaithersburg, MD: Aspen.

covered healthcare services, as well as the quality and appropriateness of these services.

    (1) Staff model (closed model): Physicians are employed by the HMO, are typically paid on a salary basis, and may receive bonus or incentive payments based on performance.

    (2) Group practice (closed model): The HMO contracts with a multispecialty physician group practice to provide all physician services to members. The physicians are employed by the group practice, not the HMO.

    (3) Network (closed or open model): The HMO contracts with more than one group practice to provide physician services to members.

    (4) Independent Practice Association (IPA) (open model): The HMO contracts with an association of physicians to provide services to enrollees. The physicians are members of the IPA, a separate legal entity, but they remain as individual providers with their own offices and identities. Participation is open to all community physicians who meet the selection criteria. The HMO compensates the IPA on an all-inclusive physician capitation basis to provide services to enrollees. The IPA also compensates its participating physicians on a fee-for-service primary care capitation basis.

    (5) Direct contract: The HMO contracts directly with individual physicians to provide medical care to enrollees. Compensation to participating physicians may be on a fee-for-service or primary care capitation basis.

    b) Preferred provider organizations (PPOs): Employer health benefit plans and insurance carriers contract with PPOs to purchase healthcare services for covered beneficiaries from a selected group of participating providers who typically agree to follow utilization management and other processes implemented by the PPO, as well as agree to the reimbursement structure and payment models. PPOs offer incentives for enrollees to use the participating providers. Enrollees are permitted to use non-PPO providers, but they typically must pay higher coinsurance or deductibles. Key attributes of a PPO include a selected provider panel, negotiated payment rates, rapid payment terms, utilization management, and consumer choice.

    c) Exclusive provider organizations (EPOs): EPOs are structured like PPOs, but enrollees are required to receive all their covered healthcare services from the providers who participate in the EPO. Some EPOs use a gatekeeper approach to authorize nonprimary care. EPOs are usually implemented by employers whose primary concern is cost savings.

    d) Point-of-service (POS) plans: POS plans offer enrollees some indemnity-type coverage, but typically incorporate high deductibles and coinsurance to this coverage to encourage members to use the HMO-type services.

    e) Managed care overlays to indemnity insurance: Managed

care overlays provide cost control for insured plans while allowing enrollees the choice of provider and coverage for out-of-plan services. Examples of managed care overlays include general utilization management, specialty utilization management, and catastrophic or large case management.

    f) Physician hospital organizations (PHOs): PHOs are jointly owned and operated by hospitals and their affiliated physicians. They contract with managed care organizations to provide both hospital and physician services and support implementation of integrated delivery systems. PHOs have achieved only limited success in contracting with managed care plans.

  c. Medicare supplemental benefits plan (Medigap): Purchased by Medicare beneficiaries to pay for those expenses that are not covered by Medicare

  d. Auto liability: Covers medical care needed as a result of an auto accident

D. Programs for Special Groups
  1. Benefits for veterans of the armed forces: Coverage provided either for treatment of a service-related illness or for needy veterans who have nonservice-related medical problems; administered by the Department for Veterans Affairs (VA)
  2. Federal government civilian employee workers' compensation programs
  3. Family and Medical Leave Act (FMLA) (Public Law [PL] 103-3): Requires employers of 50 or more employees (and all public agencies) to provide up to 12 weeks of unpaid, job-protected leave to eligible employees for the health-related problems of the employee or a family member
  4. Indian Health Service (IHS): An agency of the U.S. DHHS that provides hospital care, dental and health benefits, substance abuse counseling, public health nursing, and other services to American Indians and Alaskan Natives
  5. Railroad Retirement Act Program
  6. Black Lung Benefits Act of 1972
  7. Longshoremen and Harbor Workers' Compensation Act
  8. Life care planning: The process of mapping out short- and long-term care needs, expenses, and resources for patients with a debilitating, chronic illness or injury. A life care plan is created to ensure that the patient receives consistent, comprehensive, cost-effective care from present as well as future caregivers (Barker, 1999).

II. Reimbursement for Healthcare Services
  A. Payment Units
    1. Fee-for-service reimbursement: The unit of payment relates to the visit or procedure. The provider or hospital is paid a fee for each office visit, procedure, or other service or supply provided. This is the only form of payment that is based on individual components of healthcare services.
    2. Prospective payment system (PPS): The payment rate to the healthcare facility is predetermined based on the medical diagnosis or treatment information, regardless of the cost for care for a specific individual.
    3. Episode-of-illness reimbursement: The provider or hospital is paid one sum for all services delivered during one illness episode. The diagnosis-related groups (DRGs) classification system is an example of this model.
    4. Per-diem payments: The healthcare facility is paid one sum for all services delivered to a patient during one day.
    5. Capitation payments: One lump sum payment is made to the provider (e.g., physician) for each patient's treatment during a month or year; this method is usually associated with managed care.
  B. Medicare Prospective Payment Systems (PPS)
    1. In acute care hospitals
      a. In 1983, in an effort to control hospital costs, Medicare implemented an episode-based PPS in hospitals using a classification system known as diagnosis-related groups (DRGs).

b. Each patient's diagnosis and other variables such as age and complications are used to categorize the patient into a DRG.

c. Each DRG represents a mutually exclusive grouping that is used to assign a preset episode payment rate.

d. The provider is paid at the fixed rate based on the DRG and facility-specific adjusters, regardless of the costs that the hospital incurs while caring for the patient.

e. If the costs are lower than the preset amount, the provider makes money, but if the costs are higher, the provider loses money.

2. In skilled nursing facilities (SNFs)

a. In an attempt to balance the federal budget, Congress passed the Balanced Budget Act of 1997, which mandated the implementation of a Medicare PPS for SNF services.

b. The per-diem PPS was implemented in 1998 and is based on the Resource Utilization Groups-III (RUG-III) classification system. Each RUG represents a grouping that is used to determine the preset per-diem payment rate.

c. Data collected using the Minimum Data Set (MDS 2.0), such as treatments provided and resident characteristics are used to categorize each patient into a RUG.

d. Payment rates are all-inclusive, so facilities do not receive additional money if utilization exceeds the RUG payment rate.

e. As with the DRG system, a provider who spends more than the preset amount loses money.

f. The schedule for the collection of MDS 2.0 assessment data is provided in Table 4-2.

  1) MDS 2.0 rehabilitation categories (Baker, 1998)

    a) Ultra high (ADL index 16-18)

      (1) In the last 7 days: Received 720 or more minutes (ADL index 9-15)

      (2) At least two disciplines (one at least 5 days; second at least 3 days) (ADL index 4-8)

    b) Very high (ADL index 16-18)

      (1) In the last 7 days: Received 500 or more minutes (ADL index 9-15)

      (2) At least one discipline for at least 5 days (ADL index 4-8)

    c) High (ADL index 13-18)

      (1) In the last 7 days: Received 325 or more minutes (ADL index 8-12)

      (2) At least one discipline for at least 5 days (ADL index 4-7)

      (3) Or if this is a Medicare 5-day or a readmission assessment, then the following may apply: In the last 7 days, received 65 or more minutes and in the first 15 days from admission, 520 or more minutes of rehabilitation services are expected on 8 or more days

    d) Medium (ADL index 15-18)

      (1) In the last 7 days: Received 150 or more minutes (ADL index 8-14)

      (2) At least 5 days of any combination of the three disciplines (ADL index 4-7)

      (3) Or if this is a Medicare 5-day or a readmission/return assessment, then the following may apply: In the first 15 days from admission, 240 or more minutes of rehabilitation services are expected on 8 or more days

    e) Low (ADL index 14-18)

      (1) In the last 7 days: Received 45 or more minutes (ADL index 4-13)

      (2) At least 3 days of any combination of the three disciplines and two or more nursing rehabilitation services received for at least 15 minutes each with each administered for 6 or more days

(3) Or if this is a Medicare 5-day or a readmission/return assessment, then the following may apply: In the first 15 days from admission, 75 or more minutes of rehabilitation services are expected on 5 or more days and two or more nursing rehabilitation services will actually be received for at least 15 minutes each with each administered 2 or more days

2) RUG-III Classification System for rehabilitation patients (Baker, 1998)

   a) Bed mobility, toileting, and transferring
     (1) Independent of supervision (ADL index 1)
     (2) Limited assistance (ADL index 3)
     (3) Extensive assistance, total dependence or activity did not occur and one-person assist (ADL index 4) or two-person assist (ADL index 5)

   b) Eating
     (1) Independent of supervision (ADL index 1)
     (2) Limited assistance (ADL index 2)
     (3) Extensive assistance, total dependence, or activity did not occur (including feeding tubes or parenteral feeding [with > 25% of calories and > 500 cc per day fluid parenteral or enteral intake in the past 7 days]) (ADL index 3)
   c) ADL Sum Range = 4–18

g. MDS data collection coordinator is a new role for rehabilitation nurses.

3. In home health care

   a. Payment reform for home health services includes an interim payment system (IPS) with reduced costs and limits, and the implementation of a PPS in 2000.

   b. Data collection for the PPS classification system will be based on the Outcome and Assessment Information Set (OASIS) instrument.

4. In rehabilitation hospitals and units

   a. A PPS was expected to begin in rehabilitation hospitals and units in 2000.

   b. HCFA will use the Function Related Groups (FRGs) as the classification system and a per-episode payment system. (*Note.* FRGs may be renamed Clinic Management Groups [CMGs].)

   c. Data collection using the Minimum Data Set for Post Acute Care (MDS-PAC) instrument will be used to classify patients into groups based on factors such as diagnosis, functional status, and age.

5. In long-term care hospitals: A PPS is under development for long-term care hospitals, and implementation is expected in 2002.

Table 4-2. Schedule of Periods of Covered Services and Related Reference Dates

Medicare MDS Assessment Type	Reason for Assessment (AA8b code)	Assessment Reference Date	Applicable Medicare Payment Days*	Number of Days Authorized for Coverage and Payment**	MDS Finished
5 day	1	Days 1–8***	Days 1–14	14	Day 8***
14 day	7	Days 11–14****	Days 15–30	16	Day 14
30 day	2	Days 21–29	Days 31–60	30	Day 37
60 day	3	Days 50–59	Days 61–90	30	Day 67
90 day	4	Days 80–89	Days 91–100	10	Day 97

*Facility staff must notify resident if coverage will not continue before first day of service period.
**Unless modified by a significant change assessment.
***Including 3-day grace period.
****Resident Assessment Protocols (RAPs) follow federal rules; RAPs must be performed with either the 5-day or the 14-day assessment. The assessors have approximately 14 days from the assessment reference date to complete the assessment and determine the RUG-III group.

Reprinted from *Medicare SNF Supplementary Provider Manual, Phase III Stage II* (p. 5-5). (1997). Washington, DC: Health Care Financing Administration (HCFA).

III. Economic Barriers to Care

A. Lack of Health Insurance
   1. Overview
      a. Approximately 40 million people in the United States do not have health insurance (Kovner & Jonas, 1998).
      b. The percentage of people without health insurance varies greatly by state because of the structure and health of local economies and Medicare program coverage. For example, in 1997, in Connecticut and Minnesota, less than 10% of the nonelderly populations were uninsured, whereas in Louisiana, Texas, and Oklahoma, the rate of uninsured people was higher than 25% (Kovner & Jonas, 1998).
   2. Who does not have insurance
      a. Young adults (ages 18 to 29) are most likely not to have insurance. This is a result of the historical dependence on employer-based health insurance coverage as well as federal/state Medicaid programs. When an employer does not offer health insurance or if the person is unemployed, the risk of not having health insurance increases.
      b. The cost of purchasing individual coverage is often prohibitive for most people, especially low-income or unemployed workers. A 1997 study found that more than half of the people without insurance earned less than $10,000 per year and that 85% earned less than $20,000 (Kovner & Jonas, 1998).
      c. Young adults often have difficulty establishing eligibility for Medicaid programs. Although guidelines vary from state to state, Medicaid eligibility is restricted to people with low incomes who fall into specific categories (e.g., children, elderly people, people who are blind or disabled, pregnant women, single parents).
   3. Elderly adults: The level of uninsurance among elderly people is low (less than 2%) as a result of the Medicare program; however, underinsurance can be an economic barrier for elderly people who must supplement their insurance coverage with out-of-pocket money.

B. Underinsurance and Other Limitations of Coverage
   1. Health insurance does not always ensure financial access to care. There are often limitations on coverage for special services, such as behavioral health care, preventive care, long-term care, catastrophic illnesses or accidents, and psychiatric care. Also, exclusions or waiting periods for illnesses or conditions may exist at the time the person enrolls in the health plan.
   2. Most health insurance plans also include copayments or deductibles to discourage overutilization of services and to reduce premium costs. Copayments and deductibles can discourage some patients from seeking preventive care (e.g., immunizations, mammograms). This is particularly a problem for people with low incomes.
   3. Substantial gaps in cost-sharing provisions and coverage exist in the traditional Medicare program.
      a. There are large deductibles and copayments for hospital care, no coverage for prescription drugs, and restrictions on long-term care coverage.
      b. It is estimated that Medicare pays less than 50% of the total costs of health care for elderly people. To cover these expenses, many elderly people have supplemental coverage (e.g., Medigap plans), which are offered through employer or retirement plans or may be purchased directly. More than 20% of elderly people and 35% of low-income elderly people have no supplemental coverage (Kovner & Jonas, 1998).
   4. Low-income elderly people may qualify for Medicaid in addition to Medicare. Although Medicaid is comprehensive, many physicians do not participate in the program because of its low level of payment. Therefore, barriers still exist for low-income elderly people trying to access basic healthcare services.

C. The Effects of Economic Barriers to Care
   1. Economic barriers to health services have an impact on both patients and the healthcare delivery system.

a. When compared to people with private insurance, uninsured people are less likely to have a usual source of health care (e.g., provider, clinic), less likely to have seen a physician during the last 12 months, and make fewer visits to the physician than the average person.

b. Uninsured people are more likely to be admitted to a hospital for a preventable or avoidable condition.

2. Not having insurance may affect an individual's health status and outcomes.

a. The Rand Health Insurance Experiment found that low-income patients had more vision, blood pressure, and other health problems than insured patients (Kovner & Jonas, 1998).

b. Other studies have shown that people who are uninsured have higher mortality rates even after adjusting for differences in socioeconomic attributes, general health status, and health habits (Kovner & Jonas, 1998).

3. Uninsured patients typically receive care from a select group of providers who are willing to provide care regardless of a person's ability to pay, such as hospital-based outpatient departments, emergency rooms, and community-based clinics.

a. Costs in these institutional-based settings are often high, therefore increasing the total costs for the delivery of care.

b. To cover the costs of caring for uninsured and underinsured people, providers must either shift fees to other payers or seek government or private subsidies.

c. Current market forces, including managed care and fixed-fee schedules, make cost-shifting difficult.

IV. Funding for Assistive Technology

A. Definition: *Assistive technology* refers to any item, piece of equipment, or product system—whether acquired commercially, off the shelf, modified, or customized—that is used to increase, maintain, or improve the functional capabilities of individuals with disabilities.

B. Why Funding for Assistive Technology Is a Significant Problem

1. Insurance or health programs do not pay for many assistive devices if they are not considered medically necessary.

2. The Technology Related Assistance for Individuals with Disabilities Act of 1988 (PL 100-407) provided grants to states.

a. To increase the availability of assistive technology

b. To conduct needs assessments

c. To develop innovative programs

d. To manage public awareness

e. To identify policies that promote the availability of assistive technology

3. In 1994, an amendment (PL 103-218) expanded and strengthened the 1988 act.

V. Income Support Programs (see Table 4-3)

A. Social Security Programs

1. Old-Age and Survivors Insurance (OASI)

a. Eligibility

1) Must be a retired worker at least 65 years old (by 2009, the minimum age will be 66); reduced benefits are available to workers who retire at age 62 or to widow(er)s or surviving divorced spouses

2) Must have reached "fully insured" status (i.e., must have worked under the program for a minimum of 10 years [1 year = 4 quarters; 40 quarters are needed to be eligible])

b. Benefits

1) No means test is required

2) Benefits are paid as an earned right

3) No minimum income amount is required during active working years

4) There is no limit on other sources of income, including savings, pensions, or insurance

2. Disability insurance

a. Eligibility

1) Must be a worker younger than age 65 with a disability: "A disabling condition is one in which the worker is so severely impaired physically or mentally that he or she is not able to perform substantial gainful work" (Jehle, 1992, p. 33)

2) Must have "fully insured" status and have 20 quarters in the 40-quarter

period, ending with the quarter the disability was sustained

  b. Benefits: Applicants are referred to state departments or agencies for vocational rehabilitation services, which vary by state

B. State Income Support Programs

  1. Workers' compensation

    a. Eligibility: Condition must be work-related

    b. Benefits: Usually calculated as a percentage of the worker's weekly earnings at the time of the injury or death

      1) Restrictions

        a) Each state designates maximum amount; frequently two-thirds of gross salary.

        b) There may be a waiting period.

        c) Some states stipulate a maximum number of weeks for benefits (e.g., 500 weeks).

      2) Types of benefits

        a) Temporary total disability: Worker is disabled for temporary period but expected to recover.

        b) Permanent total disability: Worker is disabled permanently and unable to perform any type of work.

        c) Temporary partial disability:

Worker is able to work but has diminished capacity.

        d) Permanent partial disability: Worker is able to work but has a ratable partial impairment.

        e) Survivor (death): Payments are made to spouse until remarriage and to children until age 18.

  2. State or federal income programs

    a. Aid to Families with Dependent Children

    b. Food stamps

    c. Supplemental food program for women, infants, and children

    d. Public housing and subsidized housing

    e. State general assistance or welfare programs

C. Private Sector Insurance and Benefits

  1. Retirement plans (e.g., individual or group plans)

  2. Disability income insurance (e.g., individual or group plans)

  3. Automobile insurance benefits

    a. No-fault

    b. Automobile liability

  4. General liability for personal injury or wrongful death

  5. Accidental death and dismemberment insurance

	Table 4-3. Income Support Programs Pertinent to Rehabilitation		
	Programs		
	Social Security Disability Insurance	**State workers' compensation**	**Private and/or individual disability insurance**
Population	Workers disabled before the age of 65 years and "fully insured" under covered work	Injured workers who meet state criteria for work-related conditions	Injured workers with a nonoccupational disability who are defined as unable to perform either the work related to their own occupation or any reasonable occupation
Benefits	Amount payable in retirement	Temporary total benefits that are calculated by a state formula, which is usually two-thirds of salary	A percentage of previous earnings
Time Period	For as long as person is disabled; trial work period may be stipulated	Variable; could be for person's lifetime; some states stipulate a maximum number of weeks (e.g., 500)	Policy may have a maximum benefit period (e.g., 2 years)

Sources consulted

Health Care Financing Administration (HCFA). (1997). *Your Medicare desk reference* [HCFA Publication No. 10937]. Baltimore, MD: Author. Reprinted with permission by ARN from McCourt, A.E. (Ed.). (1993). *The specialty practice of rehabilitation nursing: A core curriculum* (3rd ed., p. 228). Skokie, IL: Rehabilitation Nursing Foundation of the Association of Rehabilitation Nurses.

6. Hospital indemnity insurance benefits

7. Travel accident insurance benefits

8. Mortgage and credit disability insurance benefits

VI. The Economics of Prevention

  A. Levels of Prevention

    1. Primary prevention focuses on supporting or protecting the health and well-being of society at large. Efforts are geared toward reducing susceptibility to illness and injury, controlling exposure to disease-causing agents, minimizing risky behaviors, and removing or reducing environmental factors that increase the risk of disease or injury.

    2. Secondary prevention refers to efforts directed to high-risk populations. These include early detection of potential health problems, and, if appropriate, interventions to stop, reverse, or slow down the disease progress.

    3. Tertiary prevention describes the effort to maximize function and minimize the sequela of an injury or illness.

  B. Statistics Related to Disability in Society

    1. Approximately 34 million–43 million U.S. residents have some kind of disability that affects their ability to function (Institute of Medicine, 1991).

    2. In 1991, disability was estimated to cost the U.S. almost $200 billion annually in medical care and lost productivity (Institute of Medicine, 1991).

    3. The prevalence of disability increases dramatically with advancing age (Kassner & Bectel, 1998).

      a. Among people 50-64 years of age, approximately 1% receive help with two or more ADLs.

      b. Among people 85 years and older, approximately 11% receive help with two or more ADLs.

    4. Having an activity limitation more than doubles the average number of physician visits per year.

    5. In addition to healthcare expenses, costs relate to lost productivity, lost taxes, and increased spending on expensive remediation.

  C. The Shift from Responding to Medical Conditions to Promoting Health

    1. Healthcare services that respond to medical conditions (e.g., trauma care, treatment of infection) have expanded at the expense of addressing causes or contributory factors of health problems.

    2. National initiatives support disease prevention, health promotion, and a community focus for the healthcare system.

      a. Healthy People 2000 and its follow-up program, Healthy People 2010

      b. The Centers for Disease Control (CDC) and Prevention's Disabilities Prevention Program

      c. Health America: Practitioners for 2005, an agenda for action by U.S. schools for health professionals

      d. Recommendations from the Institute of Medicine's *Disability in America: Toward a National Agenda for Prevention* (see Figure 4-2)

  D. Challenges for Health Professionals, Including Rehabilitation Nurses

    1. Determine the types of educational programs that actually prevent illnesses or injuries and how these programs should be implemented

    2. Meet increasing demands to make health promotion and disease prevention economically worthwhile by conducting cost-effectiveness analyses

Health Policy

I. Overview

  A. Reasons Why Nurses Should Get Involved in Making Health Policy

    1. Enables participation in decisions relating to the future of the profession and health care

    2. Has a positive effect on the healthcare delivery system

    3. Promotes the ability to provide input at policy-making and health-planning levels

    4. Shows a commitment to maintaining healthcare standards

  B. Emerging Healthcare Policy Issues

    1. The delivery of healthcare services

      a. Access to care: Many people have a limited ability to obtain necessary health services for two reasons.

1) Ability to pay: People have either no health insurance coverage or are underinsured.
2) Location: People may not have healthcare personnel and facilities that are close to where they live, accessible by transportation, culturally acceptable, or capable of providing appropriate care using the language with which the patients is most familiar.

  b. Costs of care
1) In 1960, the national health expenditures represented 5.1% of the gross domestic product (GDP); expenditures per capita were $141.
2) In 1997, health care represented 13.5% of the GDP (i.e., 13.5 cents of every dollar was spent on health care); average expenditures per capita were $3,925
3) As a result, various cost-containment strategies (e.g., PPS, managed care) are now used.

  c. Quality of health care: Healthcare quality may be defined as the "degree to which patient care services increase the probability of desired patient outcomes and reduce the probability of undesired health outcomes given the current state of knowledge" (Institute of Medicine Committee on Clinical Practice Guidelines, 1992).

2. Nursing services and workforce
  a. Reimbursement for nursing services, including rehabilitation nurses
  b. Scope of practice (e.g., for advanced practice nurses), as defined by state licensure laws and regulatory bodies
  c. Funding for nursing education and research

3. Social issues related to populations that rehabilitation nurses serve
  a. Community accessibility
  b. Discrimination against people with disabilities in hiring practices or in the workplace
  c. Disincentives for people with disabilities to return to work
  d. Availability of vocational rehabilitation services

4. Environmental health issues
  a. Occupational health hazards (e.g., neurotoxicity from chemicals in the workplace)
  b. Testing of food and drugs

5. Prevention of catastrophic injuries
  a. Mandating the use of seatbelts and inflatable restraints as well as helmet use while motorcycling, bicycling, skiing, and skating
  b. Providing education about substance abuse, particularly as a cause of accidents that can result in spinal cord injury or traumatic brain injury
  c. Promoting smoke-free environments

6. Women's issues
  a. Equal rights for women, including research on women's health concerns
  b. Economic equity (including child support)
  c. Child care and elder care
  d. Employers' support of family health
  e. Vocational training for women who are new or returning to the workplace because of circumstances such as divorce or death of a spouse

7. Men's issues
  a. Research on men's health concerns (e.g., prostate cancer)
  b. Child care and elder care
  c. Employers' support of family health

8. Genetics testing (including privacy)
9. Privacy and confidentiality
10. Telemedicine
11. Internet use by consumers to find healthcare information

C. Rehabilitation Legislation (Watson, 1988)
1. Education amendments (1980; PL 96-374): Provides centers, services, personnel, training, and research related to educational needs of children with disabilities
2. Social Security Disability amendments (1980: PL 96-265): Extends trial work periods for the disabled, enabling them to retain

Social Security benefits; places gainfully employed people with disabilities in a special benefits category for needed services

3. Surface Transportation Assistance Act (1982; PL 97-424): Encourages removal of architectural barriers in transportation industry

4. Individuals with Disabilities Education Act (IDEA) (1983; PL 98-199): Ensures access to educational opportunities for children with disabilities

5. Vocational Education Act (1984; PL 98-524): Requires states to provide funds for individuals with disabilities to have access to available vocational educational opportunities

6. Rehabilitation amendments (1984; PL 98-221): Modifies the definition of "severely disabled" and places a lower age limit at 16 years; extends provisions of 1973 Rehabilitation Act

7. Rehabilitation amendments (1986; PL 99-506): Emphasizes rehabilitation needs of Native Americans with disabilities; provides funding for rehabilitation engineering to develop technologically current devices for individuals with disabilities; decreases federal share of the basic state rehabilitation program; expands influence of the National Council on the Handicapped

8. Technology-Related Assistance for Individuals with Disabilities (1988; PL 100-407): Provides grants to states in an effort to increase the availability of assistive technology, conduct needs assessments, develop innovative programs, manage public awareness, and identify policies that promote the availability of assistive technology

9. Americans with Disabilities Act of 1990 (PL 101-336) (see Figure 4-3): Prohibits discrimination on the basis of disability in the areas of employment, public services, and public accommodations; addresses telecommunications and other miscellaneous provisions

10. Technology-Related Assistance for Individuals with Disabilities amendments (1994; PL 103-218): Expands and strengthens the 1988 act

11. Balanced Budget Act of 1997 (1997; PL 105-33): Mandates new Medicare PPS for SNFs, home care, and inpatient rehabilitation

by the year 2000 (*Note.* HFCA announced in early 2000 that the inpatient rehabilitation

---

Figure 4-2. Recommendations for a National Agenda for the Prevention of Disability

Organization and Coordination
- Develop leadership of National Disability Prevention Program at CDC
- Develop an enhanced role for the private sector
- Establish a national advisory committee
- Establish a federal interagency council
- Critically assess progress periodically

Surveillance
- Develop a conceptual framework and standard measures of disability
- Develop a national disability surveillance system
- Revise the National Health Interview Survey
- Conduct a comprehensive longitudinal survey of disability
- Develop disability indices

Research
- Develop a comprehensive research program
- Emphasize longitudinal research
- Conduct research on socioeconomic and psychological disadvantage
- Expand research on preventive and therapeutic interventions
- Upgrade training for research on disability prevention

Access to Care and Preventive Services
- Provide comprehensive health services to all mothers and children
- Provide effective family planning and prenatal services
- Develop new health service delivery strategies for people with disabilities
- Develop new health promotion models for people with disabilities
- Foster local capacity for building and demonstration projects
- Continue effective prevention programs
- Provide comprehensive vocational services

Professional and Public Education
- Upgrade medical education and training of physicians
- Upgrade the training of allied professionals
- Establish a program of grants for education and training
- Provide more public education on the prevention of disability
- Provide more training opportunities for family members and personal attendants of people with disabling conditions

---

PPS was rescheduled for implementation April 1, 2001.)

D. Guidelines for Taking Political Action

1. Register and vote for the candidates of your choice

2. Be informed on issues

3. Get involved in professional nursing associations and their health policy task forces

4. Obtain lists of local, state, and national legislators (available from government offices or public libraries)

5. Join the ARN Health Policy Committee

   a. Be informed about ARN's position on legislation by contacting the ARN office or the ARN Health Policy Committee Chair or by searching the ARN Web site (www.rehabnurse.org)

   b. Join the local ARN chapter's health policy committee

   c. Communicate with the ARN Health Policy Committee Chair about local and state issues and personal activities

   d. Attend legislative conferences (e.g., Nurse-in-Washington Internship [NIWI])

   e. Apply for ARN's Malcolm Maloof Memorial Scholarship to attend NIWI

6. Do not act as a spokesperson for a national or local organization unless specifically authorized to do so

7. Establish a relationship and communicate with federal, state, and local legislators to make them aware of positions on specific issues (see Figure 4-4)

   a. Write letters

   b. Make telephone calls

   c. Send faxes

   d. Send e-mail

   e. Meet in person

   f. Volunteer professional services or provide monetary support

   g. Provide expert testimony

II. The Process of Making Health Policy

A. Phases of Health Policy Making (see Figure 4-5)

1. Policy formulation (Longest, 1996)

   a. Agenda setting

1) This first stage of policy development refers to identifying problems and possible solutions given by diverse political interests.

2) Once issues become prominent in the political agenda, they can proceed to the next stage of policy formulation—the development of legislation; however, only a small percentage of issues reach that point.

   b. Development of legislation (see Figure 4-6)

1) The legislative process begins with proposals (bills), which may be drafted by senators or representatives and their staff members, by members of the executive branch, by political or special interest groups, and by individual citizens.

Figure 4-3. Americans with Disabilities Act (ADA) of 1990

Title I: Employment

Employers cannot discriminate against a qualified disabled job applicant or employee in any manner related to employment and benefits.

Employers must make their existing facilities accessible and usable by individuals with disabilities.

Accommodations in all aspects of job attainment and performance are required in order to place individuals on an equal plane with the nondisabled.

Title II: Public Services

Qualified disabled individuals must have access to all services and programs provided by state or local governments.

Public rail transportation must be made accessible to disabled individuals and supplemented with a paratransit system.

Title III: Public Accommodations and Services Operated by Private Entities

Virtually every entity open to the public must now be made accessible to the disabled.

A study is to be conducted concerning accessibility of over-the-road transportation.

Title IV: Telecommunications Relay Services

Telephone companies are required to furnish telecommunications devices to enable hearing and speech impaired individuals to communicate by wire or radio.

Reprinted with permission of ARN from Watson, P. (1990). The Americans with Disabilities Act: More rights for people with disabilities. *Rehabilitation Nursing, 15*(6), 326.

---

a) Only members of Congress can officially sponsor a bill.

b) Occasionally, identical bills are simultaneously introduced in the Senate and the House of Representatives for consideration.

2) Each bill is assigned to the appropriate committee(s) based on its content and the jurisdiction of the committees and subcommittees. Hearings are held, and the bill is "marked up." Once approved by the full committee, the House or Senate receives the bill and places it on the legislative calendar for floor action. The bill may be further amended during debate on the floor.

3) Once the bill passes either the House or the Senate, it is sent to the other chamber of Congress, where the process is repeated. If the second chamber passes the bill, any differences between the House and Senate versions must be resolved before the bill is sent to the White House for presidential action.

4) The president has the option to sign the bill to make it a law or to veto the bill and return it to Congress with an explanation for the rejection. A presidential veto may be overridden by a two-thirds vote in both houses of Congress. If the president does not sign or veto the bill after 10 days, the bill automatically becomes law.

2. Policy implementation (includes rule making and policy operation)

a. Once enacted as law, implementation of the policy rests primarily with the executive branch of the government. Cabinet departments such as DHHS and related agencies such as HCFA and the Centers for Disease Control and Prevention oversee the implementation.

b. Other agencies such as the General Accounting Office, the Congressional Budget Office, the Congressional Research Office, and the Office of Technology and Assessment have oversight responsibility.

c. Laws are often vague on implementation details, so the organization responsible for implementing the law publishes an "Advanced Notice of Proposed Rule Making" in the *Federal Register.*

d. Policy implementation involves the actual operation of programs that are described in the enacted legislation.

3. Policy modification: This stage allows all prior decisions to be modified once the outcomes, perceptions, and consequences of existing policies are discovered. Modifications to any legislation must begin with the agenda-setting stage.

Figure 4-4. Tips for Communicating with Congressional Representatives

Telephoning

Ask to speak with the aide who handles the issue on which you wish to comment.

Identify yourself and then state that you would like to leave a message, such as "Please tell Senator/Representative [name] that I support/oppose the following bill: [House bill—HR (number), or Senate bill—S (number)."

Writing Letters

State your purpose for writing in the first paragraph

If your letter pertains to specific legislation, identify it appropriately (e.g., House bill—HR ___, or Senate bill—S ___).

Be brief and courteous

Provide key information and specific examples.

Address only one issue in each letter; keep the letter to one page.

Proofread (or spell check) your letter before sending it.

Type, print, or write legibly.

Include your full name, address, and phone number.

Use this format for the introduction of your letter:

The Honorable [full name]

[room number] [name of] Senate Office Building

United States [Senate or House of Representatives]

Washington, DC 20510

Dear [Senator or Representative]:

Address chairs of committees or the Speaker of the House as "Dear Mr. Chairman or Madam Chairwoman" or "Dear Mr. Speaker"

Sending E-mail

Use the same guidelines as writing letters

Include your home address on the e-mail correspondence

Source consulted

American Nurses Association (ANA). (1999). *Hill basics: Communication tips.* Available: http://www.nursingworld.org/gova/federal/politic/hill/gcomtips.htm

---

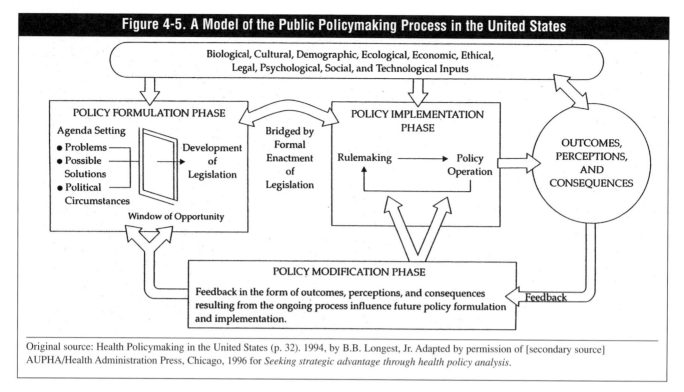

Figure 4-5. A Model of the Public Policymaking Process in the United States

Biological, Cultural, Demographic, Ecological, Economic, Ethical, Legal, Psychological, Social, and Technological Inputs

POLICY FORMULATION PHASE

Agenda Setting
● Problems
● Possible Solutions
● Political Circumstances

Development of Legislation

Window of Opportunity

Bridged by Formal Enactment of Legislation

POLICY IMPLEMENTATION PHASE

Rulemaking → Policy Operation

OUTCOMES, PERCEPTIONS, AND CONSEQUENCES

POLICY MODIFICATION PHASE

Feedback in the form of outcomes, perceptions, and consequences resulting from the ongoing process influence future policy formulation and implementation.

Feedback

Original source: Health Policymaking in the United States (p. 32). 1994, by B.B. Longest, Jr. Adapted by permission of [secondary source] AUPHA/Health Administration Press, Chicago, 1996 for *Seeking strategic advantage through health policy analysis*.

B. Opportunities for Rehabilitation Nurses to Influence Health Policy Making
  1. In policy formulation
    a. Agenda setting
      1) Define and document problems
      2) Develop and evaluate solutions to problems
      3) Shape political circumstances by lobbying and working through the legal system
    b. Legislation development
      1) Participate in drafting legislation
      2) Testify at legislative hearings
  2. In policy implementation or rule making
    a. Provide formal comments on draft rules published in the *Federal Register*
    b. Serve on and provide input to rule making advisory bodies
    c. Work on policy operation by interacting with policy operators
  3. In policy modification: Document cases for modification through operational experience and formal evaluations (i.e., research)

III. The Healthcare System's Response to Health Policy (Nosse, Friberg, & Kovacek, 1999)
  A. Growth and Development of the Healthcare Delivery System (1965–1980)
    1. The structure of the delivery system included small independent physician group practices.
    2. Larger multispecialty clinics were developing but were uncommon. Hospitals provided secondary and tertiary care.
    3. The supply of and demand for healthcare services expanded due to several factors.
      a. Introduction of Medicare and Medicaid programs
      b. An increased need for the capacity, capabilities, and the number and types of healthcare providers
      c. An increased number of people accessing the delivery system
      d. An increased amount of care provided to individuals
      e. New and improved treatments and technology
  B. Cost Containment in the Delivery of Health Care (1981–1991)
    1. Cost containment was a concern for physicians, hospitals, and public and private insurers.
    2. Acute care PPS began in 1983 and helped reduce the costs of inpatient hospital care.
      a. By decreasing the average length of stay
      b. By decreasing the use of routine diagnostic tests during inpatient hospitalizations

c. By shifting care to outpatient settings

d. By increasing the use of postacute care services (e.g., home care, rehabilitation hospitals and units, SNFs)

3. The decrease in inpatient hospital utilization resulted in excess bed capacity, decreased profits for hospitals and physicians, financial limits on purchasing new technologies and upgrading facilities.

4. These trends caused providers to compete for a larger share of the healthcare market and to react in many ways.

a. Reduced costs through reorganization and staff layoffs

b. Developed alternative care options (e.g., rehabilitation services, home care, ambulatory care, long-term care)

c. Restructured the organization through vertical and horizontal integration with other providers so that hospitals networks cover larger geographical areas and provide a full continuum of services

d. Focused new attention on marketing provider services

C. Managed Care and Assessment and Accountability (1990s)

1. Managed care enrollment increased dramatically.

2. National, publicly traded, for-profit healthcare corporations became more common.

3. Small independent providers joined together to form specialty service networks to capture and hold market shares.

4. Large physician groups joined with hospitals or contracted with managed care organizations.

5. Employers and providers looked for opportunities to bypass third-party payers.

6. Disease management and standardizing care received increased emphasis.

7. Interest in the quality of care and documenting the outcomes of health services, including publishing healthcare report cards, increased.

8. Consumerism increased.

9. Interest in providing evidence-based practice increased.

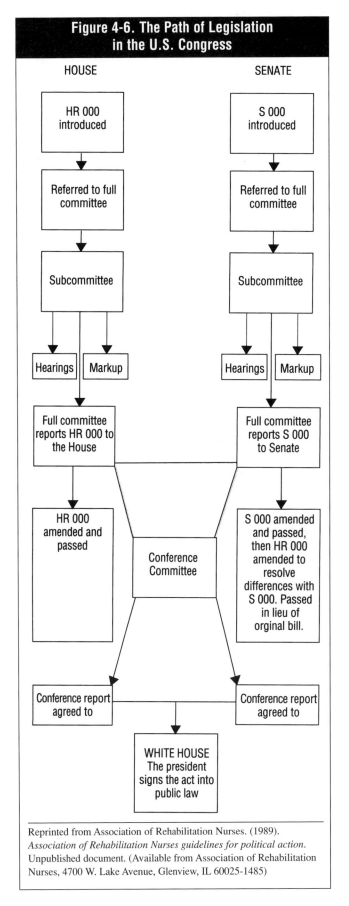

Figure 4-6. The Path of Legislation in the U.S. Congress

Reprinted from Association of Rehabilitation Nurses. (1989). *Association of Rehabilitation Nurses guidelines for political action.* Unpublished document. (Available from Association of Rehabilitation Nurses, 4700 W. Lake Avenue, Glenview, IL 60025-1485)

10. The Balanced Budget Act of 1997 mandated new Medicare PPS for SNFs, home care, and inpatient rehabilitation by the year 2000.(*Note.* HCFA announced in early 2000 that the inpatient rehabilitation PPS was rescheduled for implementation April 1, 2001.)

IV. Healthcare Reform

A. Overview

1. Concerns about the rising costs of health care, the growing number of uninsured and underinsured people, as well as the quality of care resulted in a variety of proposals for healthcare reform.

2. In 1994, the Clinton administration attempted to reform healthcare financing.

    a. Although this effort failed, the anticipation of reform caused significant changes in the delivery of healthcare services.

    b. Discussion has continued concerning the need for changes in health care.

B. Two Models for Healthcare Reform

1. Managed competition

    a. In this model, competition (not government regulation) controls healthcare costs.

    b. Insurers and consumers bid and contract for basic low-cost healthcare packages.

2. Single-payer system

    a. The federal government serves as the single payer for a basic healthcare package for all citizens and residents.

    b. Cost-containment strategies are focused on the behavior of the providers and hospitals rather than on the consumers of care.

    c. Individuals may purchase additional health coverage based on their interest and ability to pay.

References

American Nurses Association (ANA). (1999). *Hill basics: Communication tips.* Available: http://www.nursingworld.org/gova/federal/politic/hill/gcomtips.htm

Americans with Disabilities Act handbook. (1992). Washington, DC: U.S. Equal Employment Opportunity Commission and U.S. Department of Justice.

Association of Rehabilitation Nurses (ARN). (1999). *Association of Rehabilitation Nurses guidelines for political action.* Unpublished document. Available from ARN, 4700 W. Lake Avenue, Glenview, IL 60025-1485.

Baker, J. (1998). *Prospective payment for long-term care: An annual guide.* Gaithersburg, MD: Aspen.

Barker, E. (1999). Life care planning. *RN, 52*(3), 58-61.

Health Care Financing Administration (HCFA). (1997). *Your Medicare desk reference* [HCFA Publication No. 10937]. Baltimore, MD: Author.

Institute of Medicine. (1991). *Disability in America.* Washington, DC: National Academy Press.

Institute of Medicine Committee on Clinical Practice Guidelines. (1992). *Guidelines for clinical practice: From development to use.* Washington, DC: National Academy Press.

Jehle, F.F. (1992). *The complete and easy guide to Social Security and Medicare* (9th ed.). Charlotte, VT: Williamson Publishing.

Kassner, E., & Bectel, R.W. (1998). *Midlife and older Americans with disabilities: Who gets help?* Washington, DC: Public Policy Institute.

Kongstvedt, P.R. (1997). *Essentials of managed health care* (2nd ed.). Gaithersburg, MD: Aspen.

Kovner, A.R., & Jonas, S. (1998). *Jonas and Kovner's health care delivery in the United States.* New York: Springer Publishing.

Longest, B.B., Jr. (1994). *Health policymaking in the United States.* Chicago: AUPHA/Health Administration Press.

Longest, B.B., Jr. (1996). *Seeking strategic advantage through health policy analysis.* Chicago: Health Administration Press.

Medicare SNF Supplementary Provider Manual, Phase III Stage II. (1997). Washington, DC: Health Care Financing Administration.

Nosse, L.J., Friberg, D.G., & Kovacek, P.R. (1999). *Managerial and supervisory principles for physical therapists.* Baltimore: Williams & Wilkins.

Social Security programs in the United States. (1989). *Social Security Bulletin, 52*(7), 1-79.

Watson, P. (1988). Rehabilitation legislation of the 1980s: Implications for nurses as health care providers. *Rehabilitation Nursing, 13*(3), 137.

Watson, P. (1990). The Americans with Disabilities Act: More rights for people with disabilities. *Rehabilitation Nursing, 15*(6), 326.

Suggested resources

Bodenheimer, T.S., & Grumbach, K. (1995) *Understanding health policy: A clinical approach.* Norwalk, CT: Appleton & Lange.

Christiansen, C., & Baum, C. (1997). *Occupational therapy: Enabling function and well-being* (2nd ed.). Thorofare, NJ: SLACK.

Craven, G.T.A., & Gleason, C.A. (1996). Public policy and rehabilitation nursing. In S.P. Hoeman (Ed.), *Rehabilitation nursing: Process and application* (2nd ed., pp. 61-69.). St. Louis: Mosby.

Edwards, P.A. (1999). Financing health care. In P.A. Edwards (Ed.), *Pediatric rehabilitation nursing* (pp. 52-61). Philadelphia: W.B. Saunders.

Edwards, P.A. (1999). Legislation and public policy. In P.A. Edwards (Ed.), *Pediatric rehabilitation nursing* (pp. 40-51). Philadelphia: W.B. Saunders.

Mason, D.J., & Leavitt, J.K. (1998). *Policy and politics in nursing and health care* (3rd ed.). Philadelphia: W.B. Saunders.

McCourt, A.E. (Ed.). (1993). *The specialty practice of rehabilitation nursing: A core curriculum* (3rd ed.). Skokie, IL: Rehabilitation Nursing Foundation of the Association of Rehabilitation Nurses.

Milstead, J.A. (1999). *Health policy and politics: A nurse's guide.* Gaithersburg, MD: Aspen.

Rothstein, J.M., Roy, S.H., & Wolf, S.L. (1998). *The rehabilitation specialist's handbook* (2nd ed.). Philadelphia: F.A. Davis.

Section II

Functional Health Patterns and Rehabilitation Nursing

· ·

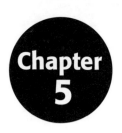

Neuroanatomy

Cynthia Kraft Fine, MSN RN CRRN

Neuroanatomy is the basis for much of the care that rehabilitation nurses provide. By understanding neuroanatomy, nurses are able to provide the most appropriate care for patients and their families. For example, if the nurse knows the specific location and the functional implications of the patient's neurologic injury, he or she can better anticipate the patient's needs, realistic goals, potential outcomes, and long-term issues that may confront the patient in the future. Also, by knowing which neurologic areas remain intact, the nurse can help the patient use these functions to compensate for the deficits and possibly function more independently.

It is important to keep in mind that trauma—whether it is vascular or from an accident—rarely affects only one part of the neurologic system. In fact, damage to any of the anatomical structures described in this chapter can affect the individual's behavior and function in many ways. Also, the patient's injury can greatly affect his or her family and significant others.

A clear understanding of neuroanatomy provides rehabilitation nurses with the foundation for providing optimal rehabilitation nursing interventions. It also provides rehabilitation nurses with a rationale for setting appropriate goals with clients and families. Rehabilitation nurses can use their knowledge of neuroanatomy to help their patients and families adapt to changes in function, use their strengths to adapt to the injury, and set realistic, outcome-based goals that can be achieved throughout the healthcare continuum.

This chapter provides an overview of neuroanatomy. Nursing interventions for neurologic injuries vary depending on the location and extent of injury. Specific interventions, planning, and evaluation are discussed in chapters devoted to specific conditions in Section III of this book.

I. Anatomy of the Brain

A. Meninges (Barker, 1994)
1. The covering of the central nervous system (CNS) that helps protect the nervous tissue (see Figure 5-1)
2. Composed of pia mater, arachnoid mater, dura mater (PAD)
   a. P: Pia mater
      1) The layer that adheres to the brain and spinal cord
      2) A highly vascularized layer that provides nourishment to the CNS
   b. A: Arachnoid mater: A thin, delicate, cobweb-like layer
   c. D: Dura mater
      1) The outermost layer that lies against the skull and vertebrae
      2) Composed of tough, white fibrous tissue
      3) Includes the tentorium cerebelli, which is the area that separates the cerebellum from the cerebrum in the occipital lobe
      4) Is the location of a condition called tentorial herniation, which occurs when intracranial pressure causes the brain to push down through the tentorial notch, compressing the brainstem
      5) Creates spaces known as sinuses, through which cerebral spinal fluid (CSF) is reabsorbed into the bloodstream

B. Spaces (Barker, 1994)
1. Subarachnoid space
   a. Space between the pia mater and arachnoid mater that is filled with CSF
   b. CSF flows from the ventricles to sinuses via the subarachnoid space.
   c. Subarachnoid hemorrhage occurs when bleeding occurs in this space.

1) Is usually caused by an arteriovenous (A-V) malformation

2) May also be the result of trauma

2. Subdural space

a. Space between the arachnoid and dura mater that is usually a potential (empty) space

b. Subdural hematoma occurs when venous blood leaks into this space.

c. Subdural hygroma occurs when CSF leaks into the subdural space: This is believed to be caused by a tear in the arachnoid mater.

3. Epidural space

a. Space between the dura mater and the bone that is usually a potential (empty) space

b. Epidural hematoma occurs when the middle meningeal artery bleeds rapidly into the epidural space.

C. Ventricles (Barker, 1994)

1. Spaces in the brain where CSF is found

2. Two lateral ventricles (one in each hemisphere) exist: CSF is formed here.

3. The third and fourth ventricles are more centrally located and allow CSF to continually flow from the brain to the spinal cord.

D. Cerebral Spinal Fluid (CSF) (Barker, 1994)

1. Cushions and protects the CNS

2. Functions similarly to blood, carrying nutrients to the CNS and removing wastes from it

E. Cerebrum (Cerebral Cortex) (Barker, 1994)

1. Believed to contain approximately 14 billion neurons, which are the building blocks of the CNS

a. Composition of neurons (Barker, 1994)

1) A cell body (perikaryon) and elongated processes that come from the body

2) Dendrites: Conduct impulses toward the perikaryon

3) Axons: Conduct impulses away from the perikaryon

b. Types of neurons

1) Pseudounipolar

a) Appear to have only one process originating from the perikaryon, which divides into two processes: One branch goes to the skin, and the other enters the CNS.

b) Typically found in the sensory ganglia of peripheral nerves

2) Bipolar

a) Have two processes originating from the perikaryon: One functions as the dendrite, the other as an axon.

b) Have limited distribution in the CNS

c) Found primarily in the visual, auditory, and olfactory systems

3) Multipolar

a) Possess one axon and many dendrites

b) Are the most plentiful type of neuron

c) Can be found throughout the CNS and peripheral nervous system (PNS)

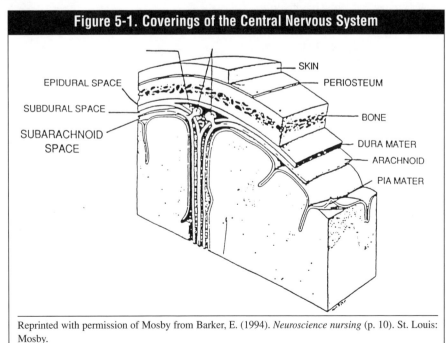

Figure 5-1. Coverings of the Central Nervous System

SKIN
EPIDURAL SPACE
PERIOSTEUM
SUBDURAL SPACE
BONE
SUBARACHNOID SPACE
DURA MATER
ARACHNOID
PIA MATER

Reprinted with permission of Mosby from Barker, E. (1994). *Neuroscience nursing* (p. 10). St. Louis: Mosby.

2. Covered with bumps (gyri) and grooves (small grooves are called sulci; large grooves are called fissures)

3. Composed of myelinated white matter, which is located deep inside the brain, and gray matter, which are cell bodies located on the outer portion of the brain

4. Divided into two halves (hemispheres)

   a. Hemispheres are connected by nerve fibers called corpus callosum that allow for communication between the two sides.

   b. One hemisphere is usually dominant.

      1) The dominant hemisphere is responsible for speech and is most often located in the left hemisphere.

      2) Dominance is also related to "handedness."

         a) 90% of the population is right-handed. 99% of these individuals have a dominant left hemisphere.

         b) 10% of the population is left-handed. 60% of these individuals have a dominant left hemisphere; however, 80% of all left-handed individuals have some mixed dominance.

5. Contains the lobes of the brain (Hickey, 1997) (see Figure 5-2)

   a. Frontal lobe(s)

      1) The anterior portion controls emotions, personality, complex intelligence (i.e., executive functions), and cognition.

      2) The posterior portion controls voluntary motor movements.

      3) Broca's area, which is responsible for the motor component of speech, is located in the left hemisphere.

      4) Injury to this area may be indicated by emotional lability, difficulty with executive functions, personality changes, difficulty initiating voluntary movements, and Broca's aphasia.

   b. Parietal lobe(s)

      1) Receives and interprets sensory input (e.g., pain, temperature, pressure, size, shape, texture, body image, left/right discrimination, and spatial orientation)

      2) Injury to this area is usually indicated by difficulty with left/right discrimination, spatial orientation, and body image perception.

   c. Occipital lobe(s)

      1) Receives and interprets visual stimuli

      2) Responsible for depth perception

      3) Injury to this area is indicated by difficulty with interpreting visual clues or stimuli.

   d. Temporal lobe(s)

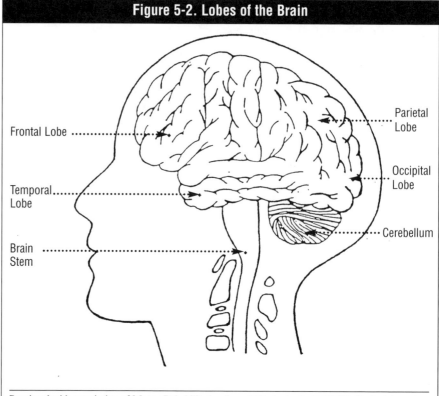

Figure 5-2. Lobes of the Brain

Frontal Lobe
Temporal Lobe
Brain Stem
Parietal Lobe
Occipital Lobe
Cerebellum

Reprinted with permission of Magee Rehabilitation from DiPaolantonio, J. (1996). *Brain injury: A family guide* (p. 8). Philadelphia: Magee Rehabilitation.

1) Controls hearing, taste, and smell
2) Includes Wernicke's area, which enables speech reception (usually in left hemisphere) and interpretation of sounds as words
3) Controls memory functions
4) Injury to this area involves loss of smell, hearing deficits, loss of taste, memory deficits, and Wernicke's aphasia.

F. Other Structures in the Brain (Barker, 1994) (see Figure 5-3)

1. Limbic system: The function and the exact structure of this system are not understood completely.

   a. Composed of a group of structures deep inside the brain associated with the hypothalamus

   b. Appears to be involved in primitive emotions (e.g., anger, rage, sexual arousal and behavior, pleasure, sadness) and the "fight or flight" response

   c. Appears to affect motivation, attention, and biological rhythm

   d. Injury to this system usually results in a hyperarousal state, which is indicated by the individual's behaviors.

2. Basal ganglia

   a. A mass of gray matter deep within the cerebrum

   b. Helps to adjust posture, allow steady voluntary movements, and suppress meaningless and

unintentional movements

c. Injury to this system usually results in dyskinesias (i.e., abnormal involuntary movements) and muscle tone alteration (i.e., rigidity and bradykinesia).

1) Tremors: Rhythmic and purposeless movements that occur at rest and disappear during intentional movements
2) Athetosis: Slow, snakelike, writhing

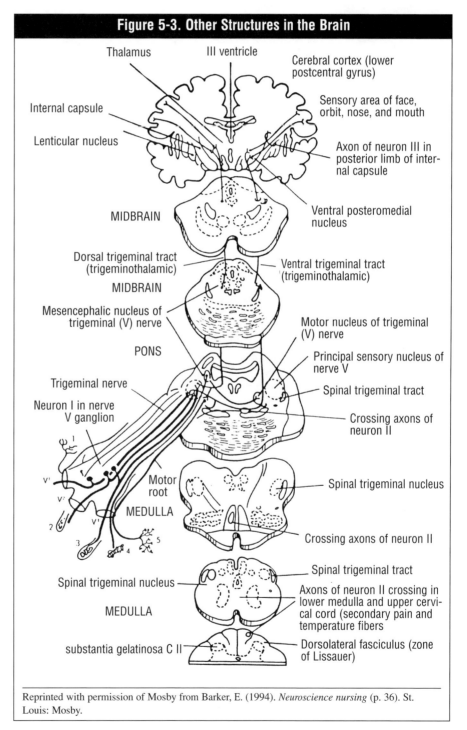

Figure 5-3. Other Structures in the Brain

Thalamus
III ventricle
Cerebral cortex (lower postcentral gyrus)
Internal capsule
Lenticular nucleus
Sensory area of face, orbit, nose, and mouth
Axon of neuron III in posterior limb of internal capsule
MIDBRAIN
Ventral posteromedial nucleus
Dorsal trigeminal tract (trigeminothalamic)
MIDBRAIN
Ventral trigeminal tract (trigeminothalamic)
Mesencephalic nucleus of trigeminal (V) nerve
Motor nucleus of trigeminal (V) nerve
PONS
Principal sensory nucleus of nerve V
Trigeminal nerve
Spinal trigeminal tract
Neuron I in nerve V ganglion
Crossing axons of neuron II
Motor root
Spinal trigeminal nucleus
MEDULLA
Crossing axons of neuron II
Spinal trigeminal nucleus
Spinal trigeminal tract
MEDULLA
Axons of neuron II crossing in lower medulla and upper cervical cord (secondary pain and temperature fibers)
substantia gelatinosa C II
Dorsolateral fasciculus (zone of Lissauer)

Reprinted with permission of Mosby from Barker, E. (1994). *Neuroscience nursing* (p. 36). St. Louis: Mosby.

movements of the extremities, face, and neck

   3) Chorea: Rapid, purposeless, jerky movements that are often associated with facial grimacing

3. Diencephalon: Composed of the thalamus and hypothalamus

  a. Thalamus

    1) Functions as a relay station for some sensory messages, particularly pain, touch, and pressure

    2) Helps to discern pleasant feelings from unpleasant feelings

    3) Lesions tend to be associated primarily with sensory loss.

    4) Thalamic syndrome is a nonspecific, spontaneous, intolerable pain that cannot be relieved pharmaceutically.

  b. Hypothalamus

    1) Located below the thalamus

    2) Is the master controller of both divisions (parasympathetic and sympathetic) of the autonomic nervous system

    3) Plays a role in producing two hormones that are stored and released from the pituitary gland

     a) Antidiuretic hormone (ADH): Enhances reabsorption of water in the kidneys

      (1) Too much ADH leads to sudden inappropriate antidiuretic hormone (SIADH), which leads to water retention. It is common to see this syndrome in trauma patients.

      (2) Too little ADH leads to diabetes insipidus and excessive water loss.

     b) Oxytocin: Stimulates uterine contractions

4. Brainstem

  a. Midbrain

    1) Is approximately 2 cm in length

    2) Composed of two structures

     a) Substantia nigra: Motor nuclei that are concerned with muscle tone. This area is impaired in patients with Parkinson's disease.

     b) Red nucleus: Large motor nuclei associated with flexor rigidity

    3) Injury to the midbrain is associated with decorticate posturing (i.e., abnormal flexion).

  b. Pons

    1) Looks like a bridge between the cerebellar hemispheres

    2) Has two areas that help control breathing

     a) Apneustic center: Initiates inspiration

     b) Pneumotaxic center: Inhibits inspiration

    3) Injury to the pons usually involves abnormal breathing patterns.

     a) Central neurogenic hyperventilation: Sustained regular, rapid deep breaths

     b) Apneustic breathing: Sustained, cramplike inspiratory efforts that pause when inspiration is complete; there also may be an expiratory pause.

    4) Involves two reflexes that are tested in comatose patients to determine pontine and brainstem involvement

     a) Oculocephalic reflex (doll's eyes): In this reflex, the eyes of the individual move in sync with head movement. In normal pontine activity, movement of the eyes lags behind.

     b) Oculovestibular reflex (calorics): To test for this reflex, water is placed in the ear canal. In pontine lesions, the eyes do not deviate toward the stimulated ear. In normal pontine function, the eyes deviate toward stimulated ear.

    5) Pontine lesions produce a "locked-in" syndrome, in which the individual has no movement except for the eyelids, but the patient is conscious and sensation is intact.

  c. Medulla oblongata

    1) Houses the respiratory center

     a) Is inspiratory dominant: The

medulla senses the need to inspire; exhalation is a passive process.

    b) Produces rhythmic breathing

    c) Involves chemoreceptors that are sensitive to CO_2 levels in the blood and cause an increase in ventilation when CO_2 is elevated

    d) Injuries to this area result in ataxic breathing in which breathing is irregular with both shallow and deep inspiratory efforts.

  2) Controls temperature, regulates hunger, thirst, and sleep-wake patterns

  3) Houses the vasodilation and vasopressor centers

  4) Originates the swallowing and vomiting centers

  d. Reticular formation

    1) Located in the brainstem

    2) Receives sensory input from all sensory organs and acts as a relay station to determine which area of the brain receives the input

    3) Is most often associated with controlling states of consciousness

    4) Is particularly susceptible to trauma

    5) Involves the following functions

      a) Motor control modulation: Coordinates (but does not inhibit) movement and plays a role in the extrapyramidal system

      b) Visceral functioning: Controls the state of consciousness

      c) Sensory filtering: Plays an inhibitory role to prevent the brain from becoming overstimulated

      d) Inhibition of stimuli: Helps to narrow down stimuli to allow selective attention and plays a major role in attention and concentration

      e) Arousal and alertness

    6) Injury to this area may cause coma.

5. Cerebellum

  a. Located below the cerebrum

  b. Involves two hemispheres and a medial portion called the vermis

  c. Contains gray matter on the outside of the cerebellar cortex and white matter on the inside of the cortex

  d. Receives sensory and motor impulses

  e. Is responsible for the following functions

    1) Coordination of all reflex activity and voluntary motor activity

    2) Regulation of muscle tone and posture

    3) Influence and maintenance of equilibrium

  f. Injury to this area can produce a variety of signs of dysfunction.

    1) Deficits on the same (ipsilateral) side of the body as the injury

    2) Hypotonia: Decreased resistance to passive movement

    3) Postural changes and wide-based gait to compensate for loss of muscle tone

    4) Ataxia (clumsy, uncoordinated movement)

      a) Intentional tremors

      b) Jerky movements

      c) Dysmetria: Inability to judge movement within space, thereby losing control of motor activity

      d) Dysdiadochokinesis: Inability to perform alternating movements rapidly or regularly

      e) Nystagmus: Disorders or ataxia of ocular movement

      f) Ataxia of speech muscles

G. Cranial Nerves (Barker, 1994)

  1. Twelve cranial nerves (CN) (see Table 5-1)

  a. CN I: Olfactory—smell

  b. CN II: Optic—vision

  c. CN III: Oculomotor—eye movement (e.g., elevating eyelids, moving eyes in and out, constricting pupil, accommodating for light)

  d. CN IV: Trochlear—eye movement down and outward

  e. CN V: Trigeminal—chewing, sensations of face, scalp, and teeth

  f. CN VI: Abducens—outward eye movement

  g. CN VII: Facial—facial expression, taste (anterior two-thirds of tongue), salivation, crying

Table 5-1. Cranial Nerves

Cranial Nerve	Origin and Course	Function
CN I: Olfactory		
Sensory	Mucosa of nasal cavity; only CN with cell body located in peripheral structure (nasal mucosa). Pass through cribriform plate of ethmoid bone and go on to olfactory bulbs at floor of frontal lobe. Final interpretation is in temporal lobe.	Smell. However, system is more than receptor/interpreter for odors; perception of smell also sensitizes other body systems and responses such as salivation, peristalsis, and even sexual stimulus. Loss of sense of smell is termed anosmia.
CN II: Optic		
Sensory	Ganglion cells of retina converge on the optic disc and form optic nerve. Nerve fibers pass to optic chiasm, which is above pituitary gland. Some fibers decussate, others do not. The two tracts then go to the lateral geniculate body near the thalamus and then on to the end station for interpretation in the occipital lobe.	Vision.
CN III: Oculomotor		
Motor	Originates in midbrain and emerges from brainstem at upper pons.	Extraocular movement of eyes.
	Motor fibers to superior, medial, inferior recti, and inferior oblique for eye movement; levator muscle of the eyelid.	Raise eyelid.
Parasympathetic	Parasympathetic fibers to ciliary muscles and iris of eye.	Constrict pupil; changes shape of lens.
CN IV: Trochlear		
Motor	Comes from lower midbrain area to innervate superior oblique eye muscle.	Allows eye to move down and inward.
CN V: Trigeminal		
Sensory	Originates in fourth ventricle and emerges at lateral parts of pons. Has three branches to face: ophthalmic, maxillary, and mandibular.	Ophthalmic branch: Sensation to cornea, ciliary body, iris, lacrimal gland, conjunctiva, nasal mucosal membranes, eyelids, eyebrows, forehead, and nose.
		Maxillary branch: Sensation to skin of cheek, lower lid, side of nose and upper jaw, teeth, mucosa of mouth, spheno-pola-tive-pterygoid region, and maxillary sinus.
		Mandibular branch: Sensation to skin of lower lip, chin, ear, mucous membrane, teeth of lower jaw and tongue.
Motor	Goes to temporalis, masseter, pterygoid gland, anterior part of digastric muscles (all for mastication), and the tensor tympani and tensor veli palatini muscles (clench jaws).	Muscles of chewing and mastication and opening jaw.
CN VI: Abducens		
Motor	Arises from a nucleus in pons to innervate lateral rectus eye muscle.	Allows eye to move outward.

Table 5-1. Cranial Nerves (Continued)

Cranial Nerve	Origin and Course	Function
CN VII: Facial		
Sensory	Lower portion of pons goes to anterior two-thirds of tongue and soft palate.	Taste anterior two-thirds of tongue. Sensation to soft palate.
Motor	Pons to muscles of forehead, eyelids, cheeks, lips, ear, nose, and neck.	Movement of facial muscles to produce facial expressions, close eyes.
Parasympathetic	Pons to salivary gland and lacrimal glands.	Secretory for salivation and tears.
CN VIII: Acoustic		
Sensory	Cochlear division: Originates in spinal ganglia of the cochlea, with peripheral fibers to the organ of Corti in the internal ear. Goes to pons, and impulses transmitted to the temporal lobe.	Hearing.
	Vestibular division: Originates in otolith organs of the semicircular canals in the inner ear and in the vestibular ganglion. Terminates in pons, with some fibers continuing to cerebellum. Only cranial nerve originating wholly within a bone, petrous portion of temporal bone.	Equilibrium.
IX: Glossopharyngeal		
Sensory	Posterior one-third of tongue for taste sensation and sensations from soft palate, tonsils, and opening to mouth in back of oral pharynx (fauces). Fibers go to medulla and then to the temporal lobe for taste and sensory cortex for other sensations.	Taste in posterior one-third of tongue. Sensation in back of throat; stimulation elicits a gag reflex.
Motor	Medulla to constrictor muscles of pharynx and stylopharyngeal muscles.	Voluntary muscles for swallowing and phonation.
Parasympathetic	Medulla to parotid salivary gland via otic ganglia.	Secretory, salivary glands. Carotid reflex.
CN X: Vagus		
Sensory	Sensory fibers in back of ear and posterior wall of external ear go to medulla oblongata and on to sensory cortex.	Sensation behind ear and part of external ear meatus.
Motor	Fibers go from medulla oblongata through jugular foramen with glossopharyngeal nerve and on to pharynx, larynx, esophagus, bronchi, lungs, heart, stomach, small intestines, liver, pancreas, kidneys.	Voluntary muscles for phonation and swallowing. Involuntary activity of visceral muscles of heart, lungs, and digestive tract.
Parasympathetic	Medulla oblongata to larynx, trachea, lungs, aorta, esophagus, stomach, small intestines, and gall bladder.	Carotid reflex. Autonomic activity of respiratory tract, digestive tract including peristalsis and secretion from organs.
CN XI: Spinal Accessory		
Motor	This nerve has two roots, cranial and spinal. Cranial portion arises at several rootlets at side of medulla, runs below vagus, and is joined by spinal portion from motor cells in cervical cord. Some fibers go along with vagus nerve to supply motor impulse to pharynx, larynx, uvula, and palate. Major portion to sternomastoid and trapezius muscles, branches to cervical spinal nerves C2-C4.	Some fibers for swallowing and phonation. Turn head and shrug shoulders.

Table 5-1. Cranial Nerves (Continued)		
Cranial Nerve	**Origin and Course**	**Function**
CN XII: Hypoglossal Motor	Arises in medulla oblongata and goes to muscles of tongue.	Movement of tongue necessary for swallowing and phonation.

Reprinted with permission of Mosby from Rudy, E. (1984). *Advanced neurological and neurosurgical nursing* (1st ed.). St Louis: Mosby. (Also reprinted in Barker, E. [1994]. *Neuroscience nursing* [pp. 78-79]. St. Louis: Mosby.)

h. CN VIII: Acoustic—hearing and sense of balance

i. CN IX: Glossopharyngeal—secretes saliva, swallowing, controls gag reflex, sensation in the throat and taste

j. CN X: Vagus—swallowing, voice production, heart rate, rate of peristalsis, sensation of throat, thoracic, and abdominal viscera

k. CN XI: Spinal accessory—shoulder and head movement

l. CN XII: Hypoglossal—tongue movement

2. Mnemonic tip for remembering the cranial nerves: On Old Olympus' Towering Top, A Finn And German Viewed Some Hops

H. Components that Provide the Vascular Supply to the Brain (Barker, 1994) (see Figure 5-4)

1. Internal carotid arteries (right and left)

   a. Supply 80% of the blood supply to the brain

   b. Divide to form the anterior cerebral artery and the middle cerebral artery

2. Vertebral arteries (right and left)

   a. Supply 20% of the blood supply to the brain

b. Join to form the basilar artery as it passes over the pons and then splits and becomes the posterior cerebral arteries at the level of the cerebrum

3. Communicating arteries

   a. Posterior: Connects the posterior cerebral and middle cerebral arteries

   b. Anterior: Connects the two anterior cerebral arteries

4. Circle of Willis

   a. Formed by the anastomosis of the two internal carotid arteries and the two

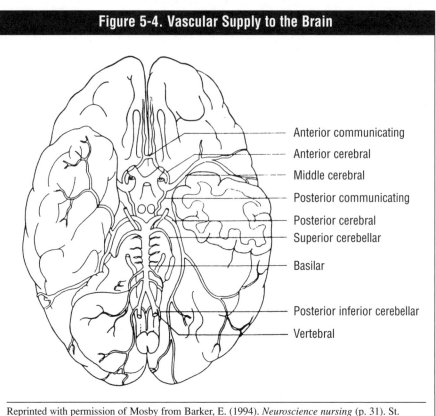

Figure 5-4. Vascular Supply to the Brain

Anterior communicating

Anterior cerebral

Middle cerebral

Posterior communicating

Posterior cerebral

Superior cerebellar

Basilar

Posterior inferior cerebellar

Vertebral

Reprinted with permission of Mosby from Barker, E. (1994). *Neuroscience nursing* (p. 31). St. Louis: Mosby.

vertebral arteries

b. Composed of the following arteries

1) Anterior cerebral
2) Posterior cerebral
3) Anterior communicating
4) Posterior communicating
5) Internal carotid

c. Allows blood that enters either the internal carotid arteries or the vertebral arteries to be distributed to any part of the brain

d. Located at the base of the skull in the subarachnoid space

1) This is the site of many congenital aneurysms.
2) If an aneurysm bursts or vessels are sheared or torn, a subarachnoid hemorrhage occurs.

II. Anatomy of the Spinal Cord

A. White and Gray Matter (Barker, 1994)

1. White matter is located in the outside portion of the spinal cord, whereas gray matter is more centrally located: This is the opposite of the brain's makeup of white and gray matter.

2. The anterior portion of the cord contains gray matter that innervates major muscle groups.

3. The spinal cord starts at the end of the brainstem and continues through the vertebral bodies to T12.

a. Conus medullaris: The cone-shaped area from T10-T12

b. Cauda equina (horse's tail): The area at the end of the conus medullaris that is not actually a part of the spinal cord, but is composed of peripheral nerves

B. Spinal Nerve Levels (Barker, 1994) (see Table 5-2)

1. Cervical (C)

a. C1: Innervates the chin for sensation
b. C2: Innervates the lateral neck muscles that provide head support
c. C3: Innervates the anterior and posterior neck muscles that provide head support
d. C4: Innervates the deltoids and diaphragm
e. C5: Innervates the biceps and deltoids
f. C6: Innervates the wrist extensor muscles
g. C7: Innervates the triceps
h. C8: Innervates the flexor profundus muscles

2. Thoracic (T)

a. T1: Innervates the intrinsic muscles of the hand
b. T1-T6: Innervates the intercostal muscles
c. T7-T12: Innervates the upper and lower

Table 5-2. Muscles and Functions Affected by Level of Spinal Cord Injury		
Spinal Nerve	**Muscle Group Movement**	**Assessment Technique**
C4-C5	Shoulder abduction	Shoulders are shrugged against downward pressure of examiner's hands
C5-C6	Elbow flexion (biceps)	Arm is pulled up from resting position against resistance
C7	Elbow extension (triceps)	From flexed position, arm is straightened out against resistance
C7	Thumb-index pinch	Index finger is held firmly to thumb against resistance to pull apart
C8	Hand grasp	Hand grasp strength is evaluated
L2-L4	Hip flexion	Leg is lifted from bed against resistance
L5-S1	Knee flexion	Knee is flexed against resistance
L2-L4	Knee extension	From flexed position, knee is extended against resistance
L5	Foot dorsiflexion	Foot pulled up toward nose against resistance
S1	Foot plantar flexion	Foot pushed down (stepping on the gas) against resistance

Reprinted with permission of Mosby from Barker, E. (1994). *Neuroscience nursing* (p. 88). St. Louis: Mosby.

abdominal muscles, thoracic muscles, quadratus lumborum flexors

3. Lumbar (L)

   a. L1-L2: Innervates the iliopsoas muscles

   b. L3: Innervates the quadriceps

   c. L4: Innervates the tibialis anterior

   d. L5: Innervates extensor hallicus longus

4. Sacral (S)

   a. S1: Innervates gastrocnemius

   b. S2-S4: Innervates specific motor and sensory functions, including anorectal muscles, perineal sensation, sphincter control, genitalia, and sexual function

C. Neurologic Levels (Zedjlik, 1992)

  1. Nerve roots

   a. The nerve roots that come from the spinal cord contain both a motor and sensory component.

   b. The cervical area has eight nerve roots. The first seven roots pass above the vertebrae. The eighth root passes below the vertebrae.

   c. All other spinal nerve roots (those originating in the thoracic, lumbar, and sacral areas) pass below the vertebrae.

   d. Nerve roots are named for the vertebral area from which they pass through.

  2. Tracts of neurons

   a. Neurons are bundled together in ascending and descending tracts, which connect the PNS with the CNS.

   b. Tracts transmit both sensory and motor impulses; their names indicate the direction that the impulses travel.

    1) If the word spinal comes first, the impulses travel from the spinal cord to the brain.

    2) If the first word is related to the brain, then the impulses descend from the brain to the spinal cord.

   c. Major sensory tracts (see Figure 5-5)

    1) Posterior columns: Sensations of deep touch, proprioception, and vibration, as well as most bowel and bladder sensations

    2) Anterior spinocerebellar: Unconscious proprioception

    3) Lateral spinothalamic: Pain and temperature

    4) Anterior spinothalamic: Touch and some pressure

   d. Major motor tracts

    1) Anterior (ventral) corticospinal: Fine tuning of muscle tone

    2) Lateral corticospinal: Major voluntary movement

  3. Spinal reflexes, which are necessary for normal neurologic function (Barker, 1994) (see Figure 5-6)

   a. The brain is able to inhibit approximately 80% of spinal reflexes to maintain voluntary control over posture and movement.

   b. A normal spinal cord reflex involves the following:

    1) Sensory input, which ascends to the cell body where it synapses with a motor neuron

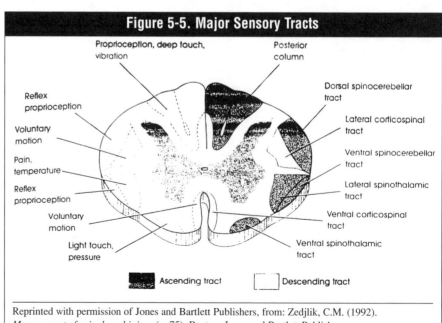

Figure 5-5. Major Sensory Tracts

Proprioception, deep touch, vibration

Posterior column

Reflex proprioception

Voluntary motion

Pain, temperature

Reflex proprioception

Voluntary motion

Light touch, pressure

Dorsal spinocerebellar tract

Lateral corticospinal tract

Ventral spinocerebellar tract

Lateral spinothalamic tract

Ventral corticospinal tract

Ventral spinothalamic tract

■ Ascending tract   □ Descending tract

Reprinted with permission of Jones and Bartlett Publishers, from: Zedjlik, C.M. (1992). *Management of spinal cord injury* (p. 75). Boston: Jones and Bartlett Publishers.

2) The motor cell body, which sends an impulse down to cause motor activity

c. The brain is able to prevent or speed up a synapse if the stimulus is anticipated (i.e., the brain maintains ultimate control over the spinal cord).

d. Sensory messages also reach the brain as a part of this process.

e. When an individual suffers a spinal cord injury (SCI), reflex activity resumes after spinal shock; however, the connection between the brain and spinal cord is missing and thus the brain can no longer inhibit or facilitate spinal reflexes, which causes spasticity.

f. Reflex activity does not return at the level of injury because the neurons are damaged or destroyed.

g. If damage occurs to the peripheral nerves or the cauda equina, reflex activity does not occur.

4. Upper motor neuron (UMN) versus lower motor neuron (LMN) (American Spinal Injury Association [ASIA], 1996)

a. UMN injury

1) Occurs when damage to the motor neuron comes from the pyramidal tracts down to the spinal cord. The lesion forces the lack of synapse between the spinal cord and the brain.

2) UMN injuries are the result of damage to CNS tissue.

3) UMN injuries usually result in spasticity below the level of injury, reflexes below the level of injury, and a spastic bowel and bladder.

b. LMN injury

1) Occurs when damage to the motor neuron

comes from the spinal cord or the axon that innervates the target muscles. The lesion forces a lack of synapse between the peripheral nerves and the spinal cord.

2) LMN injuries are the result of damage to the PNS as it exits the CNS.

3) LMN injuries usually result in the lack of preservation of spinal reflexes below the level of injury, flaccidity, and the destruction of bowel, bladder, and sexual functioning reflexes.

4) LMN injuries are most commonly seen in SCIs below T12.

D. Circulation to the Spinal Cord (Waxman, 1996)

1. The spinal cord is a highly vascularized organ that receives its blood supply from the vertebral arteries.

a. Damage to the arteries can be a result of damage to the vertebrae or vertebral alignment.

b. Damage can be caused by trauma, vascular anomalies, infarcts, or vascular surgery.

2. The anterior spinal artery provides the blood supply to the anterior two-thirds of the spinal cord.

3. The posterior spinal arteries provide the blood supply to the posterior one-third of the spinal cord: These arteries provide the needed blood supply to the posterior one-third of the white matter and some of the posterior portions of the meninges.

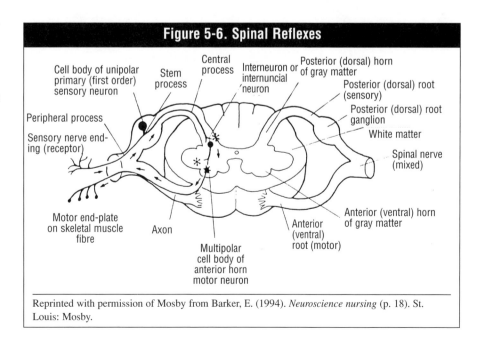

Figure 5-6. Spinal Reflexes

Cell body of unipolar primary (first order) sensory neuron

Stem process

Central process

Interneuron or internuncial neuron

Posterior (dorsal) horn of gray matter

Posterior (dorsal) root (sensory)

Posterior (dorsal) root ganglion

White matter

Peripheral process

Sensory nerve ending (receptor)

Spinal nerve (mixed)

Motor end-plate on skeletal muscle fibre

Axon

Multipolar cell body of anterior horn motor neuron

Anterior (ventral) root (motor)

Anterior (ventral) horn of gray matter

Reprinted with permission of Mosby from Barker, E. (1994). *Neuroscience nursing* (p. 18). St. Louis: Mosby.

III. The Neurological Assessment

A. Assess All Neurologic Injuries for Motor and Sensory Components

1. Types of injuries (ASIA, 1996)

   a. Tetraplegia

      1) Impairment or loss of function in the cervical segments of the cord

      2) Results in loss of function in the upper and lower extremities and the trunk, including the pelvic organs

   b. Paraplegia

      1) Impairment or loss of function in the thoracic, lumbar, or sacral segments of the cord

      2) Results in loss of function in the lower extremities and the trunk, including the pelvic organs

2. Muscle grading system: Used to quantify a muscle group's strength using a consistent terminology (ASIA, 1996)

   a. Grade 0 = Absent, no strength

   b. Grade 1 = Trace amount of strength against gravity

   c. Grade 2 = Poor amount of strength against gravity

   d. Grade 3 = Fair amount of strength against gravity

   e. Grade 4 = Good amount of strength against gravity

   f. Grade 5 = Normal amount of strength against gravity

3. Extent of damage to the cord, which can be described as complete or incomplete

   a. ASIA (1996) developed definitions of complete and incomplete injuries.

      1) ASIA A: Complete injury

         a) No preservation of sensation or motor function in S4-S5

         b) Zone of partial preservation: Refers to the neurologic levels (motor and/or sensory) caudal to the neurologic injury that remain partially innervated. This term is used only with complete injuries.

      2) ASIA B: Incomplete injury—sensation is preserved throughout the cord and includes S4-S5.

      3) ASIA C: Incomplete injury—motor function is preserved below the neurologic level of injury and the majority of the muscles are at Grade 3 or lower. Depending on the neurologic level of injury, the functional gains made by an individual with this classification may or may not be significant.

      4) ASIA D: Incomplete injury—motor function is preserved below the neurologic level of injury and the majority of the muscles are at Grade 3 or higher. Depending on the neurologic level of injury, the functional gains made by an individual with this classification usually are significant.

      5) ASIA E: Normal sensory and motor function

   b. Incomplete injuries can also be further defined by identifying the clinical picture (see Figure 5-7).

      1) Types of incomplete SCIs or clinical syndromes (ASIA, 1996): These injuries are usually the result of circulatory impairment, although they may be the result of direct trauma to the spinal cord.

         a) Anterior (spinal artery) syndrome: The most common incomplete syndrome (ASIA, 1996)

            (1) Damage occurs to the anterior spinal artery, resulting in damage to the anterior two-thirds of the spinal cord.

            (2) Damage causes a loss of major voluntary motor and sensory pathways. The posterior tracts (columns) are spared, which results in intact sensations of proprioception, vibration, and touch.

         b) Central cord syndrome (ASIA, 1996)

            (1) Damage occurs via a severe flexion or extension injury in the cervical area.

            (2) The injury causes bleeding or bruising to the central portion of the cord, resulting in a

"recovery" pattern that involves decreasing the swelling and bruising in the area.

(a) The recovery pattern involves increased sensation, ascending from the most distal portion of the body usually to the level of the injury, as well as the return of bowel and bladder sensation and voluntary control, and, finally, increased movement, ascending from the most distal portion.

(b) Due to the location of the neurons that control the upper extremities, the individual will often have increases in lower extremity function; however, the upper extremities will continue to be neurologically impaired.

c) Brown-Sequard syndrome (ASIA, 1996)

(1) Damage to one side of the cord, often caused by a violent injury (e.g., knife, ice pick, or bullet wound)

(2) Damage results in the following neurologic pattern

(a) Loss of voluntary movement below the level of injury on the injured side of the body

(b) Loss of pain and temperature sensations on the opposite side of the body

d) Conus and cauda equina injuries (ASIA, 1996)

(1) Involve loss of motor function of the nerves directly involved in the injury

(2) Minimally impair sensation

(3) Involve a variable pattern that is often asymmetrical

(4) Results in flaccid paralysis that affects bowel, bladder, and sexual functioning

B. Take a Team Approach to Neurologic Assessment

1. The assessment of the patient with neurologic impairment should be done as a team.

2. A team approach provides the patient and the team with the data that will determine the level of interventions needed.

C. Include the Following Information in the Assessment (Dimitrijevic, Hsu, & McKay, 1992)

1. Neurologic function

a. Cognitive

Figure 5-7. Incomplete Spinal Cord Injury Syndromes

Central cord syndrome: A lesion occurring almost exclusively in the cervical region, involving the central gray matter and the more medial white matter, producing greater weakness in the upper limbs than in the lower limbs and sacral sensory sparing.

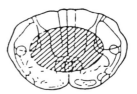

Brown-Sequard syndrome: A lesion involving primarily one side of the cord that produces ipsilateral paralysis and loss of proprioception and contralateral loss of pain and temperature sensations.

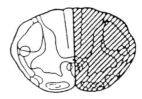

Anterior cord syndrome: A lesion involving the anterior two-thirds of the cord that produces paralysis and loss of pain and temperature sensations, while preserving proprioception.

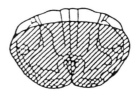

Illustrations reprinted with permission of American Spinal Injury Association (ASIA) from: ASIA. (1990). *Standards for neurological classification of spinal injury patients* (rev. ed., pp.16-19). Atlanta: Author.

Definitions reprinted with permission of American Spinal Injury Association (ASIA) from: ASIA. (1996). *International standards for neurological classification of spinal cord injury* (rev. ed., pp. 19-21). Atlanta: Author.

b. Motor

c. Sensory

2. Neurologic dysfunction

   a. Cognitive

   b. Motor

   c. Sensory

D. Document and Routinely Reevaluate the Following Areas (Mauro, 1996)

1. Rancho Los Amigos level

2. Pontine function

3. Cerebellar function

4. Motor function and its effect on activities of daily living (ADLs)

5. Sensory loss and its effect on ADLs

6. Ability to integrate new information and tasks into the daily routine

IV. Autonomic Nervous System (see Figure 5-8)

A. Overview (Barker, 1994)

1. A specialized part of the PNS that controls the viscera at an unconscious level

2. Involves major effector organs

   a. Smooth muscle

   b. Cardiac muscle

   c. Glands

3. Carries messages from the CNS to the peripheral effector organs

4. Includes two divisions: Sympathetic and parasympathetic

5. Autonomic dysfunction can result in the following conditions

   a. Autonomic dysreflexia

   b. Orthostatic hypotension

   c. Poikilothermia (inconsistent body temperature regulation)

B. Anatomy and Physiology (Barker, 1994)

1. Has two divisions that are parallel but act in an opposing manner

   a. Sympathetic division

     1) Prepares the body to meet crisis situations

     2) Produces a "fight or flight" pattern, which is characterized by elevated heart rate and blood pressure and dilatation of the pupil of the eye

     3) Slows peristalsis and closes the bladder neck

   b. Parasympathetic division

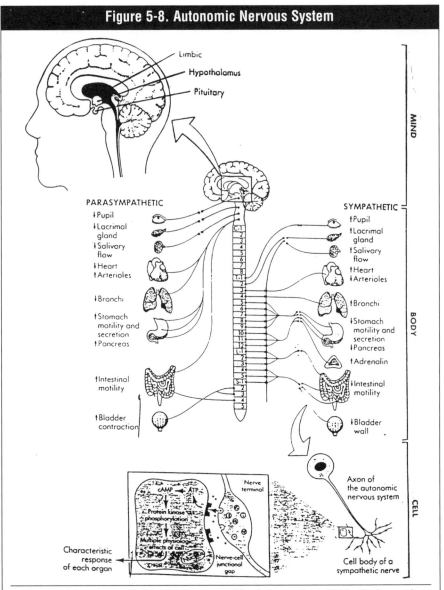

Figure 5-8. Autonomic Nervous System

Reprinted with permission of Mosby from Guzzetta, C.E., & Dassey, B.M. (1992). *Cardiovascular nursing: Holistic practice.* St. Louis: Mosby.

1) Is more vegetative in action
2) Operates in calm moments and allows the body to restore itself
3) Slows the heart rate, lowers blood pressure, increases gastrointestinal activity, and shunts blood from the periphery to the internal organs

2. Functions independently of the hypothalamus and vasomotor centers in the brainstem
3. Responds to local stimulation: Both inhibitory and facilitative influences from higher centers are blocked.

References

American Spinal Injury Association (ASIA). (1990). *Standards for neurological classification of spinal injury patients* (rev. ed.). Chicago: Author.

American Spinal Injury Association (ASIA). (1996). *International standards for neurological classification of spinal injury patients* (rev. ed.). Chicago: Author.

Barker, E. (1994). *Neuroscience nursing.* St. Louis: Mosby.

Dimitrijevic, M.R., Hsu, C.Y., & McKay, W.B. (1992). Neurophysiological assessment of spinal cord and head injury. *Journal of Neurotrauma, 9*(Suppl. 1), S293-S300.

DiPaolantonio, J. (1996). *Brain injury: A family guide.* Philadelphia: Magee Rehabilitation.

Guzetta, C.E., & Dassey, B.M. (1992). *Cardiovascular nursing: Holistic practice.* St. Louis: Mosby.

Hickey, J.V. (1997). *The clinical practice of neurological and neuroscience nursing* (4th ed.). Houston: J.B. Lippincott.

Mauro, J.A. (1996). *Instant nursing assessment: Neurologic.* New York: Delmar Publishers.

Rudy, E. (1984). *Advanced neurological and neurosurgical nursing* (1st ed.). St. Louis: Mosby.

Waxman, S.G. (1996). *Correlative neuroanatomy* (23rd ed.). Stamford, CT: Appleton & Lange.

Zedjlik, C.M. (1992). *Management of spinal cord injury.* Boston: Jones and Bartlett Publishers.

Suggested resources

Anderson, D.K., & Hall, E.D. (1993). Pathophysiology of spinal cord trauma. *Annals of Emergency Medicine, 22*(6), 48-53.

Buchanon, L.E., & Nawoczenski, D.H. (1987). *Spinal cord injury: Concepts and management approaches.* Baltimore: Williams & Wilkins.

Dolan, J.T. (1991). *Critical care nursing: Clinical management through the nursing process* (3rd ed.). Philadelphia: F.A. Davis.

Evans, M.J. (1995). *Neurologic neurosurgical nursing* (2nd ed.). Springhouse, PA: Springhouse Corporation.

McCourt, A.E. (Ed.). (1993). *The specialty practice of rehabilitation nursing: A core curriculum* (3rd ed.). Skokie, IL: Rehabilitation Nursing Foundation of the Association of Rehabilitation Nurses.

Mitchell, P.H., Hodges, L.C., Muwaswes, M., & Walleck, C.A. (1988). *Neuroscience nursing.* Norwalk, CT: Appleton & Lange.

Ricci, M.M. (Ed.). (1984). *Core curriculum for neuroscience nursing* (2nd ed.). Park Ridge, IL: American Association of Neuroscience Nurses.

Staas, W.E., Jr., Formal, C., Gershkoff, A., Freda, M., Hirschwald, J.F., Miller G.T., Forrest, L., & Burkhard, B. (1988). Rehabilitation of the spinal cord injured patient. In J. DeLisa (Ed.), *Rehabilitation medicine: Principles and practice* (pp. 635-667). Philadelphia: J.B. Lippincott.

Stover, S.L., DeLisa, J.A., & Whiteneck, G.G. (1995). *Spinal cord injury: Clinical outcomes from the model systems.* Gaithersburg, MD: Aspen.

Walleck, C.A. (1990). Neurologic considerations in the critical care phase. *Critical Care Clinics of North America, 2,* 357-361.

Whiteneck, G. (Ed.). (1989). *Management of high quadriplegia.* New York: Demos Publications.

Whiteneck, G. (Ed.). (1993). *Aging with a spinal cord injury.* New York: Demos Publications.

Chapter 6

Health Maintenance and Management of Therapeutic Regimen

Kay Viggiani, MS RN CS

"The goal of rehabilitation nursing is to assist the individual who has a disability and/or chronic illness in restoring, maintaining, and promoting his or her maximal health" (Association of Rehabilitation Nurses [ARN], 1994, p. 3). Rehabilitation clients must have effective health management to achieve and maintain an optimal quality of life. Maintenance of maximal health includes both the prevention of further loss of function as well as the prevention of secondary conditions such as cardiovascular, cardiopulmonary, and psychosocial conditions. In addition, the impact that falls and injuries can have on clients and families cannot be underestimated.

All of these conditions can prolong the rehabilitative process and increase the cost of health care. Certainly, pathological factors may contribute to the onset of these conditions. Very often they are caused by problems and changes within the healthcare system. For example, the average length of stay (LOS) for a person with a spinal cord injury (SCI) has decreased by approximately 60% since 1989. Also, people with disabilities are living longer and need long-term health promotion interventions.

Although health promotion and disease prevention interventions that focus on people with disabilities have received little attention in the past, now is the time for rehabilitation nurses to ensure that clients receive this vital information. Health promotion interventions for people with disabilities should include the entire environment, including personal and social factors. Access to needed health and community services will ensure the client's ability to successfully maintain health, prevent disease, and manage the therapeutic regimen. With the passage of the Americans with Disabilities Act (ADA) of 1990 (PL 101-336), people with disabilities have legal rights to equal access in the community.

Successful rehabilitation nursing includes the transfer of knowledge and accountability for healthcare needs from nurses to clients and their families in a manner that promotes health and wellness for the individual with a disability. This chapter examines the concepts of health promotion and disease prevention and describes strategies to obtain access to needed services.

I. Overview of Health Promotion
A. Definitions
1. Health
   a. Health describes a number of entities (Edelman & Mandle, 1998)
      1) A philosophy of care (e.g., health promotion, health maintenance)
      2) A system (e.g., the healthcare delivery system)
      3) Practice (e.g., good health practices)
      4) Behaviors (e.g., health behaviors)
      5) Costs (e.g., healthcare costs, insurance)
   b. Health relates to all aspects of a person's life, including physical well-being, social interactions, mental and emotional capacities, and spiritual beliefs and practices.
   c. "Health is created and lived by people within the settings of their everyday life, where they learn, work, play, and love. Health is created by caring for oneself and others, by being able to make decisions and have control over one's life circumstances and by ensuring that the society one lives in creates conditions that allow that attainment of health by its members" (Dines & Cribb, 1993, p. 209).

2. Wellness
   a. Wellness is dynamic. It is often conceptualized as a continuum with illness at one end and wellness at the other end. The degrees of health span the entire spectrum.
   b. Wellness is a dynamic evolving process that reflects physical, psychological, and social integration and growth within an individual and an enhanced quality of life (Hanak, 1992; Edwards et al., 1999).
   c. In the pursuit of health, a person seeks growth-producing challenges, positive and flexible relationships with others, and health-enhancing activities (Edwards et al., 1999).

B. Principles and Theories Related to Health and Wellness
   1. Actual or potential threats to health, roles, self-efficacy, or empowerment follow catastrophic events, and the loss of health is stressful: In one study, clients descriptions of powerlessness during hospitalization for acute SCI revealed that feelings of powerlessness occurred at various times during hospitalization but were significantly more intense and frequent with increased acuity. Clients who were older than 60 years of age and those whose injury resulted in quadriplegia reported the most feelings of powerlessness (Richmond, Metcalf, Daly, & Kish, 1992, as cited in Hoeman, 1996).
   2. *Nursing's Agenda for Health Care Reform* called for consumers to assume more responsibility for their own care and become better informed about the range of providers and the potential options for services (ANA, 1991).
   3. Wellness requires active participation and is based on personal experience and observation (i.e., learning through experiencing the positive or negative consequences of behavioral choices made by self or others) (Ardell & Tager, 1982).
   4. Health belief models help formulate a plan that will meet the needs and capabilities of the client in making health behavior changes. The health belief model (Rosenstock & Becker, 1988) helps assess a person's perceived state of health or threat of disease and

guides nurses who are considering factors that contribute to a client's perceived state of health risk for disease and to the probability of the client taking appropriate action (Edelman & Mandle, 1998) (see Figure 6-1)

   5. The idea of self-efficacy is that behavior is determined by expectancies and incentives (Bandura, 1977a, 1977b; Edelman & Mandle, 1998).
   a. There are three types of expectancies and incentives (Edelman & Mandle, 1998).
      1) Environmental cues or beliefs about how events are connected
      2) Outcome expectations or the consequences of personal actions
      3) Efficacy expectations or personal competence to perform the behavior required to influence outcomes.
   b. Incentives are defined as the values of a particular object or outcome.

   6. The theory of hardiness is associated with health and wellness (Kobasa, Hilker, & Maddi, 1979; Kobasa, Maddi, & Zola, 1983).
   a. People who have a high level of hardiness involve themselves in whatever they are doing (commitment), believe and act as if they can influence the events that form their lives (control), and consider change to be not only normal but also a stimulus to development (challenge) (Kobasa et al., 1983).
   b. Characteristics of people with a low level of hardiness
      1) Alienation
      2) Sense of powerlessness
      3) Sense of threat in the dynamic, changing process of life
   c. People with a high level of hardiness maintain and strive for wellness even in highly stressful situations.

   7. Locus of control is also associated with health and wellness.
   a. Locus of control is the "individual's beliefs about whether or not a contingency relationship exists between behavior (action) and reinforcements (outcomes)" (Shillinger, 1983, p. 59).

Figure 6-1. Health Belief Model							
Individual Perceptions or Readiness for Change	The value of health to the individual compared to other aspects of living	Perceived susceptibility to a disease level threatening the achievement of certain goals or aims	Perceived seriousness of the disease level threatening the achievement of certain goals or aims	Belief in the diagnosis and therapy plan			
Modifying Factors About the Person	Demographic variables (age, gender, etc.)	Socioeconomic variables (family and peer group characteristics, income and education)	Previous experience with the disease	Risk factors to a disease attributed to heredity, race or culture, medical history or other causes	Level of participation in and satisfaction with regular health care	Actual extent of change necessary	Personal aspirations in life and valued social and vocational activities
Motivating and Environmental Factors (Cues to Action)	Exposure to mass media	Advice from others	Reminders from health professionals	Illness of a family member or friend	Perceived benefits of complying with a treatment plan	Previous success at changing behaviors	
Client-Nurse Transaction Factors *(assessing the likelihood of taking preventive health actions, the nurse compares this picture of "perceived threat of disease")*	Past use of health services	Perceived benefits of health action	Perceived barriers to promotion action	Continued reassessment of the treatment plan by client and provider			

Adapted with permission of Mosby from Edelman, C. & Mandle, C. (1998). Health promotion throughout the lifespan (4th ed., p. 228). St. Louis: Mosby

b.   Types of control (Lefcourt, 1981)

1) Internal control: An individual's belief that his or her own actions influence outcomes

2) External control: An individual's belief that external forces determine outcome

a) Chance: Belief that events occur randomly and are totally divorced from individual action

b) Powerful others: Belief that outcomes are dominated by powerful authority figures

II. Prevention of Injury

A. Secondary Conditions

1. Adults with physical disabilities are at risk for a variety of secondary conditions that may reduce their health and independence. The National Council on Disability and the Centers for Disease Control and Prevention are developing efforts to prevent these health problems and help consumers maintain their health and independence (White & Seekins, 1996).

2. Pope and Tarlov (1991) and White and Seekins (1996) described secondary conditions as being causally related to a disabling condition (e.g., pathology, impairment, functional limitation, additional disability).

The Specialty Practice of Rehabilitation Nursing: A Core Curriculum, 4th Ed.

3. Examples of secondary conditions (White & Seekins, 1996)
   a. Urinary tract infections
   b. Pressure sores
   c. Psychosocial issues (e.g., depression)
   d. Cardiovascular or cardiopulmonary conditions
   e. Neuromusculoskeletal conditions

4. A secondary condition can involve environmental problems such as access to the physician's office.

5. A secondary condition can arise if the newly injured person has learned little about his or her disability and how to identify potential health risks: New strategies and channels of outreach should be identified to provide information about prevention to people who need it.

B. Levels of Prevention (Edelman & Mandle, 1998)
   1. Overview: Each level of prevention occurs at a distinct point in the development of the disease and requires specific nursing interventions.

   2. Three levels of prevention
      a. Primary prevention
         1) Description: Generalized health promotion and specific protection against disease
            a) O'Donnell (1987) defined health promotion as the science and art of helping people change their lifestyle to move toward a state of optimal health: Health promotion is therefore not just exercise and nutrition information; it is also proactive decision making at all levels of care.
            b) One aspect of health promotion is the prevention of secondary disabilities.
               (1) People with disabilities, particularly those who use wheelchairs or who are bedridden, are at great risk for acquiring other disabling conditions.
               (2) The health status of people with disabilities is continuously affected by such factors as the aging process, traumatic injuries, debilitating illnesses, burns, deleterious lifestyles behaviors and stress (Marge, 1988)
         2) Primary prevention strategies: Increase exercise, improve diet, control weight, reduce substance abuse, and screen for heart disease, cancer and diabetes (Marge, 1988)
      b. Secondary prevention
         1) Description: Emphasizes early diagnosis and prompt treatment to halt the pathological process, thereby shortening its duration and severity and enabling the individual to return to a state of health as soon as possible.
         2) Secondary prevention strategies: Use screening and early detection measures (e.g., clinical screening protocol for pressure sore prevention) to limit or reverse the effect of the impairment and the development of secondary conditions (Marge, 1988).
      c. Tertiary prevention
         1) Description: Stops the disease process and prevents complete disability. The objective is to return the individual to his or her maximum capacity of function in society within the constraints of the disability.
         2) Tertiary prevention strategies
            a) Prevent disadvantages by incorporating goals of equal opportunity, full participation, independent living, and economic self-sufficiency
            b) Build on partnerships that link the individual with family, clinical healthcare providers, community service providers, friends, and peers (Patrick, 1997; Patrick, Richardson, Starks, Rose, & Kinne, 1997).

III. Falls and Restraints

A. Review of Research Related to Falls

1. Prevention of falls and related injuries is an essential aspect of secondary prevention for people with disabilities.

2. A number of factors can potentially affect the risk for falling.

3. Numerous studies on risk factors are associated with falls in the elderly population, especially regarding risk management programs or nursing diagnoses (Hendrich, 1988a, 1988b; Porter, 1999; Robbins et al., 1989; Ross, Watson, Gyldenvand, & Reinboth, 1991).

4. A study by Mahoney (1999) produced strong evidence that older adults are at a high risk for loss of independence in walking when they are hospitalized.

   a. This study determined that 1 in 8 hospitalized older adults lost the ability to walk independently, and one-fourth did not regain their walking ability 3 months later.

   b. Previous use of assistive devices, particularly walkers, placed clients at a higher risk, as did existing visual or cognitive impairments.

   c. The clients who were most frail prior to hospitalization were at the highest risk for falls.

   d. The use of assistive devices before hospitalization was a predictor for falls it was related to a decline in functioning and a loss of walking independence with hospitalization.

5. Research that specifically addresses risk factors related to falls in rehabilitation settings has been minimal (Vlahov, Myers, & Al-Ibrahim, 1990) and report various findings.

   a. A study by Mion et al. (1989) found that altered proprioception was the only major predictor of falling in medical rehabilitation clients.

   b. A study by Arbesman and Wright (1999) found that the risk for falling for hospitalized older people is highest soon after the client is placed in a mechanical restraint.

6. A study on medical, surgical, and nursing home units (Brians, Alexander, Grota, Chen, & Dumas, 1991) at a large veterans hospital indicated that four variables were statistically related to client falls; clients with one or more of these four variables were at even greater risk if they used a wheelchair.

   a. Dizziness, unsteady gait, impaired balance

   b. Impaired memory or judgment

   c. Weakness

   d. A history of falling

B. Use of Restraints

1. Physical restraints: "Any manual method or physical or mechanical device, material, or equipment attached or adjacent to the individual's body that the individual cannot remove easily which restricts freedom of movement or normal access to one's body" (Health Care Financing Administration [HCFA], 1999).

2. Chemical restraints

   a. Defined as "drugs prescribed to control mood, mental status or behavior" (HCFA, 1999)

   b. Associated with potential side effects in elderly people (Hendrich, 1988b)

      1) Oversedation
      2) Increased confusion
      3) Orthostatic hypotension
      4) Parkinsonian syndrome-type reactions

3. Caution for using restraints: Neither physical nor chemical restraints necessarily lessen agitated and confused behavior.

   a. Restraints can increase injury.

   b. Clients continue to fall by trying to go over bedrails or getting tangled in restraints.

   c. An alternative is to create a restraint-free environment to maintain the client's safety by implementing specific interventions (McCloskey & Bulechek, 1996) (see Figure 6-2).

C. Nursing Diagnosis: Risk for Injury—Falls

1. Definition (Doenges & Moorhouse, 1998): Risk of injury as a result of environmental conditions interacting with the individual's adaptive and defensive resources

Figure 6-2. Physical Restraints

Definition

Application, monitoring, and removal of mechanical restraining devices or manual restraints which are used to limit physical mobility of patient

Activities

Obtain a physician's order, if required by institutional policy, to use a physically restrictive intervention or to reduce use

Provide patient with a private, yet adequately supervised, environment in situations where a patient's sense of dignity may be diminished by the use of physical restraints

Provide sufficient staff to assist with safe application of physical restraining devices or manual restraints

Designate one nursing staff member to direct staff and communicate with the patient during the application of physical restraints

Use appropriate hold when manually restraining patient in emergency situations or during transport

Identify for patient and significant others those behaviors which necessitated the intervention

Explain procedure, purpose, and time period of the intervention to patient and significant others in understandable and nonpunitive terms

Explain to patient and significant others the behaviors necessary for termination of the intervention

Monitor the patient's response to procedure

Avoid tying restraints to siderails of bed

Secure restraints out of patient's reach

Provide appropriate level of supervision/surveillance to monitor patient and to allow for therapeutic actions, as needed

Provide for patient's psychological comfort, as needed

Provide diversional activities (e.g., television, read to patient, visitors, mobiles), when appropriate, to facilitate patient cooperation with the intervention

Administer PRN medications for anxiety or agitation

Monitor skin condition at restraint site(s)

Monitor color, temperature, and sensation frequently in restrained extremities

Provide for movement and exercise, according to patient's level of self-control, condition, and abilities

Position patient to facilitate comfort and prevent aspiration and skin breakdown

Provide for movement of extremities in patient with multiple restraints by rotating the removal/reapplication of one restraint at a time (as safety permits)

Assist with periodic changes in body position

Provide the dependent patient with a means of summoning help (e.g., bell or call light) when caregiver is not present

Assist with needs related to nutrition, elimination, hydration, and personal hygiene

Evaluate, at regular intervals, patient's needs for continued restrictive intervention

Involve patient in activities to improve strength, coordination, judgment, and orientation

Involve patient, when appropriate, in making decisions to move to a more/less restrictive form of intervention

Remove restraints gradually (i.e., one at a time if in four-point restraints), as self-control increases

Monitor patient's response to removal of restraints

Process with the patient and staff, on termination of the restrictive intervention, the circumstances that led to the use of the intervention, as well as any patient concerns about the intervention itself

Provide the next appropriate level of restrictive action (e.g., area restriction or seclusion), as needed

Implement alternatives to restraints, such as sitting in a chair with table over lap, self-releasing waist belt, gerichair without tray table, or close observation, as appropriate

Teach family the risks and benefits of restraints and restraint reduction

Document the rationale for use of restrictive intervention, patient's response to the intervention, patient's physical condition, nursing care provided throughout the intervention, and rationale for terminating the intervention

Reprinted with permission of Mosby from McCloskey, J., & Bulechek, G. (Eds.). (1996). *Nursing Interventions Classification (NIC)* (2nd ed., pp. 432-433). St. Louis: Mosby.

2. Risk factors
   a. Knowledge deficit regarding safety techniques and proper use of equipment
   b. Impaired mobility
   c. Neuromuscular deficit
   d. Cognitive deficit
   e. Impaired sensation or perception
      1) Temperature
      2) Touch
      3) Positive sense (proprioception)
      4) Vision
      5) Hearing
   f. Environmental hazards
   g. Adverse effects of medication
   h. Unmet elimination needs
   i. Seizures, vertigo
   j. Fatigue
   k. Use of chemical or physical restraints
   l. History of falling
3. Interventions
   a. For use in institutions (McCloskey & Bulechek, 1996) (see Figure 6-3)
   b. For use in the home and community
      1) Evaluate the degree of risk by using a home safety assessment tool
      2) Assess the client's and family's knowledge of safety needs and injury prevention and motivation to prevent injury in home, community, and work settings
      3) Assess socioeconomic status and availability and use of resources
      4) Identify interventions and safety devices to promote a safe physical environment and individual safety
      5) Make referrals to occupational or physical therapists as appropriate (Doenges & Moorhouse, 1998)
      6) Teach the client and family to monitor environmental hazards and recommend changes to promote the highest level of safety
         a) Install grab bars or handrails
         b) Use mobility devices
         c) Unclutter the floors (e.g., get rid of scatter rugs)
         d) Place frequently used items in easily accessible places
         e) Ensure adequate lighting, especially at night
         f) Place the bed in a low position
      7) Help the client meet self-care needs until independence can be achieved or until the care attendant or caregiver has received appropriate education
      8) Teach the client and family about the potential side effects of medications and alcohol
      9) Ensure safety for the client who has deficits in cognitive or thought processes by changing the environment to meet safety needs
         a) Provide methods to communicate with caregivers
         b) Establish a toileting program
         c) Install door locks or an escape alarm
         d) Provide an organized, consistent, uncluttered environment
      10) Teach mechanisms to compensate for sensory-perceptual deficits
         a) Test water before bathing
         b) Use compensatory strategies for visual field deficits
         c) Prevent burns and frostbite
      11) Teach the client and family the signs and symptoms of seizure activity and ways to maintain safety during and after a seizure
      12) Teach safety factors associated with transfer techniques, gait training, and mobility devices
      13) Provide proper, well-maintained footwear
      14) Ensure that the toileting program is adequate to meet nighttime needs
      15) Teach the client and family how to decrease the effects of orthostatic hypotension (e.g., sit on edge of bed for several seconds before transferring)
      16) Provide appropriate information on community resources (e.g., emergency call devices for outside assistance when the client is alone)
      17) Use distraction, redirection, humor, and quiet areas to decrease agitated behavior and avoid the use of restraints

Figure 6-3. Fall Prevention

Definition
Instituting special precautions with patient at risk for injury from falling

Activities
Identify cognitive or physical deficits of the patient that may increase potential of falling in a particular environment
Identify characteristics of environment that may increase potential for falls (e.g., slippery floors and open stairways)
Monitor gait, balance, and fatigue level with ambulation
Assist unsteady individual with ambulation
Provide assistive devices (e.g., cane, walker) to steady gait
Maintain assistive devices in good working order
Lock wheels of wheelchair, bed, or gurney during transfer of patient
Place articles within easy reach of the patient
Instruct patient to call for assistance with movement, as appropriate
Teach patient how to fall as to minimize injury
Post signs to remind patient to call for help when getting out of bed, as appropriate
Use proper technique to transfer patient to and from wheelchair, bed, toilet, and so on
Provide elevated toilet seat for easy transfer
Provide chairs of proper height, with backrests and armrests for easy transfer
Provide bed mattress with firm edges for easy transfer
Use physical restraints to limit potentially unsafe movement, as appropriate
Use side rails of appropriate length and height to prevent falls from bed, as needed
Place a mechanical bed in lowest position
Provide a sleeping surface close to the floor, as needed
Provide seating on bean bag chair to limit mobility, as appropriate
Place a foam wedge in seat of chair to prevent patient from arising, as appropriate
Use partially filled water mattress on bed to limit mobility, as appropriate
Provide the dependent patient with a means of summoning help (e.g., bell or call light) when caregiver is not present
Answer call light immediately
Assist with toileting at frequent, scheduled intervals
Use a bed alarm to alert caretaker that individual is getting out of bed, as appropriate
Mark doorway thresholds and edges of steps, as needed
Remove low-lying furniture (e.g., footstools and tables) that present a tripping hazard
Avoid clutter on floor surface
Provide adequate lighting for increased visibility
Provide nightlight at bedside
Provide visible handrails and grab bars
Place gates in open doorways leading to stairways
Provide nonslip, nontrip floor surfaces
Provide a nonslip surface in bathtub or shower
Provide sturdy, nonslip step stools to facilitate easy reaches
Provide storage areas that are within easy reach
Provide heavy furniture that will not tip if used for support
Orient patient to physical "setup" of room
Avoid unnecessary rearrangement of physical environment
Ensure the patient wears shoes that fit properly, fasten securely, and have nonskid soles
Instruct patient to wear prescription glasses, as appropriate, when out of bed
Educate family members about risk factors that contribute to falls and how they can decrease these risks

Figure 6-3. Fall Prevention (Continued)

Instruct family on importance of handrails for stairs, bathrooms, and walkways

Assist family in identifying hazards in the home and modifying them

Instruct patient to avoid ice and other slippery outdoor surfaces

Institute a routine physical exercise program that includes walking

Post signs to alert staff that patient is at high risk for falls

Collaborate with other healthcare team members to minimize side effects of medications that contribute to falling (e.g., orthostatic hypotension and unsteady gait)

Provide close supervision and/or a restraining device (e.g., infant seat with seat belt) when placing infants/young children on elevated surfaces (e.g., table and highchair)

Remove objects that provide young child with climbing access to elevated surfaces

Maintain crib siderails in elevated position when caregiver is not present, as appropriate

Provide a "bubble top" on hospital cribs of pediatric patients who may climb over elevated siderails, as appropriate

Fasten the latches securely on access panel of incubator when leaving bedside of infant in incubator, as appropriate

Reprinted with permission of Mosby from McCloskey, J., & Bulechek, G. (Eds.). (1996). *Nursing Interventions Classification (NIC)* (2nd ed., pp. 272-273). St. Louis: Mosby.

4. Expected outcomes

   a. General

      1) Client is free of physical injury

      2) Client and family verbalize or demonstrate an awareness of risk factors related to the client's specific deficits

      3) Client and family are aware of how to seek assistance if an injury does occur

   b. Safety behavior: Fall prevention (Johnson & Maas, 1997) (see Figure 6-4)

   c. Safety behavior: Home physical environment (Johnson & Maas, 1997) (see Figure 6-5)

IV. Nursing Management of Therapeutic Regimen for Individuals

A. Effective Management Techniques

   1. A pattern of regulating and integrating into daily living a program for treatment of illness and its sequelae that is satisfactory for meeting specific health goals (Doenges & Moorhouse, 1998).

   2. Major defining characteristics

      a. Verbalized desire to manage treatment of illness and prevent sequelae

      b. Verbalized intent to reduce risk factors for progression of illness and sequelae

B. Nursing Assessment

   1. Client's coping status regarding responsibility for and access to health care

      a. Health and lifestyle prior to injury or illness

      b. Interest in a health management program

      c. Ability and motivation to take responsibility for health, including knowledge of nutritional needs

      d. Access to and availability of healthcare providers and facilities

      e. Knowledge of prescribed medications and their effects

      f. Knowledge of medical status and related treatment program

   2. Client's emotional status

      a. Resolution of grieving process related to injury or disease

      b. Chemical dependency

      c. Methods of coping

   3. Client's spirituality: A spiritual assessment extends beyond merely ascertaining religious affiliation, church attendance, or dietary restrictions (Hoeman, 1996).

      a. Assess four specific areas (Hoeman, 1996)

         1) Sources of hope and strength (support system)

The Specialty Practice of Rehabilitation Nursing: A Core Curriculum, 4th Ed.

Figure 6-4. Safety Behavior: Fall Prevention

Definition: Individual or caregiver actions to minimize risk factors that might precipitate falls

Safety Behavior: Fall Prevention	Not Adequate 1	Slightly Adequate 2	Moderately Adequate 3	Substantially Adequate 4	Totally Adequate 5
Indicators					
Correct use of assistive devices	1	2	3	4	5
Provision of personal assistance	1	2	3	4	5
Placement of barriers to prevent falls	1	2	3	4	5
Use of restraints as needed	1	2	3	4	5
Placement of handrailings as needed	1	2	3	4	5
Elimination of clutter, spills, glare from floors	1	2	3	4	5
Tacking down rugs	1	2	3	4	5
Arrangement for removal of snow and ice from walking surfaces	1	2	3	4	5
Appropriate use of stools/ladders	1	2	3	4	5
Use of well-fitting tied shoes	1	2	3	4	5
Adjustment of toilet height as needed	1	2	3	4	5
Adjustment of chair height as needed	1	2	3	4	5
Adjustment of bed height as needed	1	2	3	4	5
Use of rubber mats in tub/shower	1	2	3	4	5
Use of grab bars	1	2	3	4	5
Agitation and restlessness controlled	1	2	3	4	5
Use of precautions when taking medications that increase risk for falls	1	2	3	4	5
Use of vision-correcting devices	1	2	3	4	5
Use of safe transfer procedure	1	2	3	4	5
Compensation for physical limitations	1	2	3	4	5
Other (specify)	1	2	3	4	5

Reprinted with permission of Mosby from Johnson, M., & Maas, M. (Eds.). (1997). *Nursing Outcomes Classification (NOC)* (p. 258). St. Louis: Mosby.

2) Concept of God or other deity
3) Relationships between spiritual beliefs and health
4) Religious practices

b. Use the spiritual well-being scale as an assessment tool (Ellison, 1982, as cited in Hoeman, 1996)

4. Client's social support: An important predictor of coping effectiveness and stress tolerance (Hoeman, 1996)

a. Amount, kind, and level of supportive contact

b. Social support provided by people the client counts on, cares about, or loves

c. Social facilitative support (e.g., service organizations or agencies)

d. Cultural or ethnic values, traditions, beliefs, and expectations given context

5. Client's functional status

a. Strength and endurance

b. Self-care needs (e.g., feeding, bathing, dressing, toileting)

c. Mobility status: Use of adaptive equipment or devices

d. Continence and elimination needs

e. Communication abilities

f. Ability to monitor environment

6. Client's general health and medical status

a. History of falls, seizures, or orthostatic hypotension

b. Perception and sensation (including vision and proprioception)

c. Sleep and rest needs

d. Comorbid health problems

e. Prescription medication

f. Over-the-counter medication

g. Alternative therapies (e.g., acupuncture, herbs, vitamins)

h. Ethnic remedies

7. Client's cognitive status

a. Memory

b. Judgment

c. Reasoning

d. Problem-solving ability

8. Pain *[Refer to Chapter 13 for more information about pain.]*

a. Record pain history, including the maximum, minimum, and typical amount of

---

Figure 6-5. Safety Behavior: Home Physical Environment

Definition: Individual or caregiver actions to minimize environmental factors that might cause physical harm or injury in the home

Safety Behavior: Home Physical Environment	Not Adequate 1	Slightly Adequate 2	Moderately Adequate 3	Substantially Adequate 4	Totally Adequate 5
Indicators					
Provision of lighting	1	2	3	4	5
Placement of handrailings	1	2	3	4	5
Smoke detector maintenance	1	2	3	4	5
Use of personal alarm system	1	2	3	4	5
Provision of accessible telephone	1	2	3	4	5
Placement of appropriate hazard warning labels	1	2	3	4	5
Disposal of unused medicines	1	2	3	4	5
Provision of assistive devices in accessible location	1	2	3	4	5
Provision of equipment that meets safety standards	1	2	3	4	5
Storage of firearms to prevent accidents	1	2	3	4	5
Storage of hazardous materials to prevent injury	1	2	3	4	5
Safe disposal of hazardous materials	1	2	3	4	5
Arrangement of furniture to reduce risks	1	2	3	4	5
Provision of safe play area					
Removal of unused refrigerator and freezer doors	1	2	3	4	5
Correction of lead hazard risks	1	2	3	4	5
Provision of age-appropriate toys	1	2	3	4	5
Use of electrical outlet covers	1	2	3	4	5
Room temperature regulation	1	2	3	4	5
Elimination of harmful noise levels	1	2	3	4	5
Placement of window guards as needed	1	2	3	4	5
Other (specify)	1	2	3	4	5

Reprinted with permission of Mosby from Johnson, M., & Maas, M. (Eds.). (1997). *Nursing Outcomes Classification (NOC)* (p. 259). St. Louis: Mosby.

pain experienced (Hoeman, 1996)

   b. Determine what exacerbates the pain

   c. Determine what alleviates the pain: Use standardized scales (e.g., McGill-Melzack Pain Questionnaire)

   d. Assess chronic pain, including premorbid and postmorbid lifestyle

   e. Use the Agency for Healthcare Research and Quality (AHRQ) standards for pain control

C. Related Factors/Etiologies

  1. Physical

   a. Loss of a body part

   b. Sensory deficits

   c. Motor skill deficits

   d. Chemical dependency

   e. Debilitating disease or injury

   f. Pain

  2. Emotional/maturational

   a. Depression or prolonged or dysfunctional grieving

   b. Decreased self-esteem

   c. Lack of experience in managing wellness

   d. Lack of motivation

   e. Decisional conflicts

   f. Family conflicts

  3. Cognitive

   a. Perceptual deficits

   b. Communication deficits

   c. Inexperience with or inability to comprehend or follow a complex treatment regimen

   d. Lack of education or intellectual development

  4. Social/economic

   a. Inability to gain access to the healthcare system

   b. Nontherapeutic relationships with healthcare providers (e.g., healthcare professionals, personal care attendants)

   c. Language differences that interfere with ability to gain access to or use healthcare or self-care resources

   d. Funding resources inadequate to obtain and maintain needed equipment, supplies, and services

   e. Complexity of the healthcare system and the therapeutic regimen

D. Interventions

  1. Identify and designate person(s) responsible for the therapeutic regimen (e.g., client, parent, spouse)

   a. Direct interventions toward all responsible people to help them develop strategies to improve management of therapeutic regimen

   b. Direct responsible people to act on behalf of the client to promote the client's wellness and health management

  2. Educate the client at his or her learning level to facilitate health maintenance

   a. Determine readiness to learn: Lack of readiness occurs when physical endurance is poor or if emotional limitations exist (Viggiani, 1997).

   b. Use teaching tools (e.g., written materials, audio- or videotapes, lectures, models)

   c. Use demonstrations and return demonstrations

   d. Use memory aids (e.g., written reminders [large print when necessary], medication dispensers, consistent location of supplies, software for life skills)

   e. Provide progressive sequential learning experiences that build on skills without overwhelming the learner (e.g., help the client take on progressive responsibility for bladder management)

  3. Design a physical environment that minimizes dependency and the sick role, especially for clients living in institutions

   a. Allow clients and healthcare providers to wear street clothes

   b. Make the environment and activities as realistic or home-like as possible

    1) Encourage the client to eat meals in the dining room with other people

    2) Allow the client to have access to food and beverages between meals

c. Help the client identify and begin to resume family role responsibilities

d. Provide privacy when the client is performing physical care and interacting with others and allow time for the client to be alone

e. Introduce the client to role models (e.g., other clients who competently manage their health and wellness)

4. Establish a milieu that fosters self-reliance and wellness

   a. Encourage the client to set goals with the help of healthcare providers

   b. Encourage the client to become involved in all phases of care planning; promote the client's control of the process

   c. Negotiate to simplify or alter client behaviors and outcomes; adapt program methods or schedules to the client's preferred routine

   d. Avoid assuming a "powerful other" role that reinforces external control

   e. Create a contract with the client to define agreed-upon responsibilities, conditions, and goals for program participation

5. Help the client and caregivers manage desired health practices and promote wellness

   a. Provide anticipatory guidance to maintain and manage effective health practices during periods of wellness

   b. Identify adaptation strategies to use when progressive illness or long-term health problems occur

   c. Monitor adherence to prescribed medical regimen

   d. Help the client and family develop stress management skills

   e. Identify ways to adapt an exercise program to meet the client's changing needs, abilities, and environmental concerns

6. Refer the client to community resources and support groups

7. Involve the client's case manager (e.g., home health agency nurse, insurance nurse case manager) in long-term follow-up and assessment of transition from inpatient to outpatient settings

E. Expected Outcomes
   1. Client will be free of physical injury.
   2. Client and family verbalize or demonstrate an awareness of risk factors related to client's specific deficits.
   3. Client and family are aware of how to seek assistance if an injury does occur.
   4. Client and family can identify necessary health maintenance activities.
   5. Client assumes responsibility for own healthcare needs within level of ability.
   6. Client adapts to lifestyle changes that support healthcare goals.

V. Nursing Management of Therapeutic Regimen in the Community
   A. Overview
      1. Access to health care historically has been a challenge to those with disabilities.
      2. Healthcare providers must be able to define strategies for obtaining healthcare services, identify the available financial resources, be knowledgeable regarding public laws governing access to healthcare services, and help people with disabilities in securing and using healthcare services.

   B. Ineffective Management Techniques
      1. A pattern of regulating and integrating into community processes programs for treatment of illness and the sequelae of illness that are unsatisfactory for meeting health-related goals
      2. Major defining characteristics: Community members and agencies verbalize an inability to meet the therapeutic needs of all members (Doenges & Moorhouse, 1998).

   C. Nursing Assessment
      1. Obstacles to gaining access to healthcare services
         a. Geographic location
            1) Availability and transportation issues related to access to healthcare facilities and community resources
            2) Access to home-based care services
            3) Prohibitive cost of transportation services
            4) Limited public funds for assistance to obtain vehicle modifications or purchase a vehicle (e.g., a van with hand controls), which decreases access to

healthcare services, especially in rural areas

    b. Architectural issues related to accessibility (including buildings and grounds)

        1) Parking lot accessibility and design

        2) Sidewalk accessibility

        3) Office building accessibility and design

        4) Healthcare facility accessibility and design

    c. Discrimination, stigma, negative attitudes

    d. Lack of information about the care needs of people with disabilities

2. Economic constraints

    a. Personal finances

        1) Loss of medical benefits, Supplemental Security Income (SSI), or Social Security Disability Insurance (SSDI) for people younger than age 65 if the person with the disability is employed and earns more than the allowable amount

        2) Possible reduction in Social Security benefits

        3) Medical benefits that are tied to income criteria, which encourage people with disabilities to be dependent on the system

    b. Unavailability of medical benefits for people with disabilities under Medicare until 2 years after the onset of the disability

        1) Discourages people with disabilities who are younger than age 65 from seeking healthcare services

        2) Raises the possibility of people with disabilities being without any medical benefits if they do not qualify for state assistance or Medicaid and thus contributes to increased numbers of indigent people seeking healthcare services

        3) Raises the possibility that people with disabilities will seek healthcare services only when their healthcare needs are advanced and require hospitalization

        4) Begins a cycle that increases the burden on healthcare providers to supply free care, which contributes to an increase in the overall cost of healthcare services

    c. Limited eligibility for funding for attendant care

        1) Funding that is usually tied to eligibility for income assistance

        2) Long waiting periods that frequently last 1-2 years

        3) Minimal reimbursement for care attendants, which makes it difficult to recruit and retain qualified people

        4) Programs that require clients to manage their own workers independently and to handle training and payroll, which may not be possible for people with severe disabilities or who are elderly

        5) Strict definitions of what constitutes a disability that may disqualify many people who need services

    d. Limited funding for independent living arrangements (residential and nonresidential models)

        1) Continued limitation of funds for independent living centers despite the fact that funding is mandated by the Rehabilitation, Comprehensive Services, and Developmental Disabilities Amendments of 1978 (PL 95-602)

        2) Some state support through Medicaid Title XIX funding for attendant assistance and community support services

        3) The rarity of independent living programs in rural areas

3. Issues in attendant training

    a. On-the-job training

    b. Lack of regulations regarding worker qualifications

    c. No supervision of work performance

    d. Lack of public funding that would allow control over workers' qualifications and performance

    e. Lack of availability of care attendants

who can meet the specialized needs of the pediatric population

4. Ability to obtain needed equipment, supplies, and medications
   a. Dependence on insurance coverage
   b. Possible requirement of a down payment (in cash)
   c. Frequent limits on additional equipment covered by insurance
   d. Possible inability to obtain the necessary equipment (e.g., a padded commode chair with removable arms for a person with SCI)

5. Limited healthcare services, which might arise due to attitudes, architectural designs, or reimbursement limits
   a. Limited counseling services
      1) Medical social worker services, which are usually available only though home care agencies
      2) The low number of psychiatrists and psychologists who make home visits
      3) Limited reimbursement for counseling
   b. Special healthcare needs of people with disabilities
      1) Obstetric and gynecological services
         a) Exam tables that are accessible for women with disabilities
         b) Healthcare providers who are knowledgeable in obstetric and gynecological areas
         c) Specialized training for personnel (e.g., how to care for a person with SCI who has had a baby)
      2) Dental services
         a) Offices that are architecturally accessible
         b) Accessible, comfortable office chairs
         c) Elimination of financial obstacles to preventive care (e.g., insurance such as Medicare or Medicaid that does not cover preventive care)

D. Interventions
   1. Obtain access to community resources and healthcare services (see Figure 6-6)
      a. Provide for communication and coordination between the healthcare facility team and community healthcare providers
      b. Contact local governmental disability offices, city commissions, or city departments to determine public services available to people with disabilities
      c. Involve comprehensive specialty teams when available
      d. Make referrals as needed for community support services (e.g., Meals on Wheels™, local churches with parish nursing programs)
      e. Make referrals to organizations with support groups as appropriate (e.g., National Spinal Cord Injury Association, American Heart Association)
   2. Identify barriers to community reentry
      a. Accessible housing
         1) Established referral system in place
         2) Technical assistance
         3) Development, design, and building assistance
         4) Home mortgage loans
         5) Availability of accessible public housing
         6) Funding for adaptations in private residences
         7) "Medical home" (Sia, 1992): An integrated system of services that focuses on the well-being of the whole child within the context of the family; primary health care is continuous and comprehensive and provides coordinated care that is family-centered and community-based.
      b. Transportation
         1) Designated parking
         2) Private transportation services
         3) Public transportation (e.g., availability, accessibility)
         4) Reduced bus passes
         5) Paratransit services
         6) Parking stickers
      c. Advocacy
         a) Established advisory council
         b) Involvement of advocacy groups

with communication agencies

   c) Funding for programs

   d) Information exchange regarding disability issues (e.g., legislation)

   e) Appointment of people with disabilities to governmental boards and commissions

   f) Legal assistance

   g) Public education regarding disability issues

  d. Employment

   1) Affirmative action for hiring people with disabilities

   2) Training and placement assistance; supported employment services

   3) Funding for environmental modifications

  e. Recreation

   1) Accessible community centers and leisure programs

   2) Special events focused on people with disabilities (e.g., wheelchair division of marathons)

  f. Supportive services

   1) Information and referral

   2) Counseling

   3) Personal care assistance programs

   4) Telecommunication devices for people who are deaf; sign language interpreters (e.g., at public hearings)

   5) Homemaker services

   6) Augmentative communication aids, adaptive toys, assistive technology

   7) Health screening services

   8) Funding for rehabilitation technology services and adaptive equipment

   9) Technology access, adaptive computers *[Refer to Chapter 20 for more*

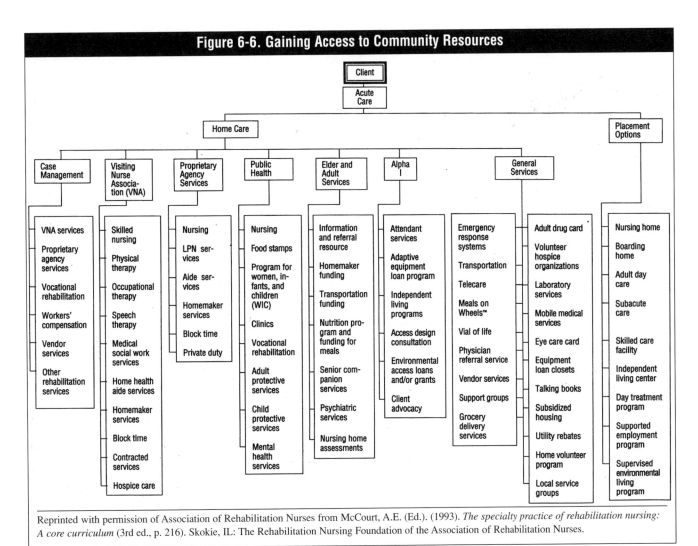

Figure 6-6. Gaining Access to Community Resources

Reprinted with permission of Association of Rehabilitation Nurses from McCourt, A.E. (Ed.). (1993). *The specialty practice of rehabilitation nursing: A core curriculum* (3rd ed., p. 216). Skokie, IL: The Rehabilitation Nursing Foundation of the Association of Rehabilitation Nurses.

information about technology and computers for people with disabilities.]

g. Education

1) Availability of educational opportunities

2) Funding

3) Building accessibility

4) Programs for disadvantaged children

5) Therapy services (e.g., occupational, physical, speech and language) available in school systems

6) Head Start program and early intervention programs

7) Bilingual education

8) Acquisition of equipment to supplement special education and related services; training in computer technology

9) Self-help groups

10) Playground accessibility and school environment modifications

11) Specialized buses, vans, cars to meet the needs of schoolchildren

h. Availability of adequate financial resources to meet healthcare needs

VI. Gaining Access to Rehabilitation and Supportive Services in the Community

A. Funding Sources

1. Agencies and sectors that receive state funding through appropriation of monies, grants, or direct reimbursement

   a. Visiting nursing associations (VNAs) and private not-for-profit home care agencies

   b. Alpha I agencies (members of National Council on Independent Living)

      1) Funded through state and federal monies

      2) Provide services to people with disabilities

         a) Peer support, attendant services, client advocacy

         b) Design consultation
            (1) Educate design professionals and the public regarding legal requirements for creating accessible environments
            (2) Provide building product information

      (3) Review designs
      (4) Assess homes after occupancy

   c) Grants and loans for environmental access

   d) Loan programs for adaptive equipment
      (1) Low interest loans
      (2) Loans for citizens and businesses to purchase technological aids that enhance independence in the home, workplace, or other environments

   e) Independent living programs: Provide instruction and hands-on experience in transitional living skills

   f) Evaluation and education for adapted vehicle driving

   g) Monitoring of access issues
      (1) Have a watchdog project to correct building code violations and publicize standards for accessible design
      (2) Mobilize statewide networks for grassroots advocacy
      (3) Inform the design and construction industries about legal requirements for building or remodeling public buildings and housing
      (4) File complaints or litigation if corrective action is not taken

2. Proprietary (for-profit) agencies

3. Public health services

   a. Nursing services
      1) Home visits for health teaching and screening
      2) Clinics for blood pressure, screening, immunizations, and flu vaccines

   b. Vocational rehabilitation

   c. Adult and child protective services

4. Elder and adult services

5. Transportation resources

   a. Public transportation

   b. Private organizations receiving state funds to purchase vans with lifts and to serve people who are elderly, have disabilities, or have state benefits (e.g., Medicaid, Paratransit)

6. Independent living programs

    a. Services vary according to the locality and program.

        1) Referral to housing and training in independent living skills

        2) Permanent residential, transitional residential, or temporary housing

        3) Attendant referrals, training, or management training

        4) Client and system advocacy

        5) Disability awareness among community

        6) Equipment repairs and referrals

        7) Reduction of environmental barriers

        8) Promotion of consumer involvement in community activities and information and referral services

    b. Program components vary with each independent living program.

7. Subacute care services, skilled nursing facilities, boarding homes

8. Vendor services

    a. Durable medical equipment

    b. Intravenous therapy (e.g., hydration, total parenteral nutrition, antibiotics, blood and blood products, pain management)

    c. Chemotherapy

    d. Medical supplies

    e. Oxygen and ventilator services

    f. Nutritional services

    g. Enteral feedings

9. Selective professional services

    a. Physicians (office and home)

    b. Inpatient and outpatient hospital services

    c. Counseling

    d. Outpatient phlebotomy services

    e. Mobile medical services (e.g., X rays, EKGs in the home)

    f. Eye care cards (e.g., funding for eye exams, glasses)

10. Programs

    a. Adult day care

    b. Day treatment programs (e.g., for people with head injuries or Alzheimer's disease)

    c. Supervised environmental living program

    d. Hospice care

    e. Prosthetic and orthotic devices

B. Agencies and Sectors That Receive Federal Funding

    1. VNAs and private not-for-profit agencies providing home care services

    2. Vendor services

    3. Some independent living programs

    4. Outpatient phlebotomy services

    5. Physicians (office and home)

    6. Extended rehabilitation facilities

    7. Hospice care

    8. Prosthetic and orthotic devices

    9. Mobile medical services

    10. Inpatient and outpatient hospital services (acute and rehabilitation)

    11. Outpatient rehabilitation services (e.g., hospital-based, VNA, private)

C. Department of Veterans Affairs (VA) Services

    1. Inpatient and outpatient hospital services

    2. Pharmacy services

    3. Vocational rehabilitation services

    4. Nursing home care

    5. Home health care

    6. Orthotic and prosthetic devices

    7. Durable medical and adaptive equipment

    8. Services for people with visual impairments

    9. Home modifications for people with disabilities

    10. Mortgage loans

D. Federal or State-Subsidized Assistance Programs Based on Income, Age, or Disability

    1. Adult drug cards

    2. Subsidized housing

    3. Utility and telephone rebates

    4. Eye care cards

a. Provide reimbursement for eye examinations and glasses

b. Are unavailable for those who have state medical cards, as the card would duplicate some coverage

5. Healthcare services at public clinics (e.g., immunizations, flu vaccines)

6. Meals on Wheels™ program

7. Books on audiotape

E. Services for Adults and Elderly People
   1. Services are funded primarily for people older than age 62.

   2. Age and income are the two main criteria for determining eligibility for programs.

   3. Services may be provided by senior companion programs.
      a. Providing respite care
      b. Running errands
      c. Taking clients out to do errands
      d. Doing light housekeeping

F. Preventive Healthcare Medicare Coverage
   1. Flu shots

   2. Screening mammogram every 12 months for all women aged 40 and older

   3. Screening pap smear and pelvic exam every 3 years or annually for women at high risk for cervical or vaginal cancer

   4. Colorectal cancer screening

   5. Blood glucose monitors, test strips, and lancets for all people with diabetes

   6. Prostate screening for all men aged 50 and older

   7. Coverage of diabetes outpatient self-management training services

   8. Pnemococcal pneumonia vaccinations

G. Rehabilitation Nursing Interventions to Help Clients Gain Access to Healthcare Resources
   1. Coordinate referrals to not-for-profit and private home care agencies

   2. Identify agencies that provide free care or sliding scale fees for services based on income and the duration of needed services

   3. Arrange for social work services to help gain access to community systems that can help provide subsidized housing, Medicaid applications, SSI, SSDI, counseling services, advocacy assistance equipment needs, and

transportation and that can help find organizations that provide community services

4. Contact the local department of human services regarding services available for rehabilitation care needs

5. Contact legislators to support funding for transferring clients to independent living centers and for training care attendants, as well as for supplemental funding that allows people with disabilities to work without a drastic reduction in or termination of medical benefits

6. Attend public hearings on issues that affect people with disabilities

7. Act as a community advocate to promote increased environmental accessibility, decreased architectural barriers, increased access to public transportation, decreased cost of services to elderly people on fixed incomes, and increased access to healthcare services

8. Make referrals to rehabilitation counselors, peer counselors, and those providing psychological services

9. Contact state disability offices, commissions, or departments for assistance

10. Promote the education of healthcare providers and caregivers within facilities and the community
    a. Provide in-service education
    b. Consult one-on-one with providers regarding healthcare issues, ways to manage individual clients' healthcare needs, and ways to promote access to healthcare services
    c. Encourage family involvement early in the rehabilitation process and teach them about equipment, procedures, medications, and ways to manage emergencies
    d. Coordinate a home visit by the rehabilitation team to evaluate the need for modifications, equipment, and ways to improve safety
    e. Promote interagency communication regarding rehabilitation needs, follow-up teaching needs, and previous nursing interventions in the event of a transfer to a different environment
    f. Periodically reassess and evaluate the client's ability to perform ADLs,

changes in level of independence, healthcare needs, and barriers to gaining access to required services

g. Contact healthcare providers in the community to determine access to buildings, cost of services, insurance coverage, ways to modify the office environment, and the availability of transportation

11. Speak at service club meetings

12. Actively participate in professional organizations that support legislation and advocacy

activities for people with disabilities (see Figure 6-7 for a list of laws governing access to rehabilitation services)

13. Promote the appointment of people with disabilities to public office and commissions and to private sector industry and business boards

14. Help clients with disabilities prepare testimony for legislative hearings

15. Participate in health planning endeavors and advocate for services that meet the needs of children and adults

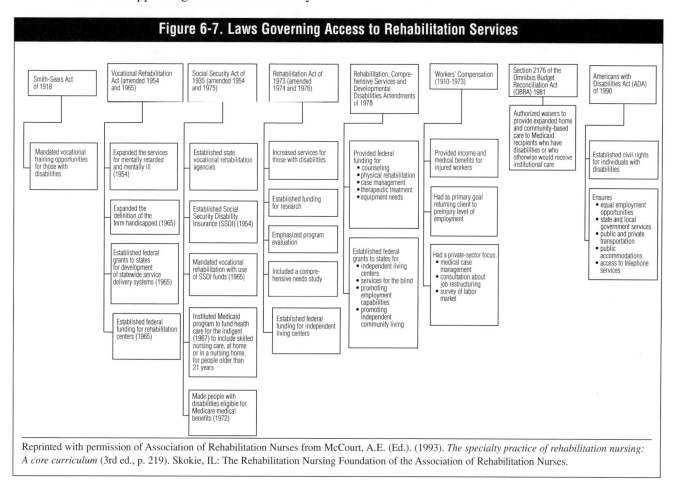

Figure 6-7. Laws Governing Access to Rehabilitation Services

Reprinted with permission of Association of Rehabilitation Nurses from McCourt, A.E. (Ed.). (1993). *The specialty practice of rehabilitation nursing: A core curriculum* (3rd ed., p. 219). Skokie, IL: The Rehabilitation Nursing Foundation of the Association of Rehabilitation Nurses.

References

American Nurses' Association (ANA). (1991). *Nursing's agenda for health care reform.* Kansas City, MO: Author.

Arbesman, M., & Wright, C. (1999). Mechanical restraints, rehabilitation therapies, and staffing adequacy as risk factors for falls in a elderly hospitalized population. *Rehabilitation Nursing, 24*(3), 122–128.

Ardell, D.B., & Tager, M.J. (1982). *Planning for wellness: A guide book for achieving optimal health* (2nd ed.). Dubuque, IA: Kendall/Hunt Publishing Company.

Association of Rehabilitation Nurses (ARN). (1994). *Standards and scope of rehabilitation nursing practice.* Skokie, IL: Author.

Bandura, A. (1977a). Self-efficacy: Toward a unifying theory of behavioral changes. *Psychological Review, 84*(2), 191–215.

Bandura, A. (1977b). *Social learning theory.* Englewood Cliffs, NJ: Prentice Hall.

Brians, L., Alexander, K., Grota, P., Chen, R., & Dumas, V. (1991). The development of the risk tool for fall prevention. *Rehabilitation Nursing, 16*, 67–69.

Dines, A., & Cribb, A. (Eds.). (1993). *Health promotion concepts and practice.* Boston: Blackwell Scientific Publications.

Doenges, M., & Moorhouse, M. (1998). *Nurse's pocket guide: Diagnoses, interventions, and rationales* (6th ed.). Philadelphia: F.A. Davis.

Edelman, C., & Mandle, C. (1998). *Health promotion throughout the lifespan* (4th ed.). St. Louis: Mosby.

Edwards, P., Hertzberg, D., Hays, S., & Youngblood, N. (Eds.). (1999). *Pediatric rehabilitation nursing.* Philadelphia: W.B. Saunders.

Hanak, M. (1992). *Rehabilitation nursing for the neurological patient.* New York: Springer.

Health Care Financing Administration (HCFA). (1999). *Medicare, preventive benefits: Empire Medical Services answer your questions.* Syracuse, NY: Empire Medicare Services.

Hendrich, A. (1988a). An effective unit-based fall prevention program. *Journal of Nursing Quality Assurance, 3*(1), 28–36.

Hendrich, A. (1988b). *Patient fall prevention.* Greencastle, IN: Ann Hendrich & Associates, Inc.

Hoeman, S. (Ed.). (1996). *Rehabilitation nursing: Process and application* (2nd ed.). St. Louis: Mosby.

Johnson, M., & Maas, M. (Eds.). (1997). *Nursing Outcomes Classification (NOC).* St. Louis: Mosby.

Kobasa, S.C., Hilker, R.R., & Maddi, S.R. (1979). Who stays health under stress. *Journal of Occupational Medicine, 21,* 595–598.

Kobasa, S.C., Maddi, S.R., & Zola, M.A. (1983). Type A and hardiness. *Journal of Behavioral Medicine, 6*(1), 41–49.

Lefcourt, H. (Ed.). (1981,). *Research with locus of control construct.* New York: Academic Press.

Mahoney, J. (1999, August 31). *Assessment of falls risk after hospitalization: Interventions to decrease the risk of falls and improve mobility* [Online]. Available: http://www.ssc.wisc.edu/aging/mahoney.htm

Marge, M. (1988). Health promotion for persons with disabilities: moving beyond rehabilitation. *American Journal of Health Promotion, 2*(4), 29–35.

McCloskey, J., & Bulechek, G. (Eds.). (1996). *Nursing Interventions Classification (NIC)* (2nd ed.). St. Louis: Mosby.

McCourt, A.E. (Ed.). (1993). *The specialty practice of rehabilitation nursing: A core curriculum* (3rd ed.). Skokie, IL: The Rehabilitation Nursing Foundation of the Association of Rehabilitation Nurses.

Mion, L., Gregor, S., Buettner, M., Chwirchak, D., Lee, O., & Paras, W. (1989). Falls in the rehabilitation setting: Incidence and characteristics. *Rehabilitation Nursing, 14,* 17–22.

O'Donnell, M. (1987). Definition of health promotion. *Journal of Health Promotion, 1*(1), 4, 14.

Patrick, D. (1997). Rethinking prevention for people with disabilities, Part I: A conceptual model for promoting health. *American Journal of Health Promotion, 11*(4), 251–260.

Patrick, D., Richardson, M., Starks, E., Rose, A., & Kinne, S. (1997). Rethinking prevention for people with disabilities, Part II: A framework for designing interventions. *American Journal of Health Promotion, 11*(4), 261–263.

Porter, E. (1999). Getting up from here: Frail older women's experiences after falling. *Rehabilitation Nursing, 24*(5), 201–206.

Robbins, A., Rubenstein, L., Josephson, K., Schulman, B., Osterweil, D., & Fine, G. (1989). Predictors of falls among elderly people. *Archives of Internal Medicine, 149,* 1628–1633.

Rosenstock, I.M., & Becker, M.H. (1988). The social learning theory and health belief model. *Health Education Quarterly, 15*(2), 175–183.

Ross, J., Watson, C., Gyldenvand, T., & Reinboth, J. (1991). Potential for trauma: Falls. In M. Maas, K. Buckwalter, & M. Hardy (Eds.), *Nursing diagnoses and interventions in the elderly* (pp. 18–31). Redwood City, CA: Addison-Wesley Nursing.

Shillinger, F. (1983). Locus of control: Implications for clinical practice. *Image: The Journal of Nursing Scholarship, 15*(2), 58–63.

Sia, C. (1992). The medical home: Pediatric practice and child advocacy in the 1990s. *Pediatrics, 90*(3), 1419–1423.

Viggiani, K. (1997). Special populations. Chapter 9 in S. Bastable (Ed.), *Nurse as educator: Principles of teaching and learning,* Boston: Jones and Bartlett Publishers, pp. 204–233.

Vlahov, D., Myers, A., & Al-Ibrahim, M. (1990). Epidemiology of falls among patients in a rehabilitation hospital. *Archives of Physical Medicine and Rehabilitation, 71,* 8–12.

White, G., & Seekins, T. (1996). Preventing and managing secondary conditions: A proposed role for independent living centers. *Journal of Rehabilitation,* pp. 14–21.

Suggested resources

Alston, R., & Leung, P. (1997). Reform laws and health care coverage: Combating exclusion of persons with disabilities. *Journal of Rehabilitation*, pp. 15-19.

Buchanan, R., & Alston, R. (1997). Medical policies and home health care provisions for persons with disabilities. *Journal of Rehabilitation*, pp. 20-23.

Fullmer, S., & Majumder, R.K. (1991). Increased access and use of disability related information for consumers. *Journal of Rehabilitation, 57*(3), 17-22.

Huntt, D., & Growick, B. (1997). Managed care for people with disabilities. *Journal of Rehabilitation*, pp. 10-14.

Kennedy, J. (1997). Personal assistance benefits and federal health care reforms: Who is eligible on the basis of ADL assistance criteria? *Journal of Rehabilitation*, pp. 40-45.

Mahoney, J., Sager, M., Danham, N., & Johnson, J. (1994). Risk of falls after hospital discharge. *Journal of American Geriatric Society, 42*(3), 269-274.

Teague, M.L., Cipriano, R.E., & McGhee, V.L. (1990). Health promotion as a rehabilitation service for people with disabilities. *Journal of Rehabilitation, 56*(1), 52-56.

U.S. Census Bureau. (1990). *National health interview survey on assistive services (NHIS-AD)*. Washington, DC: U.S. Government Printing Office.

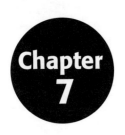

Chapter 7

Physical Healthcare Patterns and Nursing Interventions

Suzanne T. Rogers, MA RN CRRN

Maria J. Amador, BSN RN CRRN

Teresa A. Bryan, BSN RN CRRN

The physical patterns of health form the basis of rehabilitation nursing. Nutrition, elimination, sleep-rest, activity-exercise, and sexual-reproductive patterns are all affected by the major illnesses, impairments, and disabilities seen in rehabilitation practice. Rehabilitation nurses must be experts in identifying actual problems and potential problems that result from the disruption of these health patterns. Nurses also must be able to collaborate with patients in setting realistic, appropriate goals and must be astute when selecting interventions to reach these goals in a timely and cost-effective manner.

The nursing process provides the framework, the functional health patterns provide the substance, and the nurse's professional philosophy guides nursing practice. Nurses must always begin with what the patient needs, expects, or wants. They must value growth, increased independence, interaction with others, and self-actualization. Nurses must always seek ways to integrate nursing practice into the interdisciplinary team's work of restoration and rehabilitation. Although all rehabilitation professionals work together to provide interdisciplinary care, nurses coordinate the care, interact with family and other community supports, and intercede for the patient across disciplines when services need to be added, adapted, or revised.

Within this chapter, the functional patterns of health have been revised slightly to focus particular attention on the assessment and care of skin and sleep as necessary precursors to activity. Also, the content of this chapter makes distinctions within activity between mobility, self-care, and issues surrounding the physical aspects of sexuality and reproduction for individuals who have permanent disruptions to their health.

I. Nutrition: Eating, Swallowing, and Feeding
  A. Overview
    1. Adequate nutrition is necessary for all life functions, but it is of particular importance for individuals with disability, chronic illness, or developmental difficulties.
    2. Participation in therapeutic exercises and in relearning daily activities requires energy, strength, and endurance.
    3. Inadequate intake of food or fluid, as well as consumption in excess of body demands, places the individual at significant risk for multiple complications.

    4. Impaired swallowing, frequently seen in patients with neurological injuries, requires prompt and accurate identification to minimize the risk of aspiration.
    5. Rehabilitation nurses must assess nutritional adequacy, recognize signs of impaired swallowing and risk for aspiration, and select appropriate interventions to restore nutritional health.
  B. Nutritional Intake
    1. Elements of dietary intake to meet metabolic demand
      a. Protein to build tissues
      b. Carbohydrates for available energy

c. Fats for sustained energy demands

d. Vitamins, especially niacin and vitamin C

e. Minerals, especially zinc and calcium

f. Fluids, especially water

g. Fiber

h. Associated factors

　1) Taste
　2) Smell
　3) Texture and consistency
　4) Access to food
　5) Interest in food
　6) Cultural and religious relevance of food
　7) Social factors surrounding eating
　8) Selection of food (e.g., availability, cost)
　9) Medical restrictions on diet

2. Nursing assessment of nutritional adequacy

a. Body weight and height

b. Dietary history and preferences, including recent and remote past

c. Cultural and religious patterns, interests and choices, ability to select and prepare food

d. Apparent muscle wasting and absence of body fat stores (e.g., use of triceps measurement)

　1) Acute illness
　2) Comorbidities
　3) Depression

e. Presence of excessive body fat stores: The individual who is morbidly obese may have severe underlying nutritional deficiencies.

　1) Energy demands of body weight
　2) Inactivity
　3) Greater reliance for energy on fats, simple carbohydrates, and glucose
　4) Lower dietary fiber intake

f. Diagnostic laboratory data

　1) Serum albumin: Indicates available protein stores
　2) Hemoglobin: Indicates ability to transport oxygen

　3) Glycohemoglobin: Indicates blood glucose control over the past 3 months

3. Expected patient outcomes related to nutritional adequacy

a. Reestablish or maintain nutritional balance so that dietary intake is sufficient to meet metabolic demands

b. Promote maximum nutritional support by encouraging the use of the gut whenever possible

4. Nursing interventions to promote nutritional adequacy

a. Help the patient select balanced meals

　1) Adequate calories, protein, and essential nutrients
　2) Select from what is available, acceptable, and meets nutritional demands

b. Teach the patient the importance of nutrition

c. Pay attention to possible food-drug interactions

d. Encourage and support efforts to improve intake for desired weight loss or maintenance

e. Monitor weight and albumin and hemoglobin levels

f. Use nutritional supplements, vitamins, and fluids

g. Have small, frequent meals to meet calorie and vitamin needs when indicated

h. Encourage sufficient fiber intake to promote bowel peristalsis

i. Increase fluid intake for nutritional balance as well as elimination, if not contraindicated (e.g., congestive heart failure [CHF])

j. Adjust food consistency for ease of chewing and patient safety

k. Teach patient to read food labels

l. Teach patient about correct and adequate portion control of food

C. Swallowing and Aspiration
　1. Normal anatomy and physiology of swallowing

a. Structures
   1) Mouth, including teeth, lips, and tongue
   2) Throat, including pharynx, epiglottis, and trachea
   3) Esophagus and stomach
   4) Small and large intestines
b. Innervation of mouth, neck, and digestive system
   1) Voluntary component
   2) Involuntary component (e.g., cranial nerves, peristalsis)
c. Mechanics of swallowing (see Figure 7-1)
   1) Oral phase
      a) Food is chewed, tongue collects particles, moves the bolus to the back of the mouth, squeezing it up against the hard palate.
      b) This phase may take 5-30 seconds to complete, depending on the nature of the food.
   2) Pharyngeal phase
      a) Superior musculature of the pharynx constricts, preventing food from entering the nasopharynx.
      b) Respiration is inhibited.
      c) Epiglottis slides downward to seal the trachea, preventing the food bolus from entering the trachea.
      d) Tongue and pharynx constrict, enlarging the pharynx and the vallecula space and moving the bolus into the esophagus.
      e) In normal swallowing, this phase takes 1 second.
      f) This phase involves the most risk for dysfunction.
         (1) Oral regurgitation
         (2) Nasal regurgitation
         (3) Laryngeal penetration
         (4) Subglottic aspiration
         (5) Trapping of food in the vallecular or the pyriform sinuses
   3) Esophageal phase
      a) Food bolus moves into the esophagus.
      b) Peristaltic waves move the bolus toward the stomach.
      c) Lower esophagus sphincter relaxes, allowing food to enter the stomach.
      d) Lower esophagus sphincter closes to prevent regurgitation of stomach contents.
      e) In normal swallowing, this phase takes 5-10 seconds.
      f) Pressure on the upper stomach from tumors, hiatal hernia, or impaired peristalsis may delay this phase and produce symptoms of heartburn.
      g) Gastroesophageal reflux from impaired esophageal closure may damage lungs when patient positioning is compromised.
2. Nursing assessment components for impaired swallowing or patients at risk for aspiration (McHale, Phipps, Hovarth, & Schmelz, 1998)
   a. Difficulty in handling secretions: Drooling, ineffective cough, need for suctioning, drop in respiratory rate or oxygen saturation, or poor color with attempts to eat
   b. Inability to follow instructions or maintain eye contact
   c. Impaired ability to sit upright in a chair or to hold head erect
   d. Slurred speech
   e. Impaired ability to form a smile, purse lips, or move tongue on command
   f. Presence of facial droop or drooling
   g. Pocketing of food in mouth or impaired ability to chew and form a bolus of food
   h. Slowed ability to form food bolus and initiate swallowing reflex
   i. Inadequate swallowing with first attempt (i.e., food remains in oral cavity)
   j. Absent or impaired elevation of cricoid cartilage (i.e., Adam's apple) with swallowing

Figure 7-1. Phases of Deglutition

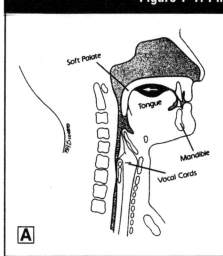

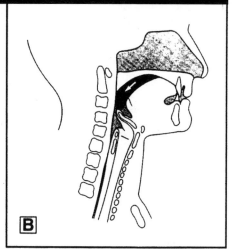

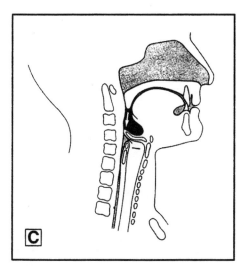

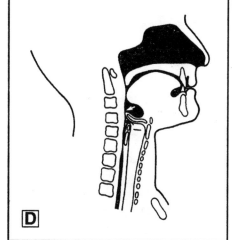

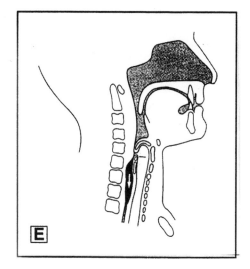

Oral (preparatory) phase (A): The food is chewed, gathered into a bolus by the tongue, and moved to the back of the oral cavity.

Pharyngeal phase (B, C, D): The bolus is pressed against the hard palate. The tongue and palate are elevated to prevent regurgitation. Laryngeal elevation, epiglottal folding, and cricopharyngeus contraction protect the tracheal opening. Vocal cord adduction and other pharyngeal constrictors relax to allow bolus transport. Potential food traps include the vallecula and the pyriform sinuses. Repeated swallowing ordinarily clears these areas. Retention allows for subsequent aspiration when the swallowing act is complete. Chin tuck widens this opening, allowing for more complete bolus transport.

Esophageal phase (E): Food bolus enters the esophagus and peristalsis begins, moving the bolus to the stomach.

Illustrations reprinted with permission of Pro-Ed from Logemann, J. (1998). *Evaluation and treatment of swallowing disorders* (2nd ed., p. 28). Austin, TX: Pro-Ed.

k. Need for more than 30 minutes to finish a simple meal

l. Gag or cough: These reflexes may be absent or depressed and should not be used solely to identify swallowing problems.

3. Expected patient outcomes related to impaired swallowing and at risk for aspiration: Patient will be able to maintain the airway, prevent aspiration, and use feeding techniques that support and encourage adequate nutrition.

4. Nursing interventions for impaired swallowing and at risk for aspiration

   a. Refer the patient for a swallowing evaluation and videofluoroscopic examination (i.e., modified barium swallow) to detect impaired deglutition and silent aspiration (McHale et al., 1998)

   b. Provide recommendations regarding appropriate strategies (McHale et al., 1998)

   c. Seat patient upright, preferably in a chair

   d. Select foods of appropriate consistency and texture

      1) Progress over time from pureed to ground to regular food

      2) With ground textured food, only gradually add food that fragments easily

      3) Stay with one food and texture at a time

      4) Do not mix solids and liquids

   e. Progress liquid intake from pudding thick to honey thick to nectar thick to thin: If necessary, use a commercial thickener to achieve the appropriate consistency.

   f. Place food on unaffected side of mouth and use small mouthfuls; encourage the patient to turn his or her head to the unaffected side to bring food into the midline (Logemann, 1998)

   g. Teach patient to concentrate fully on chewing each small mouthful, forming a food bolus, and swallowing it before taking another mouthful

   h. Use the chin tuck method to protect the airway (Welch, Logemann, Rademaker, & Karhilas, 1993)

      1) Encourage patient to do a tongue sweep of mouth to self-check for food

      2) Use compensatory strategies such as a double swallow between each mouthful to prevent aspiration

      3) Instruct patient to take small sips of water between mouthfuls or to alternate liquid and solid mouthfuls, as appropriate

   i. Visually inspect the oral cavity and use wide-mouth drinking vessels to allow visualization of progress of liquids into oral cavity

   j. Provide enough time and appropriate supervision

      1) Use adaptive devices for self-feeding and independence

      2) Give patients with impulsivity one item of food or drink at a time and limit distractions

   k. Eliminate distractions, give cues for strategies, and discourage the patient from conversing while eating

   l. Provide a calm, unhurried atmosphere

   m. Ensure that the patient remains upright for 20-30 minutes after eating a meal

   n. Do not rely on gag or cough to identify a swallowing problem

D. Typical Causes of Impaired Nutrition that Have Implications for Rehabilitation Nursing

   1. Loss of teeth

   2. Loss of sense of smell

   3. Diminished production of saliva

   4. Impaired swallowing (e.g., excessive drooling, pocketing of food)

   5. Risk of aspiration or silent aspiration

   6. Impaired digestive ability due to hiatal hernia, flattened diaphragm, or gastroesophageal reflux

   7. Impaired gastric motility

   8. Hyperglycemia (e.g., diabetes, steroids)

9. Hypoglycemia (e.g., diminished intake, insulin or other medications, exercise, vomiting)

10. Ineffective absorption of nutrients

11. Inattention to hunger from depression or isolation

12. Inability to initiate self-feeding patterns

13. Altered self-image (e.g., preexisting bulcmia, anorexia)

14. Intake of food in excess of body's caloric demands

15. Altered demands for nutrients in periodic stages of childhood growth and development

16. Exacerbated metabolic demand for nutrients resulting from trauma or disease

17. History of underlying poor nutrition, vitamin deficiencies, and dehydration

18. Medication interactions and side effects

19. Effect of comorbidities (e.g., chronic respiratory disease, cardiac disease, diabetes)

E. Nursing Care for Patients with Nutritional Access Problems

1. Patients who are fed by gastrostomy tube (G-tube) to provide either temporary or permanent access to the gut when oral intake is not possible

   a. Ensure adequate fluid intake by assessing hydration status

   b. Monitor body weight and serum albumin

   c. Regularly check gastric contents for residual

   d. Maintain head of bed at 30 degrees or higher during feeding

   e. Time feedings to be either continuous or bolus: If caloric requirements can be met, bolus is preferred with gradual return to normal patterns of intake.

   f. Use portable equipment to allow participation in therapy regimen

   g. Protect and routinely cleanse skin around gastrostomy site and use skin shields

2. Patients who are fed by hyperalimentation via central intravenous catheters when use of the gut is not possible

   a. Provide special care for access site, tubing, and solution

   b. Ensure adequate caloric intake through periodic use of lipid solutions

   c. Regularly monitor body chemistries to help in the adjustment of solution electrolytes and lipids

   d. Gradually introduce oral intake and taper hyperalimentation

F. Special Populations at Nutritional Risk

1. Children with a disability: Particular concerns are related to growth and development and the establishment of lifelong habits of healthy nutrition.

2. Geriatric patients with a disability: Particular concerns are related to energy demands of rehabilitation and presence of comorbidities as well as lifelong habits and routines.

II. **Skin Integrity, Impairments, and Interventions**

A. Overview

1. Preservation and restoration of intact skin is a major focus of rehabilitation nursing because patients present with multiple risk factors and major disruptions in health.

2. The recovery of health can be seriously impeded when pressure ulcers develop.

3. In 1994, the Agency for Health Care Policy and Research (AHCPR [now called the Agency for Healthcare Research and Quality]) published a set of practice guidelines based on extensive critique of research literature and expert review (Bergstrom, Bennett, Carlson, et al., 1994). These guidelines established the basic framework and have been modified to meet specific patient populations.

4. Rehabilitation nurses need to be skilled in maintaining intact skin and in identifying and treating pressure ulcer problems.

5. Rehabilitation nurses' major concern in skin care is to prevent and, when necessary, heal pressure wounds. All wounds should be treated with appropriate sterile techniques and dressings as necessary.

B. Anatomy and Function of the Skin (McCance & Huether, 1994)

1. Epidermis: The outermost layer, which contains keratin that protects deeper layers of the skin and is constantly being replaced by newer cells from the dermis
    a. Protects against ultraviolet radiation
    b. Protects from environmental antigens
    c. Protects the body from injury
    e. Retains moisture
    f. Excretes waste products
    g. Assists with regulating body temperature
2. Dermal layer: Fibrous connective tissue
    a. Allows elasticity of skin
    b. Permits motion
    c. Supports healing
3. Subcutaneous layer
    a. Contains sweat, oil glands, and hair follicles
    b. Provides blood supply to the skin
    c. Contains neuron receptors for touch, pain, and vasomotor response
    d. Is sustained by a layer of fat
4. Circulation
    a. Provides nutrients, oxygenation, and moisture
    b. Promotes healing through increased blood supply, phagocytosis, and tissue rebuilding
    c. Provides support and healing in response to tissue load damage
5. Nerve supply: Provides response to environment and supports homeostasis
C. Risk Factors for Loss of Skin Integrity
1. Physiological factors
    a. Altered metabolic states that increase the body's need for nutrients and may cause cellular level impairment
    b. Underlying medical conditions (e.g., diabetes, cardiopulmonary or renal disease)
    c. Low serum protein albumin or hemoglobin, which impair the body's cellular rebuilding activity
    d. Impaired circulation from peripheral neuropathies, anemia, atherosclerosis, or hypertension
    e. Prolonged pressure and immobility, which lead to pressure ulcer formation
    f. Neurological injuries that result in impaired sensation (e.g., proprioception, temperature, touch), resulting in the inability to perceive the need to move the body
    g. Medications that suppress the immune response
    h. Smoking, which decreases the effectiveness of the vascular bed by increased vasoconstriction
    i. Poor nutrition, especially inadequate intake of protein, vitamin C, and zinc
    j. Bladder and bowel incontinence
    k. Increased age: Elderly people have diminished effectiveness of skin protection, slowed healing ability, and are more likely to have comorbidities and mobility problems.
2. Mechanical factors
    a. Sustained pressure: Resting surfaces that are hard and unyielding and maintain constant pressure in one direction, particularly over bony prominences when repositioning is infrequent
    b. Shearing: The movement of muscle, subcutaneous, and fat tissues downward and compression against the bony skeleton while the epidermis does not slide (i.e., this occurs when the patient is sitting up in bed and slides down in response to gravity)
    c. Friction: Mechanical rubbing of tissue across a rough surface (i.e., this occurs with incomplete lifting or dragging a patient to pull him or her up in bed)
    d. Body moisture: Incontinence, diuresis, or sweating, especially in the skin folds of a patient who is obese
    e. Particular problems associated with stomas (e.g., G-tube, colostomy, urostomy)
    f. Incorrect fit of prostheses, braces, or orthoses, especially in the presence of neuropathy (e.g., diabetes)
3. Psychosocial factors

a. Nonconformance with recommended healthcare practices

b. Substance abuse that impairs nutrition, mobility, and sensation

c. Impaired cognitive or intellectual ability

d. Depression

e. Social isolation, particularly when the patient needs assistance in daily care

D. Nursing Assessment of Patients at Risk for Impaired Skin Integrity

1. General assessment components

   a. Underlying medical condition(s)

   b. Nutrition: Albumin and prealbumin, hemoglobin, and white blood count

   c. Circulatory support

   d. Presence of neurological injury

   e. Bladder and bowel function and body moisture

   f. Sensory-perceptual ability

   g. Mobility, activity and exercise, body positioning

   h. Pressure, shearing and friction, which may occur in the course of bedside care

   i. Age: Elderly patients are at particular risk for developing pressure ulcers as they are most likely to have substantive problems in all of these categories.

2. Assessment scales

   a. Braden scale: Contains six weighted elements, each of which is graded from 1 (very poor or very limited) to 4 (excellent, normal) and summed across all elements for a total score for individual's risk status

   b. Norton scale: Contains a simpler list of four weighted elements, scored from 1 (immobile or poor) to 4 (excellent) and summed across all elements for a total score for the individual's risk status

   c. For both scoring systems, areas of low score should prompt specific interventions to maintain or restore skin integrity. Scoring can be repeated over time to demonstrate improvement.

E. Expected Patient Outcomes Related to Potential Impaired Skin Integrity

1. Intact skin

2. Demonstrate appropriate self-efficacy measures in the management of skin integrity.

F. Nursing Interventions to Maintain Skin Integrity

1. Ensure good nutritional support and use supplements if needed

2. Manage tissue loads

   a. Turn and reposition the patient frequently (e.g., every 2-4 hours)

   b. Use good lifting, transfer, and turning techniques

   c. Cushion bony prominences

   d. Protect skin against friction and shearing

   e. Position the patient with adequate support

   f. Increase the patient's efforts toward mobility and activity

3. Care for the skin

   a. Inspect skin daily and pay special attention to all bony prominences

   b. Cleanse skin at regular intervals and use a mild cleansing agent to preserve the neutral pH of skin

   c. Apply emollients to help retain or maintain skin moisture

   d. Avoid massaging bony prominences to avoid increased tissue damage

   e. Minimize exposure to incontinence, perspiration, or wound drainage

      1) Use wicking materials to draw moisture away from the skin

      2) Use topical agents as protective barriers

      3) Institute bladder and bowel training regimes whenever possible

4. Teach patients about the importance of self-efficacy in nutrition, management of tissue loads, and general skin care

G. Normal Phases of Wound Healing

1. Vascular supply and wound stabilization (i.e., the wound bleeds and then clots)

2. Inflammation of the tissues with influx of phagocytes to remove dead tissue

3. Proliferation of fibrin and formation of a loose matrix within the wound, which supports additional tissue formation and retention

4. Maturation of the fibrin matrix into intact skin

H. Essential Elements for Planning Nursing Care for Pressure Ulcers (Bergstrom et al., 1994) and Expected Patient Outcomes

1. Nutritional assessment and support: Nutritional support will provide sufficient protein to produce serum albumin values of ≥ 3.5, and the patient's weight will be > 80% of ideal. Protein stores require several weeks of intensive therapy to demonstrate a rise in serum albumin. Prealbumin testing shows a rise in 3-5 days.

2. Management of tissue loads: Resting surfaces and positioning will provide adequate protection for tissue load to encourage healing and prevent further loss.

3. Care of the ulcer itself: Ulcer care will promote wound cleansing and healing. Response to treatment may be slow due to underlying vascular damage, comorbidities, and immobility.

I. General Nursing Interventions for Pressure Ulcers

1. Promote increased protein intake, vitamin C and zinc supplement, and adequate hydration (see Figure 7-2)

2. Keep the patient off the wound as much as possible

3. Turn and reposition the patient at least every 2-3 hours using sheets to lift (not drag) the patient; if possible, use an over-the-bed trapeze to encourage the patient to assist with lifting

4. Use positioning pillows and blocks to maintain pressure relief; consider using pressure-reducing devices (e.g., air mattresses, specialty foam surfaces, gel pads, low air-loss mattresses) (see Figure 7-3)

5. Encourage mobility

6. Keep the skin clean, dry, and lubricated; do not massage reddened bony prominences as this may increase capillary destruction

7. Change linens promptly and clean the skin after any episodes of bladder or bowel incon-

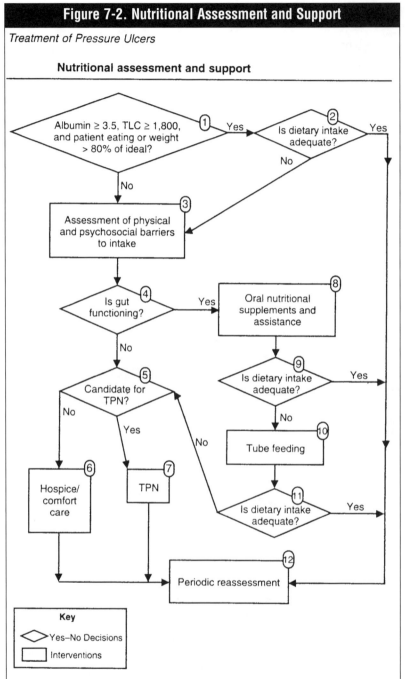

Figure 7-2. Nutritional Assessment and Support

Treatment of Pressure Ulcers

Nutritional assessment and support

① Albumin ≥ 3.5, TLC ≥ 1,800, and patient eating or weight > 80% of ideal? — Yes → ② Is dietary intake adequate? — Yes →

No ↓

③ Assessment of physical and psychosocial barriers to intake

④ Is gut functioning? — Yes → ⑧ Oral nutritional supplements and assistance

No ↓

⑤ Candidate for TPN? — No → ⑥ Hospice/comfort care

Yes → ⑦ TPN

⑨ Is dietary intake adequate? — Yes →

No ↓

⑩ Tube feeding

⑪ Is dietary intake adequate? — Yes →

⑫ Periodic reassessment

Key
◇ Yes–No Decisions
☐ Interventions

Note: TLC = total lymphocyte count; TPN = total parenteral nutrition.

Reprinted with permission from Agency for Health Care Policy and Research (AHCPR) from Bergstrom, N., Bennett, M.A., Carlson, C.E., et al. (1994). *Treatment of pressure ulcers: Clinical practice guideline no. 15* (AHCPR Publication No. 95-0652). Rockville, MD: U.S. Department of Health and Human Services Public Health Agency for Health Care Policy and Research.

tinence and provide a moisture barrier lotion for further protection

8. Provide consistent, timely treatments and document progress: Pressure ulcers become visible quickly, worsen quickly, and heal slowly.

Figure 7-3. Management of Tissue Loads

Treatment of Pressure Ulcers

Management of tissue loads

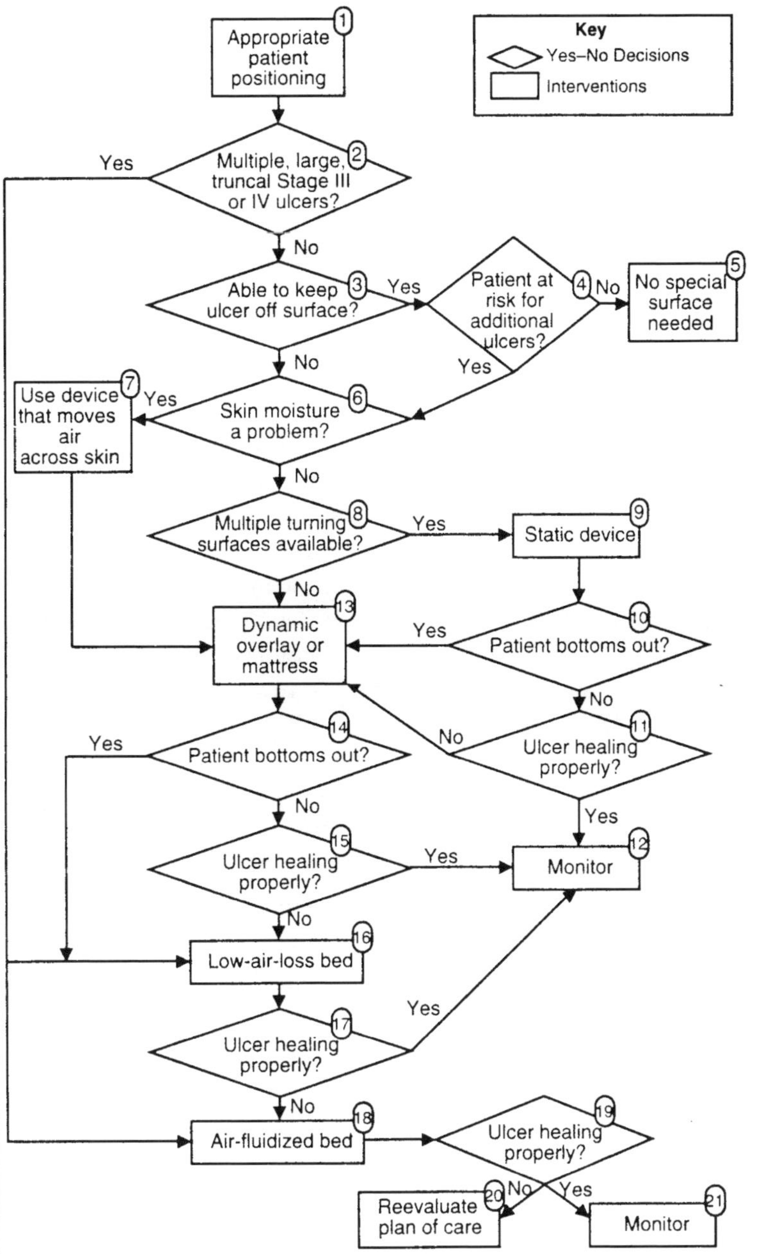

Reprinted with permission from Agency for Health Care Policy and Research (AHCPR) from Bergstrom, N., Bennett, M.A., Carlson, C.E., et al. (1994). *Treatment of pressure ulcers: Clinical practice guideline no. 15* (AHCPR Publication No. 95-0652). Rockville, MD: U.S. Department of Health and Human Services Public Health Agency for Health Care Policy and Research.

9. Focus treatment approaches on the whole person and the environment; pressure ulcers tend to be multivariant in cause.

10. Assess and reassess pressure ulcers using standard staging guidelines: Pressure ulcers are staged according to depth, characteristics of wound bed, and potential involvement of deep fascia (Bergstrom et al., 1994) (see Figure 7-4)

    a. AHCPR guidelines note that the identification of Stage I redness may be problematic in individuals with darkly pigmented skin. A reliable system for assessment should be developed (Bergstrom et al., 1994).

    b. AHCPR guidelines only indirectly address the problem of extensive tissue necrosis, which may be behind intact skin over bony prominences (Bergstrom et al., 1994), calling these Stage I wounds.

    c. Other sources recommend labeling these wounds more specifically by describing surrounding tissue carefully (Feeder, 1994; Guccione, 1993; McCulloch, Kloth, & Freedon, 1995) or even labeling them as "unable to stage."

J. Nursing Interventions for Pressure Ulcers (see Figure 7-5)

K. Documentation of Wound Healing

    1. Describe location, diameter, and depth of the wound; use transparent grids for accuracy in measurement if needed

    2. Describe wound base (e.g., color, presence or absence of moisture, slough, eschar)

    3. Evaluate undermining or sinus tract formation by gently probing the wound with sterile gauze swabs to determine the true size of the wound

    4. Note evidence of pain, induration, or inflammation and remember that redness, hardness, or discoloration around pressure areas that have poor

blood supply (e.g., heels, sacrum) can mask major tissue necrosis behind apparently intact skin

5. Include present and planned treatment regimen

6. Take pictures of the wound for baseline and repeat at periodic intervals (generally every 2 weeks) until the wound is healed: This is a helpful measure of the effectiveness of therapy; however, remember that taking such pictures may require patient consent.

7. Document pressure wounds that are healing by retaining the label of the original stage with "healing" added; do not revert back to lesser staging as the wound heals

III. Elimination: Bladder and Bowel Function

A. Overview

1. The human body eliminates the waste of metabolism through urine and stool.

2. Normal function depends on several factors.

   a. Anatomic integrity

   b. Intact neurologic components for both voluntary control and synergistic emptying

   c. A predictable pattern of waste production

Figure 7-4. Stages of Pressure Ulcers

Stage I

Nonblanchable erythema of intact skin, the heralding lesion of skin ulceration

May present as warmth, edema, induration, or hardness of soft tissues surrounding the pressure point

Stage II

Partial thickness skin loss involving epidermis, dermis or both

Presents clinically as a superficial abrasion, blister, or shallow crater

Stage III

Full thickness skin loss involving damage to or necrosis to subcutaneous tissue that may extend down to but not through underlying fascia

Stage IV

Full thickness skin loss with extensive destruction, tissue necrosis, or damage to muscle, bone, or supporting structures (e.g., tendon, joint capsule)

Undermining and sinus tracts should be assessed for depth and direction

---

d. Physical and mental ability and the psychosocial willingness to carry out toileting-related tasks

3. Incontinence is a major barrier to community living, employment, and social activity.

4. Rehabilitation nurses must be knowledgeable of the normal physiology of bladder and bowel function, clinically astute in identifying disruptions that produce incontinence and dysfunction, and expert in selecting interventions that will help the patient develop predictable, effective elimination patterns.

B. Bladder Function

1. Anatomy and physiology of bladder elimination

   a. Kidneys filter blood and selectively reabsorb electrolytes.

   b. Ureters direct urine from each kidney into the bladder.

   c. The bladder acts as a reservoir for the urine: Major muscle is the detrusor, a smooth muscle.

      1) Involves bilateral innervation by somatic and motor nerves from the sacral portion of the spinal cord

      2) Expands holding capacity to accommodate urine in response to central nervous system (CNS) inhibitory impulses (reticulospinal and corticospinal motor tracts)

      3) Empties in response to release of these inhibitory impulses

   d. Trigone muscle forms the posterior portion of the bladder wall and extends into the ureter, providing additional strength to the internal sphincter.

   e. The urethra is the passageway for urine from the bladder.

      1) Internal sphincter surrounds the bladder outlet, consists of smooth muscle, and relaxes to allow the bladder to empty.

      2) External sphincter surrounds the urethral outlet and is made of striated, skeletal muscle. It receives segmental innervation from the pudenal nerve and afferent innervation from the urethra and pelvic floor.

      3) The external sphincter relaxes as the detrusor contracts to facilitate emptying of the bladder.

f. The micturition reflex requires the coordination of several factors.

   1) Somatic (sensory) and motor neural impulses from the central and peripheral nervous system

---

Figure 7-5. Nursing Interventions for Pressure Ulcers

Stage I

Provide pressure relief for reddened areas where skin is still intact

Protect the skin from potential abrasion by applying a protective barrier lotion if necessary

Stage II

Keep the wound moist and clean to promote healing from the base up for open areas that have clean, moist, red tissue bases, no drainage, no slough (i.e., pus or white thready exudate), or eschar (i.e., black hard scabbing within the wound)

Use hydrogel ointments or hydrocolloid dressings if recommended

During dressing changes, gently, thoroughly cleanse the wound, using either normal saline or a commercial wound cleanser. Irrigation should be strong enough to clean nonadherent particles but not so strong as to cause damage to new tissue. Pressure resulting from irrigating with a 18- or 19-gauge intercath on a 30 cc syringe meets this criteria.

Adjust frequency of dressing changes to allow assessment of improvement without disruption of fibroblastic activity and the inadvertent entry of additional pathogens into the wound. In the absence of symptoms of active infection, changing the dressing every 2-3 days may be sufficient. As healing is evidenced, less frequent dressing changes are indicated.

Stage III

Clean the wound first, as Stage III wounds usually have slough or drainage and may have sinus tracts and undermining

Gently but thoroughly pack the ulcer and apply a secondary dressing

Use calcium alginates in the form of sponges or ropes or polymeric foam dressings. When using nonselective debridement (e.g., normal saline wet-to-dry dressings), take care to lessen the loss of new granulating tissue

Protect the periulcer area from maceration

Change dressings according to the amount of drainage absorbed; irrigate the ulcer with each dressing change

Decrease frequency of dressing changes as drainage slowly decreases until a clean, moist wound bed is achieved, at which point it is appropriate to change to a hydrocolloid and proceed as described for Stage II

Debride the wound if eschar (i.e., a black scab within the wound, generally at the base) is present: This can be done either through surgical sharp debridement or topical debriding enzymes. The periulcer area must be protected from maceration or unintentional damage.

Use dressings that keep the wound base moist to promote healing

Stage IV

Regularly cleanse and pack the wound, which may extend into bone, tendon, and muscle, until a clean epithelializing base is obtained (see interventions for Stage III). Stage IV wounds often require surgical closure with grafts or flaps once a clean base is obtained.

---

   2) The sympathetic and parasympathetic nervous system

   3) Muscle strength in response to neural impulses in a synergistic fashion

   4) Freedom from outlet obstruction

2. Urinary incontinence: Failure of muscle strength, detrusor instability, or obstruction; generally divided into four types, although patients may have a mixed pattern

a. Urge incontinence

   1) Related to the mechanics of micturition, an unstable detrusor muscle, urethral hypertrophy or impaired cognitive function

   2) Related to difficulty retaining urine when bladder reaches specific but low pressures

   3) Characterized by hurrying to reach the bathroom, inability to remove clothing in time, premature micturition, and soiling of underclothes: Once urination begins, the patient is unable to stop it until the bladder is empty.

b. Stress incontinence

   1) Small amounts of urine leak when there is an increase in abdominal pressure secondary to such causes as laughing, coughing, or sneezing.

   2) Individual has no warning of incontinence.

   3) Initially, small amounts of urine are lost, but the condition may progress to losing larger amounts with increasing bladder incompetence.

c. Overflow incontinence

---

1) Involves small amounts of urine that are passed in proportion to fluid intake

2) Involves a sense of abdominal pressure that is unrelieved by micturition and persistent feelings of fullness and needing to urinate

3) Caused by hypertrophy of bladder neck or enlarged prostate

4) May be aggravated by certain medications (e.g., antihistamines, alpha-adrenergics)

d. Functional incontinence

1) Related to impaired cognitive function (i.e., volitional control) and culturally and socially inappropriate voiding

2) Often occurs in patients with head injury

3) May be related to environmental inaccessibility or problems with arranging clothing

3. Nursing assessment of urinary incontinence

a. Confirm factors related to episodes and type of incontinence and select appropriate interventions (Pires & Lockhart-Pretti, 1992)

b. Determine whether a mixed pattern may be identified due to incomplete or partially damaged neural pathways rather than ablation

c. Ask specific questions of patients who have some neural control, as they may be reluctant or embarrassed to voluntarily relate episodes of incontinence

d. Determine cognitive function and the ability to participate in interventions, which will play a major role in reaching continence goals

e. Make observations during caregiving regarding the amount and frequency of loss of urine and situations surrounding incontinent episodes

f. Assess abdominal and suprapubic palpation for tenderness or fullness

g. Determine hydration status and possibility of constipation

h. Ask specific questions regarding situations that lead to urine loss

1) Do you ever find that you cannot get to the bathroom in time?

2) Do you leak urine when you cough or laugh?

3) Do you feel the need to urinate but only small amounts come out?

4) Do you need to wear pads to absorb urine? How many do you use and how often do you change them?

5) Do you feel you have no control over urination?

6) How do you manage control of urination (e.g., reduce fluids after 6 pm, eliminate caffeine, always toilet before going out, use pads or other assistive devices)?

i. Review medications for causative relationships (e.g., antihistamines may cause retention)

j. Determine sphincter response to stimulus (bulbocavernosus reflex) and use the pinprick test of pubic area and inner upper thighs for sensation and intact reflex arc

k. Assess postvoid residual to determine the bladder's ability to empty or to measure success in bladder training

l. Use specific urodynamic testing (e.g., cystometry) to assess the synergy of detrusor activity, presence of ureteral reflux, and voiding pressures

m. Assess associated variables

1) Age, mobility, and ability to get to and use a toilet

2) Hand coordination, ability to remove and readjust clothing, presence of neurologic injury

3) Pelvic floor muscle strength, particularly in women

4) Prostate enlargement in men

5) Constipation

n. Note that elderly people frequently get up from sleep to empty the bladder

1) More urine may be produced at night when vascular perfusion of the kidneys improves as a result of being in the supine position.

2) Diminished levels of antidiuretic hormone (ADH) are present in the blood.

3) Sleep cycles are less deep than in younger people.
4. Expected patient outcomes for the management of urinary incontinence
   a. Empty the bladder no more than every 3-4 hours
   b. Remain continent between emptying
   c. Sleep without interference from urinary drainage
   d. Avoid recurrent urinary tract infections and complications of bladder dysfunction
5. Nursing care plan for bladder incontinence related to mechanical or non-neurogenic factors (see Figure 7-6)
6. Urinary incontinence related to neurogenic bladder dysfunction
   a. Upper motor neuron (UMN) dysfunction (i.e., reflexic, spastic, or uninhibited bladder)
      1) Results from disruption, injury, or disease above T12-S1
      2) Prevents UMN control of voiding (intention)
      3) Involves intact reflex arc at the segmental level
      4) Involves the bladder emptying in response to stretching fibers in the bladder wall, but voiding is unpredictable and incomplete
   b. Lower motor neuron (LMN) dysfunction (i.e., areflexic, autonomous, flaccid or sacral bladder)
      1) Results from disruption, injury, or disease at or below T12-S1
      2) Involves ablation of reflex arc
      3) May spare afferent and efferent fibers
      4) Involves disorganized, ineffective

Figure 7-6. Nursing Plan of Care for Non-Neurogenic Urinary Incontinence

Stress Incontinence

Establish a voiding record
- Amount of fluid taken in
- Time and amount of voiding
- Episodes of wetting and activity associated with that episode
- Estimate of amount of incontinence each time (e.g., number of pads)

Teach pelvic (Kegel) exercises to increase control of the pelvic floor muscles
- Tighten the pubococcygeal muscle (as if to stop urine flow)
- Hold tightened position for a slow count to three
- Relax and repeat for a set of 10 times, starting with 5 times a day
- Gradually increase to sets of 15-20 times, each set done 5 times a day

(Note. Muscle tone and control should gradually increase, as evidenced in the voiding record. If exercises are not successful, a more detailed evaluation and medication or surgery may be indicated.)

Urge Incontinence

Ensure regular toileting every 2-4 hours during the day

Provide reminders to use the toilet when the urge occurs: Women particularly need to be reminded of this as they tend to delay toileting to complete other tasks.

Plan fluid intake and empty bladder prior to travel

Teach pelvic (Kegel) exercises as described above

Use voiding records, which can be helpful, especially with an ambulatory patient population: These should be set up to prompt recording of fluid intake, time of voiding, sensation of fullness, and feeling of emptying the bladder.

Overflow Incontinence

Use interventions when suprapubic palpation and postvoid catheterization reveal high residuals

Pay attention to intake and output: Adequate fluids and regular toileting may help to prevent overflow.

Try intermittent catheterization; however, if prostate is enlarged, insertion may be difficult: Use Cude tip (a special urologic catheter with a stiffened and slightly bent tip) and generous lubrication prior to attempting insertion.

Use a Foley catheter to provide constant drainage

Determine whether surgical correction may be indicated

Functional Incontinence

Provide cognitive retraining, when possible, which may help in recovery as neural pathways are intact

Train caregivers

Modify the environment

spinal segmental control and impulses

    5) Involves a bladder that is without tone and cannot fill and empty

  c. Sensory root disruption

    1) Involves an impaired sensory (afferent) nerve fibers between the bladder wall and the spinal segment at the level of the reflex arc

    2) Is usually due to diabetic polyneuropathy or peripheral vascular disease

    3) Involves the absence of the sensation of needing to urinate; however, the bladder can empty completely

  d. Motor root disruption

    1) Involves impaired motor (efferent) nerve fiber between the bladder wall and the spinal segment at the level of the reflex arc

    2) Occurs secondary to polio, trauma, or herniated disc

    3) Involves the sensation of fullness and needing to void but being unable to do so

7. Nursing assessment of neurogenic bladder dysfunction

  a. Assessment of neurologic damage

  b. Observations of voiding patterns

  c. Results of diagnostic studies regarding bladder filling capacity, reflexivity, and ureteral reflux

8. Expected patient outcomes for management of neurogenic bladder dysfunction

  a. Regular emptying of bladder

  b. Low or absent residual

  c. Absence of infection or reflux

9. Nursing care plan for neurogenic bladder dysfunction (see Figure 7-7)

10. Comparison of assessment, pathology, and nursing interventions by types of bladder dysfunction (see Table 7-1)

11. Specific techniques for handling urinary drainage

  a. Intermittent catheterization

    1) In hospital settings, use a sterile procedure; at home, use a clean procedure

    2) Use the smallest size catheter diameter possible

    3) Ensure that the patient or caregiver

can visualize or use touch to locate the urethral meatus, insert the catheter using clean technique, and empty the bladder either directly into the toilet or into a receptacle

    4) Wash and keep catheters in a clean container when not in use

  b. Condom catheters (for men)

    1) Determine the appropriate fit, both in width and length (many sizes are available)

    2) Clean the shaft of the penis first with soap and water and dry well; then, apply the condom and roll it along the length of the shaft

      a) Condoms include an adhesive applied to the inner surface to keep it in place; additional adhesives are not usually necessary.

      b) Condom catheters have a drainage tubing piece at the end that should be connected, using clean technique, either to a leg or bedside drainage bag.

  c. Indwelling urinary (Foley) catheters

    1) Adequate hydration ensures that urinary output is not concentrated or filled with sediment.

    2) Ordinary soap-and-water cleansing of the urinary meatus is usually sufficient.

    3) Assess for sediment by rolling the catheter gently between the fingers: If grit is detected, the catheter should be changed.

    4) Foley catheters should never be clamped or irrigated. Instead, remove and reinsert a new one to decrease the potential for urinary tract infection.

  d. Constant drainage systems: Should be kept closed and intact at least while the individual is in the hospital setting

    1) Drainage systems should be maintained at or below the level of the bladder to prevent backflow of urine from the tubing into the bladder.

    2) At home, where there are fewer pathogenic organisms, regular changing from a bedside drainage bag to a leg bag requires a clean technique.

The Specialty Practice of Rehabilitation Nursing: A Core Curriculum, 4th Ed.

Both bags can be rinsed and reused, as appropriate.

3) Periodic cleansing of the bag with a mild bleach solution is recommended.

e. Ileo-loop urostomy: A surgical procedure for patients with severe bladder reflux and recurrent infection. It is treated much like an ileostomy but requires extremely careful fitting of the collection appliance, scrupulous skin care, and frequent emptying.

C. Bowel Function
1. Normal anatomy and physiology of bowel elimination

a. Small and ascending large intestines absorb nutrients from liquid stool.

b. Transverse component of the large intestines absorbs some of the fluid, and stool begins to be more formed.

c. Descending large intestines and rectum absorb additional water, and kidney waste is added. Stool is compacted into a more solid form.

d. Internal sphincter retains stool in the rectum.

e. External sphincter expands to allow the passage of stool from the rectum.

f. Abdominal wall musculature assists with evacuation.

g. Peristalsis moves the stool along the gut.

h. Neurological support allows the gut to continue to function apart from CNS.

1) Voluntary and involuntary innervation occurs at the reflex, segmental, and cortical level.

2) Parasympathetic and sympathetic innervation occurs from the autonomic nervous system.

3) Enteric nervous system influences the intrinsic neural control of the mobility, absorption, and secretion activities of the gut; it is influenced by the autonomic nervous system, but is independent of it.

4) Like the bladder, the bowel is capable of emptying at a reflex level, when stretch fibers in the descending large colon stimulate the reflex arc.

Figure 7-7. Nursing Care Plan for Neurogenic Bladder Dysfunction

Upper Motor Neuron (Reflexive)

Consider timed voiding, which may be effective because motor fibers are intact, but there is no sensation

Consider the potential for kidney infection if urologic studies reveal the occurrence of reflux of urine up the ureters and into the kidneys

Use stimulation of the reflex arc (e.g., pulling pubic hair, stroking the inner thigh)

If reflux is not a problem, teach the patient to use the Credé maneuver, which puts pressure on the abdominal wall above the symphasis pubis and triggers the stretch fibers of the bladder to contract

If hypertension is not a problem, use the Valsalva maneuver, in which the individual raises the intra-abdominal pressure through glottal closure and abdominal pushing (This assists with complete emptying of the bladder.)

Use intermittent catheterization (sterile technique in the hospital; simple clean technique in the community): This requires good hand coordination or the help of an attendant.

Use timed voiding with identified maneuvers to stimulate bladder contraction

For men, attach a condom catheter to a constant drainage bag either in a leg or bedside bag

Remember that the extent of these self-management strategies depends on the patient's hand and motor control, available resources, and concerns for infection, reflux, or skin breakdown

Teach patient to understand autonomic dysreflexia, which must be treated immediately if symptoms occur [Refer to information about spinal cord injury in Chapter 10]

Lower Motor Neuron (Areflexic)

Initially, use a Foley catheter; however, switch to intermittent self-catheterization if possible

If the bladder does not fill at all but there is a constant dribbling, teach men to use a condom catheter

Pay attention to the possibility of retention and reflux of urine back up the ureters, which can lead to renal infections

Sensory Neuron Pathway Disruption

Use timed voiding and/or intermittent self-catheterization

Pay attention to fluid intake to predict urinary output patterns

Motor Neuron Pathway Disruption

Use intermittent catheterization or Valsalva or Credé maneuvers with the usual cautions regarding hypertension and/or reflux

2. Requirements for stool formation
   a. Adequate fiber in the diet: To produce bulk so that water is trapped in the stool and enough solid matter exists to allow peristalsis to move the stool and to allow the body to defecate in an organized, effective manner
   b. Adequate fluid intake: To limit the amount of liquid reabsorbed from the descending colon
   c. General activity and mobility: To support and enhance peristalsis
   d. Upright posture: To allow gravity to assist in stool formation and passage

3. Patterns of defecation through the life span
   a. Infants: Gut functions at the reflex level.
   b. Children: As the child matures, he or she develops cortical control over the time and place of defecation.
   c. Adults: Middle age is a time of intense activity and relative regularity, which may vary slightly due to diet changes, infrequent bouts of illness, or activity; however, the bowel generally responds to simple interventions.
   d. Older adults
      1) Changes occur in striated and smooth

Table 7-1. Summary of Bladder Dysfunction and Interventions

Type	Assessment	Pathology	Interventions
Stress	Onset with exercise, coughing, sneezing; easily stopped; small amounts lost; occurs only during daytime	Sphincter incompetence; urethral instability; pelvic muscle prolapsed	Pelvic muscle exercises; bladder training; regular emptying; use of voiding diary; alpha-agonist medications to relax bladder and increase capacity
Urge	Onset with handwashing or thinking about going to the bathroom; strong stream; not easily stopped until emptied; large amounts lost; occurs during night and daytime	Detrusor muscle instability. Outlet obstruction of bladder neck due to prostate enlargement, tumor, or medication side effects (e.g., antihistamines)	Pelvic muscle exercises; bladder training; regular emptying; use of voiding diary; medications and surgical correction of pelvic muscles may eventually be required if exercises are not enough
Overflow	Onset involves the inability to empty the bladder completely; continual dribbling; observable fullness of bladder	Normal bladder function	Intermittent or indwelling catheterization; surgical correction; change in medications
Functional	Leaking associated with inability or unwillingness to toilet appropriately	Disruption of impulses from UMN; incomplete synergy of associated muscles in bladder emptying	Training of caregivers; environmental modifications; cognitive retraining
UMN (Reflex neurogenic)	Unpredictable voiding; bladder capacity varies; incomplete emptying without external assistance	Loss of reflex arc at or below sacral level	Intermittent catheterization; reflex triggers (stroking inner thigh, pulling on pubic hair); condom catheterization for men
LMN (Areflexive, atonic)	Increased bladder capacity; high postvoid residual; dribbling of urine		Intermittent catheterization; Credé or Valsalva maneuvers; indwelling catheter to allow constant drainage

muscle strength.

2) Activity gradually lessens.

3) Elderly adults generally consume less roughage in the diet and have poorer dentition.

4) Self-limiting hydration may be present secondary to urinary incontinence concerns.

5) Comorbidities may begin, along with increased medication use: These give rise to problems of constipation and help explain the focus on bowel regularity by many elderly people.

4. Assessment of bowel function

   a. Patient history and prior bowel patterns, usual time of day pattern, frequency of stool, past reliance on laxatives or other aids

   b. Present status and pattern, including time and characteristics of last stool

   c. Oozing or small hard stool alternating with watery discharge, which may indicate impaction

   d. Abdominal palpation to determine abdominal discomfort, palpable obstruction, rectal exam

   e. Medications that may affect bowel function (e.g., sedatives, diuretics, antihistamines)

   f. Infection, trauma, or stress that may affect stool formation

   g. Medical problems that may affect interventions

      1) Cardiac conditions, which would preclude the use of digital stimulation or the Valsalva maneuver

      2) Renal impairment, which would preclude the use of milk of magnesia

      3) Overextended bowel, which might rupture with high soap suds enema (a precautionary X ray of the kidneys, ureters, and bladder should be requested prior to administration)

5. Identification of problems related to impaired bowel function

   a. Colonic constipation: Identified as infrequent, small hard stool or none at all in several days

      1) Chronic constipation will enlarge the

descending colon and produce dependency on laxatives and cathartics or enemas.

2) Severe constipation and impaction cause sympathetic system problems (e.g., sweating, nausea, irritability, acute abdominal discomfort, rise in blood pressure)

3) Attention must be paid to establishing and maintaining regularity.

b. Diarrhea

   1) Identified as highly frequent liquid stool with accompanying cramping

   2) May be explosive in nature, generally related to infection, irritability of the gut, or the possibility of food poisoning

   3) May be associated with ulcerative colitis if it is not self-limiting

c. UMN (reflex neurogenic) bowel

   1) Like the bladder, the bowel is capable of reflexive emptying of the rectum without cortical awareness of the need to defecate.

   2) This condition is produced by damage to the spinal cord above T12-S1 or by damage to the cerebral cortex.

   3) Because of the innervation of the sympathetic nervous system, the patient may be aware of defecation and nervous system activity but have no conscious control over it.

d. LMN (autonomous, areflexive, flaccid, atonal) bowel

   1) Subsequent to spinal cord damage at or below T12-S1

   2) No cortical control

   3) A lack of tone in the internal and external sphincters and a frequent oozing of stool, due to damage to the reflex arc

e. Sensory paralytic (afferent nerve root loss or damage)

   1) Occurs subsequent to diabetes or tabes dorsalis

   2) Produces diminished or absent ability to distinguish the need or time of defecation, but rarely produces incontinence because the motor function of the rectum is intact

f. Motor paralytic (efferent nerve root loss or damage)

   1) Occurs subsequent to poliomyelitis, intervertebral disc disease, tumor, or trauma

   2) Results in the inability to assist with defecation

   3) Is only associated with incontinence if there is widespread disease (because of the innervation of the intestines)

g. Colostomies and ileostomies: Artificial openings on the abdominal wall to provide an exit for stool

   1) Used when the colon has become obstructed and the rectum cannot be used (malignant tumors)

   2) Used when the gut is irritated beyond repair (ulcerative colitis)

   3) Used when it is necessary to rest the colon while it repairs (major abdominal resections)

6. Expected patient outcomes related to bowel elimination

   a. Establish a regular bowel regime with complete emptying of soft stool from the rectum every 1-3 days, using the least medication possible

   b. Maintain a consistent habit and time

   c. Have no incontinent episodes

7. Nursing interventions (see Figure 7-8)

   a. Because it is possible to use existing neural pathways to establish a regular bowel program, interventions for impaired bowel elimination are similar, although patients may have different clinical pictures

   b. Because constipation leads to fecal impaction, which can, in turn, produce intestinal rupture, every attempt must be made to attain and maintain adequate bowel evacuation on a regular basis.

IV. Sleep-Rest

A. Overview

1. Adequate and restful sleep is essential to maintaining health, strength, endurance, and cognitive functioning.

2. Illness—particularly neurologic injury, deep pain, the effects of medications such as sedatives and hypnotics, the comorbidities of aging, and recent intensive care hospitalization—all affect sleep patterns.

3. Rehabilitation nurses frequently care for individuals who have suffered major illnesses and subsequent disruption of normal sleep cycles.

4. To promote healing and endurance, rehabilitation nurses should assess disruptions in patients' sleep and apply specific interventions to restore restful sleep patterns.

B. Normal Sleep Patterns

1. The normal adult human body requires 7-8 hours of restful consolidated sleep during nighttime hours in every 24-hour cycle.

2. Sleep restores homeostasis, reestablishes circadian rhythms, and integrates experiences into memory.

3. Restful nighttime sleep alternates with daytime periods of wakefulness.

4. Awake time should include purposeful activity and exercise.

5. Individuals may be in situations that require wakefulness at night (e.g., night shift workers) or interrupted sleep (e.g., parents of infants); however, restful sleep in alignment with day-night rhythms is necessary to restore order to the body.

6. Sleep is an active process.

   a. Neurotransmitters in the reticular formation of the brain are withdrawn and then reactivated.

   b. The body's ability to respond to environmental stimuli is depressed.

   c. Vital signs and muscle tone decrease.

7. There are two observable phases of sleep.

   a. Nonrapid eye movement (non-REM), or slow-wave sleep: This phase has four stages that are distinguished by changes in EEG patterns, vital signs, and neurophysiology (see Figure 7-9)

      1) Stage 1: EEG shows low voltage activity and the appearance of theta waves.

         a) Individual is arousable but lightly asleep.

         b) Healthy adults spend less than 5%-10% of sleep time in this stage.

c) Individuals who are wakened from sleep return to this stage first and begin the cycle again.

2) Stage 2: EEG shows slowing of activity with occasional low-voltage bursts of activity (sleep spindles) and periodic, isolated high-voltage waves (K complexes).

   a) Individual is asleep with slowed respiration, heart beat, metabolic rate, and muscle tone.

   b) Healthy adults spend about 50% of a night's sleep in this stage.

3) Stage 3: EEG begins to show slow, high-voltage wave forms (delta waves), the respiratory rate further decreases, and deep sleep begins.

4) Stage 4 (non-REM deep sleep or delta sleep): EEG shows high-amplitude slow delta waves that are more predominant than in Stage 3.

   a) Healthy adults spend about 20% of sleep time alternating between Stages 3 and 4.

   b) The healing properties of this sleep are seen clearly in those who have had sleep deprivation; this sleep takes precedence over other stages during the first night of recovery.

b. Rapid eye movement (REM), or dream sleep

1) EEG patterns resemble waking with muscle activity, eye movements, and changes in vital signs. The pontine reticular formation in the brain appears to control this phase of sleep (McCance & Huether, 1994).

2) Skeletal muscles are not under voluntary control, muscles of the throat and neck relax, snoring may occur.

3) Blood flow increases to the cerebral cortex.

4) Respiratory rate and heart rate increase.

5) The individual can only be awakened with difficulty and, if awakened from this level, often recalls dreaming.

6) REM sleep appears to be needed for hypothalamic functioning (Kryger, Roth, & Dement, 1994).

7) Healthy adults spend about 25% of sleep time in this part of the sleep cycle.

8) The sleeping individual moves through specific, observable phases in a predictable series of cycles.

   a. Each cycle during a night's sleep rotates from Stage 1

Figure 7-8. Nursing Care Planning for Impaired Bowel Function

If assessment indicates impaction or severe constipation, clean the bowel using a decision tree that goes from the less invasive to more invasive interventions and progresses gradually over several days

- Stimulants such as milk of magnesium may be given by mouth (Note that milk of magnesium is contraindicated in patients with renal failure).
- Stimulants may be placed in the rectum (bisacodyl or glycerin suppository) to encourage complete emptying.
- Surfactants may help to keep the stool soft.
- Irritant stimulants may be given by mouth for more aggressive cleansing (bisacodyl tablets, senna, or, as a last resort, magnesium citrate).
- Soap suds enemas may be given only with great care to avoid bowel rupture.

Once the rectum and descending colon are cleared, establish a regime that promotes regular evacuation: Interventions should be geared at maintaining defecation while gradually introducing more natural methods of function.

Include dietary fiber (unprocessed bran, fruit, such as grapes or prunes): Additional medications may be used to encourage stool bulk (cellulose derivatives or unprocessed bran).

Provide sufficient hydration

Provide for privacy, warmth, comfort, and a consistent time for defecation: Planning bowel evacuation for about 20 minutes after a meal often ensures greater emptying.

Where indicated (and not contraindicated), use the sympathetic reflex through digital stimulation of the rectum to open the sphincters and subsequently evacuate stool

Maintain a balance of stool that is easy to pass while being bulky enough for peristalsis stimulation and elimination

Use manual disimpaction where indicated

Within neurogenic bowel dysfunction, UMN bowel is more receptive to suppositories and digital stimulation, whereas LMN bowel is less responsive to these interventions and may need small enemas or disimpaction: The use of mini-enemas also increases the predictability of timing and evacuation of fecal contents.

to 2 to 3 to 4 to 3 to REM, then back to Stage 2.

b. Stage 2 follows REM and marks the beginning of the next cycle.

c. Each cycle takes about 90-100 minutes.

d. If the individual is awakened at any point, the cycle begins with Stage 1 again.

9. The normal length of time in each cycle and the frequency of each cycle vary with age (see Figure 7-10).

a. Infants and children sleep longer, spend more time in REM sleep, and have large blocks of consolidated sleep.

b. Young adults have large blocks of Stages 3 and 4 deep sleep after the first 2-3 hours of sleep, as well as consolidated dream sleep toward waking.

c. Elderly people have less REM sleep, their sleep stages change more frequently during the night, and their overall sleep is more fragmented. Like infants and young children, elderly people use naps to partially compensate for the overall loss of sleep time.

C. Nursing Assessment Components

1. Current sleep pattern

2. Patient's report of how rested they feel upon

awakening (e.g., rested enough to carry out daily activities? now? in the past?)

3. Patient's description of general sleep routine and strategies used in the past to encourage sleep (e.g., naps, bedtime routines, usual bedtime, usual awakening time)

4. Presence of dark circles under eyes, lethargy, drowsiness, irritability

5. Report from caregivers regarding night sleep (e.g., Are respirations slow and deep, alternating with more shallow periods, periods of snoring or sleep apnea, sleepwalking, or being awake during the night, toileting, ease of return to sleep?)

6. Comorbidities and current medications and their possible effects on sleep

D. Disruptions to Sleep Patterns Related to Illness and Disability

1. Elderly people

a. Night waking for toileting

b. May need to get up to move stiff, sore joints

c. May have comorbidities related to pulmonary, cardiac, or renal problems

d. May experience disruptive effects of medications, especially sedatives and hypnotics

2. Traumatic brain injury and stroke: Disrupted normal patterns and initial reversal of day-night cycles, though this is usually temporary

3. Myasthenia gravis: Sleep apnea due to skeletal muscle weakness

4. Multiple sclerosis and renal disease: Muscle twitching (clonus) or restless legs syndrome

5. Rheumatoid arthritis: Stiff, aching joints that make comfortable positioning problematic and frequent repositioning necessary

6. Cardiac disease: Treatment with diuretics, necessitating nighttime toileting and disruption of sleep

7. Pulmonary disease: Orthopnea, dyspnea, disrupted ability to breathe deeply

8. Patients who are morbidly obese: Potentially partially occluded trachea due to the compressing effect on neck and jaw from facial and neck fat when supine

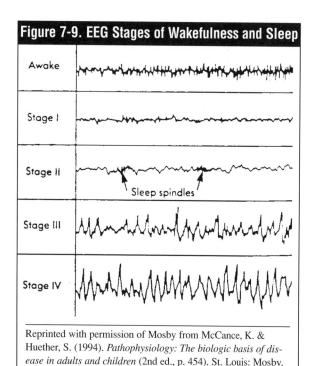

Figure 7-9. EEG Stages of Wakefulness and Sleep

Awake	
Stage I	
Stage II	Sleep spindles
Stage III	
Stage IV	

Reprinted with permission of Mosby from McCance, K. & Huether, S. (1994). *Pathophysiology: The biologic basis of disease in adults and children* (2nd ed., p. 454). St. Louis: Mosby.

The Specialty Practice of Rehabilitation Nursing: A Core Curriculum, 4th Ed.

9. Patients adjusting to permanent lifestyle changes resulting from injury and body image disruption: Depression that causes disruption of adequate restful sleep

10. Patients on medications (particularly sedatives, hypnotics, tranquilizers, and antidepressants): Disrupted normal sleep, primarily through depression of delta wave sleep. Barbiturates depress delta and REM sleep, decrease consolidated sleep, and leave the individual feeling less rested.

E. Expected Patient Outcomes Related to Sleep Patterns
   1. An established pattern that provides high-quality sleep and restoration of energy and comfort
   2. Knowledge of effective sleep-enhancing modalities

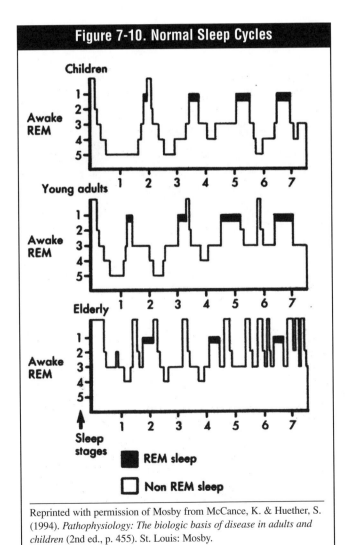

Figure 7-10. Normal Sleep Cycles

Children

Young adults

Elderly

Sleep stages

■ REM sleep

□ Non REM sleep

Reprinted with permission of Mosby from McCance, K. & Huether, S. (1994). *Pathophysiology: The biologic basis of disease in adults and children* (2nd ed., p. 455). St. Louis: Mosby.

F. Nursing Interventions
   1. Use aspects of the patient's prior bedtime routines (e.g., unwinding, relaxing activities)
   2. Play low music with gentle rhythm patterns (e.g., classical or chamber music)
   3. Provide milk or herbal decaffeinated teas and crackers
   4. Provide skin care or massage, especially using backrubs or lotions
   5. Ensure toileting before lights out
   6. Provide warmth (e.g., light blanket, bath blanket, socks)
   7. Use comfort measures (e.g., hand holding, touch therapy, prayer, guided imagery, relaxation)
   8. Ensure a quiet environment
   9. Ensure low levels of light, sound, and voices during the night
   10. Provide pain medication if indicated
   11. Use sleep medication only as a last resort because it produces artificial sleep
   12. Use available waking time whenever that occurs to consolidate nursing activities (e.g., repositioning, toileting, skin care, medications, vital signs) in ways that encourage returning to sleep
   13. Maintain a calm, unhurried demeanor that calms the patient; keep the lights low and voices hushed unless absolutely necessary
   14. Express confidence that sleep will come if the patient rests calmly

G. Interventions for Common Sleep-Related Problems
   1. Nightmares and night terrors: Use low lights to reorient the person, offer reassurances, and reestablish sleep-inducing interventions
   2. Snoring and sleep apnea: Reposition the person to a side-lying position and use pillows to retain that position
   3. Restlessness and irritability: Provide the person with a quiet, private opportunity to discuss what is troubling, offer comfort and reassurance, and then redirect to sleep
   4. Sleepwalking: Gently guide the person back to bed; it is not necessary to wake the patient
   5. Loud talking in sleep: Reposition the patient; it is not necessary to wake the patient

6. Medications
   a. Patients may rely on "sleeping pills," either prior to or while in the hospital and may have difficulty with withdrawal (rebound insomnia). The best practice is a gradual return to normal unmedicated sleep over several nights.
   b. Nurses should know the differences in available sleep-inducing medications and the contraindications for specific age groups, drug half-life, and the ability of the liver and kidneys to metabolize and excrete these drugs.

V. Mobility and Immobility

A. Overview
   1. The human body is designed to move.
   2. Mobility allows individuals to care for themselves, to interact with the environment, and to carry out purposeful activities.
   3. Balance, strength, and endurance are all components of mobility.
   4. Mobility may be lost suddenly through disease or trauma or more gradually through inactivity or illness.
   5. Prolonged immobility produces marked diminution of all body functions and places the individual in a life-threatening situation.
   6. Rehabilitation nurses identify problems of impaired mobility, set realistic goals, and collaborate with patients, families, and therapy team members to achieve these goals.

B. Nursing Assessment for Mobility
   1. Assessment of functional mobility traditionally includes four major areas.
      a. Bed mobility
      b. Transfers, including toilet transfers
      c. Wheelchair mobility
      d. Ambulation
   2. All interdisciplinary team members evaluate levels of assist (LofA) by using rankings and descriptive tools that are reliable and valid. These tools identify the amount of help or supervision needed or a device that the individual needs to perform a specific activity safely, over the required distance, and in a timely fashion.

   a. Functional Independence Measurement (FIM™) instrument, which is scored as follows:
      1) 7 = Independence
      2) 6 = Modified independence (device)
      3) 5 = Supervision or setup
      4) 4 = Minimal assistance (patient is able to do 75% or more of task)
      5) 3 = Moderate assistance (patient is able to do 50%-74% of task)
      6) 2 = Maximal assistance (patient is able to do 25%-49% of task)
      7) 1 = Total assistance (patient is able to do less than 25% of task)
   b. WeeFIM: The FIM instrument adapted for pediatric populations
   c. Other functional scales (e.g., Barthel, Katz, LORS, NANDA)
   3. Nurses assess the components of mobility.
      a. Range of motion (ROM): Evaluate range of unassisted active motion of both sides (see Figure 7-11) and distinguish between active, assisted, and passive ROM
      b. Balance: Sitting, standing, moving, amount of assistance required, and distance involved
      c. Bed mobility: Ability to turn side to side, move up in bed, move to the side of the bed, sit up in the bed, and bridge (i.e., raise hips while in the supine position)
      d. Transfer ability: Ability to move between wheelchair and bed, toilet, bath bench or shower chair, standard seating (or automobile)
      e. Wheelchair mobility
      f. Ambulation
      g. Neuromuscular problems (e.g., spasticity, rigidity, resting tremors, intention tremors, flaccidity)
      h. Coordination and proprioception
      i. Ability to follow and remember instructions
      j. Patient's expectations and past level of mobility, both recent and remote
      k. Age-appropriate growth and development and behaviors
      l. Comorbidities and general endurance

C. Expected Patient Outcomes Related to Impaired Mobility
   1. Attain optimal functional mobility using the simplest level of assistance possible
   2. Demonstrate the safe use of any needed device
D. Nursing Interventions
   1. For bed mobility
      a. Provide adequate changes in position and encourage patient's active participation
      b. Use assistive devices (e.g., siderails, trapeze, overhead frame)
   2. For transfers
      a. Provide amount of assistance required, using a consistent approach and verbal cues
      b. Use assistive devices (e.g., slide board, hydraulic [Hoyer] lift)
      c. Make adaptations for impaired transfer mobility
         1) For impaired weight-bearing mobility of one side of the body (e.g. hemiplegia, total hip precautions, fractures of the leg, unilateral leg amputation)
            a) Nurse places wheelchair on patient's strong or unaffected side (nearest armrest may need to be removed if patient is unable to come to a standing position), locks the brakes, and moves foot pedals out of the way.
            b) Patient comes to a standing position and places strong or unaffected foot forward toward chair.
            c) Patient places unaffected arm on armrest of opposite side of chair.
            d) Patient rotates body around on the ball of the unaffected foot so that body is square to the chair.
            d) Patient lowers himself or herself into chair.
            e) When another person helps the patient, the nurse explains the planned moves and encourages the patient to take sufficient time to complete each move and

maintain as much weight over his or her own feet as possible. The helper should use his or her own knees to control the patient's descent into the chair seat, while keeping one foot in front of the patient's feet to guard against slipping.
         2) For impaired weight-bearing mobility of both legs (e.g., paraplegia, bilateral amputation)
            a) Nurse places wheelchair perpendicular to the middle of the bed in the locked position.
            b) Patient raises himself or herself to sit on the bed with legs and back to the chair.
            c) Patient lifts trunk by pushing down on the mattress and hitching trunk backward.
            d) Patient grasps arms of the wheelchair and lifts self into the chair.
         3) For impaired weight-bearing mobility due to poor balance or low strength (using a slide board)
            a) Nurse places wheelchair next to the bed in the locked position and removes the armrest nearest to the bed.
            b) Patient comes to a sitting position at the side of the bed.
            c) Nurse places one end of the slide board just under the patient's buttocks and the other end on the chair.
            d) Patient hitches himself or herself toward the chair along the board by pushing down with the arms and raising the trunk or by pulling on the armrest of the wheelchair. The legs and feet follow.
            e) Once in the chair, the patient tilts away from the bed so that the slide board can be removed.
         4) For impaired weight-bearing mobility due to poor balance or low strength (using a hydraulic or Hoyer lift)

a) Nurse positions slings under the patient either in one piece or under the arms and the thighs.

b) Nurse positions the lift over the patient and lowers it so that the crossbar is accessible.

c) Nurse uses the chains to attach the slings to the crossbar, taking care to have equal length on each side and the hooks facing away from the patient.

d) With a second person available to guide the legs and torso, the nurse pumps up the lift until the patient's body clears the bed.

e) Nurse slowly moves the lift away from the bed and over the chair, which is in the locked position.

f) Nurse slowly releases the lift, allowing the patient to descend into the chair.

g) Nurse removes the chains and may leave the sling(s) in place for ease in returning the patient to bed.

3. For impaired wheelchair mobility: Wheelchairs may be used as a primary means of locomotion or for energy conservation and may be adapted to meet individual needs.

a. May be powered manually or electrically with rechargeable batteries

b. May have frame adaptations for sport participation, pediatric sizes, or body positioning requirements

c. May be controlled by one or two hands, extensions to wheel spokes or brake levers, joy sticks, pneumatic (sip and puff) switches, or voice activation

d. Wheelchair safety requires locking and unlocking brakes, controlling speed, changing direction, having appropriate body support and seating surface

4. For impaired ability to ambulate

a. Requirements for ambulation: Balance, strength, endurance, and ability to navigate various walking surfaces (e.g., floor, carpet, stairs, grass, pavement, uneven surfaces, hills)

b. Components of a normal gait: Erect balance, foot lift, push off with alternate foot, heel strike, ride-over, and heel strike of opposite foot; contralateral arms may swing to provide stability and balance.

c. Protective assistance (e.g., gait belt, hands-on supervision, verbal cues)

d. Quadricep strengthening exercises for knee and hip strength (e.g., isometric tightening of the knee and gluteus muscles, holding the contraction for 3-5 seconds,

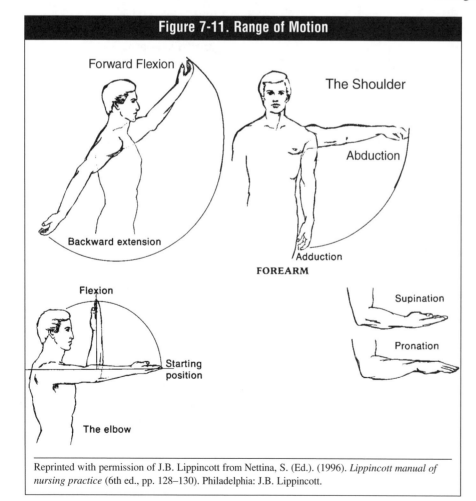

Figure 7-11. Range of Motion

Forward Flexion

Backward extension

The Shoulder

Abduction

Adduction

FOREARM

Supination

Pronation

Flexion

Starting position

The elbow

Reprinted with permission of J.B. Lippincott from Nettina, S. (Ed.). (1996). *Lippincott manual of nursing practice* (6th ed., pp. 128–130). Philadelphia: J.B. Lippincott.

The Specialty Practice of Rehabilitation Nursing: A Core Curriculum, 4th Ed.

Figure 7-11. Range of Motion (Continued)

WRIST

Radial deviation Ulnar deviation

Dorsal flexion

Palmar flexion

THUMB

Adduction

Abduction

Opposition

FINGERS

Adduction

Abduction

Extension

Neutral

ANKLE

Dorsi-flexion

Plantar flexion

Eversion

Inversion

TOES

Extension

Flexion

Adduction Abduction

Reprinted with permission of J.B. Lippincott from Nettina, S. (Ed.). (1996). *Lippincott manual of nursing practice* (6th ed., pp. 128-130). Philadelphia: J.B. Lippincott.

and then relaxing; repeated in sets of 5-10 and increased in frequency as strength returns), bicep and tricep exercises for crutch weight bearing

    e. Devices used to assist with ambulation

      1) Walkers for help with balance and forward gait: Height can be adjusted so that hands can bear some weight with elbows bent at about 30 degrees; the walker may be fitted with or without wheels; slit tennis balls may be placed over the base of the walker legs to encourage a smooth forward gait and a more normal forward progression.

      2) Hemi-walkers and platform canes for increased balance: Used with the platform extending away from the body

      3) Canes to provide stability and strength to one leg: Adjusted for fit

so that the wrist can bear some weight with the elbow slightly bent, used by placing ahead of and with the movement of the weak leg. Base tip should have a secure gripping rubber base.

    4) Crutches for protected or partial weight-bearing (two- or four-point gait) or for nonweight-bearing (three-point gait)

      a) Proper fit for standard crutches should extend from three fingers below the axilla to a point 6-8 in. to the side and out from the heel, with the handpiece allowing a 30 degree bend at the elbow and the wrist to rest on the handpiece.

      b) Base tip should have a secure wide rubber grip.

      c) Proper gait instruction includes nonweight-bearing on the axilla, careful placement of crutch tips, and caution on uneven surfaces, ice, or debris (see Figure 7-12).

      d) Forearm, Canadian, or Lofstrand crutches use the forearm for weight and are used when it is necessary to protect all joints in ambulation.

      e) Specially fitted orthoses, prostheses, and braces for support and protection: It is imperative to do skin checks before and after use.

    5. For all patients

      a. Encourage functioning at the maximally independent level that is safe

      b. Use verbal cues, reinforce learning, provide sufficient rest periods, and encourage adequate nutrition

    E. Disuse: The Hazards of Immobility (Olson, 1967)

      1. Overview

        a. Involves impairments

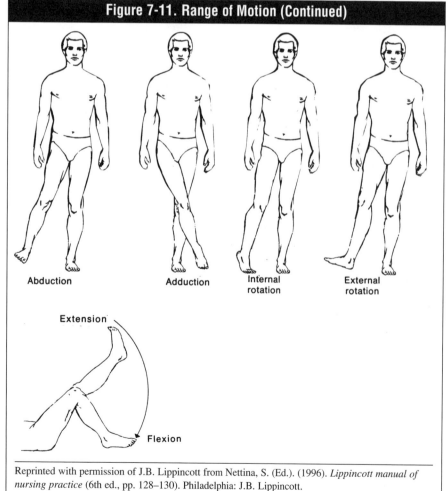

Figure 7-11. Range of Motion (Continued)

Abduction   Adduction   Internal rotation   External rotation

Extension

Flexion

Reprinted with permission of J.B. Lippincott from Nettina, S. (Ed.). (1996). *Lippincott manual of nursing practice* (6th ed., pp. 128–130). Philadelphia: J.B. Lippincott.

associated with disuse, immobility, and prolonged bed rest

   b. Affects all body systems, not just limbs affected by disease

     1) Skin breakdown and pressure ulcers from compromised circulation and pressure

     2) Bowel constipation and impaction from lowered peristalsis, inactivity, and lateral position

     3) Urinary retention, reflux, and infection from poor voiding mechanics

     4) Hypostatic pneumonia from lessened ability to clear bronchial secretions and lowered tidal volume

     5) Postural hypotension and venous thrombosis from vascular stasis

     6) Contractures of ligaments and muscle atrophy

     7) Bone demineralization from decreased stress on the bones

     8) Feelings of isolation and depression from lack of contact with others

2. Expected patient outcomes related to actual or potential hazards of immobility

   a. Prevention of as many of the sequelae of immobility as possible

   b. Early identification of impairments related to disuse

   c. Self-advocacy regarding the need to include preventive measures in daily self-care

3. Nursing interventions to prevent or limit the effects of disuse

   a. Provide frequent turning and skin care to relieve pressure and restore circulation

   b. Use pressure-relieving surfaces (e.g., air mattress, seat cushions)

   c. Pay careful attention to skin to ensure early recognition of reddened areas, wash skin gently with neutral pH soap, use lotions to lubricate skin and protect from moisture

   d. Pay attention to incontinent episodes; provide frequent checks, thorough cleaning, protective barrier creams; and adjust bowel and bladder training regimes

   e. Encourage adequate fluid intake either by mouth, G-tube, or intravenous; monitor regularly for symptoms of dehydration

   f. Establish an effective bowel program without creating long-term dependence on laxatives, cathartics, or enemas

   g. Monitor lung sounds, encourage frequent deep breathing and coughing to move and clear bronchial secretions

   h. Provide regular gentle exercise such as ROM exercises (e.g., quadricep-setting exercises)

   i. Ensure early identification of venous thrombus (e.g., fever, pain, positive Homan's sign, calf redness or warmth)

   j. Show concern for postural hypotension (e.g., quadricep-setting exercises, elastic stockings, sitting before standing)

   k. Use weight-bearing exercises to encourage retention of calcium in bones (e.g., tilt table, supported transfers)

   l. Use recreational and divisional therapy to stimulate social interaction

---

Figure 7-12. Crutch Walking Gaits

Four-Point Gait: Protected weight bearing on both feet

Right crutch followed by left foot

Left crutch followed by right foot

Repeat the pattern

Two-Point Gait: A faster version of the four-point gait

Right crutch and left foot move forward together

Left crutch and right foot move forward together

Repeat the pattern

Three-Point Gait: Full weight bearing on only one foot

Both crutches and the non-weight-bearing foot move forward together

Full weight bearing on the remaining foot

Repeat the pattern

Swing-Through Gait: A faster version of the three-point gait, also used with weight on both feet

Both crutches move forward together

Both legs are brought up to the crutches

Repeat the pattern

VI. Self-Care and Activities of Daily Living

A. Overview

1. The functional pattern of activity-exercise includes the basic elements of self-care (e.g., feeding, toileting).

    a. Activities of daily living (ADLs) include bathing, dressing, and grooming.

    b. Instrumental activities of daily living (IADLs), or more complex aspects of independence include meal preparation, household management, including finances, transportation, outdoor activities.

2. Payer sources have a major role in determining the extent of services provided and the setting in which these services are provided.

3. Rehabilitation nurses are the link between therapies, expected outcomes, and the realities of returning to community living.

B. Nursing Assessment of Self-Care Ability

1. Assess hierarchy of skills, usually learned in sequence and progress from simple to more complex (i.e., the inability to perform simpler tasks is predictive of the inability to complete more complex tasks)

2. Use rating scales to measure the level of independence or burden of care

    a. FIM instrument

        1) Is widely used by the interdisciplinary team

        2) Measures 20 discrete items (e.g., ADL, mobility, comprehension, memory) and 9 IADL items (e.g., medication administration, knowledge, compliance)

        3) Rates from 0 as maximally dependent to 5 or 7 as completely independent for each task

    b. WeeFIM: Pediatric version of FIM instrument

    c. NANDA scores for self-care and mobility: 0 = fully independent and 4 = dependent and unable (note that scoring is opposite of the FIM instrument)

    d. Mini-Mental State Exam: A short test of cognitive functions including orientation, registration, recall, calculation, language, and visual constructs

3. Assess specific motor impairments

    a. Spasticity, paralysis, flaccidity, tremors (e.g., constant, resting, intention), rigidity, contractures

    b. Energy, endurance, strength

    c. Balance while sitting and standing and the ability to self-correct alone or if pushed gently

4. Assess specific sensory impairments

    a. Visual field and acuity: Diminished or lost visual field and acuity, hemianopsia, peripheral field loss, macular degeneration, use of corrective glasses

    b. Tactile loss: Paresthesia, proprioception, temperature discrimination (needed for bathing and meal preparation)

    c. Hearing: Diminished or lost hearing, use of amplifier

5. Assess level of pain, which can interfere with learning and create additional body splinting

    a. Assess location, intensity, possible causes of pain

    b. Treat pain prior to planned therapy

C. Expected Patient Outcomes Related to Impaired Self-Care Ability

1. Complete basic self-care activities as safely and independently as possible with or without devices as appropriate

2. Demonstrate ability to use and care for assistive devices if appropriate

3. Carry out as many IADLs as is realistic as independently as possible

D. Nursing Interventions for Impaired Self-Care Ability

1. Use general teaching strategies

    a. Use the patient's preferred method of learning as much as possible

    b. Begin with simple tasks that are familiar and meaningful to the patient

    c. Repeat sequential tasks consistently

    d. Use demonstration, hand-over-hand, verbal, and written instruction

    e. Select the time of day that the patient's attention span and energy are highest

    f. Collaborate in teaching with other disciplines so that patient receives consistent, reinforcing instruction

2. Use available devices for specific losses

    a. Feeding: Plate guards, rocker knives, hand braces for utensils, nonskid place-mats for stability, drinking cups with weighted bases and wide mouths

    b. Bathing and hygiene: Face cloths, mitts, soap-on-a-rope, long-handled sponges, nailbrushes with suction cups, hand braces for toothbrush, freestanding mirrors, shower mats, grab bars, shower seats

    c. Dressing: Long-handled shoe horns, reachers, Velcro closures for clothes, elastic shoelaces, Sock Aide

    d. Grooming: Long-handled combs, adapted holders for razor, long-handled mirrors for skin inspection

    e. Toileting: Raised toilet seats, transfer bars

3. Adapt care to manage impaired energy and endurance

    a. Teach pacing techniques

    b. Provide work simplification strategies

    c. Ensure changes in workplace environment to accommodate height and sitting needs

    d. Recruit assistance

    e. Gradually increase tasks when the patient's skills and strength return

4. Provide strategies for household management and use of community resources

VII. Sexuality and Reproduction

A. Overview

1. Sexuality and reproduction are important issues for rehabilitation patients.

2. Disability and major illnesses affect sexual function, self-esteem, body image, and social relationships.

3. Rehabilitation nurses play a major role in educating patients about the effects of injury or illness on sexual function and reproduction.

4. To promote an atmosphere of permission and acceptance, rehabilitation nurses should separate their own values and attitudes in the area of sexuality in order to address the issue objectively.

5. Rehabilitation nurses should know about available methods and aids to enhance sexual expression and conception after disability.

B. Stages and Descriptions of Human Sexual Response Cycle (see Table 7-2)

C. Normal Physiology of Sexual Response

1. Men

    a. Penis is innervated by sympathetic (T10-L2), parasympathetic (S2-S4), and somatic (pudendal nerve) fibers.

    b. Erection is under parasympathetic, sympathetic, and somatic control.

    c. Psychogenic response is initiated by cortical input, including visual and tactile senses, and mediated by sympathetic pathways (T10-L2).

    d. Reflex is initiated by internal or external tactile stimulation and mediated by sacral spinal reflex (S2-S4).

    e. Emission is under sympathetic control (T10-L2), and ejaculation is under sympathetic and somatic control (S2-S4).

    f. Fertility depends on endocrine regulation, ejaculatory ability, and semen quality.

2. Women

    a. Genitalia is innervated by sympathetic (pudendal nerve and perineal nerve) and parasympathetic (splanchnic nerve) fibers.

    b. Orgasm is thought to be under parasympathetic (S2-S4) and somatic control.

    c. Fertility depends on endocrine regulation of ovulation cycles.

D. Expected Patient Outcomes Related to Sexual Function

1. Personal satisfaction with sexual function

2. Avoidance of sexually transmitted diseases

3. Pregnancy, if desired and possible

4. Ability to plan and carry out parenting roles if appropriate

E. PLISSIT Model for Sexual Counseling

1. Permission: Process of allowing questions or fears to be raised and giving permission to talk about the subject

2. Limited Information: Providing some specific information related to questions raised or concerns expressed and allowing the person to pursue the issue further if they are comfortable

3. Specific Suggestions: Assisting people with problem identification, providing specific suggestions to resolve a problem (e.g., suggestions to deal with erectile dysfunction, bowel and bladder concerns, positioning, contraception)
4. Intensive Therapy: Providing expert assistance for intensive discussion and intervention (e.g., psychotherapy for marriage and relationship counseling, medical management of impotence, infertility, childbirth)

F. Neurophysiology of Erection with Spinal Cord Injury
G. Common Classes of Medications and Their Effects on Sexual Functioning (see Table 7-3)
H. Functional Problems and Their Potential Effects

Table 7-2. Stages of Human Sexual Responses

Both Men and Women	Women	Men
Excitement Stage I		
Increased muscle tension	Clitoris swells	Penis becomes erect
Increased pulse rate	Labia majora flatten and separate	Scrotum rises
Increased blood pressure	Vaginal lubrication	Testes swell and move to body
Sex flush	Breasts enlarge	
Nipple erection	Uterus elevates and expands	
Plateau Stage II (time varies greatly)		
Muscle tension increases	Clitoris withdraws	Testes grow 2-3 times usual size
Pulse rate 100-160 beats/minute	Vaginal vasocongestion or orgasmic platform narrows	Glans color deepens, head diameter grows
Fast breathing	Vaginal opening expands inner two-thirds	Cowper's secretion
Sex flush	Uterus elevated	
	Breast areola swell	
	Vivid coloration of labia minora from bright red to deep wine	
Orgasm Stage III (lasts a few seconds)		
Rhythmic muscle contractions, then intense physical sensations, then relaxation	Clitoris retracts	Penis, urethra, and muscles at base of penis
Sex flush after pulse increases	Uterus contracts with outer third of vagina and anal sphincter	Ejaculation of initial spurts of semen; bladder neck closes; gradually tapers off
Blood pressure increases	Vaginal contractions or pelvic throbbing—may have multiple orgasms	
Respirations fast		
Relaxation Stage IV (lasts a few minutes to hours)		
Muscles relax	Clitoris descends	Loss of erection
Normal pulse	Labia, vagina, breasts, and uterus return to usual size and place	Scrotum and testes lower and return to usual size and place
Normal blood pressure		
Nipple erection reduces		
Sex flush subsides		

Reprinted with permission of Mosby from Hoeman, S. (Ed.). (1996). *Rehabilitation nursing: Process and application* (2nd ed.). St. Louis: Mosby. Originally adapted with permission from Masters, W.H., Johnson, V.E., & Kolodny, R.C. (1986). *Masters and Johnson on sex and human loving*. Boston: Little, Brown.

The Specialty Practice of Rehabilitation Nursing: A Core Curriculum, 4th Ed.

on Sexual Relationships (Table 7-4)

I. Reproductive Capabilities After Disability (Table 7-5)

J. Additional Issues Surrounding Reproduction

1. Contraception: The method should be based on the patient's physical ability, cognitive ability to comply, potential medical risks of oral contraceptive use, and personal preferences.

2. Pregnancy, childbirth, and parenting: Options vary according to the disability, available resources, and medical issues.

3. Fertility

   a. Causes of infertility: Anejaculation, impaired semen quality, impaired endocrine regulation

   b. In men with spinal cord injury, semen quality consists of normal sperm count with impaired sperm motility. Lifestyle factors such as scrotal temperatures, frequency of ejaculation, or bladder management methods were once thought to be the cause of impaired semen quality; however, research suggests that factors in the seminal plasma may be the cause of poor sperm motility (Brackett, Ferrell, Aballa, Armador, & Lynne, 1998).

   c. Treatment

      1) Vibratory stimulation and electroejaculation for anejaculation

      2) Pregnancy attempts with or without medical assistance, depending on semen quality and the couple's reproductive health

      3) Options: Intravaginal

and intrauterine inseminations (IUI), in vitro fertilization (IVF), gamete intrafallopian transfer (GIFT), and intracytoplasmic sperm injection (ICSI)

K. Safety Issues Related to Sexuality

1. Sexually transmitted diseases

   a. Syphilis, gonorrhea

   b. AIDS

   c. Hepatitis

2. Sexual abuse

L. Age-Specific Issues

1. Pediatric: Injury and congenital disorders

2. Adolescence: Concerns regarding acceptance, role, and relationships

3. Adults: Concerns regarding fertility, biological parenthood, pregnancy, and parenting

4. Older adults: Consideration of the normal effects of aging and their relationship to disability or availability of a partner

Table 7-3. Medications and Sexual Functioning

Medications	Potential Effects
Antihypertensives	Diminished sex drive, erectile ability, ejaculatory function
Anticholesterolemics	Erectile dysfunction, low sex drive
Digoxin	Decreased testosterone and luteinizing hormone in conjunction with increased estrogen; decreased desire, arousal, and erectile function
Antiarrythmics	Erectile dysfunction
Antidepressants	Erectile and ejaculatory dysfunction, anorgasm, spontaneous orgasms and ejaculation, decreased sexual desire
Benzodiazepines	Delayed orgasm or anorgasmia in women, delayed ejaculation in men, decreased sexual desire and arousal
Anticonvulsants	Erectile dysfunction, diminished sexual desire
H2 blockers	Decreased libido, erectile dysfunction, decreased sperm count
Alcohol	Transient relaxation but suppression of motor activity
Sedatives and tranquilizers	Relaxation and tranquilization, central sedation

Nurses should make patients aware of these side effects and encourage the patient to ask his or her physician to explore alternative doses or drugs as needed.

Adapted with permission of Sipski, M.L., & Alexander, C.J. (1998). Sexuality and disability. In J.A. DeLisa & B.M. Gans (Eds.), *Rehabilitation medicine: Principles and practice* (3rd ed., p. 1111). Philadelphia: Lippincott-Raven.

Table 7-4. Functional Problems and Their Potential Effects on Sexual Relationships

Functional Problem	Potential Effects	Suggestions
Sensory/Perception		
Vision	Decreased ability to appreciate visual stimuli, difficulties with depth perception	If unilateral, uninjured partner should lie on unaffected side; use other senses (e.g., verbal, touch)
Sensation	Increased sensitivity or decreased/absent tactile sensation	Define areas of tactile loss, modify stimuli to that part, modify touch to areas of hypersensitivity
Proprioception (position sense)	Injured partner may not know where body parts are without visualizing, making sexual play clumsy or uncomfortable	Allow enough light for visualization; use positioning supports for comfort
Right-left discrimination	Injured partner may not be able to follow through with directions from partner	Direct injured partner by using terms other than right or left; use hand-over-hand guidance
Neglect or denial of deficits	Injured partner may have difficulty recognizing limitation and overstate abilities; may cause embarrassment for both partners if overstated abilities are acted out	Uninjured partner take more active role and gently redirect partner; use positioning with pillows; alternate positions
Communication		
Aphasia/dysarthria	Injured partner may have difficulty correctly interpreting affect of partner or expressing own desires	Use nonverbal communication (touching, gestures)
Concrete thinking	Injured partner may miss subtle cues; sexual play may be concretely focused and one sided	Uninjured partner may need to be very direct with sexual communication and give more specific directions to focus on mutual pleasure
Disinhibition/impulse control	Injured partner may make inappropriate or offending statement to partner; may increase number of sexual partners as a result of impulse control; may show inappropriate public display of sexual impulses or activity	Uninjured partner should give feedback to partner about responses and provide suggestions for better alternatives; enforce privacy and a consistent routine; do not reinforce inappropriate behaviors; may need to implement social skills retraining in matters related to sexual behaviors with the opposite sex
Cognition		
Attention/concentration	Injured partner may be restless; unable to focus on sexual play; may affect ability to sustain an erection	Decrease external distractions during sexual play; use relaxation/imagery/ guided fantasy by uninjured partner
Memory/judgment	If short-term memory is impaired, injured partner may persevere on a sexual activity, request, or pressure partner for frequent sex; contraceptive method use should not rely on memory of injured partner	Log sexual activity; discuss contraceptive options with physician; uninjured partner may need to take responsibility for contraception
Initiative	Injured partner may lack ability to take active role in creating a supportive environment	Uninjured partner may need to initiate, provide romantic environment, encourage

Table 7-4. (Continued)

Functional Problem	Potential Effects	Suggestions
Mobility Impairment		
Paralysis	Inability to move body or a body part to position self or to respond to moves by the uninjured partner	Use pillows, alternate positioning strategies; uninjured partner may need to take more active role
Spasticity	Involuntary muscle contractions of affected parts of body; may interfere with attempts to position or reposition	Use positions that place less stress on muscles that tend to spasm; select positions so that if spasms occur, they will not disrupt activity; use reminders to tend to bowel and bladder needs before initiating foreplay; be aware that pain in another part of the body may set off spasms; pay attention to positioning
Elimination		
Bladder dysfunction	Bladder accidents during sexual activity decrease the appeal of sexual activity; presence of Foley catheter may be a hindrance to sexual activity; presence of urostomy may be a viewed as a hindrance to sexual enjoyment	Restrict fluids prior to sexual activity; complete toileting; keep towel or urinal nearby for potential accidents; if Foley catheter present, can be taped to the side (for females to the thigh, for males to the abdomen or place a condom over the shaft of penis); avoid positions that place pressure on the bladder; cover urostomy or tape to abdomen
Bowel dysfunction	Bowel accidents during sexual activity decrease the appeal of sexual activity; presence of colostomy or ileostomy may be viewed as a hindrance to sexual activity	Complete bowel regime prior to sexual activity; avoid positions that place pressure on the bowels; cover ostomy, tape to the side or remove and use an ostomy cap over stoma
Erectile Dysfunction/Anorgasm		
Male is unable to establish and/or maintain an erection	Decreased ability for penile-vaginal intercourse	Explore alternative forms of sexual satisfaction, stuffing method, exploration of erogenous zones; seek psychological counseling; get referrals for erectile dysfunction assessment; use impotence treatments and medications (e.g., topical, intraurethral, oral, injectable); use external vacuum therapy; use penile implants (e.g., semi-rigid, inflatable)
Woman is unable to achieve orgasm	Decreased ability to reach climax	Explore alternative forms of sexual satisfaction; seek psychological counseling; educate about potential to have orgasm; encourage use of clitoral stimulation

Sources consulted

Rehabilitation Nursing Foundation (RNF). (1995). *Rehabilitation nursing: Directions for practice—a basic rehabilitation nursing course* (3rd ed., pp. 164-170). Glenview, IL: Rehabilitation Nursing Foundation of the Association of Rehabilitation Nurses.

Sipski, M.L., & Alexander, C.J. (1998). Sexuality and disability. In J.A. DeLisa & B.M. Gans (Eds.), *Rehabilitation medicine: Principles and practice* (3rd ed.). Philadelphia: Lippincott-Raven.

Table 7-5. Reproductive Capabilities After Disability

Diagnosis	Fertility	Pregnancy	Childbirth	Parenting
Arthritis (includes hip and knee disease)	Unchanged	Increased pressure on joints due to weight gain	Potential need for cesarean section depending on joint involvement	Increased energy needs and pressure on joints required in child care
Brain injury	Possible premature ejaculation due to decreased attention span (men); poor libido and behavioral changes may interfere with sexual relationships (men and women)	Cognitive deficits possibly requiring assistance to ensure good prenatal care	Spasticity and sensory deficits may necessitate planned labor induction and/or cesarean section	Cognitive, temper control, memory, safety, awareness, ADL or mobility deficits possibly requiring client to obtain assistance
Stroke	Unchanged (women) (see Brain injury); possible vascular or psychogenic impotence (men) (see Brain injury)	Plan around fully stabilized CVA, especially hemorrhagic CVA, if possible	See Brain injury	See Brain injury Need for home and equipment modifications
Spinal cord injury	Temporary disruption of the menstrual cycle and ovulation (women); impaired due to anejaculation and/or poor sperm motility; cause of poor sperm quality is unknown (men)	Need for close medical supervision, possible increase in spasms due to the weight of the fetus, increased fatigue, circulation problems, edema, more difficulty with ADLs and transfers, bladder infections, or autonomic dysreflexia due to pressure of the fetus	Inability to feel contractions in injuries at or above T10, possibility of induction of a cesarean section, possibility of dysreflexia during delivery, especially with vaginal delivery	

Source consulted

McCourt, A. (Ed.). (1993). *The specialty practice of rehabilitation nursing: A core curriculum* (3rd ed.). Skokie, IL: The Rehabilitation Nursing Foundation of the Association of Rehabilitation Nurses.

References

Bergstrom, N., Bennett, M.A., Carlson, C.E., et al. (1994). *Treatment of pressure ulcers: Clinical practice guideline no. 15* (AHCPR Publication No. 95-0652). Rockville, MD: U.S. Department of Health and Human Services, Public Health Service, Agency for Health Care Policy and Research.

Brackett, N.L., Ferrell, S.M., Aballa, T.C., Amador, M.J., & Lynne, C.M. (1998). Semen quality in spinal cord injured men: Does it progressively decline post injury? *Archives of Physical Medicine and Rehabilitation, 79,* 625–628.

DeLisa, J., & Gans, B. (1998). *Rehabilitation medicine: Principles and practice* (3rd ed.). Philadelphia: Lippincott.

Feeder, J. (1994). Understanding the pressure ulcer problem. *Topics in Geriatric Medicine, 9*(4), 1–7.

Guccione, A. (Ed.). (1993). *Geriatric physical therapy.* St. Louis: Mosby.

Hoeman, S. (Ed.). (1996). *Rehabilitation nursing: Process and application* (2nd ed.). St. Louis: Mosby.

Kryger, M., Roth, T., & Dement, W.C. (1994). *Principles and practice of sleep medicine.* Philadelphia: W.B. Saunders.

Logemann, J. (1998). *Evaluation and treatment of swallowing disorders* (2nd ed.). Austin, TX: Pro-Ed.

Masters, W.H., Johnson, V.E., & Kolodny, R.C. (1986). *Masters and Johnson on sex and human loving.* Boston: Little, Brown.

McCance, K., & Huether, S. (Eds.). (1994). *Pathophysiology: The biologic basis of disease in adults and children* (2nd ed.). St. Louis: Mosby.

McCourt, A. (Ed.). (1993). *The specialty practice of rehabilitation nursing: A core curriculum* (3rd ed.). Skokie, IL: The Rehabilitation Nursing Foundation of the Association of Rehabilitation Nurses.

McCulloch, J., Kloth, L., & Freedon, J. (1995). *Wound healing: Alternatives in management* (2nd ed.). Philadelphia: F.A. Davis.

McHale, J., Phipps, M., Hovarth, K., & Schmelz, J. (1998). Expert nursing knowledge in the care of patients at risk of impaired swallowing. *Image: The Journal of Nursing Scholarship, 30*(2), 137–141.

Nettina, S. (Ed.). (1996). *Lippincott manual of nursing practice* (6th ed.). Philadelphia: J.B. Lippincott.

Olson, E.V. (1967). The hazards of immobility. *American Journal of Nursing, 67*(4), 781–797.

Pires, M., & Lockhart-Pretti, P. (1992). *Nursing management of neurogenic incontinence.* Skokie, IL: Rehabilitation Nursing Foundation of the Association of Rehabilitation Nurses.

Rehabilitation Nursing Foundation (RNF). (1995). *Rehabilitation nursing: Directions for practice—a basic rehabilitation nursing course* (3rd ed., pp. 164–170). Glenview, IL: Rehabilitation Nursing Foundation of the Association of Rehabilitation Nurses.

Sipski, M.L., & Alexander, C.J. (1998). Sexuality and disability. In J.A. DeLisa & B.M. Gans (Eds.), *Rehabilitation medicine: Principles and practice* (3rd ed., pp. 1107–1125). Philadelphia: Lippincott-Raven.

Welch, M., Logemann, J., Rademaker, A.W., & Kahrilas, P.J. (1993). Changes in pharyngeal dimensions effected by chin tuck. *Archives of Physical Medicine, 74*(2), 178–181.

Zejdilk, C.J. (1992). *Management of spinal cord injury* (2nd ed.). Boston: Jones and Bartlett.

Suggested resources

Amador, M.J., Lynne, C.M., & Brackett, N.L. (1998). Contemporary information regarding male fertility following spinal cord injury. *Spinal Cord Injury Nursing, 15,* 61–65.

Bergman-Gainea, M. (1996). Independent function: Movement and mobility. In S. Hoeman (Ed.), *Rehabilitation nursing: Process and application* (2nd ed., pp. 225–269). St. Louis: Mosby.

Brackett, N.L., & Armador, A. (in press). *Guides and resource directory to male infertility following spinal cord injury/dysfunction.* Paralyzed Veterans of America grant supported project.

Brackett, N.L., Nash, M.S., & Lynne, C.M. (1996). Male fertility following spinal cord injury: Facts and fiction. *Physical Therapy, 76,* 1221–1231.

Braddom, R.L. (Ed.). (1996). *Physical medicine and rehabilitation.* Philadelphia: W.B. Saunders.

Chang, D. (1995). Measurement of IADL in stroke. *Stroke, 26*(6), 1119–1122.

Cook, L. (1999). The value of lab values. *American Journal of Nursing, 99*(5), 66–75.

Dittmar, S., & Grecham, G. (1997). *Functional assessment and outcome measures for the rehabilitation professional.* Gaithersberg, MD: Aspen.

Edwards, P., Hertzberg, D., Hays, S., & Youngblood, N. (Eds.). (1999). *Pediatric rehabilitation nursing.* Philadelphia: W.B. Saunders.

Fine, C.K. (Ed.). (1994). *Application of rehabilitation concepts to nursing practice.* Skokie, IL: Rehabilitation Nursing Foundation.

Glenn, N. (1996). Eating and swallowing. In S. Hoeman (Ed.), *Rehabilitation nursing: Process and application* (2nd ed., pp. 347-360). St. Louis: Mosby.

Gordon, M. (1994). *Nursing diagnosis, process and application.* St. Louis: Mosby.

Greco, S. (1996). Sexuality education and counseling. In S. Hoeman (Ed.), *Rehabilitation nursing: Process and application* (2nd ed., pp. 594–627). St. Louis: Mosby.

Guenther, P. (1997). Enteral nutrition therapy. *Nursing Clinics of North America, 32*(4), 651–668.

Habel, M. (1996). Sleep, rest, and fatigue. In S. Hoeman (Ed.), *Rehabilitation nursing: Process and application* (2nd ed., pp. 508-525). St. Louis: Mosby.

Hammond, K. (1997). Physical assessment: A nutritional perspective. *Nursing Clinics of North America, 32*(4), 779–790.

Hammond, K., & Zafonte, R. (1997). Drugs for management of sleep disorders. *Physical Medicine and Rehabilitation Clinics of North America, 8*(4), 801–812.

Hays, S. (1999). Physical health care patterns and nursing interventions. In P. Edwards, D. Hertzberg, S. Hays, & N. Youngblood (Eds.), *Pediatric rehabilitation nursing* (pp. 218-257). Philadelphia: W.B. Saunders.

Johnson, E., McKenzie, S., Rosenquist, J., Lieberman, J., & Sievers, A. (1992). Dysphagia following stroke: Quantitative evaluation of pharyngeal transit times. *Archives of Physical Medicine and Rehabilitation, 73*(4), 419–423.

Johnson, K. (Ed.). (1997). *Advanced practice nursing in rehabilitation.* Glenview, IL: Rehabilitation Nursing Foundation and Association of Rehabilitation Nurses.

Kelly-Hays, M. (1996). Functional evaluation. In S. Hoeman (Ed.), *Rehabilitation nursing: Process and application* (2nd ed., pp. 144-155). St. Louis: Mosby.

Knoll, S., Bender, C., & Nelson, M. (1996). Rehabilitation of patients with swallowing disorders. In R.L. Braddom (Ed.), *Physical medicine and rehabilitation*. Philadelphia: W.B. Saunders.

LaMantia, J. (1996). Skin integrity. In S. Hoeman (Ed.), *Rehabilitation nursing: Process and application* (2nd ed., pp. 273–306). St. Louis: Mosby.

Lee, K.A. (1997). An overview of sleep and common sleep problems. *American Nephrology Nurses Association, 24*(6), 614–619.

Lewis, C. (1996). *Aging: A healthcare challenge* (3rd ed.). Philadelphia: F.A. Davis.

Mahan, L.K., & Escott-Stumps, S. (1996). *Krause's food nutrition and diet therapy* (9th ed.). Philadelphia: W.B. Saunders.

Mumma, C., & Nelson, A. (1996). Models for theory-based practice. In S. Hoeman (Ed.), *Rehabilitation nursing: Process and application* (2nd ed., pp. 21–33). St. Louis: Mosby.

Rogers, M. (1970). *An introduction to the theoretical basis of nursing*. Philadelphia: F.A. Davis.

Sipski, M.L. (1997). *Sexual function in people with disability and chronic illness: A health professional's guide*. Gaithersberg, MD: Aspen.

Theuerkauf, A. (1996). Self-care and activities of daily living. In S. Hoeman (Ed.), *Rehabilitation nursing: Process and application* (2nd ed., pp. 156–187). St. Louis: Mosby.

Urinary Incontinence Guideline Panel. (1992). *Urinary incontinence in adults: Clinical practice guidelines* (AHCPR Publication No. 92-0038). Rockville, MD: U.S. Department of Health and Human Services, Public Health Service, Agency for Health Care Policy and Research.

Youngblood, N. (1999). Models for practice and service. In P. Edwards, D. Hertzberg, S. Hays, & N. Youngblood (Eds.), *Pediatric rehabilitation nursing* (pp. 113–126). Philadelphia: W.B. Saunders.

Chapter 8

Psychosocial Healthcare Patterns and Nursing Interventions

Barbara Brillhart, PhD RN CRRN FNP-C

Rehabilitation nurses must have an understanding of the concept of psychosocial health, which involves how mental processes and social interactions influence the behavior of an individual. Theories of development, learning, and chronic illness support psychosocial healthcare patterns. Psychosocial health incorporates cognition, behaviors, sensations, perceptions, self-concept, and role attainment. Rehabilitation nurses promote psychosocial health through professional assessment and interventions. The theories and concepts presented in this chapter provide a foundation for rehabilitation nurses to promote psychosocial health over the life span.

I. Developmental Considerations Related to Psychosocial Health

A. Cognitive Maturation in Children

1. Cognitive deficits can have a profound influence on the life of a developing child; these deficits impair the input, reasoning, and thinking processes needed for normal development.

   a. Children with brain injuries can have impaired cognitive development.

   b. Delays in speech and language development related to deafness, mental deficits, or emotional disturbances can affect the child's psychosocial development

2. Piaget's (1952) and Erikson's (1963) levels of cognitive development for children provide a theoretical basis for normal development *[Refer to Chapter 15 for more on developmental stages.]*

   a. Sensorimotor period (0-2 years)

      1) Description

         a) The psychosocial development of trust vs. mistrust: Disruptions in cognitive achievement during this period impair and restrict the psychosocial development of infants and toddlers (Piaget, 1952).

      b) Examples

         (1) An 8-month-old child demonstrates goal-directed activities

         (2) A 12-month-old child understands means-to-end relationships

         (3) A 2-year-old child has the beginnings of symbolic thinking

      2) Nursing interventions: Promote sensory stimulation, security by caregivers, motor coordination, consistent personal attention, and parental education regarding growth and development

   b. Preoperative period (2-7 years)

      1) Description: The development of autonomy vs. shame, initiative vs. guilt, and the beginning of industry vs. inferiority (Erikson, 1963; Piaget, 1952)

         a) Children use representative thought to recall past events, represent the present, and anticipate the future

         b) Children ages 4-7 years use increased symbolic functioning

         c) Children with learning disabilities exhibit deficits in social skills (e.g., social perception, behavior problems, problem-solving difficulties, problems with verbal communication) (Cermak & Aberson, 1997)

    2) Nursing interventions

        a) Encourage exploration of the environment

        b) Encourage participation in age-appropriate activities

        c) Promote consistent, affectionate caregiving

        d) Diversify environmental stimuli

        e) Provide intellectual stimulation

        f) Promote peer interaction

        g) Continue parental education about age-appropriate growth and development

c. Concrete operative period (7-11 years)

    1) Description

        a) The continued development of industry vs. inferiority, which is characterized by cognitive, concrete operations

        b) Children use logical approaches to solve concrete problems

    2) Nursing interventions

        a) Promote peer interaction and socialization

        b) Encourage formal education with peers

        c) Promote creativity

        d) Continue parental education of growth and development

        e) Continue consistent interaction with parents, family, caregivers, and teachers

d. Formal operative period (11-15 years)

    1) Description: The development of identity vs. role confusion

        a) Adolescents are capable of logical thought and abstract thinking

        b) Role expectations include increasing independence, being socially successful and more mature, increasing autonomy, and increasing responsibilities

(Satir, 1988)

        c) Adolescents develop competence in self-esteem, body image, personal achievement, interpersonal relationships, and responsibility. Those with disabilities may have impaired social development if they view themselves as asexual, unattractive, or incompetent with social relationships (Sawin & Marshall, 1992)

        d) Injury or illness in late childhood necessitates creating new body and self-representativeness to correspond with changed physical being. This can be a lengthy and painful process, during which the old self is mourned. The course of adjustment is influenced by the adolescent's level of independence and the autonomy granted by the family (Voll & Poustka, 1994)

        e) Adolescents who have had a traumatic injury desire to return to their preinjury status and their school and recreational activities. Family love—in the form of physical presence, psychological or spiritual support, and motivation—is critical. The desire and motivation to regain wellness is self-initiated and requires the support of family and peers (DeWitt, 1993)

    2) Nursing interventions

        a) Treat the adolescent as a normal person

        b) Allow time for the adolescent to adjust to changes due to injury

        c) Encourage the adolescent to have close bonds with family and nurses

        d) Provide information to reduce fears and misconceptions regarding the injury

        e) Provide encouragement, peer support, and motivation (DeWitt, 1993)

The Specialty Practice of Rehabilitation Nursing: A Core Curriculum, 4th Ed.

f) Foster the adolescent's friend-
ships with peers

g) Give the adolescent
responsibilities

h) Ensure appropriate parental
protectiveness

i) Ensure that the adolescent is
involved with decision making
(Sawin & Marshall, 1992)

B. Cognitive Maturation with Adults

1. Description of social learning theory
(Bandura, 1977)

a. This theory explains human behaviors in
terms of active, dynamic interactions of
behaviors, personal factors, and
environmental influences

b. Personal interactions include the person's ability to symbolize behavioral
meanings, foresee the outcomes of
behaviors, learn through observations
and experiences, and self-determine and
self-regulate his or her life

c. Adults reflect and analyze to give
meaning to experiences

d. Young and middle-aged adult development fulfills the psychosocial phases of
intimacy vs. role confusion and generativity vs. stagnation (Erikson, 1963)

e. Cognitive and physical disability can
affect the potential and motivation to
fulfill developmental phases

f. The roles of young adults can include
positive pairing

1) Positive pairing is characterized by
willing, knowledgeable, respectful
support within the pair and includes
relationships based on equality of
value of the couple

2) Successful pairing depends on personal autonomy, emotional honesty,
expression of needs, responsibility,
accountability, freedom of choice,
and cooperation (Satir, 1988)

2. Nursing interventions

a. Promote recreational therapy

b. Encourage socialization with peers

c. Ensure access to vocational and academic counseling and education

d. Provide family counseling

e. Foster autonomy, independence, and
personal responsibility

C. Cognitive Maturation with Elderly People

1. The last psychosocial developmental phase
of ego identity vs. despair

a. Elderly people reflect on their lives and
remember worthwhile and unique
experiences

b. Disability and chronic illness can profoundly affect quality of life and
psychosocial satisfaction

c. Transition is needed to progress from the
middle-aged adult to elderly adult

1) Transitional steps start with acknowl-
edging changes that occur with aging

2) Mixed feelings are present with
changes in work status and lifestyle

3) A successful transition is characterized by the realization of the positive
aspects of aging and moving toward
new challenges.

4) A successful transition must incorporate positive attitudes feelings of
worth, flexibility, feeling of purpose,
having positive relationships, and
being part of the community (Satir,
1988)

2. Nursing interventions

a. Promote recreational therapy

b. Encourage socialization

c. Provide family counseling

d. Allow the client to reflect and reminisce

e. Foster autonomy, independence, respect,
and personal responsibility

II. A Family-Focused Care Model for Clients with Chronic Illness

A. Overview

1. Psychosocial adjustment for people with disability or chronic illness occurs in a recurrent, longitudinal sequence of stages that
involve the person with disability or illness
and his or her family and friends

2. A conceptual model, Family-Focused Care
of the Chronically Ill (Butcher, 1994) (see
Figure 8-1), can be applied to the complexity
of psychosocial healthcare patterns

B. Concepts Associated with the Model (Butcher, 1994)

1. Optimal family health: The core of the model. The concepts of development, integrity, coping, health, and interaction influence the core and all of the other concepts in an interlocking pattern

2. Development: Composed of developmental stages, developmental tasks, and family transitions. Disability can have a profound effect on the developmental capacity of the client and family

3. Coping: Composed of managing resources, problem solving, and adapting to stress and crisis. Effective coping combines family members' coping abilities in an individual and collective manner

4. Integrity: Composed of family identity and commitment; family values, history, and rituals; shared meaning of experiences; and maintenance of boundaries

5. Interaction: Contains social support, communication, and family relationships Communication is the key factor, which forms the basis of the quality of social and family relationships

6. Health: Contains health practices, health beliefs and status, and lifestyle practices, which are modified, adapted, and reformatted to meet the needs of the individual and family related to disability or chronic illness

III. Theories of Learning

A. Classical or Pavlovian Conditioning (Pavlov, 1927)

1. Initially, a neutral response is associated with another stimulus that elicits an unconditioned response

2. Eventually, the neutral stimulus elicits the response

3. Emotions are partially subject to classical learning (e.g., fear of an object or pet)

B. Operant Conditioning (Skinner, 1974)

1. Operant conditioning involves changing a child's behavior by providing a reward or reinforcement for the consequence of the child's responses

2. Reinforcement is the key element in operative learning theory

   a. People tend to repeat behaviors that have desirable outcomes

   b. Systematic reinforcement with positive reinforcers affects the rate at which responses occur

   c. Reinforcers can also be negative if they are being used to terminate an aversive behavior

   d. A conditioned behavior can be extinguished (undone) by repeatedly failing to reinforce it

   e. Behaviors can be inhibited (counteracted) by avoiding punishment

   f. Behaviors can be partially reinforced by inconsistent or random responses

C. Social Learning Theory (Bandura, 1977)

1. Positive reinforcement (e.g., food, care, attention) shapes behaviors.

2. Learning occurs when behaviors are modified in response to physical rewards (e.g.,

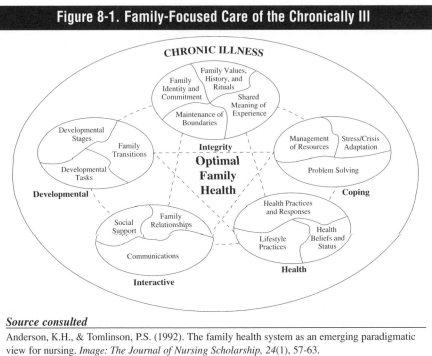

Figure 8-1. Family-Focused Care of the Chronically Ill

CHRONIC ILLNESS

Family Values, History, and Rituals
Family Identity and Commitment
Shared Meaning of Experience
Maintenance of Boundaries

Developmental Stages
Family Transitions
Developmental Tasks

Developmental

Integrity

Optimal Family Health

Management of Resources
Stress/Crisis Adaptation
Problem Solving

Coping

Social Support
Family Relationships
Communications

Interactive

Health Practices and Responses
Lifestyle Practices
Health Beliefs and Status

Health

Source consulted

Anderson, K.H., & Tomlinson, P.S. (1992). The family health system as an emerging paradigmatic view for nursing. *Image: The Journal of Nursing Scholarship, 24*(1), 57-63.

food) and indirect rewards (e.g., a smile)

3. Negative reinforcement (e.g., punishment) can be used to modify behaviors

4. Social learning theory is initiated within the family and later is influenced by the values and customs of those outside the family (e.g., peers and role models at school)

5. Desired behaviors are obtained through direct observation and imitation of another's performance

D. Gestalt Learning Theory (Wertheimer, 1959)

1. This theory defines learning as a reorganization of the person's perceptual or psychological world

2. The focus is on motivation, perception, and transference of learning

3. A person's perception is related to the total situation and involves the interactions of many factors. The interaction of the person and environment is simultaneous and mutual

4. Learning occurs when the person tries to give meaning to the environment and successfully uses objects in the environment

E. Andragogical Model of Adult Learning (Knowles, 1984)

1. Adult learners are self-directed and responsible for their own learning

2. Learners assess their own needs for learning and form their own objectives

3. Learners possess a wide range of experiences; therefore, individualized learning plans are stressed

4. Readiness to learn is determined by the need to know something in order to achieve a task

5. Positive andragogy includes the presence of interactive environments, mutual respect, collaboration, mutual trust, support, openness, authenticity, pleasure, and mutual planning

6. Learners evaluate their own level of learning by evaluating whether they have achieved their personal goals

IV. Cognitive Influences on Psychosocial Health

A. Cognition

1. Description

a. Cognition is defined as the concept of thinking and is composed of attention,

memory, abstract reasoning, generalization, concept formation, problem solving, and executive function (Grzankowski, 1997); cognitive deficits may involve one or more of these factors

b. Cognition depends on sensory input, prior experiences, learning, and recall and memory

c. An injury to the cortex of the brain or the neural pathways interferes with sensory input, cognitive integration, and planning appropriate responses

d. The cerebral cortex, internal nuclei, basal ganglia, and the cerebellum process and integrate sensory input as well as motor planning (see Table 8-1)

e. Recovery depends on the extent, quality (e.g., edema vs. destruction), and area of the injury (Grzankowski, 1997)

2. Assessment

a. Evaluate the client's ability to determine pertinent and irrelevant stimuli, to learn, to understand situations or conversations, to problem solve, and to follow a plan of action

b. Use the Rancho Los Amigos Scale (Flannery, 1998)

3. Nursing interventions

a. Use helpful cues (e.g., the client's name, pictures of familiar people or pets) to help the client identify locations

b. Encourage the client to use daily logs, written schedules, and patterns for activities of daily living (ADLs)

c. Use sensory stimulation programs (e.g., visual, auditory, olfactory, cutaneous, taste, motion) that focus on short-term interventions several times a day to increase cognition

d. Ensure a consistent schedule, staff, and environment

B. Orientation

1. Definition: The ability to know about oneself (e.g., name, age, date of birth, home), the time (e.g., current date, month, year), and facts about the environment

2. Assessment

a. Differentiate among confusion, disorientation, physical conditions (e.g., electrolyte imbalance, medications, fluid imbalance, fatigue), and sensory deficits

b. Use the Mini-Mental Status Examination (Jarvis, 1996)

3. Nursing interventions

a. Use cues to orient the client (e.g., familiar photographs of the client, family, or pets; familiar furniture; calendars; holiday decorations; clocks with large, clear numbers; schedules of daily events)

b. Clearly identify family, relatives, friends, and staff when interacting with the client

c. Ensure that the client uses intact, functional sensory aids (e.g., glasses, hearing aids)

C. Attention

1. Definition: The ability to respond to and prioritize relevant information and to ignore or put aside irrelevant information

a. Elderly people are vulnerable for attentional fatigue due to age-related physiological changes of vision, hearing, touch, and taste

b. Attentional capacity is influenced by the capacity to direct attention, attentional demands, attentional fatigue, and restorative activities

c. Attention works through global neural inhibitory mechanisms that allow the focusing that is required for prolonged or intense directed attention (Jansen & Keller, 1998)

2. Clinical example: Gregory (1995) reported

that clients with Guillain-Barré syndrome experienced attention deficits (e.g., ongoing pain, confusion between personal conversations and television programming, anger, frustration). These factors were associated with missing parts of conversations, struggling to understand the first part of the conversation as dialogue continued, being distracted by background noise, and being aware that answers did not fit the conversation. The clients' attempts to attend to conversation lead to neurological fatigue

3. Assessment

a. Assess short-term memory, planning, problem solving, incidence of accidents, irritability, impulsiveness, and frustration (Jansen & Keller, 1998)

b. Use standard questions to assess attention

Table 8-1. Cognitive Functions Affected by Brain Injury		
Area of Brain	**Function**	**Results of Injury**
Frontal lobe	Controls higher intellectual and social processing	Loss of intellect and inappropriate social behaviors
Temporal lobe	Controls new memory and learning	Impaired learning
Temporal lobe (hippocampus)	—	Temporary memory loss, lack of contralateral orientation, distractability, hyperactivity, attention deficits, perseveration
Right hemisphere	Controls recognition of geometric patterns, faces, environmental sounds, a second language, music, sense of direction, and memory for pictures	Learning impairments, memory impairments
Left hemisphere	Controls memory for language, letters, works, verbal memory (e.g., reading, writing, speech), arithmetic	Deficits with math and communication
Limbic lobe of right and left hemispheres	Controls attention that affects socialization	Deficits with socialization

Source consulted

Grzankowski, J.A. (1997). Altered thought processes related to traumatic brain injury and their nursing implications. *Rehabilitation Nursing, 22*(1), 24-28.

1) Inquire about home activities that require more or new effort (e.g., physical or environmental factors)

2) Discern the feelings that the client experiences most often

3) Identify times the client would like to but cannot express feelings and share experiences (Jansen & Keller, 1998)

   c. Differentiate among physical fatigue, neurological fatigue, and depression (Gregory, 1995)

4. Nursing interventions

   a. Use conservation and restoration measures to reduce neurological fatigue

     1) Conservation measures: Reduce or limit the extent and number of attentional demands in the internal and external environments; help the client complete necessary and desired activities in a controlled, stable environment

     2) Restoration measures: Allow rest and recovery through change in activities (e.g., taking a walk in a park, gardening, bird watching)

   b. Prioritize activities for attention

   c. Break the task into parts, focusing on step-by-step instructions

   d. Encourage daily physical activity

   e. Advise the client to avoid alcohol and drugs

   f. Individualize music selections and avoid stressful selections

   g. Modify expectations to fit the reality of the client's status

   h. Allow for growth and development

   i. Allow for variance in the client's attention throughout the day

   j. Identify triggers (e.g., situations, people, places, events) that contribute to intellectual or emotional conflict

   k. Provide client and family education

   l. Avoid denial, devaluation, or demeaning the client (Gregory, 1995)

D. Judgment

1. Description: Remembering, planning, foresight, abstraction, transference of information, and evaluating the appropriateness of an action

2. Assessment

   a. Observe the client's accuracy with money management, learning new skills, applying old knowledge in new situations, problem solving, creating and following through with realistic plans

   b. Periodically reassess the client's judgment deficits to meet his or her increasing or decreasing needs

3. Nursing interventions: Tailor interventions to match the client's level of cognition

   a. For clients with high cognitive functioning: Coordinate counseling, education, crisis management, vocational assessment and planning, and individualized self-care management

   c. For clients with moderate cognitive functioning: Provide or coordinate scheduled routines, a structured environment, counseling, individualized education, and vocational assessment and planning

   d. For clients with lower cognitive functioning: Help coordinate supervised living situations, a protective environment, sheltered vocational opportunities, case management, and legal guardians

E. Problem Solving

1. Definition: A high-level cognitive function that involves considering, recalling, and analyzing factors and selecting appropriate choices from various alternatives

2. Clinical example: People with moderate to severe traumatic brain injury (TBI) have chronic cognitive impairment during the first year after injury, even if they have good balance and can perform ADLs (Cecchini, 1998)

3. Assessment

   a. Assess the ability to plan and organize thoughts and behaviors

   b. Assess the ability to formulate alternative solutions for a problem

   c. Assess the ability to comprehend potential consequences of choices

4. Nursing interventions

a. Help the client approach problems by taking one step at a time

b. Encourage the client to differentiate between solutions to a problem and examine the consequences of solutions

c. Encourage successful problem-solving plans and build on successes

d. Examine unsuccessful problem-solving plans and discuss methods to select positive action plans

F. Motivation

1. Description

a. Motivation is the external, internal, or combined force(s) that influence behavior to satisfy needs and achieve goals

b. Motivation can be influenced by needs and wants, the cost and rewards of participating in an activity, and personal beliefs about the ability to participate and succeed (Bandura, 1977)

2. Assessment

a. Assess the amount and persistence of the client's activities toward achieving goals

b. Assess the barriers of client motivation (e.g., memory impairment, problem-solving deficits)

c. Use the Apathy Evaluation Scale (AES), which is an 18-item instrument that measures thoughts, actions, and emotions during the previous month. This instrument helps determine motivation that affects discharge function and functional levels after rehabilitation (Resnick, Zimmerman, Magaziner, & Adelman, 1998)

3. Nursing interventions

a. Help the client establish immediate and long-term goals

b. Help the client and family set a realistic plan to achieve goals

c. Break long-term goals into small, attainable goals

d. Reward successes with family and peer recognition

e. Provide resources that lead to the successful achievement of goals

G. Coping

1. Description

a. Coping is defined as cognitive and behavioral efforts directed at managing demanding and stressful situations

1) Problem-focused coping efforts are directed at lowering or eliminating threats

2) Emotional-focused coping efforts are directed at decreasing negative emotions (Lyon, 1993)

b. Personal competence with coping includes many factors (Satir, 1988)

1) The components of relationships (being content with self and others)

2) Differentiation (distinguishing between self and others)

3) Autonomy (relying on self, separate and distinct from others)

4) Self-esteem (feeling worthy about self)

5) Power (using energy to initiate and guide behaviors)

6) Productivity (manifesting competence)

7) Love (being compassionate, accepting, and giving, as well as receiving affection)

c. Antecedents of stress require coping skills

1) Personal and environmental demands that exceed resources

2) Ambiguity and uncertainty

3) Loss of control

4) Loss of social support

d. Many variables influence coping efforts (Lyon, 1993)

1) Development age

2) Severity of disability

3) Visibility of disability

4) Threat of chronicity

5) Sense of control

6) Prior coping abilities

7) Self-esteem

8) Values

9) Perceived social support

2. Clinical examples

a. A longitudinal study of people experiencing subarachnoid hemorrhages indicated that survivors continue the recovery phase for years and develop good coping skills and a positive attitude over time (Ogden, Utley, & Mee, 1997)

b. The majority of people with noninflammatory chronic pain, rheumatoid arthritis, or with good health described themselves as optimists and had similar levels of life satisfaction. Life satisfaction scores indicated effective coping with chronic illness (Bergh, Branholm, & Dahlqvist, 1997)

3. Research studies

a. In a study examining the relationships between disability severity, time use, social support, and socioeconomic status with psychosocial outcomes among people with spinal cord injury (SCI), adjustment to disability was at a moderate to high level. Satisfaction of how time was spent was a moderate predictor of psychosocial outcomes, especially life satisfaction. Financial stress and social support were strongly predictive of the level of life satisfaction (Pentland, Harvey, & Walker, 1998)

b. Coping strategies for postpolio clients that focused on controlling symptoms were more effective than attempts to maintain prior activity levels. People with postpolio syndrome experienced less anxiety, uncertainty, depression, and helplessness when dealing with increasing disability when they used symptom management interventions. The most effective symptom management interventions focused on lifestyle and personal changes (Westbrook & McIlwain, 1996)

6. Assessment

a. Assess the level and sources of stress expressed by the client and family

b. Assess the client's ability to solve problems

c. Note changes in the client's and family's abilities to meet their needs

d. Note changes in communication patterns that reflect frustration (e.g., verbal manipulation, hostility)

e. Note inappropriate behavior, activity,

and responses that reflect frustration

f. Use the Assessment Instrument of Problem-focused Coping (APC), which is a self-report instrument that focuses on a person's own assessment of competence in coping with ADLs, personal problems, and level of satisfaction with ADLs (Tollen & Ahlstrom, 1998)

7. Nursing interventions

a. Provide rehabilitation and education and locate resources beyond personal care and independence, which can allow people with SCI to expand their leisure and productive roles and promote socioeconomic integration (Pentland et al., 1998)

b. Explore the meaning of illness for the client and family, which can lead to understanding their behaviors and responses

1) The meaning the client or family associates with illness can have a profound effect on coping and adjustment and can influence relationships with the healthcare team

2) The meaning of illness is influenced by cultural beliefs, religion, values, life philosophy, and past experiences (Howell, 1998)

c. Encourage purposeful and meaningful time expenditure, which contributes to a higher quality of life—even more than the ability to be independent with ADLs (Cardol, Elvers, Oostendorp, Brandsma, & deGroot, 1996)

d. Understand the unique experience of the person with disability as influenced by his or her psychological, emotional, and spiritual needs and develop appropriate interventions to promote coping (Berman & Rose, 1998)

H. Memory

1. Description

a. Memory is crucial to all aspects of cognition and learning.

1) Short-term memory: Recall of immediate or recent events

2) Long-term memory: Storage and retrieval of information

b. Memory disorders are very distressing to

clients with head injuries and family caregivers

2. Research: Changes in a person's mental and emotional status can affect rehabilitation. A longitudinal study of stroke survivors indicated that the major mental changes after stroke were with mood, judgment, memory, and personality. Six months after the stroke, survivors experienced depression, memory loss, nervousness, irritability, frustration, low energy, and decreased initiative (Sisson, 1998)

3. Assessment
   a. Assess the client's mental status early because it is an important element in planning and determining readiness for rehabilitation
      1) Mental changes affect functional abilities, family stress levels, rehabilitation success, social activities, and employment.
      2) Early and continuing assessment is needed and family input should be encouraged (Sisson, 1998)
   b. Use the Mini-Mental State Examination (Jarvis, 1996)
   c. Assess the ability to learn new skills or facts
   d. Assess the client's ability to recall past experiences and ask family members to verify these descriptions

4. Nursing interventions: Use memory aids and strategies (e.g., family pictures, schedules, calendars, familiar environments, reminder notes), which are more effective than using rehearsal to improve the memory of people with head injuries (Thompson, 1996)

I. Self-Efficacy
1. Definition: A sense of control that is composed of coping with, appraising, and managing one's life that leads to the conviction that the person can determine behaviors that lead to desired outcomes (Bandura, 1977)
2. Assessment
   a. Investigate the client's and family's short- and long-term goals
   b. Identify fears of and barriers to self-efficacy

c. Identify learning needs associated with self-efficacy
d. Identify resources required for self-efficacy
e. Identify the client's ability to provide or direct self-care
f. Identify the client's ability to manage the vocational and recreational aspects of life

3. Nursing interventions
   a. Individualize self-care education for the client and family
   b. Encourage the client to choose activities
   c. Encourage self-responsibility
   d. Encourage behaviors and activities that lead to self-assurance
   e. Encourage alternative solutions for problem solving
   f. Provide opportunities to practice and direct self-care
   g. Provide resources for vocational development
   h. Provide opportunities for recreation and socialization
   i. Provide resources for goal achievement
   j. Encourage the client to completely evaluate the situation

V. Behaviors That Affect Psychosocial Health
A. Denial
   1. Definition: A defense mechanism in which a person is unable to admit reality or the presence of something that produces anxiety
      a. Initially, the client and family may experience shock and disbelief regarding the injury or illness and its effect on the client and family. Adjustment does not occur in even stages, but may be characterized by many approaches and avoidance adjustment measures (Davidhizar, 1997)
      b. Clients reported that denial is common until they were in formal rehabilitation programs and interacting with peers (Brillhart & Johnson, 1997) (see Research Perspective in this chapter.)
   2. Assessment
      a. Note the avoidance of discussion of the disability, injury, or illness

b. Note unrealistic discussion of the permanence or severity of the disability

c. Note unrealistic expectations of treatment or rehabilitation

d. Note inappropriate mood for the situation (e.g., extreme cheerfulness)

e. Note disregard for the need of treatment or rehabilitation

3. Nursing interventions

a. Encourage the client and family to express their feelings

b. Use a nonjudgmental attitude toward the client

c. Avoid making promises or giving false assurances

d. Communicate empathy for the client's feelings

e. Offer information about the disability, injury, illness, and the available treatment and rehabilitation

f. Encourage the client's peers to serve as role models and mentors

g. Help the client build a supportive network

h. Encourage vocational counseling and rehabilitation

i. Encourage the client to have a realistic outlook on life (Davidhizar, 1997)

B. Depression

1. Definition: A state of sadness, seen as social withdrawal, crying, anxiety, irritability, or self-degrading opinions

2. Clinical example: Depression was seen in younger clients after stroke, as indicated by their negative evaluation of the quality of life, emotional behaviors, social interactions, sexual behaviors, and recreation (Neau et al., 1998)

3. Research: Depression in stroke clients after rehabilitation was a determinant of poor social functioning during the year after the stroke; however, illness behaviors were a determinant of low functional abilities (Clark & Smith, 1998)

4. Assessment

a. Observe for overt signs of depression

b. Use the Geriatric Depression Scale for

admission and ongoing assessment (Diamond, Holroyd, Macciocchi, & Felsenthal, 1995)

c. Assess for contributing factors with depression (e.g., chronic illness, disease symptoms, lower socioeconomic status [Ai, Peterson, Dunkle, Saunders, Bolling, & Buchtel, 1997], level of social support and functioning level [Diamond et al., 1995; King, 1996])

5. Nursing interventions

a. Ensure the availability of psychological services during rehabilitation and after discharge (Scivoletto, Petrelli, Di-Lucente, & Castellano, 1997)

b. Establish a therapeutic relationship of trust

c. Use therapeutic listening and reflection techniques

d. Reinforce successful coping skills from past experiences

e. Establish short-term realistic goals and build on successes

f. Encourage family, friends, and others to provide personal support

C. Apathy

1. Definition: An attitude characterized by bland affect, lethargy, and decreased motivation. Apathetic clients may exhibit few goal-directed behaviors, a lack of productivity, decreased goal-directed thinking, decreased interest, and decreased concern about health or personal problems

2. Assessment

a. Observe mood and activity level on an ongoing basis

b. Determine lack of goal formation and follow-up on established goals

c. Assess for poor self-regulated health maintenance

d. Note lack of motivation and initiation

e. Use the Apathy Evaluation Scale, an 18-item instrument that rates a person's thoughts, actions, and emotions during 1 month. This scale has been helpful in identifying clients whose apathy is associated with stroke, dementia, or depression (Resnick et al., 1998)

3. Nursing interventions
   a. Identify the individual's short- and long-term life goals
   b. Ensure the availability of vocational counseling
   c. Encourage family involvement and cohesiveness
   d. Promote recreational therapy
   e. Promote the benefits of peer counseling

VI. Pathological-Based Behaviors That Affect Psychosocial Health

A. Confusion
   1. Definition: The inability to recall minute-to-minute, hour-to-hour, or day-to-day events
   2. Assessment
      a. Observe inaccuracies with name, date, location, and situation
      b. Observe the client's ability to understand a situation as reflected by past events
      c. Note the client's ability to follow directions
      d. Note the client's lack of recall
      e. Use the Mini-Mental State Examination (Jarvis, 1996), which is a two-part, accurate assessment instrument for baseline and ongoing mental status evaluation
         1) Part 1 focuses on name, date, season, and location
         2) Part 2 focuses on object recognition, sentence formation, the ability to follow commands, and conceptualization
         3) The entire examination can be administered in 10 minutes.
         4) A score of 27-30 indicates no mental impairment, a score of 20-26 indicates mild impairment, a score of 16-19 indicates moderate impairment, and a score of 15 or less indicates severe mental deficits
   3. Nursing interventions
      a. Help the client with reorientation: Reminders regarding name, date, and environment can be useful for clients resolving memory deficits and clients with some types of TBI
      b. Use orientation cues (e.g., printed names, personal or family pictures, calendars, seasonal decorations, schedules, clocks), especially with clients with dementia or Alzheimer's disease
      c. Ensure consistency in the environment, schedules, and staff

B. Impulsiveness
   1. Definition: The tendency to act without considering the consequences
   2. Assessment: Use a behavior flowsheet to document impulsive behaviors (e.g., pacing, banging on doors, darting across the street, getting up from the wheelchair, going over siderails)
   3. Nursing interventions
      a. Evaluate the environment for safety
      b. Use alarm doors
      c. Use alarm bracelets
      d. Establish a routine with meaningful activities
      e. Observe clients closely to prevent injury
      f. Provide family education and guidance in dealing with impulsiveness
      g. Help clients avoid fatigue by developing a sleep-awake cycle
      h. Encourage the family's involvement with the client

C. Perseveration
   1. Definition: The reflexive repetition of behaviors, vocalizations, or activities
   2. Assessment
      a. Observe the client's reflexive responses
      b. Document the onset, duration, and situational factors that aggravate perseveration
      c. Document the factors that diminish perseveration
   3. Nursing interventions
      a. Provide visual distractions
      b. Engage the client in simple activities (e.g., taking a walk)
      c. Conduct a meaningful conversation with the client
      d. Use pet therapy
      e. Help the client avoid social isolation

f. Use music therapy that involves the client (e.g., play music while exercising)

g. Gather family input about the cause and symptoms of perseveration

h. Encourage family involvement and inter-action with the client

D. Confabulation

1. Description

a. Confabulation is the invention of detail or life experiences in an attempt to compensate for memory deficits

b. The person substitutes imaginary experiences or confuses experiences with those he or she cannot recall

c. Confabulation can be quite convincing even for healthcare professionals

2. Assessment

a. Gather observations from family, relatives, or friends who know the client's life and history

b. Assess and document incidents of confabulation at frequent intervals to determine an indication of disease progression

3. Nursing interventions

a. For the family

1) Provide family education about the physiological causes of confabulation

2) Assure the family that confabulation is a symptom of memory deficits

3) Communicate frequently with the family to help them understand situations (e.g., the client's statements about a bruise, no breakfast, no one visits) and the true circumstances of the client's status and routine

4) Maintain a logbook in the client's room in which staff members record their encounters with the client: Staff and family members can use the log-book to track the day's activities and interact appropriately with the client

b. For the client

1) Provide distraction with meaningful conversation

2) Engage in simple activities

3) Avoid correcting or making negative comments to the client about confabulation

E. Emotional Lability

1. Definition: Characterized by uncontrollable, fluctuating emotional behaviors usually seen as alternating gaiety, somberness, and crying

2. Assessment

a. Observe and document emotional liability (e.g., duration, timing, cycles)

b. Observe and document factors that increase or diminish emotional lability

3. Nursing interventions

a. Provide adequate rest and sleep-wake cycles

b. Provide distraction in the early stages of emotional lability

c. Play soothing music

d. Ensure a calm atmosphere

e. Reduce situations that promote frustration or anger

f. Help staff or family members avoid overreacting to emotional episodes

g. Use reminiscence therapy

h. Encourage the client to sing familiar songs (e.g., "Row, Row, Row Your Boat")

i. Use physical activities (e.g., chair exercises)

j. Provide family education regarding emotional lability as a symptom of disease and illness and tips on managing emotional lability

F. Disinhibition

1. Definition: Uncontrolled behaviors or activities that are considered socially inappropriate. The person is unable to inhibit inappropriate behaviors, cannot foresee the consequences of inappropriate actions, and exhibits egocentric behaviors (Montgomery, Kitten, Niemiec, 1997).

2. Assessment

a. Observe inappropriate behavior (e.g., undressing in public, sexual overtures, physical or verbal abuse)

b. Evaluate the client's psychosocial status, focusing on impaired self-control and social withdrawal on an ongoing basis (Spatt, Zebenholzer, & Oder, 1997)

3. Nursing interventions
   a. Discourage behaviors involving sexual disinhibition
      1) Offer distractions that promote meaningful behavior
      2) Provide opportunities for adequate sleep and rest
      3) Encourage appropriate touch and contact by family, friends, and staff
   b. Discourage behaviors involving disrobing disinhibition
      1) Take the client to the bathroom or provide toileting routinely
      2) Maintain elimination hygiene if the client uses adult padding or diapers
      3) Provide appropriate clothing for the season and situation
      4) Provide special clothing that is difficult to remove
      5) Help the client redress himself or herself to regain dignity and privacy
   c. Discourage behaviors involving swearing
      1) Offer distractions that promote meaningful activities
      2) Avoid making the client feel shameful regarding swearing
      3) Help the family and staff avoid overreacting to client swearing
      4) Use music therapy with familiar tunes
      5) Provide family education and awareness of disease and injury processes related to swearing disinhibition
G. Agitation
   1. Definition: Uncontrolled behaviors such as restlessness, irritability, anger, vocalization, and combativeness
   2. Assessment
      a. Observe characteristic agitated behaviors (e.g., pacing, verbal aggression, physical aggression, frustration, confusion)
      b. Document the type and duration of behaviors, time of day, preceding incidence to agitation, situational influences for agitation, and response to interventions
      c. Use the Agitation Behavior Scale (ABS) (Riedel & Shaw, 1997), which was designed to evaluate people with TBI experiencing agitation

3. Nursing interventions
   a. For providing environmental control
      1) Avoid using physical restraints (e.g., Posey belts, arm restraints)
      2) Reduce environmental noise, light, and activity
      3) Provide rest periods
      4) Limit visitors
      5) Ensure the client's protection by using Craig beds or Vail beds
      6) Provide a consistent personal aide (Riedel & Shaw, 1997)
   b. For taking a specialized approach to an agitated client
      1) Provide staff education
         a) Client and staff safety
         b) Staff morale issues
         c) Phases and causes of agitation
         d) Strategies for successfully dealing with agitation
      2) Defuse the situation before it reaches physical aggression
      3) Give simple instructions (e.g., "Don't kick," "Don't hit")
      4) Avoid scolding or belittling the client
      5) Maintain a calm, controlled approach and vocalizations (Montgomery et al., 1997)
   c. For approaching the client
      1) Continue to orient the client to the environment
      2) Explain all actions to the client
      3) Allow time away from required activities if agitation is heightened
      4) Use distraction to avoid cycles of agitation
      5) Avoid reasoning with the client during a period of agitation, as the person will have difficulty processing his or her thoughts
      6) Provide physical reassurance and comfort (Flannery, 1998)

VII. Sensation and Perception Factors That Affect Psychosocial Health
   A. Deficits in Hearing
      1. Physiology of hearing: Hearing is a complex sensory perception that incorporates a stimulus, which activates the acoustic nerve (Cranial Nerve [CN] VIII), and then the cochlear nucleus, the nuclei, tracts of the

lateral lemniscus, and the inferior colliculus. The stimulus activates the structures along the brainstem's auditory pathways. Interpretation of the stimulus is based on conduction properties of various portions of the auditory tract.

2. Disruption in hearing: Disruptions of this complex system due to injury or illness can lead to partial or total deafness (see Table 8-2).

3. Assessment

   a. Use the whisper test on both ears to assess gross hearing: The examiner stands behind the client and whispers a number. The client covers one ear at a time and repeats the whispered number (Jarvis, 1996).

   b. Inspect the external ear canal, tympanic membranes, and use the Weber test (Jarvis, 1996) to assess conduction hearing loss

   c. Use the Rinne and Weber tests (Jarvis, 1996) to assess neurogenic hearing loss

   d. Evaluate the family's descriptions of the client's prior hearing status

   e. Observe the appropriateness of the client's conversational flow

   f. Observe whether the client can appropriately follow commands

   g. Note an unusual volume of the radio or television

   h. Note the condition of the client's hearing aid

4. Nursing interventions

   a. Reduce background noise

   b. Keep sentences and messages short

   c. Do not rush the client

   d. Listen and seek feedback from the client

   e. Encourage the use of bilateral hearing aides

   f. Avoid shouting to the client

   g. Use a low tone of voice

   h. Face the client when speaking to him or her

   i. Use alternative methods of communication (e.g., written notes, sign language)

B. Deficits in Vision

   1. Pathophysical factors in vision deficits involving the optic nerve: The major function of the optic nerve (CN II) is vision, which includes visual fields and visual acuity (see Table 8-3 and Figure 8-2).

      a. Assessment

         1) Test peripheral vision (i.e., visual field) using the technique of confrontation (e.g., the client gazes straight at the examiner and notes the examiner's fingers, which move into all visual fields)

Table 8-2. Pathophysiology of Hearing

Injury	Symptoms
Damage to lateral lemniscus	Partial deafness bilaterally, with more severe deafness on the side opposite of the lesion
Destruction of cortex of one hemisphere of brain	Difficulty in judging direction and distance from the source of sound

Source consulted

Pallett, P.J., & O'Brien, M.T. (1985). *Textbook of neurological nursing.* Boston: Little, Brown.

Table 8-3. Pathophysiology of Vision: Part 1 (CN II)

Injury	Symptoms
Interruptions of optic pathways to calcarine cortex in occipital lobe	Visual field deficits
Retinal tears	Visual field deficits
Damage to one optical tract before unification of the left and right tract	Monocular vision loss in ipsilateral eye associated with multiple sclerosis
Transient ischemic attacks affecting blood supply to optic nerve	Transient mononuclear vision loss
Pressure to optic chiasm	Permanent blindness associated with brain tumors
Damage to optic pathway	Homonymous hemianopia or vision loss in the same side of each eye associated with cerebral vascular accidents

Source consulted

Pallett, P.J., & O'Brien, M.T. (1985). *Textbook of neurological nursing.* Boston: Little, Brown.

2) Use the Snellen chart tests (Jarvis, 1996) and reading material (e.g., newspaper) to assess visual acuity

3) Obtain information of prior visual status from the client and family

4) Note unilateral neglect

5) Note the client's ability to read materials at near and far distances

b. Nursing interventions

1) Teach the client to scan the visual field

2) Provide environmental control for safety

3) Identify family, friends, and staff when interacting with the client

4) Ensure adequate lighting

5) Provide large-print reading materials

2. Deficits in vision involving the oculomotor (CN III), trochlear (CN IV), and abducens (CN VI) nerves: These nerves unite to control the functions of the extraocular muscles that are responsible for eye motion and binocular vision. The oculomotor nerve also controls the elevation of the upper eyelids and the constriction of the pupils (see Table 8-4).

a. Assessment

1) Inspect the eyelid for drooping (ptosis)

2) Examine the size, shape, equality, position, and light reflexes of the pupils

Figure 8-2. Visual Field Deficits Associated with Lesions of the Optic Pathway at Different Locations

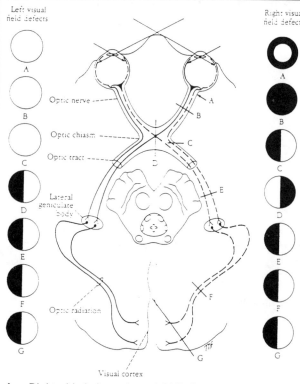

A Right-sided circumferential blindness resulting from retrobulbar neuritis

B Total blindness of right eye resulting from division of the right optic nerve

C Right nasal hemianopia resulting from a partial lesion of the right side of the optic chiasm

D Bitemporal hemianopia resulting from a complete lesion of the optic chiasm

E Left temporal and right nasal hemianopia resulting from a lesion of the right optic radiation

G Left temporal and right nasal hemianopia resulting from a lesion of the right visual cortex

Reprinted with permission of Little, Brown and Company Inc. from Snell, R.S. (1980). *Clinical neuroanatomy for medical students* (p. 382). Boston: Little, Brown. Copyright 1980 by Little, Brown and Company Inc.

Table 8-4. Pathophysiology of Vision: Part 2 (CN III, IV, VI)

Injury	Symptoms
Injury to CN III, IV, and/or VI	Marked miosis of pupils seen with brainstem strokes
	Dilation of pupils seen with increased intracranial pressure
	Ptosis of eyelid associated with multiple sclerosis or increased intracranial pressure
	Unequal pupil size associated with ipsilateral hemisphere lesions
	Nystagmus with jerking movements of eyes
Disruptions of CN III or VI	Diplopia with disruption of conjugate movements of the eye and inference with binocular vision

Source consulted

Pallett, P.J., & O'Brien, M.T. (1985). *Textbook of neurological nursing.* Boston: Little, Brown.

3) Test the ocular movements of the eye for imbalance and conjugate deviation
4) Evaluate accommodation and convergence
5) Observe ocular movements

b. Nursing interventions

1) Have the client use an eye patch to diminish double vision (diplopia)
2) Address the etiology of symptoms (e.g., increased intracranial pressure)

C. Deficits in Touch

1. Physiology of touch: The gray matter of the spinal cord has both motor and sensory components. The sensory (afferent) component consists of the dorsal (posterior) columns and the intermediate areas. Posterior horn cells remain within the central nervous system (CNS). Axons from these cells project to the anterior or ventral horn cells of the spinal cord where they divide to become ascending and descending intersegmental tracts (see Table 8-5).

2. Assessment

a. Determine whether the client can differentiate between levels of temperature

b. Evaluate the client's pain

c. Evaluate the client's sense of light touch

d. Evaluate priproception

e. Evaluate the client's sense of vibration

3. Nursing interventions

a. Ensure safety with extreme temperature exposures

b. Observe and control the sources of pain (e.g., pressure, burns, lesions)

VIII. Communication: A Function of Sensory, Cognitive, and Physiological Status

A. Communication

1. Is a complex process between sender and receiver

Table 8-5. Physiology of Touch: Spinal Cord

Region within spinal cord	Function
Gray matter	
Afferent portion composed of dorsal (posterior) columns and intermediate areas	Sensory function
	Modification of pain and temperature information
Substantia gelatinosa in dorsal horn of spinal cord	Conveys information of touch and pressure, plus proprioception to cerebellum
Nucleus dorsalis of the ventromedial portion of spinal cord	Serves as connections for spinal reflexes and transmission of sensory information to the brain
Nucleus proprius of the dorsal portion of the cord	Causes impairment of sensation on the side opposite of the lesion
White matter	
Dorsal area	Carries impulses from extremities that involve proprioceptors, tactile endings, and end organs to the medulla, to pons, to midbrain, to general sensory nucleus of thalamus, to cerebral cortex
	Transmits location of stimuli, fine gradations of stimuli intensity, modulates tactile sensations of vibration, pressure, touch, and sensation of body positioning
Spinothalamic tract	
Anterior spinothalamic tract	Conducts impulses for light touch to sensory cortex
Lateral spinothalamic tract	Conducts pain and temperature stimuli from peripheral areas to thalamus and general sensory nucleus. Responsible for crude awareness of pain and temperature, plus localization and quantitative assessment of pain and temperature
	Includes conditions such as tumors, trauma, infractions, and degenerative processes

Source consulted

Pallett, P.J., & O'Brien, M.T. (1985). *Textbook of neurological nursing.* Boston: Little, Brown.

2. Depends on the sensory, cognitive, emotional, and physical status of all components of the interaction

B. Assessment
   1. Characteristics of a person with cognitive-related communication deficits
      a. Does not speak
      b. Has problems finding words
      c. Uses inappropriate words
      d. Is unable to name familiar objects
      e. Appears confused or disoriented
      f. Displays attention deficits
      g. Is unable to speak a secondary language (if applicable)
      h. Displays emotional lability
      i. Has decreased comprehension
   2. Characteristics of a person with sensory-related communication deficits
      a. Has diminished hearing or deafness
      b. Lacks or has diminished vision
      c. Lacks appropriate responses to touch due to sensory deficits
   3. Characteristics of a person with physiological-related communication deficits
      a. Slurs speech
      b. Speaks in a whisper
      c. Has difficulty with motor planning
      d. Has difficulty with articulation

C. Nursing Interventions
   1. For cognitive-related communication problems
      a. Use short, simple sentences
      b. Use one-step commands
      c. Use nonverbal cues
      d. Use repetition and patterning when giving directions
      e. Communicate during times of peak energy and attentiveness
      f. Control the environment (e.g., background noise, light, activity, confusion)
      g. Limit the time spent on communication sessions
      h. Use a communication board with symbols

      i. Teach the family strategies for effectively communicating with the client
   2. For sensory-related communication problems
      a. Assess for intact, diminished, or absent sensation
      b. Provide sensory stimulation therapy (e.g., different textures and temperatures)
      c. Focus family education on affectionate touch in areas of intact sensation
      d. Ensure that the client uses necessary hearing aids (especially bilateral aids)
      e. Provide translators for clients who are deaf or use sign language
      f. Use nonverbal cues or gestures
      g. Ensure that the client uses necessary corrective lenses
      h. Use voice-operated computers
   3. For physiological-related communication problems
      a. Ensure that the client receives speech therapy
      b. Provide computers with word processing programs

IX. **Self-Perception and Self-Concept Issues Related to Psychosocial Health**
   A. Powerlessness
      1. Definition: The inability to use personal energy to initiate and guide personal behavior
         a. The lack of personal power makes a person powerless, which is destructive to the self (Satir, 1988).
         b. Powerlessness can be learned through negative reinforcement of dependency.
         c. Powerlessness as a reaction to threats can lead to patterns of impotence, withdrawal, and passiveness.
      2. Clinical example: Injury or illness leading to disability can destroy a person's normal level of life control and predictability. Relocation stress, experienced during the recovery and rehabilitation process, and powerlessness are influenced by decreases in biopsychosocial status, anxiety, depression, apprehension, guilt, denial, and lowered self-esteem (Nypaver, Titus, & Brugler, 1996).
      3. Assessment
         a. Note lack of initiative in goal planning and achievement

b. Note passivity

c. Note withdrawal from family, social, and vocational decisions and interactions

d. Assess apprehension and fear

4. Nursing interventions

a. Encourage the client and family to maintain control in decision making and promote environmental predictability and emotional support (Nypaver et al., 1996)

b. Help the client realize that, although the injury or illness that led to the disability cannot be changed, his or her response to the disability is a personal choice (Davidhizar, 1997)

c. Enable the client and family to recognize and mobilize their strengths and resources, feel confident, and use effective coping skills

d. Encourage the client to achieve self-direction and self-determination

e. Encourage the client and family to seek spiritual support

f. Encourage and value the client's and family's involvement as participants in the interdisciplinary team

g. Encourage the client's involvement with group and community support systems

h. Provide follow-up rehabilitation care in the home setting if applicable

B. Hopelessness
1. Definition: The reaction from feeling that a situation or condition is without solution. Associated feelings of hopelessness include powerlessness, despair, helplessness, and apathy.

2. Assessment

a. Observe for the characteristics of powerlessness, despair, apathy

b. Observe for the lack of initiative for self-help

c. Observe for depression

3. Nursing interventions

a. Enhance the client's sense of power, which precedes hopefulness

b. Establish short- and long-term goals with the client and family

c. Encourage family and social support

d. Encourage spiritual empowerment and strength

C. Helplessness
1. Definition: The belief that a person feels dependent on others for support for a situation that seems to be impossible to alter. The person may perceive that events are beyond his or her control.

2. Assessment

a. Observe for inactivity and nonparticipation in rehabilitation

b. Observe for self-isolation and withdrawal

c. Observe for general behaviors (e.g., slow movements, low voice tones, sitting alone quietly)

d. Observe for disturbances in motivation, cognition, and emotion

e. Observe for the absence of voluntary response to a situation

f. Observe for learned dependence (i.e., the inability to act and make decisions)

g. Observe for fear and depression

3. Nursing interventions

a. Foster voluntary responses and independence

b. Encourage learning and reinforce successes

c. Form the expectation of independence for the client and family (Seligman, 1975)

d. Encourage the client to evaluate his or her personal assets and affirm his or her feelings or expressions of hope

e. Encourage memory and increased coping abilities (Davidhizar, 1997)

D. Self-Perception
1. Problems with self-concept

a. Definition of self-concept: An individual's perception of himself or herself as related to others and the environment; self-concept consists of all aspects of the person

b. Assessment

1) Observe for self-criticism (e.g., negative thinking, expectations of failure)

2) Observe for self-diminution (e.g., avoiding, neglecting, or refusing to recognize personal assets) (Stuart & Laraia, 1995)

c. Nursing interventions

1) Encourage activity in community-based social integration programs to develop social skills (Burleigh, Farber, & Gillard, 1998)

2) Encourage the client to approach life with open, realistic expectations

3) Encourage and reinforce the client's evaluations of his or her personal assets

4) Encourage the client to interact with family and friends

5) Reinforce success, which can academically and vocationally increase self-concept (Brillhart & Johnson, 1997)

2. Problems with self-esteem

a. Definition of self-esteem: An attitude, feeling, and self-concept represented by behavior

1) Self-esteem is the person's sense of personal value and ability to consider himself or herself with dignity, love, and reality.

2) Self-esteem affects the inner person as well as the person's relationships with others.

3) Positive self-esteem is fostered by integrity, honesty, responsibility, compassion, and competence.

4) People with low self-worth have a "victim mentality" and expect depreciation.

b. Assessment: Observe for feelings of defeat, failure, and worthlessness (Satir, 1988), weakness, helplessness, hopelessness, fright, vulnerability, fragility, incompleteness, and inadequacy (Stuart & Laraia, 1995)

c. Nursing interventions

1) Allow time for relaxation

2) Help the client realize what is occurring and his or her reaction to the situation

3) Encourage the client to communicate with family members and share experiences

4) Encourage the client to listen to others and try to reflect how both parties perceive the communication

5) Foster relaxed, flexible family expectations

6) Encourage the client to declare, "I am unique," "I can love myself," and "I am okay" (Satir, 1988)

3. Poor body image

a. Definition of body image: A person's subjective picture of his or her own appearance that is based on observations, comparisons, and reactions by others

b. Assessment

1) Observe for grooming and hygiene status

2) Observe for initiation of self-care activities

3) Observe the functional abilities for self-care and ADLs

4) Observe the effect of the client's appearance on family, friends, and the community

c. Nursing interventions

1) Provide for independent or assisted grooming

2) Ensure that the client has appropriate street clothing for activities

3) Coordinate barber and hairdressing services

4) Encourage the use of prosthetics

5) Reinforce occupational therapy

6) Provide recreational therapy and community reentry activities

7) Encourage the client to recognize successful people with disabilities (e.g., athletes who use wheelchairs)

8) Promote positive, public images of people with disabilities in business, politics, and the media

9) Incorporate people with disabilities into play therapy (e.g., childhood books that include characters with disabilities, dolls in wheelchairs, cartoons with positive images of people with disabilities)

10) Encourage the client to attend support groups for people with disabilities

E. Unresolved Grief Associated with Disability
1. Definition: Prolonged grief and mourning that progresses beyond the initial grief associated with having an injury or illness and that incorporates the loss of function
2. Assessment
   a. Observe for appetite loss, fatigue, apathy, lack of socialization, somatic complaints, and decreased activities
   b. Observe the client's emotions (e.g., feelings of emptiness and numbness, low self-esteem, sadness, guilt) (Stuart & Laraia, 1995)
   c. Observe the client's level of willingness to participate in rehabilitation
3. Nursing interventions
   a. Encourage family and friends to reassure the client that he or she is loved for himself or herself, not for his or her appearance, physical abilities, or work capacity
   b. Foster peer modeling and mentoring (Davidhizar, 1997)
   c. Encourage the client and family to seek psychological counseling
   d. Help the client build a social, cultural, and economic network of support (Davidhizar, 1997)
   e. Help the client cultivate a positive and realistic outlook on life (Davidhizar, 1997)
   f. Allow time for adjustment, because clients often do not internalize the entire impact of a disability until the rehabilitation phase of treatment (Brillhart & Johnson, 1997)
F. Stress
1. Definition: The cognitive awareness of any external or internal unmet demands on a person that unbalances the equilibrium. Effects of stress are expressed physically, emotionally, intellectually, spiritually, and socially (Barry, 1996).
2. Assessment
   a. Observe for physiological manifestations of stress (e.g., gastrointestinal distress, cardiac palpitations, anxious facial expressions, tremors)
   b. Observe for emotional manifestations of stress (e.g., anxiety, emotional lability, restlessness, fright)
   c. Observe for intellectual manifestations of stress (e.g., difficulty in concentration and memory, poor coping strategies)
   d. Observe for spiritual manifestations of stress (e.g., value conflicts)
   e. Observe for social manifestations of stress (e.g., role conflict, status incongruity, withdrawal, antagonism, role rigidity)
3. Nursing interventions
   a. Examine the source of stress (e.g., fears of failure, lack of resources, lack of support system, role loss, ambiguity)
   b. Examine and reinforce prior successful coping measures
   c. Provide crisis management
   d. Consult with the client's case managers and social workers
   e. Encourage the client to appraise stressors and his or her responses to stress and approaches to problem solving
   f. Encourage the client and family to be flexible with roles and problem solving
   g. Promote psychological hardiness by fostering control, commitment, and challenge for growth and development
   h. Encourage the client to seek spiritual counseling and support (Barry, 1996; Lazarus & Folkman, 1984)
G. Stigma
1. Definition: The application of set attitudes and stereotypes of people with disabilities. Stigma begins in the attitudes of others but may be internalized by the person with a disability and eventually influence that person's behaviors (Goffman, 1974).
2. Assessment
   a. Observe for statements of self-depreciation
   b. Observe for self-isolationing behaviors
   c. Observe alienation and hostility by others
   d. Note family's and friends' attitudes toward people with disabilities

3. Nursing interventions
    a. Encourage the client to reevaluate the importance of physique
    b. Encourage a realistic appraisal of the difficulties of dealing with disability
    c. Encourage evaluation of personal assets and abilities
    d. Encourage the client and family to focus on the total person, not just the disability
    e. Provide counseling on dealing with stigma within the community
    f. Encourage positive images of those with disabilities in the media, business, academia, athletics, and music
    g. Ensure that children and adults with disabilities are mainstreamed into educational and recreational activities

X. Role and Relationships Related to Psychosocial Health

A. Family Roles
    1. Description *[Refer to Chapter 15 for more on family roles and theories.]*
        a. The family unit is an active, operating system.
        b. The person with disability is not in isolation, but is considered in the context of family.
        c. Family relationships are the living links that bind the family together.
        d. As a system, the family assigns roles and rules that are established for each member.
        e. Functions of the family include acquiring the means to provide for the necessities of daily life.
        g. The family is essential in dealing with internal change and external disruptions.
    2. Nurturing families
        a. Characteristics include a sense of aliveness, affection, genuineness, honesty, open communication, and love.
        b. These families make plans, adjust plans, problem solve without panic, and accept change as part of life.
    3. Troubled families
        a. Characteristics include coldness, rigidity, control, guarded communication, tolerance replacing love, and secrecy.
        b. Adjustment and problem solving are difficult as family members rigidly hold on to assigned roles and responsibilities (Satir, 1988).
    4. The effect of disability on a family
        a. A child's, adult's, or elderly person's disability can cause permanent disruptions in family patterns.
        b. Established roles and responsibilities of the family change.
        c. Life patterns continue to change as children mature, siblings marry, individuals move away, parents grow older, health status changes within the family, and members die.
        d. Problem solving and adapting to change are necessary family skills for quality family life.
    5. Assessment
        a. Observe the family members' communication patterns
        b. Observe the family's cohesiveness during change
        c. Examine the family's planning strategies
        d. Examine the family's actions, behaviors, and roles
    6. Nursing interventions
        a. Encourage family therapy with a focus on the entire family, which should include information regarding the injury or illness, strategies for handling emotional distress, assistive services, sharing concerns, and assistance with coping (Butcher, 1994)
        b. Provide training in communication skills (e.g., structured marriage enrichment programs, effective listening, self-awareness, conflict resolution) (Captain, 1995)
    7. Research
        a. People with SCI associated increased life satisfaction 1 year after injury with the closeness of the family and the level of family activities.

b. People with TBI associated life satisfaction 1 year after injury with family satisfaction, employment, intact marriage, memory, and independence (Warren, Wrigley, Yoels, & Fine, 1996).

B. Social Support

1. Definition: A multifaceted concept that includes instrumental support (e.g., equipment, services), affective support (e.g., concern, being loved, feeling important, support presence), and cognitive support (e.g., education, advice, information, role modeling, counseling) (Rintala, Young, Spencer, & Bates, 1996)

2. Clinical examples

   a. Social support was seen as a strong predictor of life satisfaction among survivors of TBI who live in the community (Smith, Magill-Evans, & Brintnell, 1998).

   b. People with TBI or SCI and their partners indicated having low availability of social support and inadequate social integration in the years after injury. This social isolation led to high levels of depression (Hammell, 1994).

   c. People with multiple sclerosis (MS) and their partners had socialization difficulties due to their inability to keep up the pace of socialization, the inability of others to understand the limitations of MS, the need for mechanical or personal assistance, the uncertainty of daily energy levels, and inadequate finances (Stuifbergen, 1992).

3. Assessment

   a. Observe for barriers in socialization (e.g., fatigue, multiple problems, isolation, lack of self-confidence, apathy) (Abjornsson, Orbaek, & Hagstadius, 1998)

   b. Observe the frequency of contact with family and friends and leisure and physical activities

   c. Use the Life Satisfaction Index (Diener, 1984)

   d. Use the Sickness Impact Profile (SIP) (Smith, Magill, Evans, & Brintnell, 1998)

   e. Use the Community Integration Questionnaire (CIQ) (Smith, Magill, Evans, & Brintnell, 1998)

   f. Use the Quality of Social Support instrument (Bethoux, Calmels, Gautheron, & Minaire, 1996)

   g. Observe the client's patterns of behaviors such as alcohol use after injury: Increased consumption of alcohol is associated with lower levels of social support (Boraz & Heinemann, 1996).

4. Nursing interventions

   a. Encourage the client to use problem- and emotion-focused coping skills

   b. Encourage social networking (Cormier-Daigle & Stewart, 1997)

   c. Involve the spouse with instrumental (task-oriented) and emotional support

   d. Encourage the client to engage in meaningful, rewarding activities

   e. Encourage social roles for identity, power, and family position (Nir, Wallhagen, Doolittle, & Galinsky, 1997)

   f. Encourage the client to attend support groups

   g. Provide crisis therapy and stress management

   h. Encourage cognitive activation and memory training (Abjornsson et al., 1998)

C. Independence and Dependence

1. Independence can be fostered when people with disabilities have responsibility for self-care and are expected to participate in family roles.

2. Assessment

   a. Observe for initiation of ADLs

   b. Assess the client's level of functional abilities

   c. Assess the client's cognitive abilities

   d. Use the Functional Independence Measure (FIM™) instrument (Kelly-Hayes, 1996) to assess both lower cognitive and functional abilities, as well as the need for supervision especially for clients with TBI (Smith & Schwirian, 1998)

Brillhart, B., & Johnson, K. (1997). Motivation and coping processes of adults with disabilities: A qualitative study. *Rehabilitation Nursing, 22*(5), 249-256.

This qualitative study was conducted through interviews with 9 men and 3 women with SCI who had completed an inpatient rehabilitation program. The participants were recruited from a freestanding rehabilitation facility in the western United States. The participants were asked the following questions:

- What helped motivate you during rehabilitation to return to an active, productive life?

- How did rehabilitation nurses and staff assist you with that process?

Analysis of the data revealed five motivational categories: independence, education, socialization, self-esteem, and realization.

Prominent concepts within the independence category included transitional family support during times of stress and change, independence and family role expectations, self-responsibility, eliminating barriers, and provision of resources for independence. Frequent concepts with education included individualized self-care instruction, client as educator, role of rehabilitation nurse as client educator, and peer educators. Prominent concepts within socialization were encouragement by friends and family, learning positive response to socialization, and seeing loved ones as family members not as attendants. Self-esteem concepts included being considered a real person and not just a client, being a self-care expert, being politically active for the disabled, and having success at school or work. Realization concepts were having progressive awareness of disability, exploring the achievement of long-term goals, accepting the disability status, and realizing the person was "still me" despite the disability.

Implications for practice

Rehabilitation nurses can foster motivation and coping for people during rehabilitation in the following ways:

- Encourage personal change and growth of the client and family

- Establish an informal, individualized approach to the client

- Enable the client and family to be knowledgeable regarding their care for self-care and direction of that care

- Foster family flexibility, involvement, and support

- Provide guides for resource management related to home care, vocational education, recreation and socialization, and independent living

- Provide client and family counseling for the adjustment to disability during inpatient and home rehabilitation

---

 e. Observe participation in academic and vocational activities

 f. Assess for initiation of recreational activities

 g. Assess for perceptions of poor health and emotional distress, which are often associated with increased dependency (Riegel, Dracup, & Glaser, 1998)

 h. Use the FAMTOOL (a family health assessment tool) to evaluate communication, shared beliefs, shared work and play, value connectedness, and effort toward physical, emotional, social, and spiritual health (Weeks & O'Connor, 1997)

 i. Assess role expectations from the different viewpoints of family members, especially those focusing on pressures, demands, personal resources, and family structure (Satir, 1988)

 j. Use the Quality of Life Scale (Ferrans, 1996)

3. Nursing interventions

 a. Encourage independence within the family unit

 b. Provide more intensive family support during transitional periods (e.g., moving from acute care to rehabilitation, rehabilitation to home, home to independence)

 c. Eliminate environmental barriers

 d. Provide resources for adaptive housing, equipment, and attendant care (Brillhart & Johnson, 1997)

 e. Encourage family counseling

  1) Appropriate support for the client

2) Education about the client's discomfort with being a unilateral receiver and burden rather than a bidirectional receiver and giver

3) The appropriate help needed by the client (Rintala et al., 1996)

f. Encourage the family to reestablish life trajectories, meet development needs, and reintegrate the survivor into the family (Brzuzy & Speziale, 1997)

4. Research: Dependence was fostered by feelings of safety within a rehabilitation unit and being reluctant to leave such security. Family attitudes that fostered dependency and the fear of risks associated with ADLs (e.g., falling during transfers) also led to dependency (Brillhart & Johnson, 1997).

5. Clinical example: Effective coping styles and strategies by rehabilitation clients at discharge included confrontation, evasion, optimism, emotional expression, palliative activities, support, and self-reliance. Generally, clients coped with discharge to home with positive thinking, a sense of humor, control of the situation and emotional control, praying, taking problems step by step, and staying active (Easton, Zemen, & Kwiatkowski, 1995).

References

Abjornsson, G., Orbaek, P., & Hagstadius, S. (1998). Chronic toxic encephalopathy: Social consequences and experiences from a rehabilitation program. *Rehabilitation Nursing, 23*(1), 38-43.

Ai, A., Peterson, C., Dunkle, R., Saunders, D., Bolling, S., & Buchtel, H. (1997). How gender affects psychological adjustment one year after coronary artery bypass graft surgery. *Women and Health, 26*(4), 45-65.

Anderson, K.H., & Tomlinson, P.S. (1992). The family health system as an emerging paradigmatic view for nursing. *Image: The Journal of Nursing Scholarship, 24*(1), 57-63.

Bandura, A. (1977). Self-efficacy: Toward an unifying theory of behavioral change. *Psychological Review, 84*, 191-215.

Barry, P.D. (1996). *Psychosocial nursing care of physically ill patients and their families* (3rd ed.). New York: Lippincott.

Bergh, G., Branholm, I., & Dahlqvist, S. (1997). On life satisfaction and perceived health in chronically ill patients. *Scandinavian Journal of Occupational Health, 4*(1-4), 37-41.

Berman, C., & Rose, L. (1998). Examination of a patient's adaptation to quadriplegia. *Physical Therapy Case Reports, 1*(3), 148-156.

Bethoux, F., Calmels, P., Gautheron, V., & Minaire, P. (1996). Quality of life of spouses of stroke patients: A preliminary study. *International Journal of Rehabilitation and Health, 2*(3), 189-198.

Boraz, M., & Heinemann, A. (1996). The relationship between social support and alcohol abuse in people with spinal cord injuries. *International Journal of Rehabilitation and Health, 2*(3), 189-199.

Brillhart, B., & Johnson, K. (1997). Motivation and the coping process of adults with disabilities: A qualitative study. *Rehabilitation Nursing, 22*(5), 249-256.

Brzuzy, S., & Speziale, B. (1997). Persons with traumatic brain injuries and their families: Living arrangements and well-being post injury. *Social Work in Health Care, 26*(1), 77-88.

Burleigh, S.A., Farber, R.S., & Gillard, M. (1998). Community integration and life satisfaction after traumatic brain injury: Long-term findings. *American Journal of Occupational Therapy, 52*(1), 45-52.

Butcher, L.A. (1994). A family-focused perspective on chronic illness. *Rehabilitation Nursing, 19*(2), 70-74.

Captain, C. (1995). The effects of communication skills training on interaction and psychosocial adjustment among couples living with spinal cord injury. *Rehabilitation Nursing Research, 4*(4), 111-118.

Cardol, M., Elvers, J., Oostendorp, R., Brandsma, J., & deGroot, I. (1996). Quality of life in patients with amyotrophic lateral sclerosis. *Journal of Rehabilitation Sciences, 9*(4), 99-103.

Cecchini, A. (1998). Functional assessment after traumatic brain injury. *Neurology Report, 22*(4), 136-143.

Cermak, S., & Aberson, J. (1997). Social skills in children with learning disabilities. *Occupational Therapy in Mental Health, 13*(4), 1-24.

Clark, M., & Smith, D. (1998). The effects of depression and abnormal illness behavior on outcome following rehabilitation from stroke. *Clinical Rehabilitation, 12*(1), 73-80.

Cormier-Daigle, M., & Stewart, M. (1997). Support and coping of male hemodialysis-dependent patients. *International Journal of Nursing Studies, 34*(6), 420-430.

Davidhizar, R. (1997). Disability does not have to be the grief that never ends: Helping patients adjust. *Rehabilitation Nursing, 22*(1), 32-35.

DeWitt, K. (1993). The experience of getting well as described by adolescents recovering from trauma: A phenomenological perspective. *Rehabilitation Nursing Research, 2*, 10, 11-16.

Diamond, P., Holroyd, S., Macciocchi, S., & Felsenthal, G. (1995). Prevalence of depression and outcome of geriatric rehabilitation unit. *American Journal of Physical Medicine and Rehabilitation, 74*(3), 214-217.

Diener, E. (1984). Subjective well-being. *Psychological Bulletin, 95*(3), 542-575.

Easton, K., Zemen, D., & Kwiatkowski, S. (1995). The effects of nursing follow-up on the coping strategies used by rehabilitation patients after discharge. *Rehabilitation Nursing Research, 4*(4), 119-126.

Erikson, E. (1963). *Childhood and society*. New York: W.W. Norton & Co.

Ferrans, C.E. (1996). Development of a conceptual model of quality of life. *Scholarly Inquiry for Nursing Practice: An International Journal, 10*(3), 293-304.

Flannery, J. (1998). Using the Levels of Cognitive Functioning Assessment Scale with patients with traumatic brain injury in an acute care setting. *Rehabilitation Nursing, 23*(3), 88-94.

Goffman, E. (1974). *Stigma*. New York: Jason Aronson.

Gregory, R. (1995). Understanding and coping with neurological impairment. *Rehabilitation Nursing, 20*(2), 74-78.

Grzankowski, J.A. (1997). Altered thought processes related to traumatic brain injury and their nursing implications. *Rehabilitation Nursing, 22*(1), 24-28.

Hammell, K. (1994). Psychosocial outcome following severe closed head injury. *International Journal of Rehabilitation Research, 17*(4), 319-332.

Howell, D. (1998). Reaching to the depths of the soul: Understanding and exploring meaning in illness. *Canadian Oncology Nursing Journal, 8*(1), 22-23.

Jansen, D., & Keller, M. (1998). Identifying the attention demands perceived by elderly people. *Rehabilitation Nursing, 23*(1), 12-19.

Jarvis, C. (1996). *Physical examination and health assessment.* Philadelphia: W.B. Saunders.

Kelly-Hayes, M. (1996). Functional evaluation. In S.P. Hoeman (Ed.), *Rehabilitation nursing: Process and application* (2nd ed., pp. 144-155). St. Louis: Mosby.

Kendall, E., & Buys, N. (1998). An integrated model of psychosocial adjustment following acquired disability. *Journal of Rehabilitation, 64*(3), 16-20.

King, R.B. (1996). Quality of life after stroke. *Stroke, 27*(9), 1467-1472.

Knowles, M.S. (1984). *Andragogy in action.* San Francisco: Jossey-Bass.

Lazarus, R.S., & Folkman, S. (1984). *Stress, appraisal, and coping.* New York: Springer Publishing.

Lyon, B. (1993). The state of nursing science: Coping with disability. *Rehabilitation Nursing Research, 2*(1), 25-31.

Montgomery, P., Kitten, M., & Niemiec, C. (1997). The agitated patient with brain injury and the rehabilitation staff: Bridging the gap of misunderstanding. *Rehabilitation Nursing, 22*(3), 20-23, 39.

Neau, J., Ingrand, P, Mouille-Brachet, C., Rosier, M., Conderq, C., Alvarez, A., & Gil, R. (1998). Functional recovery and social outcome after cerebral infarction in young adults. *Cerebrovascular Disease, 8*(5), 296-302.

Nir, Z., Wallhagen, M., Doolittle, N., & Galinsky, D. (1997). A study of the psychosocial characteristics of patients in a geriatric rehabilitation unit in Israel. *Rehabilitation Nursing, 22*(3), 143-151.

Nypaver, J., Titus, M., & Brugler, C. (1996). Patient transfer to rehabilitation: Just another move? *Rehabilitation Nursing, 21*(2), 94-97.

Ogden, J., Utley, T., & Mee, E. (1997). Neurological and psychosocial outcome 4 to 7 years after subarachnoid hemorrhage. *Neurosurgery,41*(1), 25-34.

Pallett, P.J., & O'Brien, M.T. (1985). *Textbook of neurological nursing.* Boston: Little, Brown.

Pavlov, I. (1927). *Conditioned reflexes.* London: Oxford University Press.

Pentland, W., Harvey, A., & Walker, J. (1998). The relationships between time use and health and well-being in men with spinal cord injury. *Journal of Occupational Science, 5*(1), 14-25.

Piaget, J. (1952). *The origins of intelligence in children.* New York: Norton.

Resnick, B., Zimmerman, S., Magaziner, J., & Adelman, A. (1998). Use of the Apathy Evaluation Scale as a measure of motivation in elderly people. *Rehabilitation Nursing, 23*(3), 141-147.

Riedel, D., & Shaw, V. (1997). Nursing management of patients with brain injury requiring one-on-one care. *Rehabilitation Nursing, 22*(1), 36-39.

Riegel, B., Dracup, K., & Glaser, D. (1998). A longitudinal model of cardiac invalidism following myocardial infarction. *Nursing Research, 47*(5), 285-292.

Rintala, D., Young, M., Spencer, J., & Bates, P. (1996). Family relationships and adaptation to spinal cord injury: A qualitative study. *Rehabilitation Nursing, 21*(2), 67-74.

Satir, V. (1988). *The new peoplemaker.* Mountain View, CA: Science and Behavior Books.

Sawin, K., & Marshall, J. (1992). Developmental competence in adolescents with an acquired disability. *Rehabilitation Nursing Research, 1*(1), 41-50.

Scivoletto, G., Petrelli, A., Di-Lucente, L., & Castellano, V. (1997). Psychological investigation of spinal cord injury patients. *Spinal Cord, 35*(8), 526-520.

Seligman, M.E.P. (1975). *Helpless on depression, development, and death.* San Francisco: W.H. Freeman and Company.

Sisson, R. (1998). Life after a stroke: Coping with change. *Rehabilitation Nursing, 23*(4), 198-202.

Skinner, B.F. (1974). *About behaviorism.* New York: Alfred Knoph.

Smith, A., & Schwirian, P. (1998). The relationship between caregiver burden and the TBI survivors' cognition and functional ability after discharge. *Rehabilitation Nursing, 23*(5), 252-257.

Smith, J., Magill-Evans, J., & Brintnell, S. (1998). Life satisfaction following traumatic brain injury. *Canadian Journal of Rehabilitation, 11*(3), 131-140.

Stuifbergen, A. (1992). Meeting the demands of illness: Types and sources of support for individuals with multiple sclerosis and their partners. *Rehabilitation Nursing Research, 1*(1), 14-23.

Spatt, J., Zebenholzer, K., & Oder, W. (1997). Psychosocial long-term outcome of severe head injury as perceived by patients, relatives, and professionals. *Acta Neurology Scandinavian, 95*(3), 173-179.

Stuart, G.W., & Laraia, M.T. (1995). *Principles practice of psychiatric nursing.* St. Louis: Mosby.

Thompson, S. (1996). Practical ways of improving memory storage and retrieval problems in patients with head injuries. *British Journal of Occupational Therapy, 59*(9), 418-422.

Tollen, A., & Ahlstrom, G. (1998). Assessment instrument for problem-focused coping: Reliability of APC, Part I. *Scandinavian Journal of Caring Sciences, 12*(1), 18-24.

Voll, R., & Poustka, F. (1994). Coping with illness and coping with handicap during the vocational rehabilitation of physically handicapped adolescents and young adults. *International Journal of Rehabilitation Research, 17*(4), 305-318.

Warren, L., Wrigley, J., Yoels, W., & Fine, P. (1996). Factors associated with life satisfaction among a sample of persons with neurotrauma. *Journal of Rehabilitation Research and Development, 33*(4), 404-408.

Weeks, S., & O'Connor, P. (1997). The FAMTOOL Family Assessment Tool. *Rehabilitation Nursing, 22*(4), 188-191.

Wertheimer, M. (1959). *Productive thinking.* New York: Harper & Row.

Westbrook, M., & McIlwain, D. (1996). Living with the late effects of disability: A five year follow-up survey of coping among post-polio survivors. *Australian Occupational Therapy Journal, 43*(2), 60-71.

Woodward, S. (1996). Continence clinic: Impact of neurological problems on urinary continence. *British Journal of Nursing, 5*(15), 906-913.

Worthington, A. (1996). Psychological aspects of motor neuron disease: A review. *Clinical Rehabilitation, 10* (3), 185-194.

Wyller, T., Sveen, U., Sodring, K., Petterson, A., & Bautz-Holter, E. (1997). Subjective well-being one year after stroke. *Clinical Rehabilitation, 11*(2), 139-145.

Suggested resources

Barry, J., McQuade, C., & Livingstone, T. (1998). Using nurse case management to promote self-efficacy in individuals with rheumatoid arthritis. *Rehabilitation Nursing, 23*(6), 300-308.

Cox, E., Dooley, A., Liston, M., & Miller, M. (1998). Coping with stroke: Perceptions of elderly who have experienced stroke and rehabilitation interventions. *Topics in Stroke Rehabilitation, 4*(4), 76-88.

Godgrey, H., Knight, R., & Partridge, F. (1996). Emotional adjustment following traumatic brain injury: A stress-appraisal-coping formulation. *Journal of Head Trauma Rehabilitation, 11*(6), 29-40.

Hoeman, S.P. (Ed.). (1996). *Rehabilitation nursing: Process and application* (2nd ed.). St. Louis: Mosby.

Hupcey, J. (1998). Clarifying the social support theory-research linkage. *Journal of Advanced Nursing, 27*(6), 1231-1241.

Joyce, S. (1996). Outcomes management: Measuring a restored life to recreate a valuable life for posttrauma outpatient rehabilitation. *The Interdisciplinary Journal of Rehabilitation, 9*(6), 105, 107, 116.

Kneisl, C., & Wilson, H. (1984). *Handbook of psychosocial nursing care*. Reading, MA: Addison Wesley.

Section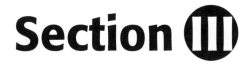

Nursing Management of Common Rehabilitation Disorders
....

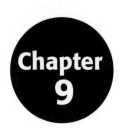

Stroke

Carla J. Howard, MS RN CRRN

Stroke or "brain attack" (also referred to as cerebrovascular accident [CVA]) affects hundreds of thousands of people on a yearly basis. The effects of stroke may be slight or severe, temporary or permanent, and can be devastating to the person as well as to the family. Patients who have had a stroke must cope with numerous sensorimotor, visual, perceptual, and language deficits. Rehabilitation should begin as soon after the stroke as possible. Rehabilitation is a team effort that focuses on regaining as much functional independence as possible. Rehabilitation also plays a major role in helping to prevent secondary complications and some long-term disabilities. To intervene effectively as a member of the rehabilitation team, nurses should have a good understanding of the physiological, perceptual, and psychological changes that occur after stroke.

I. Overview of Stroke

A. Descriptions
1. Stroke is a general term for acute brain damage caused by disease of blood vessels (Caplan, 1988).
2. Onset is rapid and produces focal injury (Gundersen, 1990).
3. When a stroke occurs, blood flow to that part of the brain is disrupted, resulting in tissue anoxia and death of brain cells (infarction).
4. The stroke process is dynamic and can have a variety of results.
    a. Persistent biochemical changes in and around the damaged cell
    b. Autolysis with accumulation of lactic acid and phosphokinase
    c. Edema: Anoxia increases blood flow to the damaged area, which can increase intracranial pressure and injure fragile cells surrounding the lesion; if edema is severe, it can cause herniation and death (Bronstein, Popovich, & Stewart-Amidei, 1991; Dolan, 1991; Gundersen, 1990; Hickey, 1992; Mumma, 1987).

B. Epidemiology (Bronstein et al., 1991; Kelly-Hayes, 1991; Millikan, McDowell, & Easton, 1987)
1. Stroke is the third most common cause of death in Western countries.

2. Mortality and incidence rates rise as age increases.
    a. Incidence has declined in recent years in the United States.
    b. Mortality rate is higher for hemorrhagic stroke.
3. Stroke occurs more commonly in elderly people, men, and African-American people.
4. Prevalence of stroke in the United States ranges from 150 to 200 per 100,000 people.
5. Approximately two-thirds of patients will survive the initial stroke. Of these, approximately half will have a residual physical and social disability (Kong, Chua, & Tow, 1998).

C. Etiology
1. Ischemic or hemorrhagic disruption of cerebral arteries is the major cause of stroke.
    a. Normal arterial blood supply to the brain involves the internal carotid artery (which ultimately becomes the middle cerebral artery) and the vertebral artery.
    b. The major arteries (i.e., internal carotid, middle cerebral, and vertebral) form the anterior and posterior circulatory systems that compose the circle of Willis
2. Systemic hypoperfusion or a cerebral compression (e.g., a tumor) less frequently produce stroke syndromes.
3. There are many potential risk factors for

stroke, many of which are preventable.

a. Hypertension

b. Obesity

c. Smoking

d. Elevated cholesterol level

e. Heavy ingestion of alcohol

f. Diabetes

g. Blood disorders (e.g., sickle-cell anemia, polycythemia)

h. Cardiac disorders

i. Family history of stroke

j. Older age: 72% of strokes occur at age 65 or older (U.S. Department of Health & Human Services, 1995)

k. Gender: Stroke is most prevalent in men; however, women who use oral contraceptives, smoke, and have migraines are at higher risk (Gundersen, 1990).

l. Race: Stroke is more common in African-American people.

m. Substance abuse (e.g., heroin, cocaine, Talwin, amphetamines) (Bronstein et al., 1991; Hickey, 1992; Licata-Gehr, 1991)

n. Transient ischemic attack (TIA)

o. Prior stroke

D. Pathophysiology

1. Ischemic stroke (about 80% of all strokes)

a. Process

1) Focal area of the brain receives little or no blood flow due to occlusion of a blood vessel.

2) Focal area of the brain and adjoining brain tissue are deprived of oxygen and glucose.

3) When the deprivation is severe enough to impair gray matter function and lasts long enough, permanent damage occurs.

b. Classifications

1) Transient ischemic attack (TIA)

a) Characteristics

(1) Short, reversible ischemic event

(2) Signs and symptoms that occur rapidly and last less than 24 hours

b) Possible precursor to major stroke, myocardial infarction (MI), or death

2) Reversible ischemic neurological deficit (RIND): A TIA process that takes a few days to resolve and is reversible

3) Systemic hypoperfusion (or ischemic-anoxic encephalopathy): Condition in which the small distal cerebral arteries do not receive enough blood flow due to cardiac pump failure or hypovolemia related to blood loss (Caplan, 1988)

4) Cerebral thrombus (Bronstein et al., 1991; Caplan, 1988; Dolan, 1991; Gundersen, 1990; Licata-Gehr, 1991)

a) Most common cause of stroke

b) A stationary clot in a large blood vessel, usually caused by atherosclerotic plaque

(1) Plaque

(a) Forms when calcium and lipids collect and attach to the vessel wall, especially in bifurcations of a large artery (see Figure 9-1)

(b) Produces narrowing that impedes or obstructs blood flow

(2) Atherosclerosis

(a) Can produce degeneration of blood vessel walls

(b) Involves tearing of a weakened wall or plaque, thus triggering the normal clotting process; such congestion further reduces circulation

5) Cerebral embolism

a) A traveling clot, which typically originates from thrombi in the heart or from plaque in the aortic arch or carotid or vertebral arteries, that becomes lodged and obstructs cerebral blood flow

b) Commonly associated with history of cardiac disease, especially atrial fibrillation in elderly people

6) Lacunar infarct (Caplan, 1988; Hickey, 1992)

a) Thrombotic occlusion in penetrating (small) cerebral arteries

b) Involves lesions that are small, oval-shaped, pitting, and deep within brain

c) Frequently develops in the pons or thalamic pathways

d) Often results in pure motor or sensory deficits

e) Commonly associated with history of diabetes and hypertension

2. Hemorrhagic stroke (about 20% of strokes) (Caplan, 1988; Dolan, 1991; Gundersen, 1990; Hickey, 1992; Loen, 1991)

a. Process

1) Spontaneous rupture of a cerebral vessel occurs; blood enters brain tissue or subarachnoid space.

2) "Because arteriosclerotic arteries lose most of their elasticity, they rupture easily. The hemorrhage occurs in areas where degenerative changes in the vessel walls permit rupture of small vessels" (Loen, 1991, p. 240).

3) Wall degeneration, especially in small cerebral vessels, is thought to stem from chronic hypertension.

b. Classifications

1) Subarachnoid hemorrhage

a) Involves blood from a ruptured vessel entering the subarachnoid space

b) Is usually related to saccular or congenital aneurysm rupture, most of which are in the carotid artery circulation

c) Can have several potential results

(1) Increased intracranial pressure

(2) Vasospasms

(3) Ischemia, which further reduces cerebral blood flow

d) Is less commonly related to arteriovenous malformation, anticoagulants, drugs, and trauma

2) Intracerebral (intraparenchymal) hemorrhage

a) Frequently caused by hypertension

b) Involves small, deep-penetrating blood vessels that rupture and release blood directly into the brain tissue

c) Usually invades deep white matter first

d) Involves the released blood putting pressure on tissue and surrounding small arterioles and capillaries, which can then tear

e) Involves resulting hematoma that acts as a space-occupying lesion and, if large enough, can cause brain shifting and/or herniation

E. Residual Deficits of Stroke (see Table 9-1)

1. Significant alterations in many psychosocial areas

a. Diminished affect

b. Increased dependence in activities of daily living (ADLs)

c. Decreased self-esteem

d. Altered role performance

e. Sexual dysfunction

f. Change in leisure and/or social activity

g. Decreased financial earning or vocational capability

2. General sequelae (all of which can influence safety)

a. Hemiplegia: Weakness or paralysis contralateral to the lesion

b. Abnormal tone, including flaccidity at first and then hypertonicity on the affected side

c. Sensorimotor problems, ataxia, imbalance

d. Language deficits if lesion is in the dominant hemisphere

e. Visuospatial perception impairments

f. Cognitive deficits

g. Memory changes

h. Emotional lability: Inability to control emotions, especially crying and laughter

i. Fatigue

j. Depression: There is controversy about whether this has an organic or an emotional basis.

k. Seizure activity

3. Left-hemispheric stroke: Common impairments and deficits

a. Right hemiparesis or hemiplegia

b. Impaired ability to think analytically

c. Inability to do mathematical computations or interpret symbols

d. Right homonymous hemianopsia

e. Behavioral changes (e.g., cautiousness, hesitancy)

f. Language problems: Language involves not only speech, but also conveying and comprehending thoughts and ideas and understanding and using symbols sequentially and grammatically (Boss, 1991) (see Table 9-2).

1) Nonfluent aphasia: Broca's (or expressive) aphasia

a) Location of damage: Occurs with lesions in the posterior part of the dominant frontal lobe (precentral gyrus) (see Figure 9-2)

b) Characteristic symptoms

(1) Speech that is slow, effortful to produce, and punctuated by long pauses between words

(2) Other language problems

(a) Anomia: Finding words and naming objects

(b) Conductive aphasia: Repeating words or phrases upon command

(c) Sentence construction

Table 9-1. Residual Deficits of Stroke (Left Versus Right Brain Injury)	Left Hemispheric Damage	Right Hemispheric Damage
Paresis/paralysis	Right side	Left side
Major deficits	Right homonymous hemianopsia; language deficits (e.g., aphasia, expression, comprehension, word-finding); confuses left and right; has trouble gesturing, reading, writing	Left homonymous hemianopsia; displays visual, spatial, perceptual deficits (e.g., gets lost, cannot dress self correctly, misjudges distance and position in space, spills things, gets stuck in doorways); has distorted body image; may have agnosia
Thought processes	Has difficulty listening and understanding; cannot process incoming language normally	Has poor judgment, may have unrealistic thoughts; has memory deficits; has difficulty with concrete thinking
Emotional style	Is easily frustrated or depressed; is aware of deficits	Is often cheerful or euphoric; will deny the illness or deficits; is unaware of problems; neglects the left side; exhibits socially inappropriate behavior
Attention span	Usually normal	Short; is highly distractible
Behavioral style	Is slow and cautious; needs encouragement	Is quick and impulsive; needs supervision to prevent injury
Strategies	Use demonstration, positive feedback; exhibit acceptance; speak slowly	Use repetition and one-step commands (it may be difficult to reeducate the patient)

Table 9-2. Language Functions of Major Classic Aphasias

Aphasia Type	Spontaneous Speech	Comprehension	Repetition	Reading	Writing
Broca's	Nonfluent	+	−	±	−
Wernicke's	Fluent	−	−	−	Paragraphic
Conduction	Fluent	+	−	+	−
Global	Mute	−	−	−	−
Anomic	Disorder of word recall	+	+	+	+
Transcortical motor	Nonfluent	+	+	+	−
Transcortical sensory	Fluent	−	+	+	−
Mixed transcortical (isolation of speech area)	Nonfluent	−	+	−	Paragraphic

Note. + = relatively intact, − = impaired

Reprinted with permission of Butterworth-Heinemann and Howard S. Kirshner, MD, Department of Neurology, Vanderbilt University School of Medicine, Nashville, TN (developer) from Love, R.J., & Webb, W.G. (1996). *Neurology for the speech-language pathologist* (3rd ed., p. 217). Newton, MA: Butterworth-Heinemann.

(d) Improper use of small words (e.g., or, and, but, if, to, from) and/or verb endings
(e) Perseveration: Unintentional repetition of a word or phrase due to impaired motor processing
(3) Impaired ability to read letters, numbers, or written material
(4) Impaired writing skills (i.e., translating one's thoughts into symbols): This should not be confused with the physical act of writing or penmanship.
(5) Altered language comprehension (Bronstein et al., 1991; Damasio, 1992)
(6) Intact automatic speech (i.e., the person may be able to express a word, phrase, profanity, or song unexpectedly and clearly)
2) Fluent aphasia: Wernicke's (or receptive) aphasia

a) Location of damage: Occurs with damage in the posterior, superior temporal dominant lobe (superior temporal gyrus) (see Figure 9-2)
b) Characteristic symptoms
(1) Problems with comprehension of words and sounds
(2) The ability to speak fluently is intact, but speech may not be correct or appropriate in the context of the conversation; mispronunciation of words and anomia can evolve because the person cannot comprehend what he or she has said and cannot detect his or her own errors
(3) Reading problems
3) Global aphasia
a) Location of damage: Frontal-temporal dominant lobes (see Figure 9-2)
b) Characteristic symptoms
(1) Comprehension and speaking problems
(2) Impaired comprehension of written language

(3) Repeating one or a few words in an effort to communicate a thought

(4) Possible intact automatic speech for routines (e.g., counting, stating days of the week, singing a song)

4) Apraxia of speech

a) Location of damage: Motor centers in the cortex that control speech

b) Characteristic symptoms

(1) Purposeful speech is hard to produce because the muscles in the mouth and throat, although not paralyzed, do not respond in the way the person intends.

(2) Speech may be clear one moment and undecipherable the next.

(3) Perseveration and inconsistency are common.

5) Dysarthria

a) Location of damage: Brainstem and/or cranial nerves

b) Characteristic symptoms

(1) Articulation problems

(2) Abnormal muscle control of the palate, tongue, labia, and/or pharynx

(3) Speech that is slow, commonly slurred, hard to understand, and may be too soft or loud

(4) Abnormal voice quality

6) Anarthria: Total loss of articulation capability due to absent muscle control; location of damage is brainstem

4. Right hemispheric stroke: Common impairments and deficits

a. Left hemiplegia or hemiparesis

b. Problems with depth perception and spatial relationships

c. Visual disturbances (including left homonymous hemianopsia)

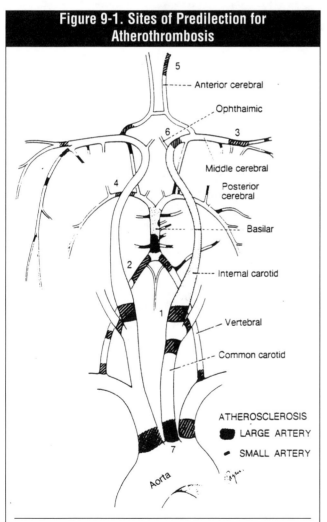

Figure 9-1. Sites of Predilection for Atherothrombosis

Source: Fisher, C.M. (1975). Anatomy and pathology of the cerebral vasculature. In Meyer, J.S. (Ed.), *Modern concepts of cerebrovascular disease*. New York: Spectrum Publications Inc.

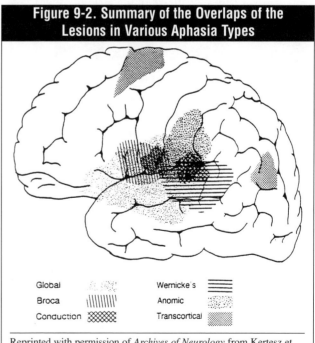

Figure 9-2. Summary of the Overlaps of the Lesions in Various Aphasia Types

Reprinted with permission of *Archives of Neurology* from Kertesz et al. (1977). Isotope localization of infarcts in aphasia. *Archives of Neurology*, 24, 590-601.

d. Inability to distinguish directional concepts such as up/down, front/back, in/out

e. Difficulty distinguishing foreground from background information (figure-ground, spatial-temporal perception)

f. Decreased ability to distinguish between similar shapes and forms (form-constancy, spatial-temporal perception)

g. Anosognosia: Denial of the extent of paralysis and physical disability and reduced insight into the ramifications of impairments

h. Somatognosia: Inability to localize and/or recognize one's own body parts and how they relate to other parts

i. Lack of awareness of others' nonverbal communication (e.g., facial expressions, tone of voice, territorial space, gestures) (pragmatic skills); display of a flat affect

j. Unilateral neglect: Inability to integrate sensory and perceptual stimuli from one side of the body or environment

k. Behavioral changes, including impulsiveness, egocentricity, quickness to try things

l. Social inappropriateness: Sexual disinhibition and inappropriate self-disclosure

m. Difficulty in finding locations, such as one's room, and understanding maps and objects (geographic-topographic memory)

5. Brainstem strokes

a. Result from ischemic or hemorrhagic process in the midbrain, pons, or medulla

b. Potential deficits: Many vital centers and nuclei of cranial nerves exist; thus, deficits can vary greatly.
   1) Dysarthria
   2) Dysphagia: Chewing and/or swallowing problems
   3) Ataxia, difficulty walking, staggered gait; quadriparesis or quadriplegia
   4) Poor balance and/or coordination
   5) Double and/or blurred vision; pinpoint pupils; horizontal gaze palsy (i.e., eye moves to the side, away from the cerebral lesion)
   6) Vertigo (with nausea)
   7) Abnormal respiratory patterns
   8) Hyperthermia

9) Coma or persistent vegetative state
10) Locked-in syndrome
    a) Characteristics
       (1) Quadriplegia and facial paralysis, except for eye and/or eyelid movement
       (2) Intact cognition
    b) Occurs when stroke is located in the pons

II. Stroke Treatment

A. Traditional Approaches

1. Several years ago, treatment for strokes was very different than it is today.

2. Healthcare professionals focused on managing the patient's medical and functional status after the stroke.

3. Supportive care included helping patients with deficits by assisting with ADLs, providing caregiver support, and obtaining needed equipment (e.g., wheelchairs, walkers).

4. Prevention of complications (e.g., pneumonia, contractures, pressure sores) were the main focus.

5. Therapy was provided to help patients improve or maintain function after the stroke.

B. Modern, Aggressive Approaches

1. Early intervention

   a. A brain attack (stroke)—like a heart attack—needs immediate medical attention.

   b. A person experiencing the warning signs of a brain attack is encouraged to get to a hospital immediately.

   c. Research and clinical trials have demonstrated some success with more aggressive stroke treatment within an early window of time following a stroke (Hill & Hachinski, 1998).

2. Thrombolytic therapy (for ischemic strokes)

   a. Recombinant tissue plasminogen activator (rtPA)

      1) Federal Drug Administration (FDA) approves this therapy for a short window of time at the onset of acute stroke.

      2) Patient is assessed for specific criteria before given this drug as a treatment.

3) Patient history must be reviewed for potential contraindications (e.g., recent previous stroke, uncontrolled hypertension at the time of treatment, seizure at onset of stroke, active internal bleeding).

4) rtPA is given only after exclusion of an intracranial hemorrhage by a cranial computerized tomography (CT) scan or other diagnostic imaging methods to rule out hemorrhage.

5) Patients are assessed using statistics combining the following outcome scales: Barthel Index (see Figure 9-3), Modified Rankin Scale (see Figure 9-4), Glasgow Outcome

Figure 9-3. Barthel Index

1. Feeding

Unable	- totally dependent	☐ 0
Needs help	- cutting, spreading butter but feeds self	☐ 5
Independent	- can eat normal food (not only soft food) provided by others but not cut up	☐ 10

2. Bathing

Dependent		☐ 0
Independent	- can get in and out unsupervised and wash self. In shower, independent if unsupervised/unaided	☐ 5

3. Grooming (personal care)

Needs help		☐ 0
Independent	- washes face, does hair, brushes teeth, shaves (implements can be provided by helper)	☐ 5 10

4. Dressing

Dependent		☐ 0
Needs help	- e.g. with buttons, zips etc. but can do about half task unaided	☐ 5
Independent	- can select and put on all clothes (including buttons, zips, laces, etc)	☐ 10

5. Bowel control (preceding week)

Incontinent		☐ 0
Occasional accident	- once a week or less often	☐ 5
Continent		☐ 10

6. Bladder Control

Incontinent	- or catheterized and unable to manage catheter	☐ 0
Occasional accident	- less than once a day (24 h)	☐ 5
Continent	- for over 7 days. If catheterized, can manage catheter alone	☐ 10

7. Toilet Use

Dependent		☐ 0
Needs some help	- can wipe self plus can do some of other tasks required of independent person	☐ 5
Independent	- can reach toilet/commode, undress. sufficiently, wipe self, dress and leave	☐ 10

8. Chair/Bed transfer

Unable	- no sitting balance, cannot sit, requires two people to lift	☐ 0
Major help	- can sit, requires one strong/skilled or two normal people to lift	☐ 5
Minor help	- one person can lift easily or needs any supervision for safety	☐ 10
Independent		☐ 15

9. Mobility

Immobile		☐ 0
Wheel chair independent	- can negotiate corners/doors unaided	☐ 5
Walks with help	- one untrained person providing physical help, supervision or moral support	☐ 10
Independent	- can walk 50 m or around house. May use any aid e.g. stick, except rolling walker	☐ 15

10. Stairs

Unable		☐ 0
Needs help	- verbal or physical help or carrying aid	☐ 5
Independent	- up and down, carrying any walking aid	☐ 10

Source: Mahoney, F.J., & Barthel, D.W. (1965). Functional evaluation: The Barthel Index. *Maryland State Medical Journal, 14*, 61-65.

Score, National Institutes of Health (NIH) Stroke Scale.

b. Time frame: rtPA is given to patients who arrive at the hospital within 3 hours of the onset of stroke and who have a blood pressure within safe parameters.

3. Thrombolytic trials in acute stroke

a. rtPA: One study tested the use for a longer time frame (i.e., a therapeutic 6-hour window), but found to be not as beneficial (Hill & Hachinski, 1998).

b. rtPA and lubeluzole: Trials of combination therapy of thrombolysis and neuroprotection have been done (Hill & Hachinski, 1998).

c. Streptokinase, urokinase, prourokinase

1) Streptokinase was studied in three large trials involving more than 1,000 patients, but the dosage was not successful. Future trials are planned (Hill & Hachinski, 1998).

2) A small series of thrombolysis tests were done with urokinase and prourokinase. Both are now being studied in Phase III trials (Hill & Hachinski, 1998).

4. Antiplatelet therapy and anticoagulation (Hill & Hachinski, 1998)

a. Aspirin: Trialed in two studies

1) Results pooled from both studies revealed a slight benefit.

2) Aspirin therapy might be given if thrombolytic therapy is contraindicated.

b. Heparin: Is widely used to prevent propagation of clot; however, it has risk of hemorrhage as do other medicines being tested.

c. Low molecular weight heparin: North American studies are in progress.

5. Management of blood pressure

a. Some fluctuation of blood pressure is expected; however, hypertension should be treated if it is > 230 mm Hg systolic or 140 mm Hg diastolic.

b. Hypertension should be treated with medications such as nitroprusside or labetalol, which can be titrated.

c. Calcium-channel blockers are likely to cause severe drops in blood pressure in some patients and should be avoided.

d. Blood pressure might be treated differently if the patient is on thrombolytic therapy.

6. Management of serum glucose

a. Not enough testing has been done on the treatment of hyperglycemia with insulin on patients who have had a stroke.

b. Experimental models suggest that hyperglycemia may increase neuronal damage, and hypoglycemia may extend an infarct.

c. Current findings suggest that intravenous (IV) solutions with glucose should be avoided and serum glucose should be monitored carefully.

7. Management of body temperature

a. In some experiments, hypothermia has been neuroprotective after focal ischemia.

b. Because fever in acute stroke worsens the prognosis, it is believed to be reasonable to use antipyretics, which are safe

---

Figure 9-4. Modified Rankin Scale

Grade	Description
0	No symptoms at all
1	No significant disability despite symptoms. Able to carry out all usual duties and activities
2	Slight disability: Unable to carry out all previous activities but able to look after own affairs without assistance
3	Moderate disability: Requiring some help, but able to walk without assistance
4	Moderately severe disability: Unable to walk without assistance, and unable to attend to own bodily needs without assistance
5	Severe disability: Bedridden, incontinent, and requiring constant nursing care and attention

Source consulted

Stroke, 1988, Vol. 19, pp. 604-607.

for fever in patients who have had a stroke.

8. Management of fluids

   a. Dysphagic patients are at risk for aspiration pneumonia and are generally not allowed to have oral fluids initially.

   b. IV fluids must be balanced carefully to give hypotensive patients enough volume to sustain cerebral perfusion and to ensure that hypertensive patients do not develop cerebral edema.

   c. Normal saline is used because dextrose and glucose solutions could cause serum glucose elevations.

9. Special stroke units

   a. Patients in special stroke units may experience a quicker recovery; however, the stroke unit may not influence survival or long-term functional outcome.

   b. Stroke units provide complex interventions including medical, nursing, and therapy professionals.

   c. Stroke units emphasize early rehabilitation (usually within 24 hours) and active participation of both the patient and family (Langhorne, Williams, Gilchrist, & Howie, 1993).

C. Future Directions in Acute Stroke Treatment: Neuroprotective Agents (Hill & Hachinski, 1998)

   1. Purpose of neuroprotective agents

      a. Neurons in the center of the infarct generally die, but surrounding neurons may be spared by neuroprotective agents currently being trialed.

      b. Neuroprotective agents are believed to preserve neurons at various stages along the cascading effect of an ischemic infarct and may decrease the size of the infarct.

      c. If treated successfully, these agents may allow time for reperfusion to be reestablished, thus reducing the volume of the infarct.

   2. Lubeluzole: Along with being trialed in combination with thrombolytic therapy, lubeluzole is also in a Phase III trial as a neuroprotective agent.

3. Clomethiazole: This drug is currently in the Phase III Clomethiazole Acute Stroke Study (CLASS) as a neuroprotective agent.

4. Other drugs: Several other drugs are also being trialed as neuroprotective agents.

D. Surgical Procedures for Acute Stroke

   1. General: Surgery is generally not the treatment of choice, but it is done in some cases (Hill & Hachinski, 1998).

   2. Middle-cerebral-artery embolectomy: Done only under rare, special circumstances

   3. Decompressive craniectomy: Done on patients with large infarctions near the middle cerebral artery; results reduce mortality rates by more than 50%.

III. Nursing Process

A. Assessment by Nurses and the Interdisciplinary Rehabilitation Team (see Figure 9-5)

   1. Medical management: Assessed by the RN and physicians (e.g., rehabilitation physiatrist and primary physician, as well as consulting physicians)

      a. Patient's medical stability: The initial primary focus in rehabilitation

      b. Assessment of medical needs that can impede rehabilitation progress if left unmanaged (e.g., hypotension, hypertension, hyperglycemia, oxygen saturation, cardiac irregularities, other chronic illnesses affecting medical stability)

   2. Communication: Assessed by speech language pathologist (SLP), RN, and registered occupational therapist (OTR)

      a. Presence of aphasia; expressive and/or receptive communication

      b. Other methods of communication (e.g., nodding, pointing, gesturing, using symbols)

      c. Premorbid communication pattern: History from family or significant other

      d. Vocalization problems from motor inability; tracheostomy

      e. Agnosia, apraxia, dysarthria

      f. Hearing aid or glasses

   3. Memory: Assessed by SLP, OTR, RN, and physical therapist (PT)

      a. Premorbid ability

b. Short-term memory

c. Long-term memory

d. Memory problems involving auditory and/or visual information

4. Problem-solving ability: Assessed by RN, SLP, OTR, PT

a. Premorbid ability

b. Ability to make appropriate choices

c. Ability to find solutions

d. Presence of planning or organizational skills

5. Sensory/visual perception: Assessed by RN, OTR, PT

a. Premorbid use of hearing aid or glasses

b. Perceptual responses; acuity of senses (e.g., vision, hearing, touch, taste, smell)

c. Medications that may alter sensation or perception

6. ADL and self-care: Assessed by RN, OTR

a. Ability to bathe, dress, or toilet self

b. Premorbid abilities

c. How much help is required

d. Ability to gather needed equipment, supplies, clothing

e. Mobility to carry out activities

f. Adaptive equipment needed (e.g., bath sponge, reacher, shoe horn)

7. Dysphagia and swallowing: Assessed by RN, SLP, OTR

a. Ability to feed self; amount of assistance needed

b. Ability to chew, drink, swallow without difficulty

c. Correct diet and consistency ordered

d. Adequate caloric and fluid intake

e. Uses correct position for eating and is awake and alert

f. Presence of drooling and pocketing, not swallowing

g. Presence of cough and gag reflex

h. Voice quality (e.g., wet, gurgly, nasal while eating)

i. Use and fit of dentures

j. Use of upper extremities (e.g., grip, able to lift utensils, able to cut and prepare food)

k. Ability to see food (e.g., hemianopsia)

8. Bowel management: Assessed by RN

a. Neurogenic bowel (sudden, involuntary defecation)

Figure 9-5. Assessment of a New Patient with Stroke

- Obtain verbal report from a nurse on the unit that sent the patient.
- Make appropriate room assignment based on deficits (e.g., turn affected side toward door for stimulation, place close to nursing station if at high risk for falls).
- When patient arrives, assist with the patient's transfer to bed: The nursing assessment begins now as the nurse observes how much the patient can do during the transfer.
- Determine if the patient can answer questions and is cognitively aware: This can be determined in a short time with conversation while welcoming the patient to the unit. If the patient is unable to provide his or her own history, ask a family member to attend the assessment.
- Assess general data (e.g., allergies, medications, identification band on).
- Obtain complete medical history and complete a head-to-toe assessment, including neurological checks (e.g., for strength, orientation). During this time, also assess communication and cognition skills.
- Assess bowel and bladder function, using information obtained from the report of other nurses, combined with information from the patient and family: This assessment may not be complete until the nurse actually toilets the patient during the first 24 hours.
- Obtain histories for sleep, nutrition, safety, and sex.
- Assess psychosocial history and educational wants, needs, and preferences for learning style.
- Assess leisure interests, community reentry needs, and discharge planning needs.
- Provide the patient and family with verbal and written orientation information about the unit and the staff.
- Communicate pertinent information to team members as soon as possible.
- Provide the patient with necessary safety equipment (e.g., bed alarm, wheelchair alarm) as soon as the assessment is complete
- Follow the assessment pattern of the unit but keep in mind that the patient may get tired or frustrated if several team members assess the same things at different times.

b. Continence history prior to stroke; bowel history (e.g., when, how often)

c. Awareness of need to defecate

d. Medication use; digital stimulation

e. Bowel sounds; abdominal tenderness or distention

f. Ability to get to bathroom; ability to don and doff clothing

g. Hygiene needs; assistance needed

h. Positioning; privacy

i. Physical activity: A study of patients with stroke (Munchiando & Kendall, 1993) discovered that as the number of hours spent in bed increased, the number of days to establish bowel program increased.

9. Bladder management: Assessed by RN

a. Neurogenic bladder: Decreased capacity and involuntary voiding as soon as urge is perceived

b. Continence history prior to stroke

c. Premorbid history (e.g., nocturia, stress incontinence)

d. Recent history (e.g., urgency, frequency, urinary tract infection [UTI])

e. Awareness of need to urinate; cognition

f. Ability to perform toileting and to get to the bathroom

g. Hygiene needs; assistance; privacy

h. Catheter (e.g., intermittent, indwelling)

i. Fluid intake

j. Medication use

10. Mobility: Assessed by RN, PT, OTR

a. Bed mobility: Moving up, down, side to side, bridging, sitting up; amount of assistance needed

b. Transfers: Bed to chair, wheelchair to toilet, to bath bench or shower chair, to car; amount of assistance needed

c. Wheelchair mobility: Type of wheelchair; ability to self-propel; amount of assistance needed

d. Gait, sitting, standing; need for devices (e.g., walker, cane, crutches)

e. Endurance, strength, balance, tone, and proprioception

f. Environment (e.g., lighting, open space)

11. Sexual functioning: Assessed by RN, physician, psychologist

a. Premorbid sexual history (e.g., preferences, frequency, initiation [partner or self])

b. Sensory deficits

c. Mobility

d. Ability to communicate; visual/perceptual deficits

e. Emotional status; fear

f. Fatigue

g. Knowledge

h. Libido

i. Need for birth control

j. Bowel and bladder management prior to sex

12. Skin integrity: Assessed by RN, PT, OTR

a. Immobility

b. Loss of sensation

c. Incontinence and hygiene

d. Presence of pressure, friction, shearing

e. Poor circulation

f. Hydration and nutrition

13. Equipment: Assessed by OTR, PT, RN, social worker (SW), discharge planner

a. Need for assistance with mobility

b. Need for assistance with ADLs

c. Financial resources available

14. Psychosocial needs: Assessed by RN, SW, psychologist

a. Role changes

b. Relationships with family members

c. Family and community support

d. Coping skills and stressors

15. Leisure: Assessed by RN and certified therapeutic recreation specialist (CTRS)

a. Premorbid leisure history

b. Current physical ability and endurance related to leisure interest

c. Cognitive status

16. Education: Assessed by each rehabilitation team member

a. Cognitive status; intellectual capacity

b. Attention span

c. Premorbid learning needs (e.g., visual, auditory, kinesthetic, combination)

d. Level of formal education

e. Ability to read or write

f. Language and cultural barriers

g. Motivation and readiness to learn

h. Environmental barriers

i. Knowledge of disability and self-care needs

j. Support and presence of caregivers

17. Safety: Assessed by each rehabilitation team member

a. Cognition and awareness

b. Risk for and prior history of falls

c. Environment (e.g., hospital, home)

d. Medication that alters level of consciousness

e. Sensory impairments

18. Comfort and pain level: Assessed by RN

a. Subluxation and shoulder pain: Subluxation is painless; however, manipulation and improper positioning of a subluxed shoulder is what causes pain.

b. Shoulder-hand syndrome

c. Pain and its location, frequency; self-reported measure of pain, using intensity scale of 1-10 for nonaphasic patients; use University of Alabama at Birmingham (UAB) Pain Behavior Scale for nonverbal, aphasic patients (Simon, 1996) [Refer to Chapter 13 for pain scales.]

d. Pain related to activity or randomly occurring

e. What relieves pain

f. Effectiveness of medicine

g. Changes in sleep pattern: Patients with large hemispheric stroke may have a temporary reversal of sleep-wake rhythms (i.e., lethargy during day and wakefulness and agitation at night) (Culebras, 1992).

h. Sleep history (e.g., normal bedtime, need for white noise, lights)

i. Sleep problems: Onset, frequent awakenings, nocturia

j. Environmental (e.g., hot, cold, comfortable bed)

19. Spiritual: Assessed by RN and chaplain

a. Sources of hope and strength

b. Religious practices

c. Scheduled time for privacy

20. Discharge planning: Assessed by discharge planner in conjunction with rehabilitation team

a. Physical deficits and need for adaptive equipment

b. Caregiver knowledge and support

c. Financial resources available

d. Need for community resources

e. Adaptations needed for home environment with rehabilitation team input

B. Nursing Diagnoses Frequently Associated with Stroke

1. Impaired physical mobility

2. Self-care deficits (specify level)

3. Sensory-perceptual alteration

4. Impaired verbal communication

5. Altered elimination (bowel and bladder)

6. High risk for aspiration and/or impaired swallowing

7. Potential for injury

8. Impaired home maintenance management and discharge planning

9. Impaired thought processes

10. Disturbance in body image

11. Altered sexuality pattern

12. Caregiver distress syndrome

13. Spiritual distress

14. Alteration in skin integrity

15. Knowledge deficit

16. Alteration in comfort

C. Planning and Patient Goals Related to Nursing Diagnoses
1. Demonstrate maximal independence in mobility
2. Perform ADLs at optimal level of independence with or without the use of assistive devices
3. Be free from injury
4. Identify diversional activities to decrease stress (by caregivers)
5. Verbalize satisfaction with sexuality
6. Identify negative feelings related to self-image
7. Verbalize understanding of the diagnosis and treatment of stroke (CVA)

D. Interventions for Each Assessed Area
1. Medical management
    a. Monitor vital signs (more frequently during early rehabilitation); medication for hypertension as needed; IV fluids for hypotension (if the patient is hypotensive, hemoconcentration can occur and cerebral perfusion decreases, potentially worsening the infarct)
    b. Monitor blood glucose and regulate with insulin as needed
    c. Use IV solutions of normal saline (NS)
    d. Provide oxygen as ordered and titrate to 90% or greater
    e. Use telemetry monitoring or electrocardiogram (EKG) for cardiac abnormalities
    f. Check lung sounds and risk of aspiration
    g. Check for fever (e.g., UTI, pneumonia)
    h. Check lab values (e.g., activated partial thromboplastin time [aPTT], hemoglobin and hematocrit [H & H], electrolytes)
    i. Measure legs daily for swelling; assess for deep vein thrombosis (DVT)
2. Communication: "Language is the most human of mental skills" (Mace & Rabins, 1981, p. 29). Without language, the person with a stroke is lonely, depends on others, and loses self-confidence.
    a. Determine communication method: All disciplines should use consistent methods.

    b. Ensure that hearing aids and glasses are available if needed
    c. Use symbols and communication boards
    d. Provide a supportive environment; be patient and calm
    e. Include the family when possible
    f. Use music therapy: The person may be unable to speak but able to sing.
    g. Speak slowly and distinctly; use short, simple sentences; maintain eye contact
    h. Establish yes/no reliability
    i. Try cueing; prompt if the direction of verbalization is understood
    j. Allow for success; offer praise
3. Memory
    a. Use memory books
    b. Use cueing and repetition
    c. Use memory games and allow the patient to reminisce
    d. Work from simple to complex concepts and promote success
    e. Present material in different ways (e.g., written, verbally, pictures, demonstration)
4. Problem-solving ability
    a. Allow the patient to make choices beginning with safe and simple options
    b. Help with planning
    c. Organize and prioritize information
    d. Break problems into steps and cue the patient through the steps
5. Sensory/visual perception
    a. Provide adaptive equipment (e.g., glasses, hearing aid)
    b. Ensure appropriate lighting and color contrast
    c. Make large-print books and materials available
    d. Place items to allow for visual cuts (homonymous hemianopsia) and teach the patient to visually scan the environment
    e. Reduce environmental noise (e.g., radio, television)
    f. Adapt environment to accommodate

hearing loss (e.g., flashing light for phone)

g. Use aromatherapy

h. Provide various textures and temperatures

i. Ensure safety (e.g., hot or cold, especially with decreased sensation)

j. Serve foods of various colors, taste, and smell

k. Review medications (e.g., sedatives)

l. Set up room to stimulate the neglected side

m. Eliminate spatial difficulties (e.g., use colored food on white plate)

6. ADLs and self-care

a. Ensure privacy and a safe environment (e.g., grab bars, tub bench)

b. Establish a bathing and toileting routine and provide adaptive equipment for bathing, dressing, and toileting

c. Involve caregivers in ADL training

d. Incorporate crossover neurodevelopmental techniques (NDTs) (i.e., the patient's uninvolved side helps the involved side during activity)

e. Provide ongoing comprehensive history and assessment for ADL training and for determining the patient's home care assistance needs (documentation of this may be required by the patient's insurance company)

f. Adapt the home environment for wheelchair, equipment, and accessibility

g. Allow the patient to choose his or her clothing; encourage use of clothing that is loose or easy to put on

h. Allow time for activity and rest between self-care activities and promote energy-saving techniques, beginning in bed and progressing throughout the day

i. Dress the patient's affected side first

7. Dysphagia and swallowing

a. Evaluate swallowing (via bedside or radiology) as identified by videofluoroscopic swallow study (VSS): Aspiration occurs in 40%–70% of patients with stroke (Daniels et al., 1998).

b. Position the patient upright for feeding and administering medication

c. Ensure the correct level of dysphagia diet and consistency (e.g., thicken if needed); ensure that dentures fit properly; obtain a dental consult

d. Observe during meals for pocketing, drooling, swallowing

e. Provide adaptive equipment (e.g., divided plate, cutout cup)

f. Crush medications into applesauce; turn the patient's head to the affected side if he or she has difficulty swallowing medications

g. Monitor weight changes and lab values

h. Consult with dietitian about the patient's food preferences

i. Monitor hydration: Patients on oral dysphagia diets may not meet fluid requirements, which can lead to dehydration (Foley, Finestone, Woodbury, Greene-Finestone).

j. Use supplemental tube feedings: Check for residual and placement of tube and position the patient upright for feedings

k. Use supplemental parental nutrition: Maintain IV site and monitor labs

8. Bowel management

a. Verify premorbid bowel evacuation routine and adapt bowel program to accommodate previous routine

b. Increase fluid intake, bulk, fiber; monitor intake and output

c. Monitor bowel sounds and abdominal distention; avoid gas-forming foods

d. Position the patient upright; use toilet or commode rather than bedpan; allow time for complete evacuation

e. Provide appropriate medications (e.g., stool softeners, enemas, suppositories)

f. Teach digital stimulation as needed

g. Encourage the patient to wear loose clothing and use good hygiene after each stool

9. Bladder management

a. Determine continence history, provide adequate lighting if the patient has a history of nocturia

b. Set up bladder program to decrease or avoid incontinence

c. Assess medications that contribute to incontinence (e.g., diuretics, sedatives, anticholinergics, antihypertensives)

d. Provide adequate hydration (i.e., fluid intake of 2,000–3,000 cc/day if tolerated) and monitor intake and output

e. Use bladder scan and catheterize for postvoid residuals > 150 cc generally, or > 300 cc if the patient is unable to void

f. Provide time, privacy, and adaptive equipment for hygiene

g. Provide medication to facilitate bladder tone and emptying

10. Mobility

a. Work with patient on bed mobility, bridging, sitting up, moving up and down, and increasing endurance

b. Use general concepts of NDTs (e.g., normalizing muscle tone, integration vs. compensation, meaningful activities vs. simulated activities) to help with proprioception

c. Increase mobility by transferring patient from bed to chair and back using transfer NDTs (see Figure 9-6)

d. Provide safe environment for mobility practice (space and lighting)

e. Encourage the patient to wear sturdy shoes to prevent foot drop

f. Ensure safety when the patient attempts to sit or stand: According to clinical experience, more than one-third of falls in patients who have had a stroke occur while rising or sitting down.

11. Sexual functioning

a. Encourage the use of times of day when the patient most is rested

b. Provide education and support with significant other

c. Teach positioning (e.g., supine or on affected side, use pillows for support)

d. Discuss fear of another stroke

e. Instruct partner on the emotional lability of the patient

f. Encourage tactile stimulation to enhance communication, especially if the patient is aphasic

g. Discuss birth control methods

h. Encourage the patient to evacuate the bowel and bladder prior to sex

12. Skin integrity

a. Inspect skin regularly for friction, shearing, pressure

b. Teach weight-shifting techniques

c. Use pressure-relieving devices

d. Keep patient clean and dry

e. Consult with dietitian for nutritional needs to promote healing

f. If the patient has sensory loss, guard for contact with extreme hot and cold temperatures (e.g., bath water)

g. Assess for medications that may alter level of consciousness, sensation, or awareness

13. Equipment

a. Provide adaptive equipment as needed; attempt to increase the patient's functional ability without equipment if possible

b. Verify insurance payment for durable medical equipment (DME)

c. Reinforce the use of equipment that therapists have obtained

14. Psychosocial needs

a. Provide time for verbalization and counseling for patient and family with psychologist

b. Facilitate team and family conferences as needed

c. Provide socialization opportunities (e.g., eating meals in dining room, group therapy, stroke support groups)

d. Discuss role changes with patient and family (e.g., adult child may take on the role of caregiver) (Fraser, 1999)

e. Allow the patient and family to grieve their losses (e.g., function, role, relationships)

f. Reduce stress when possible and allow the patient and family to have as much control over care as possible

Figure 9-6. Transfer Techniques for Patients Who Have Had a Stroke

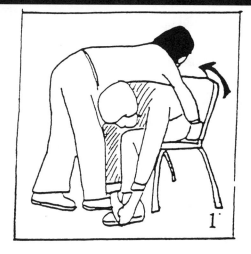

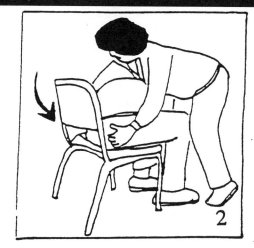

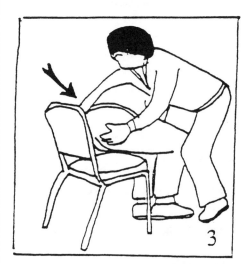

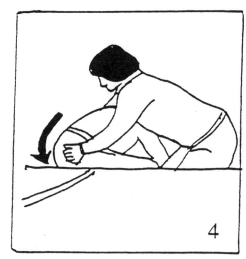

Maximal Assist

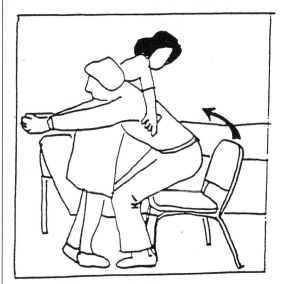

Position feet flat on floor, heels behind knees.
Bring trunk well forward prior to standing.
Encourage bilateral weight bearing.
Approximate knees through hips.
Assist by using leverage, not by lifting.

Moderate Assist

15. Leisure

   a. Incorporate the patient's leisure interests into therapy (e.g., card games)

   b. Promote community reentry using adaptive equipment (e.g., outing to a wheelchair-accessible fishing dock using a mounted fishing rod holder)

   c. Use memory games to work on cognition in group therapy

   d. Use NDTs during games (e.g., incorporate hemiplegic side using strong side hand over hand to hit balloon or reach for cards)

   e. Try to adapt the patient's leisure interests that use equipment (e.g., fasten an embroidery hoop to a wheelchair)

   f. Encourage pet therapy

16. Education

   a. Determine readiness and motivation to learn

   b. Provide information at the patient's ability and intellectual level

   c. Use a variety of teaching methods

   d. Use an interpreter if language barriers exist

   e. Plan family teaching sessions

   f. Reduce distraction and noise when teaching

   g. Make use of the time when the patient is most alert, attentive, and rested

   h. Test cognition and use return demonstration or verbalization

   i. Check awareness of current status and build knowledge base

17. Safety

   a. Ensure that the environment is free of hazards

   b. Use bed alarms, Wanderguard™, vest restraints as necessary

   c. Assess medications that may alter awareness

   d. Evaluate the patient's home (e.g., handrails, throw rugs, wheelchair ramp)

   e. Ensure kitchen and bathroom safety for patients with sensory impairments (e.g., stove, hot/cold water)

   f. Teach postmorbid impulse control and fall prevention techniques

18. Comfort and pain level

   a. Position the patient comfortably, be aware of shoulder pain (subluxation possible), and position in bed so the patient's shoulder is protracted (see Figure 9-7)

   b. Do not use the patient's arms or shoulders to move the patient up in bed

   c. Assess the intensity and location of pain and medicate as appropriate

   d. Watch for shoulder-hand syndrome: Reduce edema, maintain range of motion of metacarpal phalangeal, proximal interphalangeal, and distal interphalangeal joints, maintain wrist in slight extension, encourage movement of the involved shoulder, and maintain correct bed positioning

   e. Allow rest periods but decrease frequency if patient cannot sleep at night

   f. Provide night lighting and white noise if needed

   g. Monitor the room with cameras if the patient is impulsive at night

19. Spiritual

   a. Notify the chaplain if requested

   b. Make spiritual readings available (e.g., Bible, daily devotions)

   c. Arrange for the patient to attend chapel services if requested

   d. Schedule time for meditation and prayer

20. Discharge planning

   a. Discuss discharge goals with patient and family at conferences

   b. Set up follow-up appointments

   c. Arrange home health care, outpatient therapy, or long-term care placement

   d. Obtain DME

   e. Arrange for prescriptions

   f. Provide discharge instructions and explain medications (e.g., side effects, administration)

   g. Assist with financial and community resource information

Figure 9-7. Bed Positioning for Patients Who Have Had a Stroke

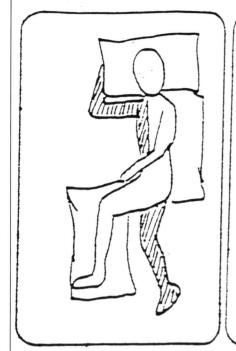 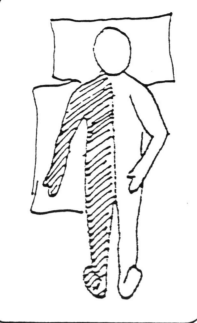 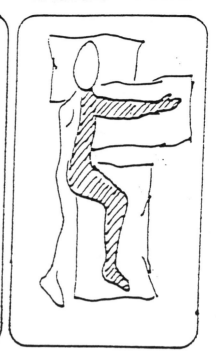

On Involved Side   Supine   On Non-involved Side

Reprinted with permission of International Clinical Educators, Inc., from Davis, J. (1997). NDT Course for Nursing. Port Townsend, WA: International Clinical Educators, Inc. Available: International Clinical Educators, Inc., PO Box 1990, Port Townsend, WA 98368, 888/665-6556, fax 360/379-1044.

E. Evaluation and Expected Outcomes
1. Evaluate the patient's optimal level of functioning
2. Individualize each patient's outcomes based on goals related to nursing diagnoses

F. Follow-Up Posthospitalization
1. 69% of stroke survivors perform self-care tasks independently and up to 80% are independently mobile; however, 70% have had significant life-changing losses related to social functioning and vocation (Johnson, Pearson, & McDivitt, 1997).
2. Studies of stroke survivors indicate that their quality of life fails to improve with time, even if their level of independence in ADLs improves drastically (Ahlsio, Britton, Murry, & Theorell, 1984).
3. Rehabilitation nurses can gain insight into the concerns and challenges facing stroke survivors who have returned to the community by assessing their learning needs and making referrals for follow-up care.
4. Many patients who have had a stroke suffer from depression, lack of concentration, nervousness, fatigue, and memory loss (Sisson, 1998).
5. It is important to refer the patient and family for counseling.

G. Future Reimbursement
1. In this time of chronic disease management, rehabilitation plays an important role in the clinical management of patients.
2. In the United States, disability-related costs total more than $170 billion a year, and the number of people with long-term disabilities is expected to double by the year 2020 (Hoenig, Horner, Duncan, Clipp, & Hamilton, 1999).

3. Reimbursement changes affect the length of stay in rehabilitation units.

4. Rehabilitation nurses will be challenged to meet the needs of patients who have had a stroke more rapidly and with fewer resources available.

References

Ahlsio, B., Britton, M., Murry, V., & Theorell, P. (1984). Disablement and quality of life after stroke. *Stroke, 15,* 886-890.

Boss, B.J. (1991). Managing communication disorders in stroke. *Nursing Clinics of North America, 26,* 985-996.

Brandstater, M.E., & Basmajian, J.V. (Eds.). (1987). *Stroke rehabilitation.* Baltimore: Williams & Wilkins.

Bronstein, K.S., Popovich, J., & Stewart-Amidei, C. (1991). *Promoting stroke recovery: A research-based approach for nurses.* St. Louis: Mosby.

Caplan, L.R. (1988). Stroke. *Clinical Symposia, 40*(4), 1-32.

Culebras, A. (1992). Neuroanatomic and neurologic correlates of sleep disturbances. *Neurology, 42*(Suppl. 6), 19-27.

Damasio, R. (1992). Medical progress: Aphasia. *The New England Journal of Medicine, 326*(8), 531-539.

Daniels, S.K., Brailey, K., Priestly, D.H., Herrington, L., Weisberg, L., & Foundas, A. (1998). Aspiration in patients with acute stroke. *Archives of Physical Medicine and Rehabilitation, 79,* 14-18.

Dolan, J.T. (1991). *Critical care nursing: Clinical management through the nursing process.* Philadelphia: F.A. Davis.

Fisher, C.M. (1975). Anatomy and pathology of the cerebral vasculature. In Meyer, J.S. (Ed.), *Modern concepts of cerebrovascular disease.* New York: Spectrum Publications Inc.

Foley, N., Finestone, H.M., Woodbury, M.G., & Greene-Finestone, L.S. (Undated abstract). Inadequate fluid intake in the dysphagic stroke patient. *Archives of Physical Medicine and Rehabilitation, 79,* 1151.

Fraser, C. (1999). The experience of transition for a daughter caregiver of a stroke survivor. *Journal of Neuroscience Nursing, 31*(1), 9-16.

Gundersen, C.H. (1990). *Essentials of clinical neurology.* New York: Raven.

Hickey, J.V. (1992). *The clinical practice of neurological and neurosurgical nursing* (3rd ed.). Philadelphia: J.B. Lippincott.

Hill, M.D., & Hachinski, V. (1998). Stroke treatment: Time is brain. *Lancet, 352*(Suppl. III), 10-14.

Hoenig, H., Horner, R.D., Duncan, P.W., Clipp, E., & Hamilton, B. (1999). New horizons in stroke rehabilitation research. *Journal of Rehabilitation Research and Development, 36*(1).

Johnson, J., Pearson, V., & McDivitt, L. (1997). Stroke rehabilitation: Assessing stroke survivors' long-term learning needs. *Rehabilitation Nursing, 22*(5), 243-248.

Kelly-Hayes, M. (1991). A preventive approach to stroke. *Nursing Clinics of North America, 26,* 931-942.

Kong, K.-H., Chua, K.S.G., & Tow, A. (1998). Clinical characteristics and functional outcome of stroke patients 75 years old and older. *Archives of Physical Medicine and Rehabilitation, 79,* 1535-1539.

Langhorne, P., Williams, B.O., Gilchrist, W., & Howie, K. (1993). Do stroke units save lives? *The Lancet, 342,* 395-397.

Licata-Gehr, E.E. (1991). Etiology of stroke subtypes. *Nursing Clinics of North America, 26,* 943-956.

Loen, M. (1991). Impairment in verbal communication. In M. Snyder (Ed.), *A guide to neurological and neurosurgical nursing* (2nd ed., pp. 235-256). Albany, NY: Delmar.

Love, R.J., & Webb, W.G. (1996). *Neurology for the speech-language pathologist* (3rd ed.). Newton, MA: Butterworth-Heinemann.

Mace, N.L., & Rabins, P.V. (1981). *The 36-hour day.* Baltimore: The Johns Hopkins University Press.

Mahoney, F.J., & Barthel, D.W. (1965). Functional evaluation: The Barthel Index. *Maryland State Medical Journal, 14,* 61-65.

Meyer, J.S. (1961). Changes in cerebral blood flow resulting from vascular occlusion. In W.S. Fields (Ed.), *Pathogenesis and treatment of cerebrovascular disease* (pp. 80-105). Springfield, IL: Charles C. Thomas.

Millikan, C.H., McDowell, F., & Easton, J.D. (1987). *Stroke.* Philadelphia: Lea & Febiger.

Mumma, C.M. (Ed.). (1987). *Rehabilitation nursing: Concepts and practice—A core curriculum* (2nd ed.). Evanston, IL: Rehabilitation Nursing Foundation.

Munchiando, J.F., & Kendall, K. (1993). Comparisons of the effectiveness of two bowel programs for CVA patients. *Rehabilitation Nursing, 18,* 168-172.

Simon, J. (1996). Chronic pain syndrome: Nursing assessment and intervention. *Rehabilitation Nursing, 21,* 13-19.

Sisson, R.A. (1998). Life after a stroke: Coping with change. *Rehabilitation Nursing, 23*(4), 198-203.

U.S. Department of Health and Human Services. (1995). *Post-stroke rehabilitation.* Rockville, MD: Agency for Health Care Policy and Research.

Suggested resources

Baggerly, J. (1991). Sensory perceptual problems following stroke: The "invisible" deficits. *Nursing Clinics of North America, 26,* 997-1005.

Black, T.M., Soltis, T., & Bartlett, C. (1999). Using the functional independence measure instrument to predict stroke rehabilitation outcomes. *Rehabilitation Nursing, 24*(3), 109-114.

Broderick, J.P. (1996). Guidelines for medical care and treatment of blood pressure in patients with acute stroke. *Proceedings of a National Symposium on Rapid Identification and Treatment of Acute Stroke.* National Institute of Neurological Disorders and Stroke, December 12-13, 1996.

Cheng, P.-T., Liaw, M.-Y., Wong, M.-K., Tang, F.-T., Lee, M.-Y., & Lin, P.-S. (1998). The sit-to-stand movement in stroke patients and it correlation with falling. *Archives of Physical Medicine and Rehabilitation, 79,* 1043-1045.

Doolittle, N.D. (1988). Stroke recovery: Review of the literature and suggestions for future research. *Journal of Neuroscience Nursing, 20*(3),169-173.

Doolittle, N.D. (1992). The experience of recovery following lacunar stroke. *Rehabilitation Nursing, 17,* 116-120.

Goldberg, G. (Ed.). (1991). Physical medicine and rehabilitation. *Clinics of North America, 2*(3).

Gorelick, P.B. (1986). Cerebrovascular disease: Pathophysiology and diagnosis. *Nursing Clinics of North America, 21,* 275-287.

Greshem, G.E. (Ed.). (1990). Methodologic issues in stroke outcome research. *Stroke: A Journal of Cerebral Circulation, 21*(Supp. II) (9), 1-73.

Hanak, M. (1992). *Rehabilitation nursing for the neurological patient.* New York: Springer Publishing.

Hayn, M.A., & Fisher, T.R. (1997). Stroke rehabilitation: Salvaging ability after the storm. *Nursing 97.*

Hoeman, S.P. (Ed.). (1996). *Rehabilitation nursing: Process and application* (2nd ed.). St. Louis: Mosby.

Kane-Carlsen, P.A. (1990). Transient ischemic attacks: Clinical features, pathophysiology and management. *Nurse Practitioner, 15*(7), 9-14.

Oden, K.E., Kevorkian, C.G., & Levy, J.K. (1998). Rehabilitation of the post-cardiac surgery stroke patient: Analysis of cognitive and functional assessment. *Archives of Physical Medicine and Rehabilitation, 79,* 67-71.

Sandstrom, R., Mokler, P.J., & Hoppe, K.M. (1998). Discharge destination and motor function outcome in severe stroke as measured by the Functional Independence Measure/Function-Related Group classification system. *Archives of Physical Medicine and Rehabilitation, 79,* 762-765.

Travers, P.L. (1999). Poststroke dysphagia: Implications for nurses. *Rehabilitation Nursing, 24*(2), 69-73.

Wertz, R.T. (1990). Communication deficits in stroke survivors: An overview of classification and treatment. *Stroke: A Journal of Cerebral Circulation, 21*(Supp. II) (9), 16-18.

Chapter 10

Traumatic Injuries: TBI and SCI

Linda Dufour, MSN RN CRRN

Joan Williams, MSN RN CRRN ARNP-C

Kelly Coleman, RN

Catastrophic injuries of the brain and spinal cord affect millions of people each year. Accidents, falls, violence, and sporting and recreational injuries are the major causes. Annually, about 10,000 new spinal cord injuries (SCI) occur, whereas an estimated 1 million people are treated in hospitals as a result of traumatic brain injury (TBI) (National Center for Injury Control and Prevention, 1999). Both injuries largely affect the younger population and tend to occur more frequently in men. Both types of injuries produce alterations that vary according to the specific location and severity of injury.

Rehabilitation nurses play an important role in enhancing patient outcomes through astute assessment, timely interventions, and thorough evaluation. The rehabilitation process is interdisciplinary in nature and works to improve all aspects of the individual's life.

I. Traumatic Brain Injury (TBI)
  A. Overview
    1. Definitions
      a. Refers to damage to brain tissue from external mechanical forces
      b. May produce altered levels of consciousness, cognition, and/or physical ability (Rosebrough, 1998)
      c. Is not degenerative or congenital (Brain Injury Association, 1999)
    2. Open and closed brain injuries
      a. Open injuries: Caused from penetration and result in communication between the intracranial structures and the environment (Rosebrough, 1998)
      b. Closed injuries: Do not involve penetration of brain but may include depressed or nondepressed skull fractures (Marion, 1996)
  B. Types of Injuries
    1. Concussion
      a. Definition: An immediate, temporary loss of consciousness resulting from a violent blow or motion to the head

      b. Symptoms: Momentary loss of reflexes or memory, headache, confusion, dizziness, irritability, visual and gait disturbances (Hickey, 1997)
    2. Contusion: Bruising of the cerebral tissue without disruption of its architecture (Adams, Victor, & Ropper, 1997)
    3. Hemorrhagic injuries
      a. Subdural hematoma (SDH)
        1) Develops as a result of blood buildup between the dura and subarachnoid space
        2) May be bilateral or unilateral, acute, or chronic (Adams et al., 1997; Rosebrough, 1998)
        3) Occurs in 29% of people with intracranial injuries and is most often caused by tearing of veins over the convexity of the brain (Hickey, 1997)
      b. Epidural hematoma (EDH)
        1) Develops as a rapid arterial or venous bleed often associated with skull fracture or a lacerated meningeal artery
        2) Is more commonly seen in children

3) Accounts for 2%–6% of traumatic intracranial insults (Hickey, 1997; Rosebrough, 1998)
   c. Intracerebral hemorrhage
   1) Develops from extravasation of blood into cerebral tissue
   2) Is associated with contusions and lacerations
   3) May act as a space-occupying lesion compressing brain tissue (Miller, Piper, & Jones, 1996; Rosebrough, 1998)
   d. Subarachnoid hemorrhage (SAH)
   1) Develops from bleeding into the subarachnoid space
   2) Is associated with severe head injury as well as aneurysmal ruptures (Adams et al., 1997; Hickey, 1997)
4. Penetrating injuries
   a. Missile injuries (high-velocity trauma)
   1) Caused by gunshots or other types of missiles: The location, path of injury, and depth of penetration directly affect the severity of the injury.
   2) May be associated with infection because bone fragments, hair, and skin may enter the brain from penetration (Marion, 1996; Winkler, 1995)
   b. Impalement
   1) Refers to the piercing of the scalp, skull, or brain by a foreign object (e.g., knife, ice pick, pencil, scissors)
   2) May cause severe neurologic impairment depending on the location of the insult (Marion, 1996)

C. Epidemiology
   1. Incidence
   a. Based on the preliminary 1996–1997 data from the Colorado TBI Registry, the National Center for Injury Prevention and Control (NCIPC) reported that 5.3 million Americans have had a TBI (NCIPC, 1999).
   b. NCIPC (1999) also reported the following 1995–1996 data:
   1) 1 million people were treated and released for TBI from hospital emergency departments.
   2) 230,000 people were hospitalized and survive TBI, whereas 50,000 did not survive.

3) People at highest risk for TBI are adolescents, young adults, and people older than age 75.
4) Men of all ages face twice the risk of TBI than women.
5) Men ages 14–24 years are at the highest risk (Brain Injury Association, 1999).

D. Etiology/Causes of TBI
   1. Motor vehicle accidents (MVAs) (50%): Leading cause among people ages 5–64 years old (NCIPC, 1999)
   2. Falls (21%): Leading cause among people older than age 65 (NCIPC, 1999)
   3. Firearm violence (12%)
   4. Sporting injuries (10%): An estimated 300,000 sports-related mild to moderate brain injuries occur annually (Sosin, Sniezek, & Thurman, 1996).
   5. Other (7%) (Brain Injury Association, 1999)

E. Pathophysiology
   1. Primary injuries
   a. Primary injury: Damage to the brain that occurs at the moment of impact (Brontke & Boake, 1996); the physiological and anatomic change to the cranium from rapid acceleration or deformation (Marion, 1996)
   b. Acceleration and deceleration injuries: Produced from MVAs or falls from heights > 6 ft; cause damage from shearing and tension forces to brain tissue and the surrounding cerebral vasculature (Katz, 1997)
   c. Diffuse axonal injuries (DAI)
   1) DAIs are caused by microscopic damage to neuronal axons in which the axons swell and cause the involved segments to separate.
   2) Destruction occurs in the cerebral hemispheres, corpus callosum, and brainstem.
   3) Severity depends on the magnitude of the acceleration forces involved in the traumatic event (Katz, 1997).
   d. Focal injuries: Areas damaged by a localized trauma, involving consolidated areas of tissue destruction, hemorrhage, and edema to the brain and varying depths of white matter (Katz, 1997)

2. Secondary injuries
   a. Complications following a primary event (Brontke & Boake, 1996; Marion, 1996)
   b. Causes
      1) Brain swelling, increased intracranial pressure (Hickey, 1997)
      2) Intracranial bleeding, hypoxemia, ischemia (Winkler, 1995)
      3) Hypotension (Mackay, Chapman, & Morgan, 1998)
      4) Focal hypoperfusion, electrolyte imbalance, infections (Hickey, 1997)
      5) Excitotoxity and production of free radicals (Brontke & Boake, 1996; Marion, 1996; Zafonte, Muizelaar, & Peterson, 1998)

F. Assessment
   1. Classification
      a. Mild brain injury
         1) Description
            a) Occurs from direct contact or acceleration/deceleration injuries
            b) May result in a loss of consciousness for 20 minutes or less
            c) Involves Glasgow Coma Scale (GCS) scores of > 13 and negative neuroimaging
            d) May take weeks to months of recovery without specific treatment
         2) Symptoms, which often go unrecognized until they interfere with activities of daily living (ADLs): Dizziness, headache, insomnia, fatigue, and decreased memory (Gatens & Hebert, 1996; Rosebrough, 1998)
      b. Moderate brain injury
         1) Description
            a) Occurs from direct contact and acceleration/deceleration injuries
            b) Involves GCS scores ranging from 9–12
            c) Loss of consciousness may last more than 20 minutes and involve cerebral edema and/or several small hemorrhages
            d) Requires rehabilitation and leaves long-term neurologic deficits
         2) Symptoms: Difficulties with balance and coordination, amnesia, agitation, seizures, dysphagia, and/or soft speech (Rosebrough, 1998)
   c. Severe brain injury
      1) Description
         a) Loss of consciousness lasting more than 6 hours
         b) GCS scores < 8
         c) May involve contusions, tearing, and shearing of brain tissue
         d) Requires long-term rehabilitation for neurologic deficits
      2) Symptoms
         a) Alterations in cognition, perception, and physical and behavioral functioning (Rosebrough, 1998)
         b) Coma (Giacino et al., 1997; Phipps, DiPasquale, & Whyte, 1997)
            (1) Arousal: Eyes do not open spontaneously or in response to stimulation
            (2) Awareness: No evidence of perception, communication ability, or purposeful motor activity (e.g., command following)
            (3) Communication: No evidence of yes/no responses, verbalizing, or gesture
         c) Vegetative state (Giacino et al., 1997; Phipps, DiPasquale, & Whyte, 1997)
            (1) Arousal: Eyes open spontaneously; sleep-wake cycle resumes; arousal often sluggish, poorly sustained
            (2) Awareness: No evidence of perception, communication ability, or purposeful motor activity
            (3) Communication No evidence of yes/no responses, verbalization, or gesture
         d) Minimally conscious state (Giacino et al., 1997; Phipps,

DiPasquale, & Whyte, 1997)

(1) Arousal: Eyes open spontaneously; normal to abnormal sleep-wake cycle; arousal level ranges from obtunded to normal

(2) Awareness: Reproducible but inconsistent evidence of perception, communication ability, or purposeful motor activity; visual tracking often intact

(3) Communication: Ranges from none to unreliable and inconsistent yes/no responses, verbalization, and gesture

2. Assessment instruments and tools

a. Rancho Los Amigos Levels of Cognitive Function Scale: Used to interpret the cognitive recovery process after a brain injury (Rancho Los Amigos Medical Center, Adult Brain Injury Service, 1979) (see Figure 10-1)

b. Glasgow Coma Scale (GCS) (see Figure 10-2)

1) Used to assess the level of consciousness following a brain injury

2) Categorized into three main assessment areas: motor, verbal, and eye-opening responses

3) Is very useful in the acute care setting (Rosebrough, 1998)

c. Disability Rating Scale (DRS)

1) Designed to quantitatively assess severe brain injury

2) Composed of eight items that are divided into four categories, including arousability, cognitive ability for self-care, and employability (Grosswasser, Schwab, & Salazar, 1997; Rappaport, Halls, Hopkins, Belleza, & Cope, 1982)

d. Functional Independence Measure (FIM™) instrument

1) Constructed to provide a uniform measure of function in rehabilitation settings

2) Measures items of self-care, sphincter control, mobility, locomotion, communication, and social cognition

(Grosswasser et al., 1997)

e. Glasgow Outcome Scale: Developed to assess outcomes after brain injury; categories include *good recovery, moderate disability, severe disability, persistent vegetative state,* and *death* (Rosebrough, 1998)

f. Coma Recovery Scale (CRS): Designed to assess subtle gains and predict outcomes in individuals with a severe brain injury (Giacino, Kezmarsky, DeLuca, & Cicerone, 1991)

g. Neuropsychological Battery

1) Designed to measure attention, concentration, memory, problem-solving, and language functions

2) Available in several versions and configurations to assess an individual's neuropsychological functioning following a brain injury (Therapeutics and Technology Assessment Subcommittee, 1996)

Figure 10-1. Rancho Los Amigos Levels of Cognitive Function Scale (adapted version, 1979)

I.   No response to pain, touch, sound, or sight

II. Generalized reflex response to stimulation/pain

III. Localized response—blinks to strong light, turns toward/away from sound, responds to physical discomfort, gives inconsistent response to commands

IV. Confused-agitated—alert; very active, aggressive, or bizarre behaviors; performs motor activities but behavior is nonpurposeful; extremely short attention span

V.   Confused-nonagitated—gross attention to environment, highly distractible, requires continual redirection, difficulty learning new tasks, agitated by too much stimulation

VI. Confused-appropriate—inconsistent orientation to time and place, retention span/recent memory impaired, begins to recall past, consistently follows simple directions, goal-directed behavior with assistance

VII. Automatic-appropriate—performs daily routine in highly familiar environment in a nonconfused but automatic robot-like manner, skills noticeably deteriorate in unfamiliar surroundings, lack of realistic planning for own future

VIII. Purposeful-appropriate

Reprinted with permission of Rancho Los Amigos Medical Center from Rancho Los Amigos Medical Center, Adult Brain Injury Service. (1979). *Levels of cognitive function scale* (adapted version) (pp. 78-80). Downey, CA: Author.

h. Coma Near-Coma

1) Designed to expand the upper range of the DRS

2) Includes measures of vegetative state and persistent vegetative state

3) Has eight items grouped into five categories ranging from *extreme coma* to *coma* (O'Dell & Riggs, 1996; Rappaport, Dougherty, & Kelting, 1992)

i. Sensory Stimulation Assessment Measure (SSAM): Designed to expand the GCS and used to standardize sensory presentation (Duff & Wells, 1997; O'Dell & Riggs, 1996; Rader, Alston, & Ellis, 1989)

j. Western Neuro Sensory Stimulation Profile (WNSSP)

1) Used to assess auditory and visual comprehension, tracking, object manipulation, attention, arousal, tactile, and olfactory function

2) Contains 33 items in 6 areas (Ansell & Keenan, 1989)

k. Galveston Orientation and Amnesia Test (GOAT): Used to assess cognition and orientation after a brain injury (Levin, O'Donald, & Grossman, 1975)

l. Children's Coma Scale (CCS): Designed as a pediatric version of the GCS (Melvin, Lacy & Swafford-Ten Eyck, 1998)

3. Physical assessment

a. General: Determine location of brain injury and corresponding symptomatology (see Table 10-1)

b. Neurologic

1) Assess cognitive, motor, and sensory status, reflexes, and cranial nerves

2) Monitor anticonvulsant levels

3) Monitor for signs and symptoms of increased intracranial pressure

c. Respiratory: Assess patency of airway, oxygen saturation, nature of sputum, lung fields, and potential for aspiration

d. Cardiovascular: Assess blood pressure, pulse, heart rate, rhythm, risk for or

---

Figure 10-2. Glasgow Coma Scale

Scoring of Eye Opening

4 Opens eyes spontaneously when the nurse approaches

3 Opens eyes in response to speech (normal or shout)

2 Opens eyes only to painful stimuli (e.g., squeezing of nail beds)

1 Does not open eyes to painful stimuli

Scoring of Best Motor Response

6 Can obey a simple command, such as "Lift your left hand off the bed"

5 Localizes to painful stimuli and attempts to remove source

4 Purposeless movement in response to pain

3 Flexes elbows and wrists while extending lower legs to pain

2 Extends upper and lower extremities to pain

1 No motor response to pain on any limb

Scoring of Best Verbal Response

5 Oriented to time, place, and person

4 Converses, although confused

3 Speaks only in words or phrases that make little or no sense

2 Responds with incomprehensible sounds (e.g., groans)

1 No verbal response

Reprinted with permission of J.B. Lippincott from Hickey, J. (1997). *The clinical practice of neurological and neurosurgical nursing* (4th ed., p. 139). Philadelphia: J.B. Lippincott.

Table 10-1. Location of Injury and Corresponding Symptomatology

Frontal lobe	Impaired voluntary movement, social functioning, short-term memory, initiative, self-awareness and executive functions, expressive aphasia, inhibition of impulse and emotions
Temporal lobe	Impaired hearing, smell, long-term memory and musical awareness, receptive aphasia, and agnosia
Parietal lobe	Impaired spatial relationships and sensation
Occipital lobe	Impaired visual perception
Brainstem	Impaired wakefulness and regulation of life-sustaining systems, impaired taste, smell, eyelid movements and vision
Cerebellum	Impaired gait, balance, coordination

Sources consulted

Gatens, C., & Hebert, A.R. (1996). Cognition and behavior patterns. In S.P. Hoeman (Ed.), *Rehabilitation nursing: Process and application* (2nd ed., pp. 572-593). St. Louis: Mosby.

Hickey, J. (1997). *Clinical practice of neurological and neurosurgical nursing* (4th ed.). Philadelphia: Lippincott.

Rosebrough, A. (1998). Acquired brain injury: traumatic brain injury. In P. Chin, D. Finocchiaro, & A. Rosebrough (Eds.), *Rehabilitation nursing practice* (pp. 223-246). New York: McGraw-Hill.

existence of deep vein thrombosis (DVT), and risk factors for emboli (atrial fibrillation)

   e. Nutritional: Assess weekly weights, daily hydration status, and dietary intake

   f. Sensory/perceptual: Assess responses to various types of stimuli, sleep/wake cycles, and level of consciousness

   g. Elimination

     1) Assess bowel sounds and premorbid bowel patterns

     2) Assess premorbid voiding habits and history, urinary output, and bowel movements

     3) Assess bowel and bladder continence and effectiveness of bowel and bladder programs

     4) Monitor for potential alterations in elimination (e.g., constipation, diarrhea, urinary tract infection)

   h. Musculoskeletal

     1) Assess for heterotropic ossification, orthopedic injuries, premorbid history, contractures, tone, spasticity, range of motion (ROM), need for adaptive equipment

     2) Observe gait and mobility if appropriate

   i. Communication: Assess for expressive, receptive, and/or global aphasias, dysarthria, and alternative communication strategies (e.g., augmentative communication devices)

   j. Behavior: Assess for behavior excesses (e.g., agitation, disinhibition, impulsivity, poor judgment, motor restlessness, perseveration, emotional lability) and deficits (e.g., apathy, poor initiation)

   k. Safety

     1) Assess for risk of falls, wandering, impulsivity, balance, strength, and judgment

     2) Assess need for least restrictive restraint if necessary (see Figure 10-3)

   l. Psychosocial: Assess family support, coping mechanisms, and potential response to fear and anxiety

   m. Sexual: Assess level of function related to physical and/or behavioral alterations

   n. Vocational: Assess potential for returning to work or school

G. Planning: Patient and Family Goals

  1. Set individualized goals upon admission

   a. Bowel and bladder continence

   b. Improved cognition

   c. Improved mobility

   d. Improved functional independence

   e. Improved safety

   f. Improved judgment

   g. Manageable behavior

Figure 10-3. Safety Tips

TEACHING TOPICS

Don't	Do
Leave sharp objects within reach	Provide supervision with meals, toileting, ADLs
Leave poisons, chemicals, and households cleaners within reach	Communicate with patient as an adult
Leave car keys or other types of keys to heavy equipment within reach	Speak to patient in regular tone (it is not necessary to speak louder than usual)
Leave patient alone near fire sources (e.g., stove, BBQ, matches, lighters, cigarettes)	Celebrate small accomplishments
Assume the patient has his or her previous role performance or expectations	Provide brain injury awareness information to the patient's neighbors and fire and police departments
Leave patient alone near water areas (e.g., lakes, swimming pools)	Provide structure and quiet times
Leave patient alone and at risk for wandering, falls, or other injuries	Provide positive strategies in coping with changes in family roles
Leave patient alone with heavy machinery	Provide opportunities to integrate patient into leisure and recreational activities
Provide meals outside of the prescribed diet plan	Maintain a safe environment (by properly storing sharps, chemicals, car keys)
	Maintain dietary prescription and provide ready-made meals to decrease choking risk

h. Increased knowledge to care for self or patient

i. Resolution of medical issues

2. Meet at regular intervals to evaluate status of goal achievement

3. Add or delete goals based on patient's progress and condition

H. Nursing Plan of Care and Interventions for Cognitive Rehabilitation (see Table 10-2)

I. Evaluation

1. Evaluate patient and family goals and progress

    a. Continence

    b. Cognition (e.g., memory, thinking, decision making, attention span)

    c. Mobility

    d. Functional independence

    e. Safety and judgment

    f. Behavior

    g. Resolution of medical issues

    h. Family preparedness to assume care of patient (if applicable)

2. Use instruments described in Section I.F. of this chapter

J. Discharge Planning and Community Resources

1. Discharge planning should begin before admission to the rehabilitation facility.

2. Discharge planning should incorporate extensive exploration of community resources for a lifetime of disability management.

    a. Financial resources

        1) Private insurance

        2) Auto insurance

        3) Medicare and Medicaid

        4) Social Security Disability Insurance (SSDI)

        5) Litigation awards

        6) Donations

    b. Continuum of care options

        1) Skilled nursing facilities

        2) Long-term care facilities

        3) Residential programs

        4) Day therapy programs

        5) Assisted living facilities

        6) Clubhouse programs

        7) Cognitive-based centers and neurobehavioral units

        8) Home

    c. Healthcare resources

        1) Home health services

        2) Outpatient programs

        3) Local hospital network

        4) Primary care provider

        5) Durable medical equipment (DME) supplier

        6) Telemedicine programs

    d. Community resources

        1) Brain Injury Association

        2) American Heart Association

        3) National Stroke Association

        4) Epilepsy Foundation of America

        5) Local library

K. Research (see Research Perspective in this chapter)

II. Spinal Cord Injury (SCI)

A. Definitions

1. SCI: Traumatic insult to the spinal cord resulting in alterations or complete disruption of normal motor, sensory, and autonomic function

2. Tetraplegia

    a. Impairment or loss of motor and/or sensory function in cervical segments causing impairment in arms, trunk, legs, and pelvic organs

    b. Usually occurs as a result of injuries at T1 or above

3. Paraplegia

    a. Impairment or loss of motor and/or sensory function in the thoracic, lumbar, or sacral segments causing impairment in trunk, legs, and pelvic organs

    b. Usually occurs as a result of injuries at T2 or below

B. Epidemiology (National Spinal Cord Injury Statistical Center [NSCISC], 1999)

1. Incidence of SCI

    a. Approximately 40 cases per million in the United States or approximately 10,000 new cases per year

    b. Occurs primarily in young adults 16-30 years of age (56% of new injuries)

    c. 82% of patients with SCI are men

Table 10-2. Plan of Care for Cognitive Rehabilitation

Cognitive Level	Description	Nursing Diagnoses	Nursing Management
I. No Response	Is unresponsive to touch, pain, or auditory or verbal stimuli	• Alteration in sensory perception	• Increase purposeful sensory input by incorporating olfactory, visual, auditory, and tactile stimulation into daily therapy to initiate some response • Decrease "environmental noise" stimulation • Monitor cardiovascular effects of pharmacological management, which may include agents such as bromocriptine, amantadine, levodopa/carbidopa, and methylphenidate hydrochloride for neurostimulation • Schedule medications to promote sleep/wake cycles; pharmacological management may also be used to establish sleep/wake cycles (e.g., Trazadone Q HS)
II. Generalized Response	Displays inconsistent, nonpurposeful, reflexic responses to stimuli or pain	Potential for • Alteration in family coping* • Alteration in awareness • Knowledge deficit: Family related to outcome(s)* • Sleep pattern disturbance • Impaired verbal communication	• Carefully listen to/observe family when discussing the event of the patient's injuries, provide emotional support* • Provide educational materials related to injury* • Explain procedures to patient before completing them; talk in a normal tone • Provide range of motion (ROM) exercises as well as turning and positioning • Monitor cardiovascular effects of pharmacological management, which may include agents such as bromocriptine, amantadine, levodopa/carbidopa, and methylphenidate hydrochloride for neurostimulation • Schedule medications to promote sleep/wake cycles; pharmacological management may also be used to establish sleep/wake cycles (e.g., Trazadone Q HS)
III. Localized Response	Responds in a more focused manner to certain types of stimuli (e.g., turns to sound, withdraws from pain, tracks); may follow simple commands inconsistently	• Alteration in thought process, memory, thinking • Alteration in activity tolerance • Potential for impaired swallowing	• Provide methods of getting patient out of bed to increase tolerance • Provide structured rest periods • Orient patient to day, time, month, and tasks as necessary • Provide ROM exercises to increase muscle mass and tone • Decrease environmental stress and monitor stimuli • Encourage participation in self-care by directing with simple commands • Monitor cardiovascular effects of pharmacological management, which may include agents such as bromocriptine, amantadine, levodopa/carbidopa, and methylphenidate hydrochloride for neurostimulation

The Specialty Practice of Rehabilitation Nursing: A Core Curriculum, 4th Ed.

Table 10-2. Plan of Care for Cognitive Rehabilitation (Continued)

Cognitive Level	Description	Nursing Diagnoses	Nursing Management
			• Schedule medications to promote sleep/wake cycles; pharmacological management may also be used to establish sleep/wake cycles (e.g., Trazodone Q HS)
IV. Confused-Agitated	Is alert, very active, disoriented, possibly aggressive; may display inappropriate behavior in response to internal confusion; has a short attention span	• Potential for injury relating to poor judgment • Alternating in sensory perception: Overload • Acute confusion	• Maintain respectful care • Orient as necessary • Explain care to be performed in simple, concrete terms • Maintain a low tone of voice • Decrease environmental stimulation, including existing stimulation (e.g., turn off TV, decrease lighting, limit visitors, find a private room, provide one-on-one therapies with cotreatment with a behavior specialist) • Maintain structure • Decrease fatigue and anxiety • Monitor pharmacological management, which may include agents such as Buspirone hydrochloride or risperidone to maintain lower levels of agitation; lorazepam may be given for episodes of acute agitation
V. Confused-Inappropriate Nonagitated	Is alert, easily distracted, responsive to commands; pays gross attention to environment; displays absent carryover from one situation to another	• Alteration in memory, thinking • Self-care deficit	• Identify areas of motivation for self-care tasks • Monitor medication regimen • Monitor nutritional necessities with increased activity • Provide tasks that are appropriate to level (e.g., hygiene, simple meal preparation—cold cereal) • Assess sleep patterns • Decrease environmental stimulation • Establish bowel and bladder continence • Provide maximal cues for self-care tasks • Introduce memory aids (e.g., calendars, schedules)
VI. Confused Appropriate	Follows commands consistently but is inconsistently oriented to time and place; has short-term memory deficits; begins to participate in self-care	• Knowledge deficit • Impaired adjustment	• Provide education to patient regarding injury and outcomes • Support the anger involved in this stage of recovery • Provide adaptive equipment to perform ADLs • Provide daily structure • Provide cues and memory strategies when encouraging independent activities
VII. Automatic Appropriate	May perform tasks in familiar environment but	• Alteration in thought processes	• Reduce environmental structure as necessary

Table 10-2. Plan of Care for Cognitive Rehabilitation (Continued)

Cognitive Level	Description	Nursing Diagnoses	Nursing Management
	in a very robot-like manner; begins to have insight into deficits; continues to have poor judgment and problem-solving skills	• Potential for injury relating to judgment • Altered growth and development	• Provide community outings to integrate patient back into social environment • Support the patient and family in the developmental processes throughout the course of the illness • Stimulate the developmental process by interacting with patient at the appropriate level • Support the patient to problem solve
VIII. Purposeful-Appropriate	Is consistently oriented; has correct responses, intact memory; requires no supervision; has realistic planning skills	• Knowledge deficit • Social isolation (potential for loneliness) • Alteration in sexual patterns • Risk for altered parenting	• Help the patient recognize the need to anticipate concerns relating to social interaction, sexuality • Help the patient identify new roles within the family unit • Discuss aspects of meaningful conversation • Refer the patient to community-based programs that support his or her condition • Decrease barriers that contribute to isolation; transportation, and esthetics

*May be present at all Rancho levels

Sources consulted

Carpenito, L. (1997). *Nursing diagnosis: Application to clinical practice* (7th ed., pp. 112-115). Philadelphia: Lippincott.

Hickey, J. (1997). *The clinical practice of neurological and neurosurgical nursing* (4th ed., p. 139). Philadelphia: Lippincott.

2. Prognosis
    a. Life expectancy after SCI is slightly less than normal with tetraplegia and approximately the same as normal with paraplegia.
    b. Mortality rates are significantly higher during the first year after injury.
    c. Causes of death that have the greatest effect on reduced life expectancy are pneumonia, pulmonary emboli, and septicemia.

C. Etiology (NSCISC, 1999)
    1. Accidents, including MVAs (37.2%)
    2. Falls (21%)
    3. Violence (26.8%)
    4. Sports and recreational injuries (7.1%)
    5. Other (7.9%)

D. Mechanism of Injury
    1. Flexion
        a. Occurs when head is thrown violently forward
        b. Occurs when head is struck from behind
        c. Occurs commonly in MVAs and falls
    2. Flexion with rotation: Occurs when the combination of forces causes severe twisting, resulting in ruptured ligaments and dislocation
    3. Hyperextension: Occurs in forward falls in which the face or chin is struck
    4. Compression
        a. Flexion-axial
            1) Occurs when vertebral bodies are wedged and compressed
            2) Occurs in the thoracic and lumbar region
            3) Caused by a fall onto the buttocks
        b. Vertical
            1) Occurs when vertebral bodies are shattered and burst into the spinal cord
            2) Occurs typically in the cervical region

3) Caused by a high velocity blow to the top of the head (e.g., diving)

5. Penetration: Injuries that directly pierce the cord (e.g., gunshot wound, knife wound)

E. Pathophysiology

1. Varying degrees of damage associated with SCI

   a. Severity of bony injury does not always correspond to the extent of neurological impairment.

   b. Common sites of injury—the cervical and thoracolumbar junctures—are the most mobile parts of the spine.

   c. The spinal cord itself may sustain contusion without vertebral fractures or dislocations.

   d. Progressive tissue destruction occurs in the cord within hours and may involve several responses.

      1) Decrease of microperfusion at site of injury

      2) Hemorrhage in the gray matter

      3) Development of hematoma and edema

      4) Release of biochemicals at site of injury

      5) Ischemia and necrosis in the cord, causing neurological damage

2. Levels of SCI

   a. Upper motor neuron (UMN) injury

      1) Is evident in lesions above T12-L1 vertebrae

      2) Causes loss of cerebral control over all reflex activity below the level of lesion

      3) Causes spastic paralysis

   b. Lower motor neuron (LMN) injury

      1) Is evident in lesions below T12-L1 level (i.e., conus medullaris, cauda equina)

      2) Causes destruction of the reflex arc

      3) Causes flaccid paralysis

3. Clinical syndromes

   a. Central cord syndrome

      1) Caused by damage to the central part of the cord

      2) Is usually in the cervical region

      3) Produces loss of motor power and sensation that affects upper limbs more than lower limbs

   b. Brown-Sequard syndrome

      1) Caused by damage to one side (hemisection) of the cord

      2) Produces loss of motor function and position sense on the same side as the damage, and a loss of pain and temperature sensation on the opposite side

   c. Anterior cord syndrome

      1) Caused by damage to the anterior artery, affecting the anterior two-thirds of the cord

      2) Produces paralysis and loss of pain and temperature sensation below the lesion with preservation of position sense

   d. Conus medullaris syndrome

      1) Caused by damage to the conus and lumbar nerve roots

      2) May produce areflexia (flaccidity) in bladder, bowel, and/or lower limbs

   e. Cauda equina syndrome

      1) Caused by damage below conus to lumbar-sacral nerve roots

      2) May produce areflexia in bladder, bowel, and/or lower limbs

F. Assessment

1. Classification

   a. Skeletal level of injury: The level at which, by radiographic examination, the greatest vertebral damage is found

      1) Stable injury: Occurs when the bone and/or ligaments support the injured cord area, preventing progression of neurological deficit

      2) Unstable injury: Occurs when the bone and ligaments are disrupted and unable to support and protect the injured cord area, possibly causing further neurological deficit

   b. Neurological level of injury: The most caudal segment of the spinal cord with normal sensory and motor function on each side of the body (American Spinal Injury Association [ASIA], 1996)

      1) Sensory level

         a) Refers to the most caudal

segment of the spinal cord with normal sensory function on each side of the body

   b) Evaluated at a key sensory point within each of 28 dermatomes on the right and 28 dermatomes on the left side of the body

   2) Motor level (see Table 10-3)

   a) Refers to the most caudal segment of the spinal cord with normal motor function on each side of the body

   b) Evaluated at a key muscle within each of 10 myotomes on the right and 10 myotomes on the left side of the body

c. Complete injury: An absence of motor and sensory function in the lowest sacral segment

d. Incomplete injury

   1) Results in partial preservation of sensory and/or motor function below the neurological level and includes the lowest sacral segment

   2) Includes sacral sensation at the anal mucocutaneous junction as well as deep anal sensation

   3) Includes motor function of voluntary contraction of the external anal sphincter upon digital examination

e. Zone of partial preservation (ASIA, 1996)

   1) Consists of the dermatomes and myotomes that are caudal to the neurological level and that remain partially innervated

   2) Term used only with complete injuries (e.g., a person with a complete C5 injury may have patchy sensation at C6 or C7 but not have any anal reflexes, such as sacral sparing, and thus still be classified as a complete C5 injury)

2. Assessment instruments and tools

   a. Assessing impairment: ASIA Impairment Scale (1996)

   1) Frequently used scale that reflects severity of impairment

   2) Modified version of Frankel Grading System for SCI

   3) Levels of ASIA scale

   a) A—Complete: No sensory or motor function preserved in S4-S5

   b) B—Incomplete: Sensory function (but not motor function) preserved below the neurological level and extends through S4-S5

Table 10-3. Spinal Cord Segments and Corresponding Muscle and Movements		
Spinal Cord Segment	**Muscle(s)**	**Movement**
C1-3	Neck muscle	Limited head control
C4	Diaphragm	Diaphragmatic breathing
	Trapezius	Shoulder shrug
C5	Deltoid	Shoulder abduction
	Partial biceps	Partial elbow flexion
C6	Extensor carpi radialis	Wrist extension
	Biceps	Elbow flexion
C7	Triceps	Elbow extension
	Extensor digitorum	Finger extension
C8	Flexor digitorum	Finger flexion
T1	Hand intrinsics	Finger abduction
		Finger adduction
T2-T12	Intercostals	Deeper inhalation
T6-T1	Abdominals	Forceful exhalation
		Increased trunk stability
L1-L2	Iliopsoas	Hip flexion
L2-L3	Hip adductors	Hip adduction
L3-L4	Quadriceps femoris	Knee extension
L4-L5	Tibialis anterior	Ankle extension
L5	Extensor hallucis longus	Great toe extension
S1	Gastrocnemius/soleus	Plantar flexion
	Hamstrings	Knee flexion
S1-S2	Flexor digitorum	Toe flexion
S2-S4	Bladder, lower bowel	Elimination

Reprinted with permission of Springer Publishing Co. from Hanak, M. (1993). *Spinal cord injury: An illustrated guide for health care professionals* (2nd ed., p. 91). New York: Springer Publishing.

c) C—Incomplete: Motor function preserved below the neurological level; the majority of muscles below the level are grade 3 or lower

d) D—Incomplete: Motor function preserved below the neurological level; the majority of muscles below the level are grade 3 or higher

e) E—Normal: Normal sensory and motor function

b. Motor grading scale (see Table 10-4)

c. Sensory impairment scale scores: 0 = absent, 1 = impaired, 2 = normal, NT = not tested

3. Physical assessment

a. Neurologic

1) Assess cognitive, motor, and sensory status, reflexes, and cranial nerves

2) Monitor for signs and symptoms of increase or decrease in function, pain, and abnormal sensations

b. Respiratory: Assess breath sounds, patency of airway, oxygen saturation, diaphragm movement, nature of sputum and potential for aspiration, and pulmonary emboli

c. Cardiovascular: Assess blood pressure, pulse, heart rate, rhythm, edema, DVT, and signs and symptoms of orthostatic hypotension

d. Nutritional

1) Assess weekly weight, daily hydration status, and dietary intake

2) Monitor CBC, electrolytes, albumin and pre-albumin levels for anemia, electrolyte imbalance, and nutritional status

e. Elimination

1) Assess abdomen for tenderness, distension, masses, and bowel sounds, premorbid and current bowel patterns, urine for color, odor, clarity, and amount

2) Review effectiveness of bowel and bladder programs

f. Musculoskeletal: Assess for swelling, spasticity, ROM, tone, contractures, orthopedic injuries, and heterotopic ossification

g. Integumentary

1) Assess entire body for skin breakdown, especially bony prominences for redness, warmth, and blanching

2) Assess and record size, appearance, and location of any skin breakdown

h. Psychosocial: Assess family support, coping mechanisms, adjustment to disability, and potential response to fear and anxiety

i. Sexual

1) Assess level of injury in relation to physical capabilities, emotional state, behavior consistent with denial, anger, or depression

2) Monitor for suicidal themes

G. Planning

1. Setting goals (Hoeman, 1996)

a. Goals should be developed with the patient's individual strengths and limitations in mind.

Table 10-4. Motor Grading Scale

Grade	Rating of Level of Movement	Description of Motor Abilities
0	Absent	Total paralysis
1	Trace	Palpable and/or visible contraction
2	Poor	Active movement and full range of motion (ROM) when gravity is eliminated
3	Fair	Active movement and full ROM against gravity
4	Good	Active movement and full ROM against moderate resistance
5	Normal	Active movement and full ROM against full resistance

Sources consulted

American Spinal Injury Association (ASIA). (1996). *International standards for neurological and functional classification of spinal injury patients* (rev. ed.). Atlanta, GA: Author.

Zedjlik, C.P. (1992). *Management of spinal cord injury* (2nd ed.). Boston: Jones and Bartlett.

b. Rehabilitation goals should be directed toward helping the patient achieve and maintain maximum independence and safe performance of self-care activities.

c. Goals should focus on the person, not the disability.

d. Family involvement with goals from the beginning can influence the success of the patient's rehabilitation.

e. Support and instructions from rehabilitation team members can help the family assist the patient in achieving maximum independence throughout life.

2. Functional outcomes of SCI (see Table 10-5)

H. Interventions (Hoeman, 1996)

1. Interventions are determined with the patient's and family's input to promote maximum health, independence, and safety.

2. Interventions may involve teaching the patient and family about the problem-solving process, providing adaptive devices as necessary, and educating the patient and family regarding safe and effective performance of skills.

3. Rehabilitation nurses must encourage the patient and family to work toward achieving goals and to continue to perform goals that have already been accomplished.

4. Additional suggestions for providing patient care (Hickey, 1997, p.

464)

a. Establish a therapeutic nurse-patient relationship

b. Cultivate a climate of trust

c. Allow the patient to verbalize feelings

d. Accept the patient's behavior without being judgmental

e. Let the patient know that it will take time to adjust to the disability

Table 10-5. Neurological Levels and Functional Potential	
Level	**Activity**
C1-C4	Dependent in feeding, grooming, dressing, bathing, bowel and bladder routines, bed mobility, transfers, and transportation
	Independent wheelchair propulsion with pneumatic or chin control and with electronically adapted communication and environmental control devices
C1-C3	Dependent on ventilation support
C5	Independent feeding and grooming with adapted equipment
	Dependent in dressing, bathing, bowel and bladder routines, and transportation
	Requires assistance for bed mobility and transfers
	Independent wheelchair propulsion in motorized chair and with electronically adapted communication and environmental control devices
C6	Independent feeding, grooming, upper extremity dressing, bathing, bowel routine, and bed mobility—all with adapted equipment
	Requires assistance for lower extremity dressing and bladder routine
	Potentially independent transfers with transfer board
	Independent manual wheelchair propulsion with plastic rims and lugs indoors
	Independent driving with adapted van
	Independent phone operation and page turning with equipment
C7	Independent feeding, grooming, and bathing with equipment
	Potentially independent in upper and lower extremity dressing and bowel and bladder routines
	Independent in bed mobility, transfers with and without board, manual wheelchair propulsion, driving with adapted car or van and in communication activities
C8-T1	Independent in all personal care activities, bed mobility, transfers, wheelchair propulsion, driving with adapted car or van, and in communication activities
T2-T10	Independent in all activities
	Ambulation with long leg braces and crutches or walker for exercise only (nonfunctional)
T11-L2	Independent in all activities
	Potentially independent functional ambulation indoors with long leg braces and crutches
L2-S3	Independent in all activities
	Independent ambulation indoors and outdoors with short leg braces and crutches or canes

Reprinted with permission of Springer Publishing Co., from Hanak, M. (1993). *Spinal cord injury: An illustrated guide for health care professionals* (2nd ed., p. 92). New York: Springer Publishing.

f. Answer questions, referring those that you are unable to answer to the appropriate source

g. Include written reports of the patient's emotional and psychological reactions in the chart

h. Incorporate steps for meeting the emotional and psychological needs of the patient into the care plan

i. Promote a good self-concept and body image by encouraging the patient to use good grooming habits

j. Use team conferences to discuss the patient's emotional and psychological status

k. Involve the patient in the decision-making process related to his or her care so as to foster a feeling of self-control on the part of the patient

5. Nursing plan of care (see Table 10-6)

I. Evaluation

1. ASIA Impairment Scale

2. FIM instrument

3. Residual deficits and systemic dysfunction that may occur after SCI (Mandzak-McCarron, 1988; McCourt, 1993; Staas et al., 1988; Walleck, 1988)

   a. Neurological manifestations

      1) Loss or decrease of voluntary motor function below level of injury

      2) Loss or decrease of sensation

      3) Loss of normal reflex activity

      4) Autonomic dysfunction due to loss of normal sympathetic nervous system functioning

         a) Autonomic dysreflexia

         b) Hypotension

         c) Loss of thermoregulation

         d) Loss of vasomotor tone and/or control

   b. Cardiovascular manifestations

      1) Hypotension and vasodilation, causing decreased cardiac output

         a) Orthostatic hypotension: Rapid drop in blood pressure when the erect position is assumed; patients with cervical or high thoracic injury have poor vaso-motor control so there is difficulty getting blood out of the lower extremities and back to the heart.

         b) Vasodilation: Occurs as a result of loss of sympathetically induced vasoconstriction, which triggers pooling of blood in abdomen and lower extremities

      2) Bradycardia due to unopposed vagal tone (10th cranial nerve)

      3) Impaired temperature regulation manifested by poikilothermia, a condition in which the body assumes the environmental temperature due to the inability to sweat or shiver below the injury

   c. Respiratory manifestations

      1) Injury above C4: Results in paralysis of respiratory muscles, including the diaphragm; patient is dependent on a ventilator.

      2) Injury between C4-T6: Results in paralysis of the intercostal and abdominal muscles; patient usually is weaned from the ventilator but requires aggressive pulmonary management.

      3) Injury between T6-T12: Results in paralysis of some abdominal muscles; patient does not require a daily respiratory program unless an upper respiratory infection is present.

   d. Metabolic manifestations

      1) Negative nitrogen balance

      2) Decreased basal metabolic rate and expenditure of energy

      3) Hypercalcemia and/or hypercalciuria

      4) Altered secretion of pituitary-derived hormones

      5) Heterotopic ossification

   e. Gastrointestinal manifestations

      1) Peristaltic slowing, causing paralytic ileus

      2) Increased acidity, causing GI bleeding

      3) Pancreatitis after injury (Sugarman, 1985)

Table 10-6. Plan of Care for Patients with SCI

System-Specific Considerations	Nursing Diagnosis/ Collaborative Problems	Nursing Management	Level of Injury Affected
Respiratory system If possible, wean the patient from the ventilator. If weaning is not possible, plan for long-term ventilation management options (discharge home on ventilator, diaphragmatic pacer, or other options). Patients with cervical injuries usually have decreased volumes of air exchange in tidal volumes, movement of the chest with each respiration, forced expiration volume, and responsiveness to chemical stimuli for respirations resulting in chronic alveolar hypoventilation.	Ineffective airway clearance High risk for aspiration Ineffective breathing pattern High risk for respiratory infection Impaired gas exchange Risk of altered respiratory function Hypoxemia Atelectasis, pneumonia	Continue with the pulmonary program initiated in the acute phase (e.g., chest physical therapy, deep breathing and assistive coughing, use of incentive spirometer). Begin a patient/family teaching program (e.g., respiratory care, breathing exercises, assisted coughing, suction technique, oxygen, intermittent positive pressure breathing and other therapy treatments)	Cervical injuries
Cardiovascular system Bradycardia and orthostatic hypotension may occur. Orthostatic hypotension may be a problem when the head of the bed is raised or when the patient is in a wheelchair.	Risk of peripheral neurovascular dysfunction Impaired gas exchange Dysrhythmias Deep vein thrombosis Pulmonary embolus Hypovolemia Orthostatic hypotension	Apply abdominal binder and thigh-high elastic stockings Continue with air boots Slowly position patient from supine to sitting (e.g., first sit patient upright in bed, then sit patient on edge of bed with support; if patient becomes hypotensive in wheelchair, tilt wheelchair into recline position and elevate legs)	Cervical injuries High-thoracic injuries May occur in low-thoracic injuries
Nervous system Autonomic hyperreflexia can occur with injuries at the level of T6 or above. Initially, pain may be experienced at the level of injury. Some sensation (ranging from mild tingling to severe pain) may return if the lesion is incomplete. Pain may be caused by scar tissue or posttraumatic sympathetic dystrophy. Parathesias and hyperthesias may be noted.	Dysreflexia Pain Knowledge deficit Impaired physical mobility Self care deficit Sensory/perceptual alterations Sexual dysfunction Sleep pattern disturbance Risk of injury	Manage autonomic hyperreflexia Assess pain and use pain control strategies Provide information to patient and family Provide for total care needs of patient Begin patient/family teaching related to prevention and treatment of dysreflexia, comfort measures, and prevention of injury to tissue.	Autonomic dysreflexia (T-6 and above) Pain (all levels of injury) Parathesias and hyperthesias (all levels of injury)

Table 10-6. Plan of Care for Patients with SCI (Continued)

System-Specific Considerations	Nursing Diagnosis/ Collaborative Problems	Nursing Management	Level of Injury Affected
Integumentary system Skin pressure problems are a concern, although there is decreased sensation below the level of injury.	Impaired skin integrity Risk of peripheral neurovascular dysfunction Impaired tissue integrity Altered tissue perfusion peripheral Pressure ulcers Osteomyelitis	Provide skin care and turn the patient every 2 hours Inspect skin, especially bony prominences twice a day Provide for weight shifts in wheelchair every 15-30 minutes Provide for ROM exercises once daily Begin patient and family education regarding the potential and prevention of skin breakdown	Skin breakdown (all levels of injury)
Musculoskeletal system Prolonged immobility and paralysis have significant effects on bone, joints, and muscles. Spasticity may be present.	Impaired physical mobility Disuse syndrome Contractures Ankylosis Muscle atrophy Osteoporosis Spasticity		
Gastrointestinal (GI) system Neurogenic bowel may be present. Peristalsis returns but is sluggish. Other GI reflexes are sluggish. The development of gastric ulcers or hemorrhage remains a concern.	Altered bowel elimination Paralytic ileus GI bleeding Constipation	Implement aggressive physical therapy program Provide for ROM exercises once daily Position the patient's extremities in proper body alignment Monitor spasticity	Bones, joints, and muscles (all levels of injuries can have significant effects) Spasticity (T12 and above)
Genitourinary system Neurogenic bladder may be present. Altered sexual function may be present.	Altered urinary elimination High risk for infection Sexual dysfunction Renal calculi Kidney disease	Initiate a bowel program	Neurogenic bowel (potentially all levels of injury)
Metabolic system A high-fluid, high-carbohydrate, and high-protein diet is still needed for energy and tissue repair.	Fluid volume deficit Altered nutrition, less than body requirements Electrolyte imbalances	Initiate a bladder program	Neurogenic bladder (potentially all levels of injury)
Psychological and emotional responses The effect of the injury on the patient's previous functional level and lifestyle begins to be realized.	Impaired adjustment Body image disturbance Ineffective denial Grieving	Provide adequate fluid and nutritional intake	Altered nutrition (all levels of injury)

Table 10-6. Plan of Care for Patients with SCI (Continued)

System-Specific Considerations	Nursing Diagnosis/ Collaborative Problems	Nursing Management	Level of Injury Affected
The patient begins the loss, grief, and bereavement process. The effect of the injury on the family and significant other(s) begins to be realized.	Anxiety Fear Depression Altered family processes Hopelessness Powerlessness Impaired social interaction Social isolation Spiritual distress High risk for self-directed violence	Communicate with the patient and the family Be supportive Set realistic goals	Altered psychological and emotional response (all levels of injury)

Source consulted

Hickey, J. (1997). *The clinical practice of neurological and neurosurgical nursing* (4th ed.). Philadelphia: J.B. Lippincott.

4) Abnormal liver function due to trauma
5) Neurogenic bowel *[Refer to Chapter 7]*

f. Genitourinary manifestations

1) Neurogenic bladder *[Refer to Chapter 7]*
2) Urinary outlet sphincter dysfunctioning

g. Sexual manifestations *[Refer to Chapter 7]*

h. Psychosocial manifestations

1) Stressors and losses

a) Stressors
(1) Survival
(2) Quality of life
(3) Lifestyle alterations
(4) Occupational changes
(5) Participation in recreational activities

b) Losses
(1) Sensation
(2) Mobility
(3) Bowel and bladder control
(4) Sexual function
(5) Control and independence
(6) Former roles
(7) Self-esteem

2) Emotions and behaviors
a) Anxiety
b) Frustration
c) Anger
d) Hostility
e) Fear
f) Sarcasm
g) Regression
h) Denial
i) Guilt
j) Depression
k) Sensory overload

J. Discharge Planning

1. Begins prior to admission to rehabilitation
2. Is a collaborative effort between the patient, family, and interdisciplinary team
3. Includes the following considerations

a. Identify key family members who will be learning and/or performing care
b. Provide education using return demonstration by the patient and family throughout the rehabilitation stay
c. Identify the location or setting to which the patient is being discharged
d. Perform a home evaluation
e. Identify and order necessary DME
f. Identify funding sources

4. Ensure that the patient is discharged to a safe environment

K. Research Involving SCI and Aging (Gerhart, Charlifue, Metner, Weitzenkamp, & Whiteneck, 1999)

1. Overview

a. This longitudinal study began in 1990 in Great Britain to track more than 800 individuals with SCI.
b. Three phases have been completed: 1990, 1993, and 1996.

2. Death rates and causes of death

   a. SCI survivors have a higher death rate than the general population.

   b. Causes of death include cardiovascular disease, pneumonia, septicemia, cancer, and suicide.

3. Morbidity: Illnesses and complications

   a. Urinary tract infections

   b. Pressure sores

   c. Problems with chest infections, spasticity, perceived abdominal pain, and general malaise (more likely in people with tetraplegia)

   d. Musculoskeletal problems such as joint pain, stiffness, pressure sores, diarrhea, and constipation (especially in people with paraplegia)

   e. Increased fractures, cystitis, and motor and sensory changes (especially in people with incomplete injuries)

   f. Functional decline or decreasing physical independence

4. General health and life satisfaction

   a. More than 75% reported feeling generally healthy.

   b. 74% were generally satisfied with their lives.

   c. Stress and depression seemed to decrease as more years passed since the injury.

5. Risk factors

   a. Pressure sores

      1) More likely in people with paraplegia
      2) More likely in people who had already developed one pressure sore
      3) Increased risk for those with abnormal pulses in feet and lower extremities
      4) Increased risk with unemployment

   b. Upper extremity pain

      1) Decreased psychosocial well-being coincided with an increase in upper extremity pain.
      2) Limitations in ROM increased the risk of upper extremity pain.

   c. Life satisfaction

      1) Younger participants who had increased psychosocial well-being

and increased finances reported a higher life satisfaction.

      2) Participants who reported social involvement had less fatigue and were less likely to be overweight.

   d. Factors related to decreased physical independence

      1) Increased age, especially among people with paraplegia
      2) Changes in DME
      3) Changes in bladder management program
      4) Increased fatigue over time

   e. Fatigue: Those with a poor self-perception of health had more fatigue.

6. Conclusions

   a. Pressure sores and respiratory problems appear to be more of an issue with age.

   b. Musculoskeletal problems are associated more with longer durations of injury.

   c. Life satisfaction and quality of life are vital concepts, neither of which is totally dependent upon the level or severity of the disability or on the number of medical complications; however, each seems to be very important as a predictor of future outcomes.

   d. Fatigue appears to be an important predictor of future problems.

   e. Fatigue, depression, and decreased life satisfaction should not go unaddressed, as they may lead to costly and compromising complications.

L. Clinical Research (The Miami Project, 1999a, 1999b)

   1. Clinical and rehabilitative research: Focusing on understanding the nature of SCI and defining the nervous system's response to injury

      a. Study of the pathology of human SCI: A detailed analysis of postmortem human spinal cords is underway to compare actual spinal cord anatomy with diagnostic radiography (e.g., magnetic resonance images) and define the nature of the cellular damage that results from SCI.

      b. Electrophysiology of the spinal cord: Researchers have identified the appearance of a newly formed reflex, which demonstrates that nerve circuits may be altered and new connections formed after injury in humans.

   c. Spasticity and fatigue in paralyzed muscle: These factors provide essential information for designing exercise programs that optimize function in muscles that have lost some or all of their nerve supply.

   d. Central pattern generator (CPG): This group of nerve cells synchronizes muscle activity during alternating stepping of the legs.

   e. Pain research group: This group is evaluating the effect of SCI pain on quality of life.

2. Basic science research: Concentrating on techniques that hold the promise of repairing different types of spinal cord damage. Studies are underway to document the cellular nature of SCI in humans and animals.

   a. Neuroprotection to preserve as many cells as possible

   b. Regeneration of damaged axons to reestablish connection of nerve circuits

   c. Remyelination of axons

3. General notes

   a. No one theory or approach will encompass all of the effects of SCI.

   b. Many scientists believe that significant new treatments will not be found in a single approach but, rather, in a combination of techniques.

Research Perspective

Cooper, J.B., Jane, J., Alves, W., & Cooper, E. (1999). Right median nerve electrical stimulation to hasten awakening from coma. *Brain Injury, 13*(4), 261-267.

This pilot study described electrical stimulation as a promising modality to facilitate the awakening of comatose patients. The authors described the physiology of nerve conduction as a basis to familiarize the reader with the rationale for selecting this type of electrical stimulation modality. The median nerve serves as a peripheral gateway to the central nervous system, and the ascending reticular activating system (ARAS) maintains wakefulness in the brainstem. The right medial nerve was then used as a portal to stimulate the brainstem and cerebrum because an increased alertness and better speech have been observed after right medial nerve stimulation.

Comatose patients with TBI were screened for inclusion in the study. Patients receiving a postresuscitation Glasgow Coma Scale (GCS) score between 4 and 8 were enrolled after consent. All patients received the neurosurgical standard of care and were included with or without a craniotomy. Certain patients were excluded based on age or other medical conditions. Patients were randomly assigned to a control or treatment group. Each day for 2 weeks, patients in the treatment group received 8-12 hours of stimulation to the volar aspect of the right distal forearm.

At 1 week, the treatment group's GCS score had improved by an average of 4, and the control group's score had improved by an average of .7. At 2 weeks, the treatment group's score had improved by an average of 6.4, and the control group's score had improved by an average of 1.3. Patients in the treatment group stayed in the ICU for an average of 7.7 days, and patients in the control group stayed for an average of 17 days.

Implications for practice

Electrical stimulation of the right median nerve may help patients with acute brain injury recover from coma more rapidly. The burden of proof in establishing cause and effect in this population is very difficult. The observations gained from this study show promise that peripheral electrical stimulation may have positive effects on brain-injured comatose patients. Replication and larger trials may be indicated to further substantiate this important work. Right median nerve stimulation may improve outcomes, be easily instituted, carry little risk, and be cost effective.

References

Adams, R., Victor, M., & Ropper, A. (1997). *Principles of neurology*. New York: McGraw-Hill.

Ansell, B., & Keenan, J. (1989). The Western neuro sensory stimulation profile: A tool for assessing slow-to-recover head injured patients. *Archives of Physical Medicine and Rehabilitation, 70,* 104-108.

American Spinal Injury Association (ASIA). (1996). *International standards for neurological and functional classification of spinal injury patients* (Rev. ed.). Atlanta: Author.

Brain Injury Association. (1999, March 24). *The costs and causes of traumatic brain injury* [Online]. Available: http://www.biausa.org/costand.htm

Brontke, C., & Boake, C. (1996). Principles of brain injury rehabilitation. In R. Braddon (Ed.), *Physical medicine and rehabilitation* (pp. 1027-1052). Philadelphia: W.B. Saunders.

Carpenito, L. (1997). *Nursing diagnosis: Application to clinical practice* (7th ed.). Philadelphia: Lippincott.

Cooper, J.B., Jane, J., Alves, W., & Cooper, E. (1999). Right median nerve electrical stimulation to hasten awakening from coma. *Brain Injury, 13*(4), 261-267.

Duff, D., & Wells, D. (1997). Postcomatose unawareness/vegetative state following severe brain injury: A content methodology. *Journal of Neuroscience Nursing, 29*(5), 305-317.

Gatens, C., & Hebert, A.R. (1996). Cognition and behavior patterns. In S.P. Hoeman (Ed.), *Rehabilitation nursing: Process and application* (2nd ed., pp. 572-593). St. Louis: Mosby.

Gerhart, K., Charlifue, S., Menter, R., Weitzenkamp, D., & Whiteneck, G. (1999, August 10). *Aging with spinal cord injury* [Online]. Available: http://www.ed.gov/pubs/AmericanRehab/spring97/sp9706.html

Giacino, J., Kezmarsky, M., DeLuca, J., & Cicerone, K. (1991). Monitoring rate of recovery to predict outcome in minimally responsive patients. *Archives of Physical Medicine and Rehabilitation, 72*(11), 897-901.

Giacino, J., Zasler, N., Katz, D., Kelly, J., Rosenberg, J., & Filley, C. (1997). Development of practice guidelines for assessment and management of the vegetative and minimally conscious state. *Journal of Head Trauma Rehabilitation, 12*(4), 79-89.

Grosswasser, Z., Schwab, K., & Salazar, A. (1997). Assessment of outcome following traumatic brain injury in adults. In R. Herndon (Ed.), *Handbook of neurologic rating scales* (pp. 187-208). New York: Demos Vermande.

Hanak, M. (1993). *Spinal cord injury: An illustrated guide for health care professionals* (2nd ed.). New York: Springer Publishing.

Hickey, J. (1997). *Clinical practice of neurological and neurosurgical nursing* (4th ed.). Philadelphia: Lippincott.

Hoeman, S.P. (Ed.) (1996). *Rehabilitation nursing: Process and application* (2nd ed.). St. Louis: Mosby.

Katz, D. (1997). Traumatic brain injury. In V. Mills, J. Cassidy, & D. Katz (Eds.), *Neurologic rehabilitation: A guide to diagnosis, prognosis and treatment planning* (pp. 105-144). Malden, MA: Blackwell Science.

Levin, H., O'Donald, V., & Grossman, R. (1975). The Galveston orientation and amnesia test: A practical scale to assess cognition after head injury. *Journal of Nervous and Mental Disease, 167,* 675-686.

Mackay, L., Chapman, P., & Morgan, S. (1998). *Maximizing brain injury recovery* (pp. 574-575). Gaithersburg, MD: Aspen.

Marion, D. (1996). Pathophysiology and initial neurosurgical care: Future directions. In L. Horn & N. Zasler (Eds.), *Medical rehabilitation of traumatic brain injury* (pp. 28-52). Philadelphia: Hanley & Belfus.

Mandzak-McCarron, K. (1988). Rehabilitation of the patient with spinal cord injury. *Trauma Quarterly, 4*(3), 45-57.

Melvin, C., Lacy, M., & Swafford-Ten Eyck, L. (1998). Pediatric rehabilitation. In P. Chin, D. Finocchiaro, & A. Rosebrough (Eds.), *Rehabilitation nursing practice* (pp. 671-704). New York: McGraw Hill.

McCourt, A.E. (Ed.). (1993). *The specialty practice of rehabilitation nursing: A core curriculum* (3rd ed.). Skokie, IL: Rehabilitation Nursing Foundation of the Association of Rehabilitation Nurses.

The Miami Project. (1999a). *Basic science research* [Brochure]. Miami, FL: Author.

The Miami Project. (1999b). *Clinical and rehabilitative research* [Brochure]. Miami, FL: Author.

Miller, J., Piper, I., & Jones, P. (1996). Pathophysiology of head injury. In R.K. Narayan, J. Wilberger, & J. Povlishock (Eds.), *Neurotrauma* (pp. 61-70). New York: McGraw-Hill.

National Center for Injury Prevention and Control (NCIPC). (1999, April 15). *Division of acute care, rehabilitation research, and disability prevention* [Online]. Available: http://www.cdc.gov/ncipc/dacrrdp/dacrrdp.htm

National Spinal Cord Injury Statistical Center (NSCISC). (1999). *Spinal cord injury: The facts and figures*. Birmingham, AL: The University of Alabama at Birmingham.

O'Dell, M., & Riggs, R. (1996). Management of the minimally responsive patient. In L. Horn & N. Zasler (Eds.), *Medical rehabilitation of traumatic brain injury* (pp. 103-132). Philadelphia: Hanley & Belfus.

Phipps, E., DiPasquale, M., & Whyte, J. (1997). Interpreting responsiveness in person's with traumatic brain injury: Beliefs in families and quantitative evaluations. *Journal of Head Trauma Rehabilitation, 12*(4), 52-69.

Rader, M., Alston, J., & Ellis, D. (1989). Sensory stimulation of severely brain injured patients. *Brain Injury, 3,* 141-147.

Rancho Los Amigos Medical Center, Adult Brain Injury Service. (1979). *Levels of cognitive function scale* (adapted version). Downey, CA: Author.

Rappaport, M., Dougherty, A., & Kelting, D. (1992). Evaluation of coma and vegetative states. *Archives of Physical Medicine and Rehabilitation, 73,* 628-634.

Rappaport, M., Hall, K., Hopkins, H., Belleza, T., & Cope, D. (1982). Disability rating scale for severe head trauma patients: Coma to community. *Archives of Physical Medicine and Rehabilitation, 63,* 118-123.

Rosebrough, A. (1998). Acquired brain injury: traumatic brain injury. In P. Chin, D. Finocchiaro, & A. Rosebrough (Eds.), *Rehabilitation nursing practice* (pp. 223-246). New York: McGraw-Hill.

Sosin, D.M., Sniezek, J.E., & Thurman, D.J. (1996). Incidence of mild and moderate brain injury in the United States, 1991. *Brain Injury, 10,* 47-54.

Staas, W.J., Formal, C.S., Gershkoff, A.M., Freda, M., Hirshwald, J.F., Miller, G.T., Forrest, L., & Burkhard, B.A. (1988). Rehabilitation of the spinal cord injured patient. In J. DeLisa (Ed.), *Rehabilitation medicine: Principles and practice* (pp. 635-667). Philadelphia: J.B. Lippincott.

Sugarman, B. (1985). Medical complications of spinal cord injury. *Quarterly Journal of Medicine, 54*(213), 3-18.

Therapeutics and Technology Assessment Subcommittee. (1996). Assessment: Neurological testing of adults—Considerations for neurologists. *Neurology, 47*, 592-599.

Walleck, C.A. (1988). Central nervous system II: Spinal cord injury. In V.D. Cadona, P.D. Hurn, P.J. Mason, A.M. Scanlon-Schlipp, & S.W. Veise-Berry (Eds.), *Trauma nursing from resuscitation through rehabilitation* (pp. 419-448). Philadelphia: W.B. Saunders.

Winkler, P. (1995). Head injury. In D. Umphred (Ed.), *Neurological rehabilitation* (pp. 421-453). St. Louis: Mosby.

Zafonte, R., Muizelaar, J.P., & Peterson, P.L. (1998). The pathophysiology of brain injury: Understanding innovative drug therapies. *Journal of Head Trauma Rehabilitation, 13*(1), 1-10.

Zedjlik, C.P. (1992). *Management of spinal cord injury* (2nd ed.). Boston: Jones and Bartlett.

Suggested resources

American Speech-Language-Hearing Association. (1995). Guidelines for the structure and function of an interdisciplinary team for persons with brain injury. *ASHA, 37*, 23-24.

Boake, C. (1996). Supervision rating scale: A measure of functional outcome from brain injury. *Archives of Physical Medicine and Rehabilitation, 77*(8),765-772.

Berly, M.H., & Wilmot, C.B. (1984). Acute abdominal emergencies during the first four weeks after spinal cord injury. *Archives of Physical Medicine and Rehabilitation, 65*, 687-690.

Bracken, M.B., Shepard, M.J., Collins, W.F., Holford, T.R., Young, W., Baskin, D.S., Eisenberg, H.M., Flamm, E., Leo-Summers, L., Maroon, J., Marshall, L.F., Perot, P.L., Jr., Piepmeier, J., Sonntag, V.K.H., Wagner, F.C., Wilberger, J.E., & Winn, H.R. (1990). A randomized, controlled trial of methylprednisolone or naxolone in the treatment of acute spinal cord injury: Results of the second national acute spinal cord injury study. *The New England Journal of Medicine, 322*, 1405-1422.

Brain Injury Association, & Defense and Veterans Head Injury Program. (1998). *A guide to selecting and monitoring brain injry rehabilitation services.* [Online]. Available: http://www.biausa.org

Buchanan, L.E., & Nawoczenski, D.H. (1987). *Spinal cord injury concepts and management approaches.* Baltimore: Williams and Wilkins.

Costello, M., Pedersen, C., Tan, T., Devaux, R., Tan, S., Dixon, P., Lee, L., & Cahuya, E. (1997). Acquired brain injuries demanding nursing excellence. *Australian Nursing Journal, 5*(2), 24-27.

Dolan, J.T. (1991). *Critical care nursing: Clinical management through the nursing process.* Philadelphia: F.A. Davis.

Duckett, S. (1996). Staff stress in head injury rehabilitation. *Brain Injury, 10*(2), 779.

Elovic, E., & Antionette, T. (1996). Epidemiology and primary prevention of traumatic brain injury. In L. Horn & N. Zasler (Eds.), *Medical rehabilitation of traumatic brain injury* (pp. 1-28). Philadelphia: Hanley & Belfus.

Geisler, F.H., Dorsey, F.C., & Coleman, W.P. (1991). Recovery of motor function after spinal cord injury: a randomized, placebo-controlled trial with CM1-ganglioside. *The New England Journal of Medicine, 324*, 1829-1838.

Gines, D.J. (1988). Long-term nutrition care for the client with spinal cord injury. *Topics in Clinical Nutrition, 3*(3), 61-69.

Goldberg, G. (1998). What happens after brain injury? *Postgraduate Medicine, 104*(2), 99-105.

Gregory, H.H., & Bonfiglio, R.P. (1995). Limiting restraint use for behavior control: The brain injury rehabilitation unit as a model. *Maryland Medical Journal, 44*(4), 279-283.

Grzankowski, J.A. (1997). Altered thought processes related to traumatic brain injury and their nursing implications. *Rehabilitation Nursing, 22*(1), 24-31.

Palmer, C.D. (1985, January/February). The brain trauma rehabilitation program Southfield Rehabilitation Center. *Cognitive Rehabilitation*, pp. 4-9.

Prigatano, G.P. (1997). Learning from our successes and failures: Reflections and comments on "Cognitive rehabilitation: How it is and how it might be." *Journal of International Neuropsychological Society, 3*(5), 497-509.

Semlyen, J.K., Summers, S.J., & Barnes, M.P. (1998). Traumatic brain injury: Efficacy of multidisciplinary rehabilitation. *Archives of Physical Medicine and Rehabilitation, 79*(6). 678-683.

Tesio, L., & Cantagallo, A. (1998). The Functional Assessment Measure (FAM) in closed traumatic brain injury outpatients: A rasch-based psychometric study. *Journal of Outcome Measurement, 2*(2), 79-96.

Theuerkauf, A. (1996). Self-care and activities of daily living. In S.P. Hoeman (Ed.), *Rehabilitation nursing: Process and application* (2nd ed., pp. 156-187). St. Louis: Mosby.

Whiteneck, G. (Ed.). (1993). *Aging with spinal cord injury.* New York: Demos.

Yuen, H.K., & Benzing, P. (1996). Treatment methodology: Guiding of behavior through redirection in brain injury rehabilitation. *Brain Injury, 10*(3), 229-238.

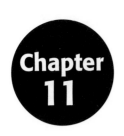

Chapter 11

Musculoskeletal and Orthopedic Disorders

Barbara A. Naden, MSN RN CRRN ONC

Rehabilitation nurses frequently come into contact with clients who have musculoskeletal disorders. Whether the client has a chronic condition (e.g., rheumatoid arthritis) or a fracture related to a fall, rehabilitation nurses are members of an interdisciplinary team that treats the whole person. Rehabilitation nurses take on the essential roles of care provider, educator, and counselor to achieve a well-rounded plan of care for these clients.

By the year 2020, it is expected that the number of people older than age 65 will be 51 million. With age can come chronic illness. Chronic illnesses can take several forms and can occur suddenly or very slowly. Chronic illnesses can involve periodic flare-ups or remain in remission with an absence of symptoms for many years.

Osteoporosis is a chronic illness that comes on very slowly and is frequently not diagnosed until after a sudden acute event, such as a fracture. Osteoporosis has only recently become an international issue, partially due to the increased growth and aging of the world's population and to the recent improvements in diagnostic testing capacity. Financial considerations related to osteoporosis also have become a concern. It has been estimated that one in two women and one in five men older than age 65 will have an osteoporotic-related fracture at some time in their life span, with an estimated annual cost of $14 million per year in the United States alone. The National Hospital Discharge Survey reported that more than 250,000 hip fractures are related to osteoporosis per year. By 2040, this number is expected to rise to 840,000 per year.

One of the objectives of the Healthy People 2000 initiative is to decrease the incidence of osteoporotic fractures. One way of achieving this is by taking a comprehensive, interdisciplinary approach in which prevention is of primary concern. Preventive programs should target infants, children, adolescents, and young adults, as they are still building up calcium stores. For people older than 30 years old, the focus should be to prevent further loss of calcium and build existing stores of calcium. Preventable safety programs should be stressed especially with people older than 65 years.

In 1992, arthritis and rheumatic diseases (chronic illnesses involving the musculoskeletal system) were the leading cause of disability, affecting 42.7 million people at an annual cost of $65 billion. Many people who have arthritis do not seek medical attention for it; instead, they use nonprescription pain relievers and arthritis ointments and liniments.

Another musculoskeletal-related objective of Healthy People 2000 is to decrease the rate of amputations in people with diabetes mellitus by 40% (i.e., from 8.2 of every 1,000 people to 4.9 of every 1,000 people) (U.S. Department of Health and Human Services [DHHS], 1998). The ability to achieve this objective lies heavily on healthcare providers. Client education and preventive health programs must be stressed, especially for diabetic clients. In recent years, revisions in Medicare have made it possible for these clients to receive therapeutic shoes that decrease the risk of skin breakdown. Also, Medicare now subsidizes podiatric care for diabetic clients with vascular and nervous system pathology involving the lower extremities.

In recent years, preventive health care has taken a much larger role. In fact, statistics show that people are already living longer, healthier, and more productive lives. However, health workers are still seeing chronic illnesses in older Americans. This is due, in part, to a lifetime of unhealthy habits. Advances in medical science and technology have shown us that once-unknown disease processes are amenable to preventive treatments and that complications can be decreased with good medical management and preventive care.

By performing accurate, thorough assessments, rehabilitation nurses can monitor chronic illnesses such as arthritis over time and adjust treatments to meet each client's symptoms and needs. Client and family education are essential elements of care, especially with musculoskeletal disorders. The client must understand the diagnosis (e.g., what it is, how it affects the body, what the natural progression is) to make informed decisions about treatment plans. Client "buy-in" is needed because the treatment plan is often long and requires a great deal of effort to achieve functional outcomes. Rehabilitation nurses play many roles in the treatment plan, which is designed to return the client to functional independence.

I. Osteoporosis

A. Overview

1. A degenerative disease that causes bones to become fragile and break with minimal to no trauma
2. Affects more than 28 million people (mostly women) in the United States
3. Leads to 1.5 million fractures (i.e., 500,000 spinal fractures, 300,000 hip fractures [Woodhead & Moss, 1998]) at an annual cost of $14 billion per year to the healthcare system (Watts, 1997)
4. A leading cause of disability in the aging population
5. Affects not only the ability to perform activities of daily living (ADLs) but also social and psychological functioning
6. Leads to a decrease in quality of life
7. A common metabolic bone disease that involves severe generalized reduction in skeletal bone mass and micro-architectural deterioration of the bone tissue (Klippel, 1997; Salmond, Mooney, & Verdisco, 1996)
8. Is associated with an increased risk for fractures of the hip, wrist, spine, ribs, and pelvis
9. Occurs when bone reabsorption is greater than bone formation
10. Is frequently not diagnosed until a fracture is sustained

B. Etiology

1. Cause: Remains unknown
2. Contributing risk factors (Kessenich, 1997; Tomaski, 1996)
   a. Genetic factors
      1) Female
      2) Asian or Caucasian, especially Northern European ancestry
      3) Family history of hip fracture, kyphosis (Dowager's Hump), osteoporosis
      4) Red or blond hair
      5) Fair skin
      6) Scoliosis
      7) Rheumatoid arthritis
      8) Small-framed body
   b. Nutritional problems
      1) Limited calcium and vitamin D intake
      2) High protein diet
      3) Poor gastrointestinal absorption
      4) Eating disorders (e.g., anorexia, bulimia)
      5) Heavy alcohol use
      6) High caffeine intake
   c. Lifestyle factors
      1) Low level of activity
      2) Immobilization
      3) Previous falls
      4) Heavy cigarette smoking
   d. Endocrine disorders
      1) Hyperthyroidism
      2) Diabetes mellitus
      3) Gonadal dysfunction in men
      4) Early or surgically induced menopause
      5) Exercise-induced amenorrhea
      6) Nulliparity
      7) Abnormally low weight or leanness
      8) Low bone density
   e. Pharmacological factors
      1) Antacids containing aluminum: Cause calcium loss in stool
      2) Antiseizure medications (e.g., phenytoin, phenobarbital, primidone): Interfere with the metabolism of vitamin D and decrease calcium absorption
      3) Tetracycline, Isoniazid, Lasix: Cause increased calcium loss in urine
      4) Vitamin A: In excess of 5,000 IU/day, increases calcium loss in the urine
      5) Corticosteroids (e.g., prednisone, dexamethasone): Long-term use results in severe osteoporosis.
      6) Thyroid hormones in excessive doses
      7) Heparin

8) Lithium

f. Other risk factors

   1) Hyperparathyroidism

   2) Neoplasm

   3) Renal dysfunction

   4) Increased vitamin D intake

   5) Increased calcium carbonate intake

   6) Previous fracture

   7) Selected chemotherapy agents

   8) Osteomalacia

3. Incidence

a. Osteoporotic fractures most often involve the hip, vertebrae, or wrist.

b. One of five women will sustain a hip fracture by age 80 (Thorngren, 1994).

c. The morbidity rate is 12%–20% within the first year after the fracture (Cummings, Rubin, & Black, 1990).

d. Half of the people with osteoporosis will become partially dependent, and 33% will require long-term care (Watts, 1997).

e. Most deaths resulting from a hip fracture occur within 6 months of the event (McClung, 1999).

4. Types of osteoporosis (Kassem, Melton, & Riggs, 1995)

a. Type I (postmenopausal)

   1) Related to rapid drop in estrogen production around the time of menopause: Estrogen is essential for normal calcium absorption.

   2) Diet low in calcium and vitamin D

b. Type II (senile or age-related)

   1) Occurs in men and women older than age 70

   2) Is the result of the normal aging process and chronic lack of calcium

   3) May be due to renal dysfunction, which affects the conversion of vitamin D to a form usable for calcium absorption

c. Disuse osteoporosis

   1) Seen with paraplegia, quadriplegia, and other disorders that limit mobility

   2) Involves an initial rapid decrease in bone mass due to increased bone reabsorption and decreased bone formation (National Institutes of Health

[NIH] Consensus Development Panel on Optimal Calcium Intake, 1994)

   3) Associated with increased calcium intake, which must be monitored carefully due to potential risks (NIH Consensus Development Panel, 1994)

     a) Hypercalcemia

     b) Ectopic ossification

     c) Ectopic calcification

     d) Nephrolithiasis

C. Pathophysiology

1. Skeletal system influence

a. The normal bone remodeling cycle is constant and is governed by reabsorption activities of osteoclasts and bone-forming osteoblasts (Kessenich, 1997).

   1) There are two basic types of bone.

     a) Cortical bone: Dense and less metabolically active; forms the outer shell of the bone

     b) Trabecular bone: Metabolically active; is concentrated in the flat bones of the pelvis, vertebrae, forearms, and ribs

   2) All bones are made of both types, but the proportions differ.

b. Normally, 10% of bone is undergoing a remodeling cycle at a given time (Kessenich, 1997).

c. The cycle is balanced until approximately age 30, when bone loss outweighs bone growth at a rate of 3%–5% per decade (World Health Organization [WHO], 1994).

2. Endocrine system involvement

a. Bone reabsorption is affected by parathyroid hormone, 1,25 dihydroxyvitamin D, and calcitonin.

b. Each affects the regulation of serum calcium (see Figure 11-1).

c. Parathyroid hormone increases the reabsorption of bone by increasing osteoclast activity and, ultimately, bone breakdown.

d. Release of parathyroid hormone activates vitamin D to 1,25 dihydroxyvitamin D_3 and allows calcium to be absorbed in the gastrointestinal tract.

e. Release of calcitonin inhibits osteoclasts,

thus decreasing bone resorption and causing a decrease in serum calcium levels.

    f. Estrogen may affect these hormones and has been noted to increase the osteoblastic cells available for new bone growth (DeCherney, 1993).

   3. Menopausal influence

    a. Menopause begins a marked acceleration in bone loss—as much as 15% during the perimenopausal period.

      1) Bone loss begins approximately 1.5 years before the last menstrual period.

      2) Continued rapid bone loss continues until about 1.5 years after the last menstrual period.

    b. Bone loss is due to a decrease in natural estrogen.

    c. Estrogen replacement decreases the effects of menopause on bone loss.

D. Diagnosis

   1. Thorough history (Salmond et al., 1996)

    a. Family history

    b. Excessive height loss (more than 2 in.)

    c. Fractures from minimal trauma before age 40

    d. Complaints of bone pain, particularly in the back

    e. Onset of menopause and estrogen deficiency: The single most common cause of osteoporosis (Biskobing, 1997)

    f. Low intake of calcium, lactose intolerance

    g. Steroid use

    h. Northern European heritage

    i. Gum disease or tooth decay

    j. Excessive caffeine use

    k. Cigarette use

    l. High alcohol intake

    m. Sedentary lifestyle or long-term immobilization

    n. History of specific conditions

      1) Thyroid problems

      2) Liver problems

      3) Diabetes mellitus

      4) Renal failure

      5) Malignancies (Watts, 1997)

      6) Other endocrine disorders

    o. Medication history

      1) Corticosteroids

      2) Isoniazid

      3) Heparin

      4) Tetracycline

      5) Anticonvulsants

      6) Thyroid supplements

   2. Physical examination (Salmond et al., 1996)

    a. Fracture of wrist, femur, vertebral compression fractures

    b. Marked kyphosis, Dowager's hump

    c. Shortened status

    d. Muscle atrophy

    e. Muscle spasms in back

Figure 11-1. Hypocalcemia and Hypercalcemia

Hypocalcemia

⇓ Calcium blood level
⇓
Release of parathyroid hormone from parathyroid gland
⇓
⇑ Release of calcium from bones
⇑ Calcium reabsorption from kidneys
⇑ Calcium absorption from the gut
(requires presence of Vitamin D)
⇓
⇑ Blood calcium levels normal

Signs and symptoms
- Nerve excitability
- Paresthesias
- Muscle cramping
- Muscle spasm
- Tetany
- Death

Hypercalcemia

⇑ Calcium blood levels
⇓
Release of calcitonin from thyroid gland
⇓
⇓ Release of calcium from bones
⇓ Calcium reabsorption from kidneys and gut
⇓
⇓ Blood calcium levels normal

Signs and symptoms
- Muscle weakness
- Ataxia, coma
- Arrhythmia, cardiac arrest
- Fractures
- Extreme polyuria

---

f. Difficulty bending forward

g. Impaired breathing

h. Poor dentition

3. Laboratory tests (Salmond et al., 1996)

a. 24-hour urine calcium level

b. Serum calcium, phosphorus, alkaline phosphatase levels

c. Serum osteocalcin

d. Thyroid tests

e. Fasting urine sample for calcium and hydroxyproline, corrected for creatinine (Woodhead & Moss, 1998)

4. Bone mineral density evaluation ("AACE Clinical Practice Guidelines," 1996)

a. Results are measured against two standard norms.

1) Age-matched readings (the z-score): Compare an individual's results (the t-score) and what is expected in someone of the same age and body size.

2) Young-normal readings: Compare an individual's results to the estimated peak bone density of a healthy young adult

b. WHO has established diagnostic criteria for women who have not experienced fractures, based on the bone mineral density t-scores.

1) Normal: 0 to 1 standard deviation (*SD*) below the young normal mean

2) Osteopenia or low bone mass: 1 to 2.5 *SD* below the young normal mean

3) Osteoporosis: Greater than 2.5 *SD* below the young normal mean

4) For every decrease in bone mass of 1 *SD*, the relative risk of fracture increases 1.5 to 3 times.

5) A client with one or more low trauma fractures is considered to be osteoporotic regardless of the bone mineral density measurement.

5. Radiographic studies

a. Looking for diffuse radiolucency

b. Presence of vertebral compression fractures and bone spurs

E. Resulting Disabilities

1. Hip fracture

a. By the age of 80 years, one of every five women has suffered a hip fracture (Thorngren, 1994).

b. The lifetime risk of hip fracture for white women is 16%–18%. For white men, it is 5%–6%; for black women, it is 6%; for black men age 50 or older, it is 3% (McClung, 1999).

c. The incidence of hip fracture in women is twice that of men worldwide (Kannus et al., 1996).

d. The incidence of hip fracture is greater in elderly people who are institutionalized.

e. A woman has twice the risk of a fracture if her mother had a hip fracture (Cummings et al., 1995).

f. Prompt surgical fixation allows for earlier ambulation, which helps to decrease the complications of immobility.

g. The cause of the hip fracture must be investigated; it may be a sign of an underlying medical problem (e.g., cardiac, neurological, malignancy).

2. Vertebral compression fractures

a. Usually occur in cervical and lumbar regions and may not be accompanied by pain

b. Usually seen in younger postmenopausal women

c. May lose up to 6 in. in height as a result of kyphosis (Darovic, 1997)

d. Conservative treatment

1) Cervical collar
2) Lumbar corset
3) Jewett brace
4) Thoracolumbarsacral orthosis (TLSO)

e. Surgical management

1) Decompression laminectomy
2) Spinal fusion

3. Wrist fracture: Usually seen in younger postmenopausal women

4. Balance disturbances as a result of kyphosis and scoliosis

5. Falls resulting from balance disturbances

F. Client Education
1. Ensure a balanced diet with calcium-rich foods and vitamin D and calcium supplements when indicated
2. Promote a regular weight-bearing exercise program
3. Decrease or eliminate risk factors (e.g., smoking, consuming caffeine or alcohol)
4. Instruct in home and community safety measures
5. Evaluate bone mineral density
6. Maintain a record of client's height
7. Discuss with physician hormone replacement therapy or other osteoporosis medication
8. Manage medications

G. Interventions After Diagnosis
1. Pharmacological management
   a. Calcium
      1) Adequate calcium intake is essential to achieving optimal peak bone mass (NIH Consensus Development Panel, 1994).
      2) Most Americans do not get the recommended daily allowance (RDA) of calcium based on their age and physiologic need (Heany, 1998).
      3) Optimal recommended calcium requirements are as follows (NIH Consensus Development Panel, 1994).
         a) Children: 800–1,200 mg/day
         b) Adolescents: 1,200–1,500 mg/day
         c) Premenopausal adult women: 1,000–1,500 mg/day
         d) Postmenopausal women not taking hormone replacement: 1,500 mg/day
         e) Postmenopausal women taking hormone replacement: 1,200–1,500 mg/day
         f) Men aged 60 and older: 1,300 mg/day
         g) Elderly people: 1,000–1,500 mg/day
         h) Average RDA: 1,400–1,500 mg/day
      4) There are many sources of calcium.
         a) Milk, yogurt, cheese, cottage cheese, ice cream, tofu, salmon, broccoli, spinach, kale, eggs, beans, sardines, clams, oysters
         b) Calcium-fortified foods (e.g., cereal)
         c) Supplements
            (1) Calcium carbonate: Inexpensive and efficient (e.g., Tums)
            (2) Tricalcium phosphate or calcium citrate (e.g., Os-Cal): Effective alternatives if GI symptoms occur (McClung, 1999)
            (3) Alka: Two antacids
   b. Estrogen replacement therapy
      1) The most effective treatment for postmenopausal osteoporosis
      2) Slows the rate of bone loss
      3) Is surrounded by controversy: The decision to supplement must be explored carefully.
   c. Vitamin D: Needed for adequate calcium absorption
      1) Deficiency occurs when there is inadequate exposure to the sun, inadequate dietary intake, and acquired resistance to vitamin D (NIH Consensus Development Panel, 1994).
      2) Deficiency can be relieved by eating foods that are fortified with vitamin D and supplementing the diet with 600-800 IU/day of vitamin D (NIH Consensus Development Panel, 1994).
   d. Alendronate (Fosamax)
      1) Proven to prevent bone resorption, reduce the risk of fractures, and slow the course of disease (Spratto & Woods, 1998)
      2) Requires special precautions for ingestion (see Figure 11-2)
   e. Calcitonin (Miacalcin) nasal spray
      1) Indicated for women who are 5 or more years postmenopausal
      2) Has been shown to increase spinal bone mass

3) Must be taken with 1,200 to 1,500 mg calcium and 400 IU of vitamin D (Heaney, 1998; Solomon, 1998)

   f. Raloxifen (Evista) (Eli Lilly, 1998)

      1) A selective estrogen receptor modulator that imitates some of estrogen's positive effects

      2) Prevents bone loss through the body

2. Exercise and weight bearing

   a. Walk, jog, swim, use a stationary bike, do theraband or aerobic exercise on a regular basis to promote bone remodeling and increase bone density

   b. Limit, as much as possible, any event that may cause prolonged immobilization

3. Pain management: Manage pain resulting from changes in the musculoskeletal system and compression fractures to allow for early and progressive activity

4. Safety issues: Conduct a fall prevention safety assessment, asking the following questions (Mosby Great Performance, 1995, pp. 6–7)

   a. "Is there adequate lighting in each room?

   b. Are night-lights placed throughout the house where they're needed?

   c. Are stairways adequately lighted?

   d. Are light switches within reach and easy to use?

   e. If the person uses a wheelchair, can he or she still reach the light switches?

Figure 11-2. Client Education: Precautions for Fosamax Therapy

Instruct the client to take the medication correctly
- Take on an empty stomach, first thing in the morning
- Take with a full 8 oz. of tap water (not bottled water, coffee, or juice)
- Take with 1,200–1,500 mg of calcium and 400 IU of vitamin D
- Wait at least 30 minutes before eating or drinking anything, including taking any other medication
- If possible, wait 60 minutes before eating or drinking to ensure an enhanced absorption of the medication
- Do not lie down after taking the medication

Provide information about therapeutic side effects of the medication

Explain the safety issues for proper storage of the medication

TEACHING TOPICS

---

   f. Are you using 'warm' incandescent light rather than 'cold' florescent light that may produce glare?

   g. Have you removed throw rugs that might cause falls?

   h. Do carpets have worn areas or places that have come loose or untacked?

   i. Are floors free of phone and extension cords?

   j. Are walkways clear of clutter, boxes, or low furniture that might cause a fall?

   k. Are there nonskid strips in potentially dangerous areas such as stairs, bathroom floors, in front of the toilet, and in the bath or shower?

   l. Are the stairs free of cracks and sagging carpeting?

   m. Are there sturdy railings on both sides of the stairway?

   n. Are carpets low-pile monotone rather than shag?

   o. Does the bathroom have grab bars around the toilet, and in the tub or shower, capable of supporting a 250-lb load?

   p. Does the house have heat sources such as radiators and space heaters that may be obstacles for a person using a cane?

   q. Is there a possibility that the person's medications may affect his or her movement, balance, or consciousness?"

H. Prevention Strategies

1. Set a goal to have the optimal level of bone mass by the time menopause begins

2. Manage diet to take in the RDA of calcium and vitamin D throughout the life span

3. Exercise and continue an active healthy lifestyle throughout life

4. Decrease or eliminate risk factors

   a. Stop smoking

   b. Decrease caffeine intake

   c. Decrease alcohol intake

   d. Maintain a balanced diet

   e. Limit medications that affect bone mass

   f. Maintain an ideal weight

   g. Prevent falling episodes

I. Research Topics
  1. Differing requirements for bone mass and calcium for different races and ethnic backgrounds (NIH Consensus Development Panel, 1994)
  2. Long-term effects related to calcium supplementation in postmenopausal women and in older men (NIH Consensus Development Panel, 1994)
  3. New medications: Clinical trials (Woodhead & Moss, 1998)

II. Arthritis
  A. Overview of Arthritis
    1. The inflammation of a joint
    2. Affects connective tissues (e.g., muscle, tendons, bursa, fibrous tissue)
    3. A term that the public uses to describe pain and stiffness of the musculoskeletal system (sometimes referred to as rheumatism)
    4. A medical term that is restricted to rheumatic diseases that involve inflammatory conditions affecting the joints
    5. Has more than 100 different Arthritis Foundation classifications
    6. The second leading cause of limitation of movement (after heart disease)
    7. The leading cause of absenteeism in the workplace and the second leading reason for disability payments (after mental illness)
    8. Involves an excess of $8.6 billion in annual lost wages and medical bills
    9. An increasing problem for the growing older population in the United States that is putting an increased strain on Medicare
  B. Classification of Arthritis (see Figure 11-3)
    1. Inflammatory
    2. Degenerative
    3. Metabolic
  C. Rheumatoid Arthritis (RA)
    1. Definition
      a. A chronic inflammatory systemic condition that primarily affects joints, but can also damage muscles, lungs, skin, blood vessels, nerves, and eyes
      b. Associated with a symmetrical involvement of the peripheral joints
      c. Common symptoms: Fatigue and weight loss
    2. Etiology
      a. Remains unknown
      b. Theories

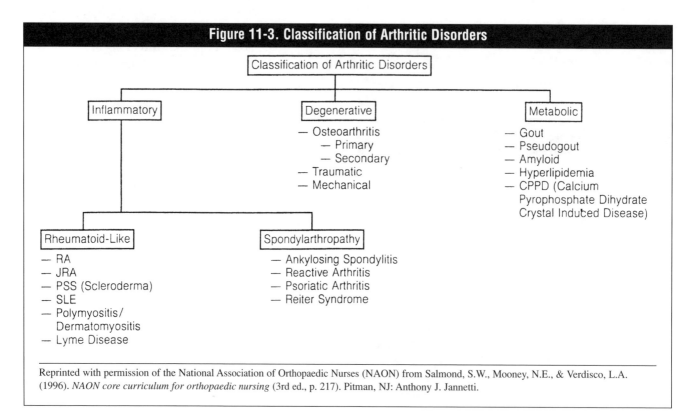

Figure 11-3. Classification of Arthritic Disorders

Classification of Arthritic Disorders

Inflammatory
  Rheumatoid-Like
    — RA
    — JRA
    — PSS (Scleroderma)
    — SLE
    — Polymyositis/ Dermatomyositis
    — Lyme Disease
  Spondylarthropathy
    — Ankylosing Spondylitis
    — Reactive Arthritis
    — Psoriatic Arthritis
    — Reiter Syndrome

Degenerative
  — Osteoarthritis
    — Primary
    — Secondary
  — Traumatic
  — Mechanical

Metabolic
  — Gout
  — Pseudogout
  — Amyloid
  — Hyperlipidemia
  — CPPD (Calcium Pyrophosphate Dihydrate Crystal Induced Disease)

Reprinted with permission of the National Association of Orthopaedic Nurses (NAON) from Salmond, S.W., Mooney, N.E., & Verdisco, L.A. (1996). *NAON core curriculum for orthopaedic nursing* (3rd ed., p. 217). Pitman, NJ: Anthony J. Jannetti.

1) A genetically controlled host immune response to an unknown stimulus (Thalgott, LaRocca, & Gardner, 1993)
2) An infectious microorganism (which has not been isolated yet)
3) Genetic predisposition
   a) Affects more women than men by a 3:1 ratio
   b) Tends to be seen in families with a history of RA
4) Trauma
5) Alteration of the normal peripheral vascular bed by an autonomic influence (Salmond et al, 1996)
6) Increased stress (emotional and physical): Known to cause acute exacerbations

3. Pathophysiology
   a. Process (Thalgott et al., 1993)
      1) Involves synovial proliferation, joint effusion, and edema in the small joints
      2) Causes cartilage to erode and be destroyed
      3) Forms pannus in the articular cartilage and destroys the joint: Pannus is the inflammatory cells and granulation tissue that covers and erodes the articular cartilage (Salmond et al., 1996).
      4) Affects ligaments and the joint capsule, making it impossible to maintain proper alignment and position, which causes the deformity
      5) Results in a generalized osteoporosis that develops in these areas and makes surgical stabilization difficult
      6) Produces fibrous adhesions, bony alkylosis, and uniting of opposing joint surfaces, which occur in the later stages of RA
      7) Involves irreversible effects
   b. Effects of RA on the joint
      1) Joint destruction
      2) Joint inflammation and effusion, particularly in the feet, hands, fingers, wrists, and elbows
      3) Redness, swelling, and pain with motion

   c. Effects of RA on the body
      1) General: Fatigue, anorexia, weight loss, aching, and stiffness
      2) Lymph: Enlarged glands
      3) Pulmonary
         a) Caplan's syndrome (i.e., rheumatic nodules with cavitation)
         b) Pleuritis
         c) Interstitial fibrosis
         d) Pleural effusion
         e) Interstitial pneumonia
      4) Neurologic: Localized neuropathy
         a) Foot drop, as a result of nerve injury secondary to ischemia, compression, or obstruction of the nerves going to the ankle
         b) Entrapment neuropathy
         c) Spinal cord compression
      5) Ocular: Uveitus, Sjögren's syndrome
      6) Cardiovascular
         a) Fibrous pericarditis in 10% of cases
         b) Cardiomyopathy
         c) Vasculitis
      7) Skin: Thinning
      8) Rheumatic: Nodules may occur.
         a) Present in 20% of cases
         b) Presence is associated with a poor prognosis
         c) Firm, nontender, oval mass up to 2 cm diameter
         d) Found in subcutaneous tissue over pressure points (e.g., elbows, sacrum, dorsal surface of the hand)
         e) Found in other areas (e.g., lungs, heart valves, vocal cords, eyes)

4. Incidence (Salmond et al., 1996)
   a. Affects 3%–5% of the population
   b. Affects RA clients: 85%–90% of RA clients have a positive rheumatoid factor (RF).
   c. Affects women more frequently than men
   d. Affects people of all races
   e. Is not affected by climate

f. Has an onset age that is usually between 20 and 50 years: Most cases are diagnosed when people are in their 40s.

g. Can affect elderly people: 25% of elderly people will develop RA with sudden onset when they are affected by another severe disease. RA is best managed in these clients aggressively with disease-modifying antirheumatic drugs (DMARDs).

5. Types of RA

   a. Juvenile arthritis (JA)

      1) A chronic inflammatory condition that has an onset before age 16 years

      2) Includes three types of onset, which are classified during the first 6 months of the illness (Youngblood & Edwards, 1999)
         a) Systemic onset
         b) Pauciarticular arthritis
         c) Polyarticular onset
            (1) Rheumatoid factor (RF) negative
            (2) RF positive

      3) Aspects of classification (see Table 11-1)

      4) Affects approximately 1 in 1,000 children

      5) Affects slightly more girls than boys

      6) Is generally mild in form

   b. Adult rheumatoid arthritis (RA)

6. Classification: Four or more criteria (Arnett, Edworthy, & Bloch, 1988)

      1) Morning stiffness for at least 1 hour, present for at least 6 weeks

      2) Arthritis of three or more joints
         a) Soft tissue swelling or fluid
         b) Affects joints such as right/left proximal interphalangeal (PIP) joint, metacarpophalangeal (MCP) joint, metatarsophalangeal (MTP) joint, wrist, elbow, knee, or ankle
         c) Present for at least 6 weeks

      3) Arthritis of hand joints
         a) Soft tissue swelling or fluid
         b) Affects at least one area in a wrist, PIP, or MCP
         c) Present for at least 6 weeks

      4) Symmetric arthritis
         a) Bilateral involvement of the same joint
         b) Affects PIPs, MCPs, or MTPs, but may not be absolutely symmetric
         c) Present for at least 6 weeks

Table 11-1. Juvenile Arthritis: Onset Types and Clinical Aspects	
Systemic Onset	Any age; female = male; about 20% of cases Recurrent, intermittent fever greater than 103° F, usually high once or twice each day Rheumatoid rash—pale red, nonpruritic, macular on trunk and extremities Joint manifestations vary and lag behind systemic symptoms Internal organ involvement—liver, spleen, heart
Polyarticular Onset RF Negative	Females 4:1, any age but peaks 1–3 years and 8–10 years Involves four joints or more—wrists, knees, ankles, elbows, feet Insidious or precipitated by infection—progression early, tends to get worse over time Morning sickness—systemic distribution
Polyarticular Onset RF Positive	Female, younger than 10 years of age Family history Clinical features as adult form—more likely to develop severe chronic arthritis Fever usually less than 103° F, rash, anemia, fatigue, anorexia, failure to gain weight
Pauciarticular Arthritis	Most common type, females younger than 4 years of age Four or less joints; knee most common, also ankles and hips Painless swelling, child is walking "funny" Few systemic signs—irritable, tired, poor weight gain, chronic eye inflammation

Reprinted with permission of W.B. Saunders from Youngblood, N.M., & Edwards, P.A. (1999). Autoimmune and endocrine conditions. In P.A. Edwards, D.L. Hertzberg, S.R. Hays, & N.M. Youngblood (Eds.), *Pediatric rehabilitation nursing* (pp. 414). Philadelphia: W.B. Saunders.

5) Rheumatoid nodules: Subcutaneous, over bony prominences, extensor surfaces, or juxta-articular regions

6) Serum RF: Determined by a method that is positive in fewer than 5% of normal control subjects

7) Radiologic changes: Posterior and anterior (PA) hand and wrist roentgenograms will show erosions or unequivocal bony decalcifications.

7. Diagnosis (Salmond et al., 1996)

   a. Thorough history and physical assessment

      1) Assess for fatigue, malaise, and weakness

      2) Note reports of vague arthralgias, myalgias, joint pain and stiffness, decreased range of motion (ROM)

      3) Note joint size, shape, color, symmetry

      4) Assess for presence and history of joint swelling, redness, cyanosis, warmth, tenderness, family history of arthritis

      5) Note shiny, taut skin over joint

      6) Assess for muscle atrophy and flexion contractures

      7) Note subluxation in metacarpal and metatarsal joints and ulnar deviation of fingers

      8) Assess for deformities or fibrous or bony ankylosis

         a) Spindle-shaped fingers

         b) "Swan neck," "boutonniere," "cock-up toes"

         c) Broadening of the forefoot, clawing of the toes, plantar calluses

      9) Assess for side effects of steroid therapy

         a) Buffalo hump, moon face

         b) Abdominal distention

         c) Ecchymosis after minimal trauma

         d) Impotence

         e) Amenorrhea

         f) Hypertension

         g) Generalized weakness

         h) Muscle atrophy

      10) Cutaneous nodules over bony prominences

      11) Assess for vascular deficits

      12) Assess muscle strength and presence of muscle spasm and sensation

      13) Note joint mobility, crepitus, function, and sensation

      14) In children, look for longer, shorter, or larger bones than normal: Inflammation can affect the growth plates in the bones.

      15) In children, behavioral and physical changes (Youngblood & Edwards, 1999)

         a) Irritability

         b) Morning stiffness

         c) Pain

         d) Limping or walking funny

         e) Heat and swelling in a joint

         f) Intermittent rash

         g) Altered posture

      16) Recent trauma or infection

      17) In children, changes in facial appearance and dental problems

   b. Laboratory studies

      1) Anemia

      2) Elevated white blood cell (WBC) count

      3) Erythrocyte sedimentation rate (ESR)

      4) Protein electrophoresis

      5) Rheumatoid factor (RF)

      6) Antinuclear antibodies (ANA)

      7) C-reactive protein (CRP)

      8) Urinalysis

   c. Radiologic studies

      1) Early signs

         a) Soft tissue swelling

         b) Periarticular osteoporosis

         c) New bone formation

         d) Subchondral cyst formation

      2) Late signs

         a) Subchondral erosions

         b) Narrowing of joint spaces

         c) Diffuse osteoporosis

   d. Other

      1) Arthroscopy

      2) Thermograph and bone scan

      3) Joint aspirations

8. Resulting disabilities: JA is the primary cause of disability in children.

   a. Deforming contractures of joints

   b. Joint instability

   c. Spinal cord compression, usually cervical

   d. Depression and anxiety

e. Deficits in ADLs and instrumental activities of daily living (IADLs)

f. Mobility deficits

g. Chronic pain

9. Client education

a. What does RA/JA mean?

b. How will it affect the body?

c. Why me?

d. How is it diagnosed?

e. What causes RA/JA?

10. Interventions after diagnosis: Early arrest of the disease process

a. Goal: To maintain joint function and prevent deformities

b. Pharmacologic management

1) Anti-inflammatory agents

a) Salicylates

b) Nonsteroidal anti-inflammatory drugs (NSAIDs)

c) Phenylbutazone

d) COX-2 specific inhibitors (e.g., Celebrex/Celecoxib)

2) Glucocorticoids: Infrequently used in JA, secondary to the effects on growth

3) Intra-articular steroids

4) Remission-inducing agents

a) Gold salts

b) Hydroxychloroquine

c) D-penicillinamine

5) Immunosuppressants

a) Azathioprine (Imuran)

b) Cyclophosphamide (Cytoxin)

c) Chlorambucil (Leukeran)

d) Leuamisole (Tetramisole)

e) Sulfasalazine (Azulfidine)

f) Methotrexate (Mexate)

g) Leflunomide (Arava)

6) Antitumor, necrosing-factor agents

a) Enbrel (Etanercept)

b) Remicade (Infliximab)

7) Baseline urine and blood studies prior to initiating these medications

c. Physical therapy: Encourage participation in an exercise program and use of assistive devices to keep mobile and remain flexible (e.g., hydrotherapy)

d. Occupational therapy: Help make ADLs and IADLs easier by using adaptive aids

e. Splints: Use to give joints rest, correct deformity, and provide physical support to unstable joints

f. Psychological support

1) Antidepressants

2) Support groups

g. Vitamins, minerals, and herbs (e.g., Echinacea, Ginkgo, St. John's wort)

h. Cartilage matrix enhancers (e.g., Osteo-Bi-Flex, Cosamin DS, Glucosamine)

i. Client education

1) Choose a treatment regimen

2) Teach how to incorporate it into life

3) Manage medication

4) Teach how to prevent complications

5) Explain the importance of physical and occupational therapy

6) Explain how to properly use assistive devices

7) Teach joint conservation techniques

8) Teach energy conservation techniques

9) Explain what happens if techniques do not work

11. Surgical interventions after diagnosis

a. Goals: To relieve pain, stabilize the joint, and correct deformity of the joint

b. Total joint replacement

1) Areas include hips, knees, ankles, shoulders, elbows, phalanges.

2) Aggressive rehabilitation in acute care, rehabilitation facilities, or subacute care settings is essential to successful outcomes.

3) For children, joint replacement is delayed as long as possible until bone growth has finished.

c. Arthrodesis or fusion of the bony joint

d. Laminectomy and spinal fusion for cord compressions

e. Tendon repair (if done within 2 days of rupture)

f. Tenosynovectomies and synovectomies

12. Research topics

a. The actual causes of RA (e.g., genetic or immunologic component) ("New Drugs," 1999)

b. Clinical trials on new anti-inflammatory medications that have decreased side effects

c. Clinical trials on medications that affect the immune system component of the disease ("New Drugs," 1999)

d. The use of oral type II collagen to treat JA (Youngblood & Edwards, 1999)

e. The role of immunology in the etiology and pathogenesis of RA and JA (Youngblood & Edwards, 1999)

D. Degenerative Joint Disease (DJD) or Osteoarthritis (OA)

1. Definition

a. A progressive, noninflammatory process that affects weight-bearing joints in particular

b. Characterized by degeneration of the articular cartilage at the joint

2. Etiology

a. Unknown at this time

b. Contributing risk factors

1) Age

a) Strongest risk factor, but not solely responsible for causing OA

b) Changes related to aging in cells and tissues: May induce development of the disease

2) Trauma

a) Injury to articular cartilage leaving fragments in the joint

b) Recurrent dislocation of the patella

c) Congenital dislocation of the hip

3) Obesity: Increases the load on the joints that causes changes in posture and gait

4) Lifestyle

a) Athlete's knee

b) Dancer's ankle

c) Tennis elbow

5) Intra-articular sepsis

6) Primary diagnoses affecting joints

a) Hemophilia

b) Paget's disease

c) Diabetes mellitus

d) Charcot-Marie-Tooth disease

7) Menopause

8) Immune response

9) Preexisting joint abnormalities

a) RA

b) Legg-Calvé-Perthes disease

c) Avascular necrosis

3. Pathophysiology (Salmond et al., 1996)

a. Articular cartilage pits, softens, and frays, losing elasticity and becoming more susceptible to stress damage.

b. Gradually, full thickness loss of the articular cartilage occurs, leaving exposed subchondral bone that then goes through a remodeling process.

c. This bone hypertrophies and forms spurs at the joint margins and at ligaments, tendons, and the joint capsule.

d. Spurs or osteophytes break off into the joint.

e. A secondary synovitis occurs later in the process, helping to further affect the joint's function.

f. With advanced disease, all the cartilage may be destroyed.

4. Incidence

a. DJD/OA is the most common form of arthritis.

b. The disease may begin when the person is in his or her 20s, but it peaks when the person is in his or her 50s or 60s.

c. 40 million Americans have radiologic evidence of OA; more than one-third exhibit signs and symptoms.

d. Incidence is higher in Caucasians.

e. The disease affects women twice as often as men who are older than age 55.

f. Hip, knee, cervical, and lumbosacral joints are most frequently involved.

g. Women's hands are affected most after menopause.

h. Lifestyle and occupation may be factors.

5. Diagnosis

a. History

1) Early stages: Joint stiffness, relieved with activity

2) Later: Pain on movement, relieved with rest

3) Advanced stages
    a) Night pain and pain at rest
    b) Limping
    c) Parasthesias
b. Physical
    1) Localized symptoms
    2) Enlarged joints
    3) Decreased ROM
    4) Crepitus
    5) Joint instability
    6) Changes in alignment with flexion deformity
    7) Pain on movement
c. Diagnostic tests
    1) Radiologic tests (see Figure 11-4)
        a) An X ray of involved joint will not necessarily show the severity of the clinical symptoms.
        b) X rays taken during weight bearing may show deformity.

Figure 11-4. Cartilage Destruction in Osteoarthritis

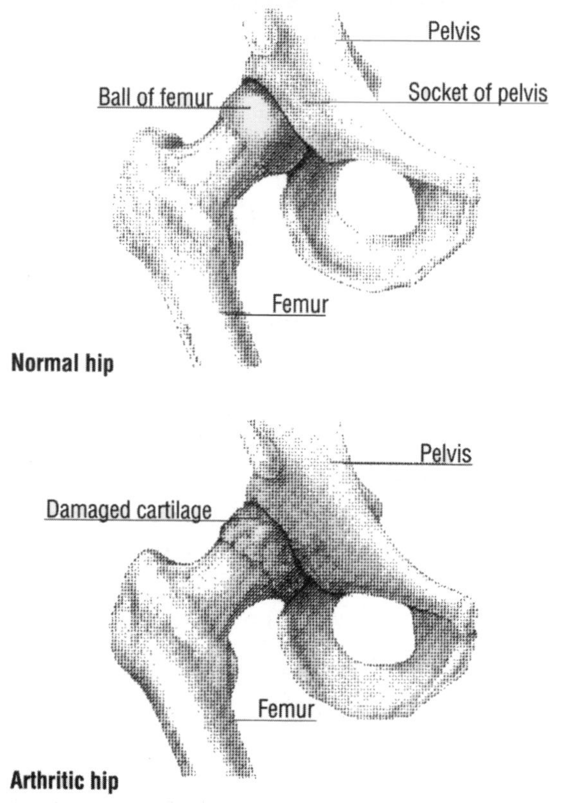

Pelvis
Ball of femur
Socket of pelvis
Femur
Normal hip

Pelvis
Damaged cartilage
Femur
Arthritic hip

Reprinted with permission the American Academy of Orthopaedic Surgeons from American Academy of Orthopaedic Surgeons. (1988). *Arthritis* [Public Information brochure] (p. 3). Park Ridge, IL: Author. (Available from American Academy of Orthopaedic Surgeons, 6300 N. River Road, Rosemont, IL 60018)

2) Laboratory tests
    a) Sedimentation rate: May be minimally elevated
    b) Analysis of synovial fluid after aspiration of the involved joint
6. Resulting disabilities
    a. Pain with rest and movement
    b. Joint contractures
    c. Loss of joint function
    d. Loss of independence
    e. Depression and anxiety
7. Client education
    a. What does DJD mean?
    b. How will it affect the body?
    c. Why me?
    d. How is it diagnosed?
    e. What causes it?
    f. How can it be prevented?
8. Interventions
    a. Goals of treatment
        1) Reduce pain
        2) Regain joint ROM
        3) Regain independence with mobility and ADLs
    b. Pharmacological management
        1) Administer early in the morning and before activity
        2) Aspirin
        3) NSAIDs: Used when aspirin is no longer effective
        4) Adrenocorticoids: Local intra-articular injection for severely symptomatic joints
        5) Analgesics
        6) Vitamins, minerals, and herbal remedies
    c. Interdisciplinary approaches
        1) Physical therapy to establish an exercise program
            a) Pool therapy
            b) Home exercise program
        2) Heat/cold applications
        3) Splinting or bracing
        4) Use of assistive devices
        5) Use of TENS unit for pain reduction
        6) Weight loss
        7) Nontraditional remedies

a) Meditation

b) Relaxation exercises

c) Massage

d) Biofeedback

d. Surgical interventions

1) Arthroscopy of joint to remove osteophytes and loose bodies (e.g., particles and fragments of cartilage and bone floating freely within the synovial fluid of the joint)

2) Total joint replacement: Relieves pain, restores motion, and increases joint stability

a) Contraindications to elective surgery

(1) Acute or chronic infection

(2) Major bone loss

(3) Poor muscle function

(4) History of noncompliance

(5) Age

(6) Malnutrition

(7) Bone marrow disease

b) Possible complications

(1) Wound or joint infection

(2) Dehiscence of incision line

(3) Hematoma

(4) Deep vein thrombosis (DVT) or pulmonary embolism (PE)

(5) Neurovascular compromise

(6) Dislocation

(7) Loosening or fracture of components

(8) Wear on components

3) Laminectomy and spinal fusion

4) Arthrodesis: Surgical fusion of the joint

e. Psychological support

9. Trends in total joint replacement

a. Use of critical pathways, which begin 3–4 weeks before surgery and include the following components:

1) Total joint classes to educate the client and coach about what to expect

2) Preoperative therapy session to teach total joint exercises

3) Home evaluation, if necessary, before surgery

4) Preadmission coordination of all equipment and follow-up services

b. Decreased length of stay; on average, 3 days of acute care

c. Discharge with home therapy or outpatient therapy or transfer to a rehabilitation facility or subacute care unit for the remainder of rehabilitation (usually less than 1 week)

10. Client education

a. Choice of treatment regimen

b. How to incorporate it into lifestyle

c. Medication management

d. The importance of physical and occupational therapy and assistive devices

e. Other options for treatment

1) Arthroscopy

2) Arthroplasty

3) Arthrodesis

f. Complications and risks of surgery

g. Precautions after surgery

h. Life with an artificial joint

11. Future research

a. Outcome studies on the use of critical pathways

b. Improvements in the components used in total joint arthroplasty

c. Debates about which protocol best prevents DVT (Hyers, Hull, & Weg, 1995)

E. Metabolic Arthritis (Gout)

1. Definition: A disturbance in the uric acid metabolism in which urate salts are deposited into joints and subcutaneous tissues

2. Etiology

a. Remains unknown

b. Primary gout: Results from a genetic defect in purine metabolism and leads to an increased uric acid production and/or retention of uric acid

c. Secondary gout

1) Hydrochlorothiazide and pyrazinamide, which affect urate excretion

2) Malignant disease, myeloproliferation psoriasis, and sickle-cell anemia: May lead to gout because of the increased cell turnover, breakdown, or renal dysfunction

3) Caused by overindulgence in foods

high in protein (e.g., organ meat, shellfish, alcohol)
3. Pathophysiology
   a. Four stages of gout (Salmond et al., 1996)
      1) Asymptomatic: Urate levels increase but no signs or symptoms are present.
      2) Acute attack: First attack is sudden.
         a) Involves extreme pain in one or more joint, usually the great toe
         b) Characterized by tissue damage and inflammation
      3) Intercritical period: Between attacks, symptom free
      4) Chronic gout: Persistent pain and renal dysfunction
         a) Tophi: Uric acid crystal lumps found in joints and cartilage (usually the earlobe, fingers, hands, knees, and feet) that lead to the erosion of surrounding tissues similar to RA
         b) Renal tubules: Affected due to kidney stone formation
   b. Uric acid crystal deposits: Surrounded by an inflammatory process that leads to fibrous tissue, giant cells, and local necrosis
4. Incidence
   a. Affects up to 20 million Americans
   b. Affects men in 95% of all cases, with the first attack happening after age 30
   c. Affects the foot and great toe in 90% of diagnosed cases
5. Diagnosis
   a. History
      1) Frequency of attacks and severity and location of symptoms
      2) Pain history
      3) Dietary history (e.g., high protein intake)
   b. Physical assessment of specific signs and symptoms
      1) Red, swollen, deformed, tender, dusty cyanotic joints, especially in the great toe, ankles, fingers, and wrists
      2) Fever
      3) Tachycardia, hypertension
      4) Headache

      5) Joint effusion
      6) Severe pain in the joint
      7) Decreased ROM
      8) Severe back pain
   c. Diagnostic tests
      1) Laboratory tests
         a) Serum uric acid levels: Elevated
         b) Urinary uric acid levels: Elevated in secondary gout
         c) Urinalysis: Albuminuria
         d) Complete blood count (CBC): Leukocytosis
         e) Sedimentation rate: Elevated
      2) Radiological examination of the affected joint
         a) Initially, the joint looks normal.
         b) Later, the joint looks punched out, as urate crystals replace bony structures (Salmond et al., 1996).
         c) Eventually, a narrowing of the joint space is apparent, degenerative arthritic changes occur, and cartilage is destroyed.
      3) Aspiration of synovial fluid: See crystals
      4) Renal studies to determine if the kidneys are affected
6. Resulting disabilities
   a. Deformation of the involved joint
   b. Renal dysfunction
   c. Cardiovascular lesions
   d. Tophi deposits leading to infection
   e. Thrombosis
   f. Hypertension
   g. Chronic pain
7. Interventions
   a. Goals of treatment: To control symptoms and decrease the frequency of acute attacks
   b. Pharmacological management
      1) Aspirin and acetaminophen for pain management of mild attacks
      2) Colchicine
         a) Prevents or relieves acute attacks
         b) Does not affect uric acid synthesis

c) Is a prophylactic agent

d) Is taken at the first sign of an acute attack

e) Involves side effects (e.g., B12 deficiency, diarrhea)

   3) Uricosurics: Probenecid, Anturane

    a) Inhibits reabsorption of uric acid

    b) Is not effective in an acute attack

   4) Allopurinal

    a) Reduces synthesis of uric acid

    b) Is not effective in acute attack

    c) Increases activity of anticoagulants and hypoglycemics

   5) Corticosteroids: Used for inflammation resistant to colchicine therapy

   6) Sodium bicarbonate, citrate solutions: Used to increase urine pH that increases uric acid excretion by the kidney

c. Nutrition

  1) Protein-limited diet

  2) Alcohol and purine restriction

  3) Weight loss encouraged

d. Joint protection

e. Pain and symptom management

  1) Acute attack

   a) Bed rest during episode and until 24 hours after

   b) Immobilization of affected joint

   c) Joint protection

   d) Pain management

  2) Chronic attack

   a) Treat with uricosurics

   b) Increase fluids

f. Surgical

  1) Inject corticosteroids into the joint

  2) Aspirate joints

  3) Excise and drain joint to remove crystals

  4) Use surgery to improve function and decrease deformity

g. Psychological support

8. Client education

a. What is gout?

b. What are the stages of gout?

c. What are the symptoms and signs of gout?

d. What do you do when you see the signs of gout?

e. How do you decrease the chances of an attack?

  1) Medication management

  2) Diet education

  3) Weight loss

f. What are joint conservation techniques?

g. How do you manage the pain of an attack?

9. Future research: Clinical drug trials

III. Amputation

A. Overview

1. Clients with amputations account for a significant part of the population in most rehabilitation facilities.

2. Loss of a body part is permanent, leaving the individual with alterations in mobility and body image, as well as self-care deficits.

3. Rehabilitation interventions are critical for successful adaptation and reintegration into the community.

4. A national health objective for 2000 is to decrease diabetes-related amputations by 40%, from 6.2 per 1,000 people, to 4.9 per 1,000 people with diabetes (U.S. DHHS, 1998): To achieve this goal, regular foot assessments and client education on proper foot care must be stressed long before any problem is noted.

B. Prevention of Amputations

1. Get regular foot assessments by a medical practitioner or podiatrist

2. Check daily for cracks, sores, blisters, with prompt medical attention if anything is noted

3. Cleanse with a mild soap and water daily and dry well

4. Get special care if the person is diabetic

C. Types of Amputation

1. Congenital: Absence of part or all of an extremity at birth

2. Acquired: Loss of part or all of an extremity as a direct result of disease, trauma, or surgery

D. Incidence

1. Age

  a. Rate of amputation increases with age.

  b. Peak incidence occurs between 41 and 71 years of age; 75% of all amputations occur in people age 65 or older.

2. Sex: Incidence of amputations is higher in men.

3. Race: African Americans with diabetes have an increased amputation rate compared with Caucasians with diabetes.

4. Type: Lower extremity amputations are usually related to disease, and upper extremity amputations are usually related to trauma.

E. Etiology
   1. Disease-related amputations
      a. Diabetes mellitus *[Refer to Chapter 14 for more information about diabetes.]*
         1) Diabetes is the leading cause of non-traumatic amputation in the U.S., accounting for 45%–70% of all non-traumatic amputations (U.S. DHHS, 1998).
         2) 50% of these clients are older than age 65 and have vascular, peripheral nerve, cardiac, respiratory, visual, and kidney problems (U.S. DHHS, 1998).
      b. Peripheral vascular disease (PVD)
         1) In the past, 80% of clients with amputations had PVD, and 75% had diabetes (Burgess, 1983).
         2) PVD is 2.5 to 3 times more common in diabetic clients.
         3) PVD advances more rapidly in diabetic clients.
         4) A diabetic client with PVD is unable to form collateral circulation (Spollett, 1998).
      c. Osteomyelitis
         1) Inflammation of the bone (localized or generalized) due to a pyrogenic infection
         2) Causes bone destruction, acute pain, and fever
         3) Can be aggravated by diabetes and PVD
      d. Gangrene
         1) The death of body tissue, usually associated with a loss of vascular supply and followed by bacterial invasion
         2) Dry gangrene: Common because of the gradual reduction in blood flow to the area
      e. Thrombosis: Results from an atherosclerotic event

2. Trauma-related amputations
   a. Account for 75% of upper extremity amputations and 30% of all amputations
   b. Result from motor vehicle accidents (MVA), gunshot wounds, falls, frostbite, explosions, war injuries, burns, and industrial and farm accidents
   c. Occur more commonly in men 17 to 55 years of age

3. Tumor-related amputations: 5% are due to sarcomas and are most common in children 10 to 20 years of age.

F. Presurgical Interventions
   1. Preamputation interventions
      a. Local treatment of wound
      b. Intravenous antibiotics
      c. Debridement procedures
         1) Wet to dry dressings
         2) Whirlpool treatments
         3) Surgical debridement
      d. Revascularization procedures
      e. Hyperbaric oxygen treatments
      f. Pain management: Pain must be aggressively managed before the amputation procedure to decrease phantom limb pain after surgery (Jensen, Krebs, Nielsen, & Rasmussen, 1983).
   2. Client and family education
      a. What to expect from the preamputation interventions
      b. What happens when conservative treatment fails
      c. What to expect after the amputation
      d. What is phantom pain?
      e. The rehabilitation process
      f. Therapy before surgery (Yetzer, 1996)
         1) Transfer training
         2) Strengthening exercises
         3) Use of assistive devices
      g. The grieving process, which is normal

G. Surgery
   1. Types of surgery
      a. Closed procedure
         1) A full-thickness flap of skin covers the distal end of bone
         2) Accounts for most amputations

b. Open procedure (or guillotine procedure)

   1) Performed when infection is present or likely to develop

   2) Leaves the end of the residual limb open

2. Level of amputation

  a. Based on the level of viable tissue, the amputation is usually done as low as possible.

  b. Preservation of the knee joint is preferred for optimal mobility and function.

  c. Energy expenditure is an issue (Friedmann, 1988).

    1) Using a unilateral below-knee prosthesis requires 10%–40% more energy than normal.

    2) Using an above-knee prosthesis requires 60%–100% more energy than normal.

    3) Energy requirements are compounded if the client is a bilateral amputee: A person with a bilateral below-knee amputation uses less energy for walking than a person with a unilateral above-knee amputation.

3. Presence of comorbidities that affect outcomes

  a. Cardiopulmonary deconditioning

    1) Occurs as a result of presurgical treatments (e.g., bed rest)

    2) Increases if the client also has a severe cardiac and/or pulmonary history

    3) Can best be limited with presurgical therapy interventions that are continued after surgery

  b. Peripheral vascular disease: Determines level of amputation required

  c. Diabetes: Affects wound healing

4. Replantation, which has high success rates with upper extremities and digits and is considered in the following cases (O'Hare & LineaWeaver, 1990):

  a. Amputation of thumbs or multiple digits

  b. Amputations in children

  c. Clean amputations at the palm, wrist, or forearm

  d. Complex injuries that might benefit from acute microsurgical reconstruction (e.g., revascularization, free flap coverage)

5. Tumor-related surgery (Piasecki, 1991)

  a. An alternative treatment done less frequently due to advances in limb salvage surgical procedures

  b. Indicated when tumor margins are not microscopically clean or local resection is not possible

H. Postoperative Interventions

1. Complications after amputation surgery (see Figure 11-5)

2. Pain management

  a. Acute postoperative pain: Early intervention has been shown to decrease phantom pain the most; the use of epidural analgesia both pre- and postoperatively has shown promise (Williams & Deaton, 1997).

  b. Phantom limb pain

    1) Painful sensations perceived in the missing limb

    2) Often described as knifelike, burning, or squeezing sensations

---

Figure 11-5. Potential Complications After Amputation Surgery

Pressure ulcers and skin breakdown (e.g., buttocks, heels)

Nonhealing surgical incisions requiring revision surgery healing by secondary intention

Infection

Osteomyelitis

Gangrene

Falls without injury

Falls with injuries (e.g., fractures, dehiscence of incision)

Postoperative confusion related to anesthesia, medication, sepsis

Altered mental status, which can worsen dementia, Alzheimer's disease

Depression, anxiety, fear, and adjustment disorders

Embolism (e.g., pulmonary embolism, deep vein thrombosis)

Heart attack or stroke

Diabetic reactions

Flexion contracture

Deconditioning secondary to decreased mobility prior to surgery

---

3) Frequently described as similar to presurgery pain
4) Occurs to some extent in all amputees
5) Has no known cure, but involves many theories as to why it occurs

3. Contracture prevention
   a. Goal: To keep the joint above the site of the amputation in full extension to allow for a more functional gait
   b. Lying in prone position
      1) Stretches the hip muscles into full extension
      2) Usually done three or four times a day for 20 minutes each time
      3) Counteracts decreased mobility and increased chair dependency
   c. Knee extension
      1) Prevents contracture of the knee joint and allows for a more functional gait
         a) Some surgeons cast the extremity immediately after surgery to decrease the chance of a flexion contracture: A disadvantage of this method is that the surgical incision cannot be examined.
         b) Some surgeons place a knee immobilizer over the top of the surgical dressing: A benefit to this method is that wound checks can be done.
      2) Splints, boards, wheelchair extensions: All attempt to keep the limb in extension and allow for wound checks.
   d. Elbow extension: Usually done with a splint made specifically for the client

4. Psychological support
   a. Allow the client to grieve at his or her own pace
   b. Watch for signs of disturbance: Along with the physical discomfort, psychological distress has been cited as a major reason for nonuse of the prosthesis (Medhat, Huber, & Medhat, 1990).
      1) Refusal to look at or touch residual limb
      2) Unwillingness to discuss predicted limitations or use of prosthesis

      3) Refusal to participate in self-care
      4) Social withdrawal
   c. Make referrals to support groups for amputees

5. Therapy
   a. Transfer training
      1) Standing pivot transfers
      2) Sliding board transfers
   b. Ambulation training
      1) Begin with parallel bars and progress to a walker
      2) Balance training (sitting and standing)
   c. Preprosthetic training
      1) Teach client to be functional at the wheelchair level
      2) Condition the residual limb
      3) Practice ROM exercises
   d. Deconditioning and strengthening exercises for the entire body
   e. Functional activity training
   f. Prosthetic evaluation and recommendation

6. Wound management
   a. For clients with immediate postoperative casting: Monitor for signs of increased edema, drainage, and odor
   b. For clients without casting: Monitor the following:
      1) Dehiscence
      2) Nonhealing
      3) Infection
      4) Progressive gangrene
      5) Lack of pulse in the next joint proximally
   c. For clients with residual limb edema
      1) Decrease pain and prepare limb for prosthetic fitting
      2) Use appropriate methods of shrinkage and bandaging (see Figure 11–6)
         a) Ace wrap: Rewrap limb every 3–4 hours
         b) Residual limb (stump) shrinker: Remove every 3-4 hours to assess incision line
         c) Jobst compression boot: Use for 20 minutes, three or four times a day, along with an ace wrap or shrinker

d) Elevation: Do not allow limb to hang down for extended periods of time

7. Desensitization to decrease pain

   a. Tap the distal aspect

   b. Rub the distal aspect

   c. Stroke the distal aspect

   d. Massage the residual limb

I. Prosthetic Management

1. Remember that prostheses can be functional or cosmetic

2. Develop a wearing schedule

   a. Usually start with 2 hours on, 2 hours off, one or two times a day when sitting

   b. Perform pre- and postwearing skin check, looking for areas of redness, irritation, skin breakdown, which means the prosthesis needs adjustment

3. Build up wearing times as tolerated

4. May need to use numerous prostheses over the long term due to specific requirements related to work, school, home, sports, and leisure activities

5. Provide prosthetic care prior to donning the prosthesis

   a. Check prosthesis for mechanical stability

   b. Wipe off with damp cloth daily

   c. Wipe off socket and allow to dry before donning the prosthesis

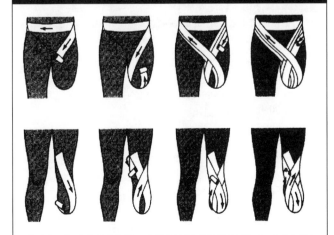

Figure 11-6. Bandaging a Residual Limb

Reprinted with permission of Mosby from Beare, P.G., & Myers, J.L. (1990). *Principles and practice of adult health nursing* (p. 1398). St. Louis: Mosby.

d. Apply clean, dry socks to the residual limb

   1) Sock size depends on amount of shrinkage.

   2) Weight loss or gain of as little as 5 lbs can affect the prosthesis' fit and function.

J. Geriatric Considerations

1. Many amputees are older than age 65, and the effects of the aging process can affect their rehabilitation.

2. Dual diagnoses and rehabilitation problems are common in this population (Lee & Itoh, 1988).

   a. Cardiopulmonary capacity

   b. Poor neuromuscular coordination

   c. Visual impairments

   d. Weakened musculature

   e. Limited ROM

K. Research Topics

1. The causes of phantom limb pain and phantom sensations (Davis, 1993)

2. Preoperative education and pain management's effects on outcomes after surgery (Jahangiri, Jayatunga, Bradley, & Dark, 1994)

3. Client outcome studies: Inpatient rehabilitation, home care, outpatient rehabilitation—which helps the client become more functional faster

IV. **Nursing Diagnoses Associated with Musculoskeletal and Orthopedic Disorders**

A. Overview

1. Rehabilitation nurses work in many settings: Acute care hospitals, rehabilitation hospitals, home care, schools, long-term care facilities, ambulatory care centers, and insurance companies.

2. Nearly every rehabilitation nurse will someday care for a person with musculoskeletal and orthopedic disorders no matter what practice setting he or she works in.

3. As the population ages, nurses will see more clients with these chronic illnesses in everyday practice.

B. Assessment

1. Thorough health history

2. Thorough physical examination

3. Functional assessment, focusing on the musculoskeletal and neuromuscular systems

4. Psychological assessment

C. Nursing Diagnoses and Plans of Care

1. Impaired physical mobility (see Table 11-2): Adjust for client's age, physical ability, and support systems available for assistance

2. Knowledge deficit (see Table 11-3)

   a. Adjust based on the following factors
      1) Client's diagnosis
      2) Prior knowledge about the disease
      3) Age of the client
      4) Educational level

   b. Provide information in several forms (e.g., verbal, written) at numerous times

3. Self-care deficit (see Table 11-4): Tailor to the client's abilities and disabilities, but do not encourage dependency on others

D. Other Potential Nursing Diagnoses

1. Ineffective individual coping: Denial

   a. Lack of comprehension of the seriousness of the diagnosis

   b. Denial used as a defense mechanism

2. Alterations in comfort: Pain

   a. Surgical procedures

Table 11-2. Nursing Plan of Care: Impaired Physical Mobility

Nursing Diagnosis: Impaired Physical Mobility

Related to the following:
- Limited movement ability
- Activity restrictions
- Need to use assistive devices
- Need for assistance for ambulation and transfers
- Intolerance to activity
- Pain and discomfort
- Limited strength

Goals	Interventions
Demonstrate optimal independence in mobility skills and ADLs	Teach safe use of assistive devices (e.g., walkers, canes)
	Encourage participation in self-care tasks with or without assistive devices
	Consult physical therapist (PT) and occupational therapist (OT) for a prescribed exercise program
	Encourage participation in recreational activities and community outings
	Teach home safety and fall prevention
Help client and family with activity restrictions	Determine prescribed activity education restrictions and length of the restrictions
	Educate client and family about why restrictions are needed
	Teach client and family how to maintain restrictions in real-life situations
	Educate client and family on what to do if restrictions are broken (e.g., notify physician)
Improve tolerance to activity	Encourage the use of assistive devices
	Provide adequate rest periods between activities
	Teach ways to combine activities
	Teach client to pace activities to allow for rest periods
	Encourage compliance with exercise program created by PT and OT
	Educate about the need to adapt environment to maximize independence
Manage pain	Teach about prescribed pain medications and the best times to take them
	Provide nonpharmacological options for pain management (e.g., heat, ice)
	Provide comfort measures
	Educate about the need to stay active to avoid further complications of deconditioning

Expected Outcomes

Maintain a level of independence with mobility and ADLs

Understand and adhere to activity restrictions as prescribed

Report improved tolerance to activity

Report effective pain management program

Maintain safety precautions with all activities

The Specialty Practice of Rehabilitation Nursing: A Core Curriculum, 4th Ed.

b. Joint destruction

c. Pathology of the injury or disease

d. Therapy procedures and exercises

e. Medical treatment plan

f. Activity restrictions

3. Alteration in family processes

    a. Role changes required by the disability

    b. Diagnosis of a chronic illness with disabling features

4. Potential for injury

    a. Activity restrictions

    b. Balance changes created by weight-bearing restrictions

    c. Use of assistive devices

    d. Rushing to get things done and not thinking about safety

    e. Unsafe environment

5. Noncompliance: Medical

    a. Medication regimen

    b. Diet restrictions

    c. Failure to comply with therapy's exercise program

    d. Failure to obtain preventive medical care

6. Alteration in skin integrity

    a. Surgical procedures

    b. Immobility

    c. Pressure sores

    d. Nutritional deficits

    e. Nodule development in RA

Table 11-3. Nursing Plan of Care: Knowledge Deficit

Nursing Diagnosis: Knowledge Deficit

Related to the following:
- Chronic illness diagnosis
- Prescribed treatment regimen
- Possible complications

Goals	Interventions
Verbalize understanding about diagnosis and prescribed treatment plan	Teach client and family about the diagnosis • What does the diagnosis mean? • How will it affect the body? • Why me? • How is it diagnosed? • What causes the disease? • What does the future look like? Explain the treatment options presented by the physician Teach the specifics of the treatment plan • Medication management • Nutritional management • Activity restrictions, use of assistive devices, need for regular exercise • Consult PT or OT for exercise program • Encourage proper health maintenance (e.g., eye exams, foot assessments) • Community resources available • The importance of complying with the treatment plan Tailor information to the client's and family's educational level Integrate cultural and religious differences Be creative when presenting information Use age-appropriate education principles Progress from simple to complex topics Repeat information to reinforce learning Provide written information if possible
Verbalize understanding of possible complications and what to do about them	Offer information frequently about complications associated with the diagnosis Teach the client and family what to do if signs and symptoms develop Teach the consequences of complications that are not addressed in a timely manner
Verbalize understanding of the disease process and what the future may hold	Explain the natural progression of the disease Describe treatment changes that may occur as the result of the disease progression (e.g., more aggressive medications, surgical procedures, need for more assistance with mobility and ADLs) Describe possible comorbidities that may occur as a result of the disease

Expected Outcomes

Actively participate in the prescribed treatment plan
Understand the disease condition and possible complications and comorbidities
Know what to do if signs and symptoms of complications arise

Table 11-4. Nursing Plan of Care: Self-Care Deficit

Nursing Diagnosis: Self-Care Deficit

Related to the following:
- Decreased activity tolerance
- Pain and discomfort
- Fear, anxiety, and depression
- Lack of motivation
- Inability to perform or complete bathing
- Inability to perform or complete dressing and grooming self-care activities
- Inability to perform toileting self-care activities

Goals	Interventions
Demonstrate the ability to use adaptive equipment	Teach or reinforce the use of assistive devices provided by therapy (e.g., plate guards, swivel utensils, universal cuffs, reachers, long-handled sponges, wash mitts, grab bars, tub or shower seats, walkers, crutches, canes) Educate the family about what the client can do and what he or she may need help with
Perform toileting, bathing, and dressing activities at optimal level of independence	Set up the environment so the client has easy access to all equipment, hygiene products, and clothing Allow extra time to complete tasks Encourage the use of safety measures Provide privacy based on the client's safety level
Maintain safe bathing practices	Teach and reinforce safety measures often (e.g., adequate lighting, no-slip strips on floors and tub or shower floors, electric appliances placed away from water sources, need for rails and grab bars) Provide a means of calling for help as needed (e.g., call bells, panic buttons) Teach how to test water temperature to prevent burns if the client has neurological problems
Improve tolerance in performing self-care activities	Teach the client how to pace himself or herself during ADLs Provide rest periods between activities as necessary Educate the client and family about energy conservation techniques Provide assistance to the client to prevent exhaustion Encourage the client to choose loose-fitting clothes that are easy to put on
Show an interest in hygiene and wear own clothes	Encourage the client to see himself or herself as becoming healthier Encourage the client to wear his or her own clothes as much as possible Adapt clothing for easier application as necessary (e.g., Velcro closures, adjustments to clothing to fit over bulky appliances) Provide assistance with hair, makeup, or shaving as needed Foster an atmosphere that promotes wellness Provide psychological counseling as necessary (e.g., for adjustment disorders, depression, anxiety)

Expected Outcomes

Use assistive devices for eating, grooming, dressing, and toileting in a correct, safe, and efficient manner
Maintain an independent level of functioning for toileting, bathing, grooming, and dressing activities
Maintain a safe environment
Demonstrate improved tolerance to performing ADLs
Demonstrate improved motivation to perform ADLs

The Specialty Practice of Rehabilitation Nursing: A Core Curriculum, 4th Ed.

f.   Crystal development in gout

g.   Use of splints, casts, braces, orthotics, and prosthetics

7. Social isolation

a.   Prescribed activity restrictions

b.   Lack of transportation

c.   Lack of social support network

d.   Self-imposed isolation

e.   Self-esteem issues

f.   Lack of motivation

g.   Chronic pain issues

E. Diagnoses Specifically Relevant for Children
1. Alteration in self-esteem

2. Alteration in body image

3. Alteration in growth and development

4. Ineffective family coping

5. Knowledge deficit related to community resources

References

AACE clinical practice guidelines for the prevention and treatment of postmenopausal osteoporosis. (1996, March/April). *Endocrine Practice, 2*, 155-177.

American Academy of Orthopaedic Surgeons. (1988). *Arthritis* [Public Information brochure] (p. 3). Park Ridge, IL: Author.

Arnett, F.C., Edworthy, S.M., Bloch, D.A. (1988). The American Rheumatism Association 1987 revised criteria for the classification of rheumatoid arthritis. *Arthritis Rheumatology, 31*, 315-324.

Beare, P.G., & Myers, J.L. (1990). *Principles and practice of adult health nursing.* St. Louis: Mosby.

Biskobing, D. (1997, December). *Postmenopausal osteoporosis: Pathogenesis, diagnosis and treatment.* Lecture presented at the Osteoporosis and Bone Densitometry Conference, Emory University, Atlanta, GA.

Burgess, E.M. (1983). Amputations: Symposium on orthopaedic surgery. *Surgical Clinics of North America, 63*(3), 749-770.

Cummings, S.R., Rubin, S.M., & Black, D. (1995). The future of hip fractures in the United States numbers, costs, and potential effects of postmenopausal estrogen. *Clinical Orthopaedics, 252*, 163-166.

Darovic, G. (1997). Caring for patients with osteoporosis. *Nursing '97, 27*(5), 50-51.

Davis, R.W. (1993). Phantom sensation, phantom pain, and stump pain. *Archives of Physical Medicine and Rehabilitation, 74*, 243-256.

DeCherney, A. (1993). Physiologic and pharmacologic effects of estrogen and progestins on bone. *Journal of Reproductive Medicine, 38*, 1007-1014.

Edwards, P.A., Hertzberg, , D.L., Hays, S.R., & Youngblood, N.M. (Eds.). (1999). *Pediatric rehabilitation nursing.* Philadelphia: W.B. Saunders.

Eli Lilly. (1998). *Evista (Raloxifene hydrochloride).* Indianapolis, IN: Author.

Friedmann, L.W. (1988). Rehabilitation of the amputee. In J. Goodgold (Ed.), *Rehabilitation medicine* (pp. 601-645). St. Louis: Mosby.

Heaney, R.P. (1998). Recommended calcium intakes revisited: Round table. In P. Burckhardt, B. Dawson-Hughes, & R.P. Heaney (Eds.), *Nutritional aspects of osteoporosis* (pp. 317-325). New York: Springer-Verlag.

Hyers, T.M., Hull, R.D., & Weg, J.G. (1995). Anti-thrombotic therapy for venous thrombo-embolic disease. *Chest, 108*(4), 335S-351S.

Jahangiri, M., Jayatunga, A.P., Bradley, J.W., & Dark, C.H. (1994). Prevention of phantom pain after major lower limb amputation by epidural infusion of Diamorphine, Clonidinell and Bupivacaine. *Annals of the Royal College of Surgeons of England, 76*, 324-326.

Jensen, T.S., Krebs, B., Nielsen, J. & Rasmussen, P. (1983). Phantom limb pain, and stump pain in amputees during the first 6 months following limb amputation. *Pain, 17*, 243-256.

Kannus, P., Parkkari, J., Sievanen, H., Heinonen, A., Vuori, I., & Jarvinen, M. (1996). Epidemiology of hip fracture. *Bone, 18*(Suppl. 1), 57S-63S.

Kassem, M., Melton, L.J., & Riggs, B.L. (1995). The type I/II model for involutional osteoporosis. In R. Marcus, D. Feldman, & J. Kelsey (Eds.), *Osteoporosis.* San Diego, CA: Academic Press.

Kessenich, C.R. (1997). The pathophysiology of osteoporotic vertebral fractures. *Rehabilitation Nursing, 22*(4), 192-195.

Klippel, J.H. (1997). *Primer on the rheumatic diseases* (11th ed.). Atlanta: Arthritis Foundation.

Lee, M., & Itoh, M. (1988). Geriatric rehabilitation management. In J. Goodgold (Ed.), *Rehabilitation medicine* (pp. 393-406). St. Louis: Mosby.

McClung, B.L. (1999). Using osteoporosis management to reduce fractures in elderly women. *The Nurse Practitioner, 24*(3), 26-42.

Medhat, A., Huber, P.M., & Medhat, M.A. (1990). Factors that influence the level of activities in persons with lower extremity amputation. *Rehabilitation Nursing, 15*, 13-18.

Mosby Great Performance. (1995). *Helping at home, preventing falls* [Pamphlet]. (Available 14964 NW Greenbrier Parkway, Beaverton, OR 97006)

National Institutes of Health (NIH) Consensus Development Panel on Optimal Calcium Intake. (1994). Optimal calcium intake. *Journal of the American Medical Association, 272*, 1942-1948.

New drugs: Etanercept (Enbrel). (1999, February). *American Journal of Nursing, 99*(2), 60.

O'Hare, M., & LineaWeaver, W.C. (1990). Microsurgical replantation: Development and current status. *Critical Care Nursing Quarterly, 13*(1), 1-11.

Piasecki, P. (1991). Limb salvage procedures for osteosarcoma. *Nursing Clinics of North America, 26*, 33-41.

Salmond, S.W., Mooney, N.E., & Verdisco, L.A. (1996). *NAON core curriculum for orthopaedic nursing* (3rd ed.). Pitman, NJ: Anthony J. Jannetti.

Solomon, J. (1998). Osteoporosis: When supports weaken. *RN, 61*(5), 37-40.

Spollett, G.R. (1998). Preventing amputations in the diabetic population. *Nursing Clinics of North America, 33*(4), 629-637.

Spratto, G.R., & Woods, A.L. (1998). *PDR nurses' handbook* (3rd ed.). Montvale, NJ: Medical Economics.

Thalgott, J., LaRocca, H., & Gardner, V.O. (1993). Arthritides affecting the spinal column. In S.H. Hochschuler, H.B. Cotler, & R.D. Guyer (Eds.), *Rehabilitation of the spine*. St. Louis: Mosby.

Thorngren, K. (1994). Fractures in older persons. *Disability Rehabilitation, 16*, 119-126.

Tomaski, A.M. (1996). Metabolic bone disease. In S.W. Salmond, N.E. Mooney, L.A. Verdisco (Eds.), *NAON core curriculum for orthopaedic nursing* (pp. 297-313). Pitman, NJ: Anthony J. Jannetti, Inc.

U.S. Department of Health and Human Services (DHHS). (1998, August 14). Diabetes-related amputations of lower extremities in the Medicare population: Minnesota, 1993-1995. *Morbidity and Mortality Weekly Report (MMWR), 47*(31), 649-652.

Watts, N.B. (1997, September). Osteoporosis: Prevention, detection and treatment. *Journal of the Medical Association of Georgia*, pp. 224-226.

Williams, A.M., & Deaton, S.B. (1997). Phantom limb pain: Elusive, yet real. *Rehabilitation Nursing, 22*(2), 73-77.

Woodhead, G.A., & Moss, M.M. (1998). Osteoporosis: Diagnosis and prevention. *The Nurse Practitioner, 23*(11), 18-35.

World Health Organization (WHO). (1994). *Assessment of fracture risk and its application to screening for postmenopausal osteoporosis* (WHO Technical Report Series 843). Geneva: Author.

Yetzer, E.A. (1996). Helping the patient through the experience of an amputation. *Orthopaedic Nursing, 15*(6), 45-49.

Youngblood, N.M., & Edwards, P.A. (1999). Autoimmune and endocrine conditions. In P.A. Edwards, D.L. Hertzberg, S.R. Hays, & N.M. Youngblood (Eds.), *Pediatric rehabilitation nursing* (pp. 412-419). Philadelphia: W.B. Saunders.

Suggested resources

Arthritis Health Professions Association. (1989). *A core curriculum in rheumatology for health professionals*. Atlanta, GA: Professional Education Department, Arthritis Foundation.

Bellantoni, M.F. (1996). Osteoporosis prevention and treatment. *American Family Physician, 54*(30), 986-991.

Bichler, L. (1999). Foot ulcers in diabetes. *Advance for Nurse Practitioners, 7*(1), 49-52.

Cosman, F., Nieves, J., Horton, J., Shen, V., & Lindsay, R. (1994). Effects of estrogen on response to edetic acid infusion in postmenopausal osteoporotic women. *Journal of Clinical Endocrinology and Metabolism, 78*, 939-943.

Heaney, R.P. (1987). Prevention of osteoporotic fracture in women. In L.V. Avioli (Ed.), *The osteoporotic syndrome: Detection, prevention, and treatment* (pp. 67-90). Orlando, FL: Grune & Stratton.

Levin, M. (1993). Diabetic foot ulcers: Pathogenesis and management. *Journal of ET Nursing, 20*, 191-198.

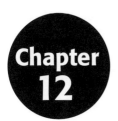

Chapter 12

Cardiovascular and Pulmonary Rehabilitation: Acute and Long-Term Management

Lynn M. Carbone, BSN RN CRRN

Cardiovascular heart disease affects 12 million Americans (American Heart Association [AHA], 1999j), and 30 million Americans experience some form of chronic lung disease. Heart diseases are the leading causes of death, and chronic obstructive lung diseases are the fourth leading causes of death in the United States (Connors & Hilling, 1998). Complications of cardiovascular disease and pulmonary disease greatly affect quality of life and the economy (see Table 12-1). Pulmonary disease is the leading cause of disability in the United States according to the American Lung Association (ALA). Chronic obstructive pulmonary disease (COPD) is the third ranking condition after congestive heart failure and stroke in necessitating home care services (Connors & Hilling, 1998).

Early detection and rehabilitation can prevent the progression of cardiac and lung diseases to a disabling state. Cardiac and pulmonary rehabilitation programs use a comprehensive interdisciplinary approach to achieve positive patient outcomes. These programs have a comprehensive approach focused on individualized preventive and therapeutic interventions. Rehabilitation programs help patients make lifestyle adjustments, decrease risky health behaviors, maximize physical status without endangering life, and reduce the rate of morbidity and mortality. Rehabilitation is a continuous process that begins in the critical care period and extends to a lifelong program of lifestyle adaptation (Connors & Hilling, 1998; Huang, Kessler, McCulloch, & Dasher, 1989). Acute care and home health rehabilitation nurses may adapt the information in this chapter for their patients' health promotion and disease prevention needs. Assessments, interventions, and goals should be individualized according to the patient as well as the practice setting.

Cardiac rehabilitation programs serve patients with manifestations of congenital or acquired heart disease (e.g., myocardial infarction, chronic angina, cardiomyopathy) and those who have multiple uncontrolled risk factors or have had cardiac surgery (AHA, 1999d). There are four phases of cardiac rehabilitation programs (Huang et al., 1989):

- Phase I: Usually the first 4 days in the coronary care unit
- Phase II: Next 14 days of the hospital stay
- Phase III: Outpatient phase of 6–8 weeks
- Phase IV: The lifelong recovery phase

Pulmonary rehabilitation programs serve patients with manifestations of COPD, nonobstructive lung disease, and other lung disorders. Assessment, patient training, exercise, psychosocial intervention, and follow-up are essential components of a pulmonary rehabilitation program (Connors & Hilling, 1998).

According to the AHA, risk factor interventions significantly improve clinical outcomes but their application is inconsistent across medical care settings. Scientific evidence demonstrates that comprehensive risk factor interventions extend overall survival, improve quality of life, decrease need for interventional procedures, and reduce the incidence of subsequent myocardial infarction (AHA, 1999l).

I. Cardiovascular Heart Disease (CVD)

A. Overview

1. The nation's Number 1 killer, claiming 959,227 lives in 1996, or 41.4% of all deaths.

2. One-sixth of those who die from CVD are younger than 65 years of age.

3. Per 100,000 deaths, 215.6 are white men, 315.9 are black men, 125.3 are white women, and 209.3 are black women (AHA, 1999c).

B. Types of CVD

1. Coronary artery disease (CAD): Disorder of the coronary arteries that leads to disruption of the blood flow that supplies oxygen and nutrients to the myocardium

2. Congestive heart failure (CHF): Complex syndrome that results from the heart's inability to increase cardiac output sufficiently to meet the body's metabolic demands

3. Cardiomyopathy: Disease that diffusely affects the myocardium, resulting in enlargement or restriction and leads to ventricular dysfunction

4. Congenital heart defects (CHDs): Structural or functional abnormalities of the heart or great vessels existing from birth that obstruct blood flow in and to the heart and cause the blood to flow abnormally through the heart (AHA, 1999f; Canobbio, 1990; Glanze, 1987; Huang et al., 1989; Tierney, McPhee, & Papadakis, 1994)

   a. Aortic stenosis (AS)

   b. Atrial septal defect (ASD)

   c. Atrioventricular (A-V) canal defect

   d. Bicuspid aortic valve

   e. Coarctation of the aorta

   f. Ebstein's anomaly

   g. Eisenmenger's complex

   h. Hypoplastic left heart syndrome

   i. Patent ductus arteriosus (PDA)

   j. Pulmonary atresia

   k. Subaortic stenosis

   l. Tetralogy of Fallot

   m. Total anomalous pulmonary venous (P-V) connection

   n. Transposition of the great arteries

   o. Tricuspid atresia

   p. Truncus arteriosus

   q. Ventricular septal defect (VSD)

C. Epidemiology/Incidence

1. CAD

   a. Leading cause of morbidity and mortality in United States

   b. Accounts for 476,124 deaths per year, or 1 of every 4.9 deaths

   c. Involves 1.1 million new and recurrent cases of attack yearly

---

Table 12-1. Estimated Direct and Indirect Economic Costs

Cardiovascular Disease

Type of cost	Cost in billions of dollars
Heart disease	$183.1
Coronary artery disease	$99.8
Stroke	$45.3
Hypertensive disease	$33.3
Congestive heart failure	$21.0
Total	$286.5*

Pulmonary Disease

Type of cost	Cost in billions of dollars
Total direct**	$33.4
Total indirect**	$51.0
Total (direct and indirect)	$84.4

Examples

Chronic obstructive pulmonary disease	$23.5
(direct cost = $14.7; indirect cost = $8.8)	
Asthma	$12.4
(direct cost = $9.8; indirect cost = $2.6)	

* *Totals may not add up evenly due to overlap and rounding (e.g., someone with coronary artery disease may also have hyptertensive disease).*

** *Direct costs include cost of physicians and nursing services, hospital and nursing home services, medications, home health, and other medical services. Indirect costs include lost productivity resulting from morbidity and mortality*

Sources consulted

American Heart Association (AHA). (1999i). *Economic cost of cardiovascular diseases* [Online]. Available: www.americanheart.org/statistics/10econom.html.

Connors, G., & Hilling, L. (Ed.). (1998). *Guidelines for pulmonary rehabilitation programs: American Association of Cardiovascular and Pulmonary Rehabilitation—Promoting health and preventing disease* (2nd ed.). Champaign, IL: Human Kinetics.

---

d. 12 million people who have angina, heart attack, or other forms of CAD are alive (approximately 5.8 million men and 6.1 million women) (AHA, 1999j)

2. CHF

   a. Affects 4.6 million Americans: 2.2 million men and 2.3 million women

   b. Mortality in 1996 was 43,837: 16,695 men and 27,142 women

   c. Involves 400,000 new cases annually

   d. Increased hospital discharges from 377,000 in 1979 to 870,000 in 1996

   e. Caused $3.4 billion ($5,153 per discharge) to be paid by Medicare to beneficiaries in 1995, according to data from the Health Care Financing Administration (HCFA) (AHA, 1996b)

3. Cardiomyopathy

   a. Mortality: 27,501 people. Prevalence: approximately 50,000 people

      1) 87% of cardiomyopathies are a dilated form of the disease: 50% of patients are alive 5 years after diagnosis, and 25% are alive 10 years after diagnosis.

      2) 36% of young athletes who die suddenly may have hypertrophic cardiomyopathy.

      3) Highest mortality is among elderly people, especially elderly men and African Americans (AHA, 1996b).

4. CHD

   a. Affects approximately 32,000 births yearly (i.e., about 1% of live births)

   b. Affects 1 million Americans

   c. Affects infants younger than 1 year of age: 58.7 of 100,000 deaths in white children, and 76.1 of 100,000 deaths in black children.

   d. Involves 4,820 American deaths in 1996 (AHA, 1999g)

D. Etiology

   1. Causes

      a. CAD: Atherosclerosis

      b. CHF (AHA, 1999h; Canobbio, 1990)

         1) Decreased myocardial contractility

            a) CAD

            b) Myocarditis

            c) Cardiomyopathy

            d) Infiltrative diseases (e.g., amyloidosis, tumors, sarcoidosis)

            e) Collagen-vascular diseases (e.g., systemic lupus erythematosus, scleroderma)

            f) Drugs (e.g., beta-adrenergic blocking agents, calcium antagonists)

         2) Increased myocardial workload

            a) Hypertension

            b) Pulmonary hypertension

            c) Vascular disease

            d) Cardiomyopathy

            e) Intra-aortic shunting

            f) Hyperthyroidism

         3) Congenital heart disease

      c. Cardiomyopathy (Canobbio, 1990; Huang et al., 1989)

         1) Dilated

            a) Excessive alcohol use

            b) Third trimester pregnancy

            c) Infections (e.g., bacterial, viral, fungal)

            d) Immunological abnormalities (e.g., thiamine deficiency, thyrotoxicosis, diabetes mellitus)

            e) Ischemia

            f) Noninfectious conditions (e.g., rheumatic heart disease, scleroderma, systemic lupus erythematosus, polyarteritis)

         2) Hypertrophic (idiopathic): Genetic

         3) Restrictive

            a) Infiltrative or fibrotic processes within the myocardium

            b) Amyloidosis

            c) Hemachromatosis

            d) Glycogen storage disease

            e) Sarcoidosis

            f) Neoplasm

      d. Congenital heart defects

         1) Unknown causes

         2) Genetics

         3) Environment

         4) Teratogens

            a) Drugs

b) Alcohol

c) Viral infections (AHA, 1999f; Canobbio, 1990)

2. Risk factors for cardiovascular disease (AHA, 1999m; Canobbio, 1990; Huang et al., 1989)

  a. Nonmodifiable

    1) Heredity

    2) Race

    3) Sex

    4) Age

  b. Modifiable

    1) Smoking

    2) Hypertension

    3) Elevated serum cholesterol

    4) Diabetes mellitus

    5) Sedentary lifestyle

    6) Stress

    7) Oral contraceptives

    8) Alcohol

    9) Obesity

E. Pathophysiology

1. CAD: Involves formation of plaque inside a vessel, impeding the flow of blood (see Figure 12-1)

  a. Theories

    1) Plaque formation

      a) Endothelium becomes damaged due to a variety of factors.

        (1) Elevated serum cholesterol and triglycerides

        (2) Hypertension

        (3) Cigarette smoke

Figure 12-1. Lesions of the Atherosclerotic Process

LONGITUDINAL   CROSS   CELLULAR

LUMEN · Endothelium · Internal Elastic Membrane · INTIMA · MEDIA · ADVENTITIA

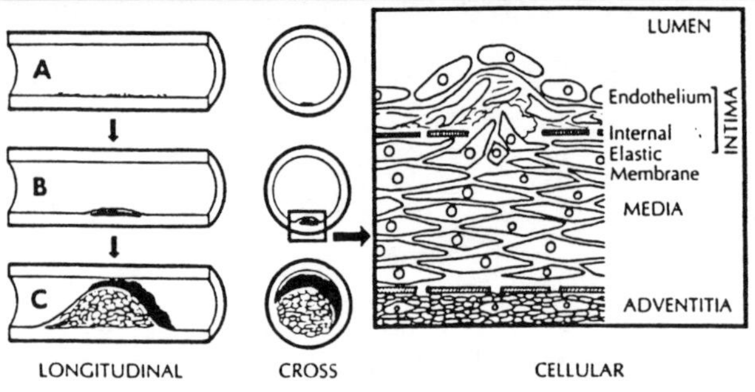

Reprinted with permission of Mosby from Huang, S., Kessler, C., McCulloch, C., & Dasher, L. (1989). Cardiac rehabilitation of the myocardial patient. In *Coronary care nursing* (2nd ed., p. 133). Philadelphia: W.B. Saunders.

      b) Fats, cholesterol, fibrin, platelets, cellular debris, and calcium deposit in arterial wall.

      c) Thickened endothelium narrows arterial lumen, impeding blood flow and decreasing oxygen supply to myocardium.

      d) Formation of thrombus or hemorrhage around plaque blocks blood flow.

    2) Abnormal growth of smooth muscle cells

      a) Platelets form prostaglandins that may destroy the walls of arteries.

      b) Platelets also contain platelet growth factor, which stimulates the growth of smooth muscle cells.

      c) Abnormal growth of smooth muscle cells may be one of the earliest events in the artherosclerotic process.

    3) Deposition of connective tissue cells

      a) Lipoproteins from the blood that are trapped in the arterial wall accumulate and become oxidized.

      b) Lipoproteins become modified and are absorbed by smooth muscle cells.

      c) Foam cells are formed, causing connective tissue cells to become deposited (AHA, 1999b).

  b. Severity of disease

    1) Measured by degree of obstruction in each coronary artery and the number of arteries involved

    2) Involves an increased risk of death with arterial lumen obstructions exceeding 75% of one or more coronary arteries (Canobbio, 1990)

2. CHF (functional defects): Impaired cardiac output

  a. Left-sided heart failure

    1) Increased left ventricular end diastolic pressure (LVEDP)

    2) Increased fluid pressure in pulmonary vessels

b. Right-sided heart failure

    1) Persistent increased LVEDP, which increases venous congestion

    2) Tricuspid valve regurgitation

    3) Right ventricular infarct

    4) Pulmonary disease

c. Decreased ability of kidneys to dispose of sodium and water

3. Cardiomyopathy (structural defects) (see Figure 12-2)

  a. Dilated

    1) Gross dilation of heart chambers with normal to decreased myocardium wall thickness

    2) Poor contractility

    3) Decreased ejection fraction

  b. Restrictive

    1) Endocardium and myocardium infiltrated with fibroelastic tissue

    2) Impaired relaxation function

  c. Hypertrophic

    1) Thickened interventricular septum causing rigidity of myocardium

    2) Impeded ventricular contractility

4. Congenital heart defects

  a. Severity of symptoms depends on the type of the defect.

  b. Obstruction of right ventricular outflow creates hypertrophied right ventricle and right-to-left shunt (i.e., decreased systemic

arterial oxygen saturation, cyanosis, and reduced pulmonary blood flow) (Canobbio, 1990).

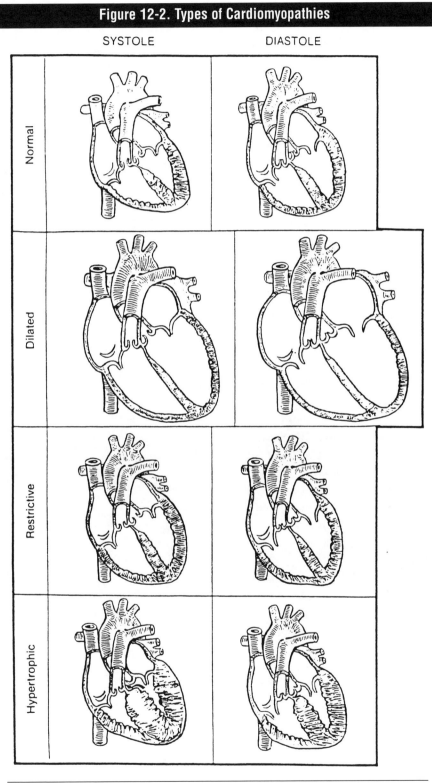

Figure 12-2. Types of Cardiomyopathies

SYSTOLE   DIASTOLE

Normal

Dilated

Restrictive

Hypertrophic

Reprinted with permission of Mosby from Canobbio, M. (1990). *Cardiovascular disorders* (p. 93). St Louis: Mosby.

F. Residual Deficits
1. Dysrhythmias
   a. Cardiac arrest
   b. Sudden death
2. Ischemia: Manifested as chest pain (i.e., angina pectoris) (Canobbio, 1990; Tierney et al., 1994)
   a. Stable angina (precordial chest pain)
      1) Precipitated by hypertension, tachycardia, other dysrhythmia, strenuous activity, cold temperature, emotional stress, or a large meal
      2) Has a short duration that subsides completely when the aggravating factor is removed (e.g., rest after exertion): If attack is precipitated by anger or a large meal, it may last as long as 15-20 minutes.
      3) Involves substernal sensation (chest pain), which is often characterized as aching, sharp, tingling, burning, or pressure radiating to the left arm and shoulder, neck, jaw, or scapular inner aspects of both arms
   b. Unstable angina
      1) Occurs with minimal activity or at rest
      2) Involves chest pain lasting longer than 30 minutes
      3) Is less responsive to medications and may progress to infarction
      4) Involves sensations similar to stable angina but may be more severe
   c. Variant (Prinzmetal's) angina
      1) Characteristically occurs in early morning and awakens patient
      2) Involves chest pain that intensifies quickly and lasts longer than stable angina
      3) Involves sensations similar to stable angina
3. Myocardial infarction (MI): Death of myocardial tissue from inadequate coronary perfusion; blood supply to heart is severely reduced or stopped (Canobbio, 1989; Tierney et al., 1994)
   a. May occur at rest or with exertion
   b. Lasts longer than 30 minutes, is continuous and unrelieved by rest, position change, or nitroglycerin tablets
   c. Involves chest pain characterized as crushing, squeezing, stabbing, or heavy pressure that radiates down the left arm and to neck, jaws, teeth, epigastric area, and back
   d. Is associated with other symptoms (e.g., diaphoresis, weakness, apprehension, lightheadedness, syncope, dyspnea, orthopnea, nausea, vomiting)
4. Emboli formation from diminished blood flow
   a. Stroke
   b. Pulmonary emboli
5. Psychosocial effects
   a. Sense of helplessness
   b. Fear of dying
   c. Anxiety
   d. Apathy
   e. Depression
   f. Social withdrawal
   g. Guilt
6. Poor tissue perfusion
   a. Renal failure from diminished blood flow
      1) Fluid retention
      2) CHF
      3) Edema (e.g., peripheral, sacral, genitalia, abdominal)
      4) Electrolyte imbalance
   b. Malnutrition
      1) Decreased nutrient absorption
      2) Decreased gastrointestinal motility
      3) Nausea, vomiting, fatigue (Canobbio, 1990; Huang et al., 1989)
   c. Hypoxic encephalopathy from diminished cerebral blood flow
   d. Hypoxemia

G. Management Measures
1. Risk factor modification
   a. Stop smoking
   b. Control blood pressure
   c. Control cholesterol
      1) AHA-recommended cholesterol levels
         a) Lower low-density lipoproteins (LDLs) to < 130 mg/dl

b) Raise high-density lipoproteins (HDLs) to > 35 mg/dl

c) Maintain total cholesterol level of < 200 mg/dl (AHA, 1999e; National Heart, Lung and Blood Institute [NHLBI], 1998a)

2) Ways to lower elevated cholesterol levels (see Figure 12-3)

a) Diet

b) Exercise

c) Weight control

d) Medications

e) Smoking cessation

d. Control diabetes

1) Control weight

2) Modify diet

3) Administer medication properly

e. Perform physical activity (see Figure 12-4)

1) Monitor metabolic equivalents (METs): Exercise programs are written in METs of an activity. MET is the rate of energy expended that requires oxygen to be consumed at 3.5

Figure 12-3. Ways to Lower Cholesterol Levels
Diet (AHA dietary guidelines)

Step I Diet: Primary Prevention (no presence of disease)

8%–10% of total daily calories from saturated fat

No more than 30% of total calories from fat

Up to 10% of total calories from polyunsaturated fats

Up to 15% of total calories from monounsaturated fat

Less than 300 mg of cholesterol per day

Less than 2,400 mg of sodium per day (1 1/4 teaspoons of salt)

55%–60% or more of calories should come from carbohydrates, especially complex carbohydrates

Total calories should help achieve and maintain a healthy weight

Step II Diet: Secondary Prevention (presence of disease and elevated cholesterol levels)

7% or less of total calories per day from saturated fat

30% or less of total calories per day from fat

Less than 200 mg of dietary cholesterol per day

Just enough calories to maintain a healthy weight

Food Options

Poultry, fish, and lean cuts of meat (remove skin from chicken and trim fat)

Skim milk or 1% milk

Cheese with less than 3 g of fat per ounce

Liquid vegetable oils that are high in unsaturated fat

Foods high in starch and fiber (e.g., whole grain breads and cereals, pasta, rice, dry beans and peas, vegetables, fruits)

Fewer commercially prepared and processed foods made with saturated or hydrogenated fat

Physical Activity

Lowers LDL levels

Raises HDL levels

Lowers blood pressure

Lowers triglyceride levels

Reduces weight

Improves fitness of the heart and lungs

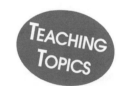

Weight Control

Eat fewer calories

Burn more calories with more physical activity

Medications

If LDL levels remain high after changing eating habits, the physician may introduce medications

Bile acid sequestrants (e.g., cholestyramine, colestipol)

Nicotinic acid

HMG CoA reductase inhibitors (e.g., lovastatin, pravastatin, simvastatin)

Fibric acid derivatives (e.g., gemfibrozil)

Probucol

Estrogen replacement therapy for postmenopausal women

Smoking Cessation

Smoking lowers HDL

Sources consulted

American Heart Association (AHA). (1999k). *Prevention, primary* [Online]. Available: www.americanheart.org/Heart_and_Stroke_A_Z_Guide/prevpri.html.

American Heart Association (AHA). (1999l). *Prevention, secondary* [Online]. Available: www.americanheart.org/Heart_and_Stroke_A_Z_Guide/prevsec.html.

National Heart, Lung and Blood Institute (NHLBI). (1998b). *Lowering blood cholesterol levels: Diet, exercise and weight control* [Online]. Available: www.healthtouch.com/level1/leaflets/nhlbi/nhlbi014.htm.

Figure 12-4. Physical Activity Teaching Guide

General Guidelines

Check with physician before beginning an exercise program
Follow appropriate physical activity guidelines, which vary according to the type and extent of heart disease
Gradually increase exercise
Do warm-up exercises
Pace exercise efforts so as not to tire too quickly
Schedule rest breaks into program
Follow guidelines for heart rhythm and rate, blood pressure, and body signals

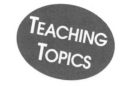

Target Heart Rate
If unable to count heart rate:

Conversation pace refers to the ability to walk and talk at the same time and indicates adequate pace
Becoming short of breath quickly indicates working too hard

If able to count heart rate:

(For the deconditioned cardiac patient, a target heart rate may be set by the physical therapist or physician)
Start by assessing the resting heart rate
After approximately 2 minutes of exercise, assess heart rate: It should be no more than 20 beats above the resting heart rate per MET level.
Assess heart rate after resting 2 minutes: The heart rate should return to resting.
Monitor blood pressure in the same manner: It should not exceed 20 mmHg over resting blood pressure per MET level
Body signals for rest: Shortness of breath, diaphoresis, fatigue, nausea, dizziness, chest pain

Walking Program
General guidelines

Be well rested
Record resting and activity heart rates, distance, time walked, and any symptoms
Walk in a continual and rhythmic motion
Wear loose-fitting clothing and comfortable shoes
Do not walk after meals; wait at least a half hour
Decrease walking speed if the heart rate exceeds the target heart rate
Walk on level surfaces
Avoid extremes of heat or cold
Walk daily

Step-by-step program

Step 1: Walk 4–5 minutes four times daily, trying to increase 1–2 minutes each day. When walking 10 minutes, walk only twice daily. When able to walk 15 minutes at a time for 2 days, go on to Step 2.
Step 2: Walk slowly for 5 minutes, then briskly for 5 minutes, then slowly for 5 minutes once daily for 1 week. If no adverse symptoms, the target heart rate is not exceeded and can walk the brisk pace for the time indicated, go on to Step 3.
Step 3: Following the previous guidelines, slowly progress by increasing the brisk portion of the walk by 2 minutes each week. For example, the following week would be walking slowly for 5 minutes, briskly for 7 minutes, then slowly for 5 minutes.

Activities to Avoid (until appropriate MET level is reached)

Lifting greater than 10 lbs.
Heavy household chores
Activities that cause stress
Driving, until approved by physician
Climbing stairs (initially)

Sources consulted

American Heart Association (AHA). (1999n). *Target heart rate* [Online]. Available: www.americanheart.org/Heart_and_Stroke_A_Z_Guide/target.html.
Huang, S., Kessler, C., McCulloch, C., & Dasher, L. (1989). Cardiac rehabilitation of the myocardial patient. In *Coronary care nursing*. Philadelphia: W.B. Saunders.
Saint Joseph's Regional Medical Center (SJRMC). (1996). *The beat goes on: Educational materials for the cardiac patient and family*. South Bend, IN: Author.

Table 12-2. Examples of Metabolic Equivalents (METs) in Daily Activities

MET	Self-Care	Work	Recreation
1.0-2.0	Sitting Standing Eating Bathing seated Using bed pan	Knitting Typing Hand sewing Machine sewing	Sitting, painting Driving car Playing cards Playing piano
2.0-4.0	Dressing Bathing (standing) Showering Using bedside commode	Shopping Kneading dough Washing dishes Welding Cleaning windows or floors Painting walls Assembly-line work	Light woodworking Playing horseshoes Playing billiards Fishing

4.0-6.0	Full grooming
	Walking downstairs
		Painting, hanging wallpaper,
		  plastering, masonry
		Mechanic
		Carpentry
		Gardening
		Shoveling (light earth)
		Chopping wood
		Doing "handyman" activities
		  (shoveling, carpentry)
			Golfing (with cart)
			Walking
			Fly fishing
			Playing badminton
			Playing table tennis
			
			Walking
			Cycling (8 mph)
			Playing softball or baseball
			Canoeing
			Horseback riding
			Light hiking
			Hunting
			Water-skiing
			Playing water volleyball

6.0-8.0		Splitting wood Felling trees Mowing lawn by hand	Playing tennis (singles) Light downhill skiing Scuba diving Playing touch football Playing light basketball Swimming
8.0-10.0		Heavy shoveling Moving, pushing objects Carrying heavy objects	Running Swimming Ski touring Doing gymnastics Aerobic dancing Playing handball, racquetball, squash

Source consulted

Huang, S., Kessler, C., McCulloch, C., & Dasher, L. (1989). Cardiac rehabilitation of the myocardial patient. In *Coronary care nursing* (p. 431). Philadelphia: W.B. Saunders.

ml/minute/kg of body weight (Huang et al., 1989) (see Table 12-2)

2) Gradually increase exercise
3) Monitor target heart rate
4) Follow walking program
5) Take appropriate precautions

f. Manage stress
   1) Identify stressors
   2) Use relaxation techniques
   3) Educate about disease process and prognosis

4) Offer spiritual support
5) Identify support groups
6) Offer counseling
7) Encourage lifestyle changes (Carbone, 1999)
   a) Returning to work
     (1) The decision to return to work should be made with the cardiologist.
     (2) Returning to work depends upon the patient's stamina, postoperative complications, and job demands.
   b) Resuming sexual activity
     (1) Be able to climb two flights of stairs (6.0-8.0 METs) (Huang et al., 1989) without the following problems:
       (a) Shortness of breath
       (b) Angina
       (c) Palpitations
       (d) Fatigue
     (2) Follow these guidelines when engaging in sexual activity
       (a) Be well rested
       (b) Wait until at least 30 minutes after a meal
       (c) Stay relaxed
       (d) Avoid straining the upper arms and sternum; try new positions

       (e) Avoid sexual activity in hot, humid, or very cold conditions
       (f) Cease activity if angina occurs and call cardiologist
       (g) Ask cardiologist about using prophylactic sublingual nitroglycerin, which can be prescribed before sex if angina is a problem
   8) Teach cardiopulmonary resuscitation (CPR)
  g. Control weight
2. Invasive interventions
  a. Percutaneous transluminal coronary angioplasty (PTCA)
   1) PCTA is an invasive nonsurgical therapeutic procedure via a catheter introduced into the coronary artery.
   2) Patency is restored to the coronary artery by inflating and deflating a balloon at the distal end of the catheter to compress plaques within the arteries (Canobbio, 1990; Saint Joseph's Regional Medical Center [SJRMC], 1996).
    a) Athrectomy: A rotary device either slices or pulverizes plaques within the arterial lumen.
    b) Stent placement: After angioplasty, a small metal stent is inserted to maintain patency of the arterial lumen (SJRMC, 1996).
   3) According to the AHA, 666,000 angioplasties were done in 1996 (452,000 on men; 214,000 on women) (AHA, 1999a) at a cost of approximately $20,730 per procedure (AHA, 1996a).
  b. Surgical procedures
   1) Open heart
    a) Coronary artery bypass graft (CABG): According to the AHA, 598,000

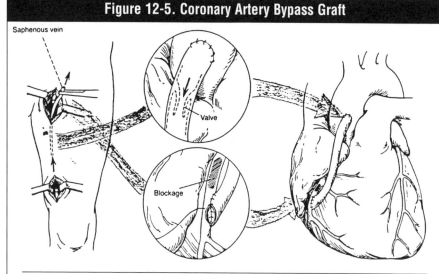

Figure 12-5. Coronary Artery Bypass Graft

Saphenous vein

Valve

Blockage

Reprinted with permission of Mosby from Huang, S., Kessler, C., McCulloch, C., & Dasher, L. (1989). Cardiac rehabilitation of the myocardial patient. In *Coronary care nursing* (2nd ed., p. 408). Philadelphia: W.B. Saunders.

CABGs were performed in 1995 (AHA, 1999a) at a cost of $44,820 per procedure (AHA, 1996a) (see Figure 12-5).

    b) Valve replacement

  2) Heart transplant

  3) Pacemaker or automatic intracardio-defibrillator (AICD) placement

  4) Ablation: Laser procedure that focuses on an area of the heart causing a dysrhythmia; the area is lysed to stop the cycle.

  5) Correction of congenital defects

3. Medications, which can be used alone or in combinations (depending upon the CVD and the severity of symptoms) (Canobbio, 1990; Huang et al., 1989)

  a. Vasodilators

  b. Beta-adrenergic blocking agents

  c. Angiotensin-converting enzyme (ACE) inhibitors

  d. Anticoagulation/antiplatelets

  e. Antiarrhythmics

  f. Calcium antagonists

  g. Antihyperlipidemic agents

  h. Stool softeners

  i. Cardiac glycosides

  j. Diuretics

  k. Nitrates

  l. Oxygen

H. Nursing Process

  1. Assessment

    a. Subjective elements

      1) Palpitations, dizziness, lightheadedness, syncope, shortness of breath, fatigue, poor appetite, insomnia, restlessness, anxiety and fear, nausea

      2) Chest discomfort: Quality, location, precipitating factors, duration, alleviating factors

    b. Objective elements

      1) Skin: Presence of pallor, diaphoresis

      2) Cardiac output: Tachycardia, bradycardia, irregular heart rhythm, heart murmur, hypotension, hypertension, confusion, decreased urine output, peripheral edema, sacral or genitalia edema, weight gain, abdominal distention, electrocardiogram changes, elevated cardiac serum enzymes (CK-MB) and muscle proteins (T[cTNT] and 1[cTN1])

      3) Pulmonary status: Crackles, wheezes, dyspnea, labored breathing, frothy, blood-tinged sputum, cyanosis

      4) Nutritional: Anorexia, decreased skin turgor and integrity

    c. History

      1) Health habits

      2) Medical

      3) Social support

      4) Previous independence level

      5) Medications

  2. Diagnoses (North American Nursing Diagnosis Association [NANDA], 1999)

    a. Activity intolerance

    b. Pain

    c. Impaired home maintenance management

    d. Altered nutrition (less than body requirements)

    e. Altered thought processes

    f. Altered tissue perfusion (cardiopulmonary)

    g. Anxiety

    h. Fluid volume excess

    i. Knowledge deficit: Disease process, medications, self-care, compliance

    j. Impaired gas exchange

    k. Impaired skin integrity

    l. Ineffective individual coping

    m. Ineffective family coping (compromised)

    n. Self-care deficits (e.g., feeding, bathing, grooming, dressing, toileting)

    o. Noncompliance to therapeutic regimen

  3. Plan: Goals for patient and family

    a. Demonstrate understanding of exercise plan and verbalize understanding of activity intolerance by modifying activity and rest to prevent fatigue, palpitations, shortness of breath, and diaphoresis

    b. Verbalize pain relief after measures are taken

    c. Demonstrate understanding of and

participation in self-care management including activities of daily living (ADLs), exercise programs, dietary management, lifestyle changes

    d. Maintain adequate nutritional status to lower risks of further cardiac events and promote healing

    e. Maintain adequate urine output, mentation, heart rate, and rhythm

    f. Demonstrate decreased anxiety and verbalize understanding of disease, procedures, and expected outcomes

    g. Identify stressors and develop strategies to decrease stress

    h. Verbalize an understanding of the importance of taking medications as prescribed, actions of medications, how to administer medications, and potential side effects

    i. Maintain skin integrity without breakdown

    j. Verbalize and demonstrate an understanding of the importance of following therapeutic and medical treatment recommendations

4. Implementation

    a. Activity intolerance

      1) Monitor activities that aggravate condition: Type of activity, intensity, and frequency of symptoms

      2) Monitor blood pressure, heart rate, and respiratory rate before, during, and after exercise, staying within target heart rate parameters

      3) Coordinate rest periods into program

      4) Increase activities gradually

    b. Cardiac pain management

      1) Administer vasodilators for chest pain as ordered

      2) Administer oxygen therapy as ordered to enhance oxygen to myocardium

      3) Monitor vital signs

      4) Assess effectiveness of analgesia

    c. Nutrition

      1) Consult with dietitian for special dietary instructions and meal planning

      2) Weigh daily

      3) Offer caloric supplements

      4) Offer measures to improve appetite (e.g., appropriate environment, good oral care, small frequent meals)

      5) Administer antiemetics before meals

      6) Administer medications so they do not interfere with meals

    d. Tissue perfusion

      1) Monitor level of consciousness, signs and symptoms of hypoxemia

      2) Monitor laboratory values of BUN, creatinine, electrolytes

      3) Monitor vital signs for changes

      4) Have baseline electrocardiogram available

      5) Document changes in the patient's condition

    e. Anxiety

      1) Explain procedures, disease process, and expected outcomes

      2) Allow the patient to express feelings

      3) Involve family, significant other, and spiritual counselor

      4) Encourage participation in decision-making process into lifestyle changes

      5) Offer information about support groups, social services, and vocational counseling

    f. Fluid volume excess

      1) Administer diuretics as ordered and monitor their effectiveness (e.g., increased urine output, decreased edema, clear lung sounds)

      2) Monitor weight daily and report weight gain of 2 lbs in 24 hours

      3) Restrict sodium and fluid intake

    g. Knowledge deficit

      1) Instruct about disease process and expected outcomes

      2) Instruct about medications: Purpose, dosage, how to administer, potential side effects, take only as prescribed (do not use previous medications unless approved by physician), and the importance of follow-up with physician

      3) Practice energy conservation techniques, teaching signs and symptoms of overexertion

      4) Instruct on dietary restrictions and

infection prevention

5) Offer counseling for school, sports, employment, genetics, marriage, child bearing, contraceptive use, resuming sexual relations, and learning CPR

6) Instruct about oxygen safety

7) Instruct about proper protection of sternum and grafts if the patient has had open-heart surgery (see Figure 12-6)

8) Instruct on modification of risk factors

9) Include significant other and family members in all instructions

h. Gas exchange

1) Monitor chest X ray

2) Elevate head of the bed

3) Monitor breath sounds and for changes in respiratory function

4) Encourage coughing and deep breathing

i. Self-care

1) Perform ADLs in seated position to conserve energy

2) Teach proper incisional care for surgical patients

j. Compliance

1) Assess patient's and family members' readiness to learn and follow therapeutic regimen

2) Stress importance of administering medications as prescribed, reporting untoward reactions or responses to medications, difficulties in obtaining recommended medications (e.g., expenses, accessibility)

3) Assess understanding and willingness to comply

5. Evaluation

a. Patient and family should achieve goals set with the nurse.

b. If goals are not met as originally designed, then reassessment should be done and revisions to the plan of care developed.

II. Pulmonary Disease

A. Types

1. Obstructive pulmonary diseases (Connors & Hilling, 1998)

a. Chronic obstructive pulmonary disease (COPD): Persistent airway obstruction that decreases the lung's capacity to take in and excrete oxygen (Wilson & Thompson, 1990)

1) Chronic bronchitis: Excessive secretion of bronchial mucous obstructing air flow and causing chronic coughing

2) Emphysema: Abnormal alterations of the air spaces distal to the terminal bronchiole; destruction of alveolar walls increases lung compliance, which decreases oxygen/carbon monoxide exchange (Tierney et al., 1994; Wilson & Thompson, 1990)

b. Asthma: Inflammation of the trachea and bronchi in response to various stimuli, causing narrowing of the airway passages (Wilson & Thompson, 1990)

c. Cystic fibrosis: Genetic disorder of the exocrine glands, causing secretion of abnormal mucus that obstructs glands and ducts of various organs (Tierney et al., 1994), most commonly the respiratory, pancreatic, and sweat glands (Wilson & Thompson, 1990)

d. Alpha 1 antitrypsin (a1AT) deficiency

e. Bronchiectasis

f. Bronchiolitis obliterans

2. Restrictive pulmonary diseases (Connors & Hilling, 1998)

a. Interstitial lung disease (ILD)

1) Description: Damaged lung tissue causes the walls of the air sacs to become inflamed. The inflammation leads to scarring or fibrosis (pulmonary fibrosis) of the interstitium, causing the lung to become stiff (ALA, 1998g).

2) Examples: Interstitial fibrosis, occupational lung disease, sarcoidosis

b. Neuromuscular and neurologic conditions: Parkinson's disease, postpolio syndrome, amyotrophic lateral sclerosis (ALS), multiple sclerosis (MS), Guillian-Barré syndrome, myasthenia gravis, Duchenne's muscular dystrophy, spinal cord injury (SCI), diaphragm dysfunction (Connors & Hilling, 1998)

Figure 12-6. Instructions for Open-Heart Surgical Patients

Incision Care
Wash the incisions every day with warm water and antibacterial soap
Wash hands first and use separate clean washcloths for each incision to prevent cross infections
Do not use lotions, creams, or oils on the incisions (they can cause infection)
Watch the incisions daily and report any signs of infection (e.g., change in amount or color of drainage, bright red color, increased swelling or tenderness, or edges that pull apart) to the surgeon

Bathing
Take a shower at home if it has been approved by the occupational therapist
Have the water stream on the back, not directly on the incisions
Wait to take tub baths for at least 3–4 weeks after the operation and then only if the therapist feels it is safe

Leg Elevation
Wear antiembolism hose until the follow-up visit with the surgeon
Put hose on in the morning, take them off at night, and clean them on a daily basis
Have someone help put them on
Put legs up on a stool when resting if the ankles and feet begin to swell and at frequent intervals throughout the day

Incentive Spirometer
Use the incentive spirometer every 2 hours while awake (this helps to prevent pneumonia or other breathing problems)
Check with the surgeon at follow-up visits about continuing use

Diet
If using a specific diet before surgery, continue it at home; however, adhere to any modifications made by the dietitian or speech therapist
Be aware that loss of appetite is normal after surgery and that will gradually return

Bowel Activity
Prevent constipation by eating fresh fruits, vegetables, and whole-grain foods
Exercise
Avoid straining
Drink adequate amounts of water
Add prune juice to breakfast
Call the family physician if no bowel movement for 3 days

Activity
Follow the home exercise program described by the physical and occupational therapists
Walk as an excellent form of exercise
Alternate periods of activity with rest
Stop and rest if experiencing extreme fatigue, excessive sweating, shortness of breath, light-headedness, nausea, or a pounding heart
Do not lift more than 10 lbs to protect the breastbone and the grafts on the heart while they heal

Smoking
Please quit smoking: Smoking decreases the oxygen in the blood, damages the arteries and the new bypass grafts, and increases the risk for needing another bypass operation.

Driving
Do not drive until the physiatrist and/or surgeon recommends it: Conditions requiring patients to come to the rehabilitation unit may put them at risk for injury.
Remember that it is okay to be a passenger
Continue to use seat belts; pad the shoulder strap if necessary

Warning Signs
Call the surgeon if any of the following occur: A temperature of 101° or higher, chills, shortness of breath, abnormal pain, changes in pulse rate, palpitations, a weight gain of 2–3 lbs or more in 1 day, signs of infection at the incision sites, diarrhea for more than 24 hours

Emotions
Realize that being emotional or having difficulty concentrating or remembering is common after surgery: This should improve each day and disappear as strength and rest is regained (within about 4–6 weeks).

Source consulted

Carbone, L. (1999). An interdisciplinary approach to the rehabilitation of open-heart surgical patients. *Rehabilitation Nursing, 24*(2), 55-61.

c. Chest wall diseases: Kyphoscoliosis, spondylitis

3. Other conditions (Connors & Hilling, 1998)

a. Lung cancer

b. Lung transplantation

d. Morbid obesity

e. Primary pulmonary hypertension

f. Post-thoracic surgery

g. Sleep apnea

h. Ventilator dependency

i. Volume reduction surgery

B. Epidemiology

1. Incidence

a. Obstructive pulmonary diseases

1) COPD (includes chronic bronchitis and emphysema)

a) Leading cause of disability in the United States (Connors & Hilling, 1998)

b) Fourth leading cause of death: 97,262 deaths in 1995

c) Affects 16 million people

(1) 14 million people have chronic bronchitis: It affects more women than men and more Alaskan natives than white or African Americans (ALA, 1998h).

(2) 2 million people have emphysema: It affects 54% more men than women (ALA, 1998e).

d) Involves $23.5 billion in total healthcare costs: $14.7 billion in direct costs, $8.8 billion in indirect costs

e) COPD: Third ranking condition after CHF and stroke that requires home health care

2) Asthma

a) 14.6 million people have asthma.

(1) This is an increase of 61% between 1982–1994.

(2) 4.8 million are under the age of 18 (ALA, 1998i).

b) 5,600 people die each year from asthma.

(1) Mortality rates increased by 45.3% between 1985 and 1995.

(2) The death rate is higher for African Americans than for whites.

c) Hospitalizations increased by 284% since 1979: Asthma is the Number 1 cause of school absences, and it causes an estimated 3 million lost work days per year (ALA, 1998b).

d) Asthma affects male children more than females: 25% become symptom free as adults (ALA, 1998b; Wilson & Thompson, 1990).

e) Asthma affects more Puerto Ricans than any other ethnic group (ALA, 1998i).

f) 85% of women and 72% of men have asthma into adulthood (ALA, 1998b).

g) Asthma costs $12.4 billion in total healthcare costs: $9.8 billion in direct care and $2.6 in indirect care (Connors & Hilling, 1998).

3) Cystic fibrosis

a) Most common life-threatening pulmonary disease of children

b) Seen in one of every 2,000 live births

c) Affects white children most frequently, and more males than females (Wilson & Thompson, 1990)

b. Restrictive pulmonary diseases: Sarcoidosis

1) African Americans are three times more likely to develop this disease than whites.

2) In the U.S. Navy, between 1990–1993, 16 African Americans to 2.5 whites in 100,000 people had sarcoidosis (ALA, 1998k).

c. Other conditions: Lung cancer

1) Lung cancer is the most common, fatal, malignant cause of cancer death.

2) An estimated 160,400 Americans died in 1997 because of lung cancer.

3) Lung cancer occurs more often in people older than age 50 who have a long history of smoking, in more African American men than white men, and in more white women than in African American women (ALA, 1998j).

C. Etiology/Causes

1. Obstructive pulmonary diseases

    a. Chronic bronchitis

       1) Smoking

       2) Recurrent infections

       3) Environmental irritants: Coal mines, industrial pollutants, grain handlers, metal molders, dust (ALA, 1998c)

       4) Abnormal growth of bronchi (Glanze, 1987)

    b. Emphysema

       1) Smoking

       2) Recurrent infections

       3) Environmental irritants

       4) Alpha1-Antitripsin: a1AT is an inherited form of emphysema. People with this pulmonary disease have inherited the two genes, one from the mother and one from the father, that lack the protein a1AT, which neutralizes the natural enzyme neutrophil elastase that helps destroy and remove bacteria and dead lung tissue. When this enzyme is not neutralized after its job is completed, then damage to the lung tissue occurs (ALA, 1998a).

    c. Asthma

       1) Exercise-induced: Occurs during exercise and may be related to heat or water loss from bronchioles

       2) Occupational-induced: Triggered by agents found in the workplace and occurs within a few weeks to many years after exposure to the irritant

       3) Cardiac-induced: Bronchospasm associated with CHF

       4) Medication-induced: May be caused by medications (e.g., beta-blocking agents, aspirin, nonsteroidal anti-inflammatory drugs [NSAIDs], histamine, methacholine, acetylcysteine, nebulized medications)

       5) Environmental irritants (Tierney et al., 1994)

    d. Cystic fibrosis: Genetic

2. Restrictive pulmonary diseases

    a. ILD: Inflammation

       1) Occupational and environmental irritants

       2) Sarcoidosis

       3) Drugs

       4) Radiation

       5) Connective tissue or collagen diseases

          a) Rheumatoid arthritis

          b) Systemic sclerosis

       6) Genetics (ALA, 1998g)

    b. Neuromuscular and neurologic disease: ALS, diaphragm dysfunction, MS, Parkinson's disease, postpolio syndrome (Connors & Hilling, 1998)

3. Other conditions

    a. Lung cancer

       1) Smoking and second-hand smoke

       2) Exposure to radon

       3) Exposure to occupational carcinogens

    b. Lung transplantation: ILD, emphysema, a1AT, cystic fibrosis

D. Pathophysiology

1. Obstructive pulmonary diseases

    a. COPD

       1) Chronic bronchitis

          a) Hypertrophy and hypersecretion of goblet and mucous gland cells in bronchioles causes extension into terminal bronchioles.

          b) Increased secretions cause bronchial congestion and narrowing of the bronchioles and small bronchi.

          c) Lower respiratory tract becomes colonized by bacteria and stimulates secretions by leukocytes.

          d) Leukocytes cause swelling and tissue destruction of the bronchial walls so that they become granulated and fibrotic, leading to stenosis and obstruction that impair the exchange of oxygen to and from the lungs (Wilson & Thompson, 1990).

    (1) Acute: Not associated with fever

    (2) Chronic: Mucus-producing cough most days of the month for 3 months out of a year for 2 successive years without underlying disease

    (3) May precede or accompany emphysema (ALA, 1998c)

  2) Emphysema

    a) Recurrent infections, history of smoking, and exposure to environmental irritants cause deficiency in the protease inhibitor a1AT.

    b) Elastase, a neutral protease, which is produced by leukocytes and alveolar macrophages, proliferates and destroys lung elastin as it becomes uninhibited due to the deficiency of a1AT (Wilson & Thompson, 1990).

    c) Alveoli become destroyed, causing permanent holes in the lower lung tissues.

    d) Oxygen/carbon dioxide transfer in the blood is inhibited.

    e) Lungs lose their elasticity and bronchial tubes collapse, trapping air in the lungs (ALA, 1998e).

b. Asthma: Irritants stimulate bronchoconstriction of the smooth muscles that line the bronchial tubes, causing fluid to leak from blood vessels and stimulating inflammation. The inflammation narrows the airways and mucus forms so thick that the cilia are unable to remove it from the airways effectively. This impairs oxygen delivery to the blood and lungs, trapping carbon monoxide (Allergy and Asthma Network/Mothers of Asthmatics [AAN/MA], 1998).

  1) Extrinsic-inhaled allergens, infection, physical exertion, stress

    a) Beta cells are stimulated and differentiate into plasma cells that produce immunoglobulin E antibodies (IgE).

    b) IgE attaches to mast cells and basophils in bronchial walls. Mast cells release histamine, prostaglandins, bradykinin, and slow-reacting substance (SRS) of anaphylaxis.

    c) Histamine stimulates bronchial small muscle contraction and vascular permeability, causing leakage of proteins and fluids into bronchial mucosa thus constricting and obstructing bronchial tubes.

  2) Intrinsic: Parasympathetic-stimulated vagal nerves, whether mechanical or chemical, cause release of acetylcholine and cause bronchoconstriction and production of histamine, prostaglandins, bradykinin, and SRS (Wilson & Thompson, 1990).

c. Cystic fibrosis

  1) Genetic disorder of the exocrine glands

  2) Dysfunctional exocrine gland production of abnormal secretions of mucus by the goblet cells

  3) Involves thick mucoproteins that coagulate in glands and ducts, causing obstruction (Wilson & Thompson, 1990)

2. Restrictive pulmonary disease: ILD

a. There are a variety of chronic lung disorders—some with known causes and some with unknown causes (idiopathic)—whose progress and symptoms vary from one person to another.

b. All ILDs begin with inflammation. Areas of inflammation heal and may lead to permanent scarring of the lung tissue, causing pulmonary fibrosis. The fibrosis causes permanent loss of the tissue's ability to transport oxygen.

  1) Bronchiolitis: Inflammation of the bronchioles

  2) Alveolitis: Inflammation of the alveoli

  3) Vasculitis: Inflammation of the

capillaries of the lungs (ALA, 1998g)

3. Other conditions: Lung cancer

    a. Develops when the genes responsible for sequential cell division, proto-oncogenes, change to oncogenes.

       1) This causes cells to indiscriminately divide.

       2) This division and proliferation is without regard to the needs of the body.

       3) These undifferentiated cells do not function normally and impede the functions of healthy cells.

    b. Types of lung cancer (National Cancer Institute [NCI], 1998; Wilson & Thompson, 1990)

       1) Adenocarcinoma

          a) Occurs in 40% of cases

          b) Begins along periphery of lungs and under the lining of bronchi

          c) Affects peripheral lung tissue or areas scarred from pulmonary infarct, infection, or fibrosis

          d) Affects more women and nonsmokers

       2) Squamous cell carcinoma

          a) Occurs 30% of cases

          b) Begins in bronchi

          c) Occludes airways and causes lungs to collapse

          d) Spreads to intrathoracic sites

          e) Affects more men

       3) Small cell/oat cell carcinoma

          a) Occurs in 20% of cases

          b) Spreads quickly to nodes, intrathoracic structures, and other organs

       4) Large cell, or bronchioloalveolar cell carcinoma: Occurs in 5%–8% of cases

       5) Giant cell, clear cell, or pulmonary blastoma: Occurs in less than 2% of cases

E. Residual Effects

1. Obstructive pulmonary diseases

    a. COPD: Chronic bronchitis and emphysema

       1) Factors that worsen the condition

          a) Acute bronchitis

          b) Pneumonia

          c) Pulmonary embolus

          d) Left ventricular failure

       2) Common complications

          a) Pulmonary hypertension

          b) Cor pulmonale

          c) Chronic respiratory failure

       3) Symptoms

          a) Shortness of breath

          b) Cough

          c) Sputum production

          d) Weight loss (with emphysema)

          e) Obesity (with chronic bronchitis) (Tierney et al., 1994)

    b. Asthma

       1) Mediastinal or subcutaneous emphysema

       2) Bronchitis

       3) Pulmonary hypertension

       4) Cor pulmonale

       5) Respiratory failure (Wilson & Thompson, 1990)

    c. Cystic fibrosis

       1) Systemic effects

          a) Reproductive tract: Causes sterility by obstructing the vas deferens in men and blocking sperm from entering the uterus due to thick cervical secretions

          b) Pancreatic duct obstruction: Inability of pancreatic enzymes to be released, causing malabsorption, nutritional deficiencies, diabetes mellitus

          c) Bile duct obstruction: Causes portal hypertension and liver failure

          d) Blocked sweat glands: Decrease absorption of sodium and chloride leading to dehydration

          e) Bronchial obstruction: Causes infections, respiratory disease, and cor pulmonale

          f) Electrolyte imbalance: Causes decreased absorption of sodium and chloride and increased perspiration leading to dehydration (Wilson & Thompson, 1990)

2) Intestinal obstruction

3) Esophageal varices

4) Pulmonary hypertension

5) Cor pulmonale

6) Lung abscess

7) Pulmonary insufficiency

8) Atelectasis

9) Pneumothorax (Wilson & Thompson, 1990)

2. Restrictive pulmonary disease: ILD—respiratory distress

3. Other lung disease: Lung cancer

a. Chronic cough

b. Hemoptysis

c. Wheezing

d. Chest pain (ALA, 1998f)

e. Residual effects of treatments

1) Surgical treatment: Weakened arm and chest muscle; fluid may build up in space left after resection.

2) Radiation therapy: Loss of appetite related to nausea, vomiting, loss of taste, oral and throat sores affecting swallow, weight loss, pulmonary fibrosis, dry, itching, tender skin

3) Chemotherapy: Immunosuppression, decreased clotting time, fatigue, aloplecia, nausea, vomiting, and oral sores affecting appetite (NCI, 1998)

F. Management Measures

1. For all respiratory diseases

a. Maximize breathing

b. Maintain or improve functional status

c. Enhance coping skills, identify stressors, and modify behavior

d. Maintain or improve nutritional status

e. Educate about disease process and prognosis

f. Use mechanical ventilation as needed

2. For specific diseases

a. Obstructive pulmonary disease

1) COPD

a) Goal: To stop the progression of the disease, to maximize breathing, to reduce airway secretions, inflammation, and bronchospasm

b) Identify and manage precipitating factors

c) Encourage smoking cessation

d) Encourage prevention and early treatment of airway infections and vaccinations against influenza and pneumococcal disease (Tierney et al., 1994)

e) Encourage use of chest physiotherapy techniques (see Figure 12-7)

f) Provide medications

(1) Ipratropium bromide

(2) Theophylline

(3) Corticosteroids

(4) Ampicillin or tetracycline (Tierney et al., 1994; Wilson & Thompson, 1990)

g) Use supplemental oxygen

2) Asthma

a) Include interventions as above, except chest physiotherapy

b) Control environmental and emotional triggers

c) Medications

(1) Bronchodilators and sympathomimetics (e.g., albuterol, metaproterenol, bitolterol, pirbuterol, terbutaline, isoetharine, isoproterenol, epinephrine)

(2) Anticholinergics (e.g., ipratropium bromide, atropine sulfate)

(3) Theophylline

(4) Corticosteroids (e.g., beclomethasone dipropionate, triamcinolone acetonide, flunisolide, prednisone, methylprednisolone sodium succinate, hydrocortisone sodium succinate)

(5) Antimediators: Cromolyn sodium (Tierney et al., 1994)

(6) Use of peak flow meter

(a) Inexpensive handheld device that measures air flow from the lungs

(b) Benefits: Asthma management, medication adjustment, indication of worsening or improvement of symptoms, reassurance (ALA, 1998b)

3) Cystic fibrosis
   a) Goal: Early diagnosis and comprehensive interdisciplinary therapy are important in lengthening survival time and alleviating symptoms.
   b) Psychological, genetic, and occupational counseling
   c) Chest physiotherapy (Tierney et al., 1994)
   d) Medications
      (1) Treat infections based on results of culture and sensitivity testing
      (2) Expectorants (e.g., iodinated glycerol, potassium iodide)
      (3) Bronchodilators (e.g., salbutaonol, theophylline, fenoterol aerosol)
      (4) Steroids (e.g., prednisone)
      (5) Agents that help digest carbohydrates, fats, and proteins (e.g., pancreatin with meals or snacks, pancrelipase before or with meals or snacks)
      (6) Immunizations against influenza and pneumonia
   e) Oxygen therapy
   f) Surgical procedures
      (1) Pulmonary lavage or bronchial washing
      (2) Resection of blebs and pleural scars
      (3) Lung transplantation (Wilson & Thompson, 1990)
   b. Restrictive pulmonary disease
      1) Goal: Prevent inflammation and relieve symptoms
      2) Medications
         a) Corticosteroids (combination therapy of drugs with corticosteroids is still under investigation)
         b) Immunizations against influenza and pneumonia
      3) Oxygen therapy (ALA, 1998g)
   c. Other conditions: Lung cancer
      1) Surgery: Lobectomy, pneumonectomy, segmental resection
      2) Radiation therapy
      3) Chemotherapy
      4) Strengthening program
      5) Weight loss management
   G. Nursing Process
      1. Assessment

Figure 12-7. Patient Teaching for Home Management of Chest Physiotherapy

General Information

Chest physiotherapy (e.g., postural drainage, chest percussion, coughing) may be recommended by the physician for use with chronic bronchitis, emphysema, or cystic fibrosis to help loosen and remove mucus from the lungs.
Techniques may be done in the morning, before bedtime, or when secretions are more than usual as recommended by the physician. Oral fluids will help to thin the mucus.

TEACHING TOPICS

Postural Drainage

Lie on bed with chest over side, resting head on a pillow on the floor
For 10–20 minutes each, lie on stomach, left side, then right side

Chest Percussion (requires a second person)

While the patient is in the postural drainage position, the second person cups his or her hands and rhythmically pats the patient's back, alternating hands for 3–4 minutes

Cough

While in the postural drainage position, take slow deep breath through the nose
Open the mouth and, while breathing out, cough three times to help bring up the mucus
Repeat several times
Cough mucus out of the mouth as swallowing may cause nausea

Contraindications

Cyanosis or dyspnea caused by technique, increased pain or discomfort, prolonged bleeding or clotting times, extreme obesity, predisposition to pathological fractures

Sources consulted

Loeb, S. (Ed.). (1992). Teaching patients with chronic conditions. Bethlehem Pike, PA: Springhouse Corp.

Wilson, S.F., & Thompson, J.M. (1990). *Respiratory disorders*. St. Louis: Mosby.

---

a. Medical and family history

1) Use of supplemental oxygen, medical devices, and knowl edge of appropriate usage
2) Medications: Allergies and drug intolerance
3) Triggers in work and home environments
4) Lifestyle
   a) Smoking history
   b) Work and home activities
5) Recent illnesses: Complete blood count to monitor white blood cells for signs of infection and hematocrit to follow anemia, bleeding, cirrhosis, and dehydration (Fischbach, 1988)
6) Self-care skills
7) Knowledge and use of medications

b. Physical (Tierney et al., 1994; Wilson & Thompson, 1990)

1) Exercise
   a) Physical limitations (e.g., strength, functional ability, orthopedic limitations)
   b) Exercise tolerance, need for supplemental oxygen, cardiac function (Connors & Hilling, 1998)
2) Neurological: Cognition changes, lethargy, restlessness
3) Pulmonary: Dyspnea, tachypnea, wheezes, crackles, rhonchi, decreased breath sounds, cough, hoarseness, clubbed fingers, chest retractions, barrel chest, decreased chest wall movement, productive thick sputum that may be odorous, hemoptysis, postnasal drainage
4) Cardiovascular: Tachycardia, dysrhythmia, fatigue, chest pain, edema
5) GI
   a) General: Weight loss or gain, appetite, oral sores, constipation, dehydration, reflux
   b) Special GI considerations for CF patients: Bulky, foul-smelling, pale, or watery stool; intestinal obstruction, fecal impaction, and tarry stools if bleeding; jaundice; ascites; abnormal liver function;

laboratory results
6) Skin: Decreased skin turgor with dehydration, diaphoresis
7) Psychosocial: Fear of suffocation, sleep disturbance, depression, anxiety

c. Nutritional: Weight loss, lack of appetite, loss of taste, swallowing difficulties, constipation, hydration, serum albumin

d. Psychosocial
1) Support systems
2) Individual and family coping

e. Knowledge of disease process

2. Diagnoses (NANDA, 1999)

a. Ineffective breathing pattern
b. Ineffective airway clearance
c. Impaired gas exchange
d. Activity intolerance
e. Altered nutrition (less than body requirements)
f. Risk for constipation
g. Risk for infection
h. Sleep pattern disturbance
i. Risk for spiritual distress
j. Ineffective individual coping
k. Ineffective family coping (compromised)
l. Anxiety
m. Sexual dysfunction
n. Self-care deficits (e.g., feeding, bathing, grooming, dressing, toileting)
o. Impaired home maintenance management
p. Knowledge deficit
q. Ineffective management of therapeutic regimen (individual or family)

3. Plan

a. Goals for the patient
1) Demonstrate effective breathing patterns without fatigue
2) Demonstrate improved airway clearance through use of postural drainage when appropriate, coughing, deep breathing, and taking medications as directed
3) Demonstrate resolution of cognitive changes if they have not become permanent; resolve cyanosis
4) Demonstrate ability to do ADLs

using compensation measures when necessary to prevent dyspnea or fatigue; for children, demonstrate ability to participate in normal activities using preactivity medications

   5) Demonstrate stable weight for age and size, take adequate caloric intake daily, and have a normal albumin level

   6) Have regular bowel movements without constipation or dehydration and take in adequate amounts of fluid daily

   7) Remain free of infection and prevent influenza and pneumonia

   8) Demonstrate adequate sleep patterns for rest and rejuvenation

   9) Verbalize decreased spiritual distress and measures to prevent recurrence

   b. Goals for the family

   1) Demonstrate support for the person with the disability and verbalize resources available for family support

   2) Acknowledge fear and anxiety and demonstrate ways to decrease anxiety (e.g., hobbies, social activities, relaxation techniques)

   3) Verbalize understanding of compensation measures while engaging in sexual activity

   4) Verbalize knowledge of disease process, precipitating factors of respiratory difficulties and how to avoid or minimize effects, how to administer medication and oxygen therapy properly, and when to call the physician

   5) Verbalize and demonstrate understanding of the therapeutic regimen and the importance of self-monitoring and compliance with therapeutic recommendations

4. Interventions

   a. Observe respiration depth and rate, dyspnea, nasal flaring

   b. Inspect thorax or symmetry of respiratory movement, chest muscle retractions, changes in skin color and capillary refill, changes in mentation or behavior

   c. Auscultate lungs for adventitious sounds

   d. Administer oxygen, bronchodilators,

antibiotics, corticosteroids, and other medications as directed

   e. Teach breathing techniques and exercises to conserve energy (see Figure 12-8)

   f. Identify ways to conserve energy in daily activities

   g. Adapt ways to enhance endurance and conserve energy

   h. Slowly increase activity as tolerance allows, promoting as much independence as possible

   i. Encourage adherence to a regular exercise program with planned rest periods between activities: Teach patients receiving intermittent, continuous, or nocturnal ventilator support to do the following (Connors & Hilling, 1998):

   1) Strengthen skeletal muscles that have atrophied from critical illness, less than optimal nutritional support, or corticosteroid use

   2) Strengthen skeletal muscles by beginning exercises during periods while the patient is receiving ventilator support, adjusting ventilator settings as required, and including strengthening techniques (e.g., free weights, gravity, manual resistance, elastic bands)

   3) Improve nutritional support through supplements, considering the possibility of using a feeding tube to increase muscle strength and endurance: Patients with a tracheotomy have limited speech and are at risk of aspiration.

      a) Assist with speech through the use of cuffless or fenestrated tracheotomy tubes or Passe Muir valves

      b) Prevent aspiration by teaching compensatory swallowing techniques

   j. Provide uninterrupted periods of rest

   k. Identify sources of irritants (Tierney et al., 1994)

   1) Triggers

      a) Air particles (indoor and outdoor)

b) Cold air or sudden temperature change

c) Tobacco or smoke from burning wood or leaves

d) Perfume, paint, hair spray

e) Strong odors or fumes

f) Allergens (e.g., dust mites, pollen, pollution, animal dander)

g) Common cold, flu, or respiratory illness

h) Vigorous exercise

i) Stress or excitement

j) Certain foods

2) Control measures

a) Do a skin test to identify allergens

b) Keep an asthma diary to list triggers (ALA, 1998b)

c) Use pillow and mattress covers

d) Remove carpets

e) Use air-filtering devices or air conditioning

f) Wash pets (especially dogs) weekly

g) Ensure early detection of respiratory infections

h) Manage nasal disorders

i) Stop smoking

l. Monitor pollution index and adjust outdoor activities accordingly (ALA, 1998d)

m. Avoid exposure to colds and flu and encourage vaccinations against influenza and pneumonia (ALA, 1998c)

n. Promote caloric intake to support adequate growth (e.g., exceeding daily requirements by 25%, high in protein, low in fat, vitamin supplements for CF patients)

o. Provide frequent small meals to lessen fatigue

p. Provide appropriate food consistency to enhance energy conservation during meals

q. Offer antiemetics before meals to reduce nausea

r. Maintain good oral care

s. Monitor for swallowing difficulties and risk for aspiration

t. Monitor for nutritional risk

Figure 12-8. Breathing Tips and Exercises

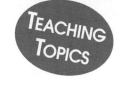

Things to Avoid to Help Make Breathing Easier
Heavy traffic and smog
  Aerosol spray
Products that produce fumes
Cold weather
Very dry air
Exercise

Pursed-Lip Breathing
Can be done anywhere
Helps get rid of air trapped in the lungs
Slows breathing to make it more efficient
Must be practiced so that when an episode of shortness of breath occurs, the exercise is familiar

Technique
Breathe in slowly through the nose holding for 3 seconds
Purse the lips as if whistling
Breathe out slowly through the pursed lips for 6 seconds

Abdominal Breathing
Must be done lying down
Slows breathing to become more efficient
Helps relax the body

Technique
Lie on back in a comfortable position with a pillow under the head
Place one hand on abdomen below the ribs and the other on the chest
Slowly breathe in and out through the nose using abdominal muscles
Watch the hand on the abdomen, which should rise and fall with breathing, and the hand on the chest, which should remain still

Sources consulted

Connors, G., & Hilling, L. (Ed.). (1998). *Guidelines for pulmonary rehabilitation programs: American Association of Cardiovascular and Pulmonary Rehabilitation—Promoting health and preventing disease* (2nd ed.). Champaign, IL: Human Kinetics.
Wilson, S.F., & Thompson, J.M. (1990). *Respiratory disorders.* St. Louis: Mosby.

---

1) Weight loss (weigh daily), dehydration (keep records of intake and output and skin turgor)
2) Appetite (count calories)
3) Loss of taste, oral sores, nausea, or vomiting
4) Monitor albumin levels and offer protein supplements as needed for healing and weight maintenance
5) Administer vitamins and pancreatic enzymes for CF patients as ordered

u. Monitor stools
1) Be alert for constipation
   a) Encourage fluids, fiber, stool softeners, or laxatives
   b) Encourage ambulation
2) Note color, amount, consistency, consistency, frequency, and presence of blood

v. Teach about medications
1) Explain usage, symptoms of effectiveness, ineffectiveness, and toxicity
2) Monitor theophylline levels
3) Maintain inhalation equipment
4) Teach about safe oxygen use in the home (Wilson & Thompson, 1990)
   a) Explain that oxygen is very combustible
      (1) Keep away from open flames and heat
      (2) Stay away from smokers
      (3) Stay out of rooms with a running gas stove or gas or kerosene space heater
   b) Prevent leakage
      (1) Keep tank upright
      (2) Turn off system when not in use
      (3) Do not place anything over the tubing
      (4) Keep an all-purpose fire extinguisher available
      (5) In case of fire, turn off the oxygen and leave the home
      (6) Notify the fire department that there is oxygen in the home: Many fire departments offer free safety inspections.
   c) Watch for symptoms of not enough or too much oxygen
      (1) Breathing becomes difficult, irregular, or slow
      (2) Restlessness or anxiousness
      (3) Tiredness or drowsiness
      (4) Difficulty waking up
      (5) Persistent headache
      (6) Confusion, difficulty concentrating, or slurred speech
      (7) Cyanotic fingertips or lips
   d) Teach the patient to notify the physician if any of these symptoms occur: Never change the flow rate without guidance from the physician

w. Teach about diagnostic tests, disease process, prognosis, and therapies

x. Assist the patient and family with coping and stress reduction
1) Develop trust with patient and family, encourage family members to express feelings, assist in problem solving, identify support systems, offer support network as needed
2) Promote normal growth and development
3) Discuss financial concerns and make appropriate referrals
4) Encourage personal control
5) Maintain privacy
6) Teach relaxation and stress reduction techniques

y. Consult with chaplain or the patient's spiritual guide to offer spiritual support

z. Offer education on sexual activity (Loeb, 1992; Tierney et al., 1994; Wilson & Thompson, 1990)
1) Determine knowledge of effects of illness and treatment on sexual functioning
2) Provide an atmosphere to discuss sexual concerns
3) Perform airway clearance therapies 1 hour before sexual activity
4) Help the patient plan sexual activity at optimal times
5) Avoid sexual activity after meals
6) Encourage alternative positions that are less stressful

7) Encourage frequent rest during sexual activity to minimize pulmonary compromise while increasing partner satisfaction by prolonged stimulation

aa. Stress the importance of adhering to the medical and therapeutic regimen: Ensure that the patient and family understand and follow through with the treatment plan

5. Evaluation

a. Remember that patient follow-up is very important

b. Evaluate the patient's understanding of instructions and how the interventions are affecting them, positively or negatively

c. Revise goals and interventions with the patient and the physician as needed

References

Allergy & Asthma Network/Mothers of Asthmatics. (AAN/MA). (1998). *What is asthma?* [Online]. Available: www.health-touch.com/level1/leaflets/aan/aan096.htm.

American Heart Association (AHA). (1996a). *Medical procedures, facilities and cost* [Online]. Available: www.americanheart.org/statistics/09medicl.html.

American Heart Association (AHA). (1996b). *Other cardiovascular diseases* [Online]. Available: www.americanheart.org/statistics/07other.html.

American Heart Association (AHA). (1999a). *Angioplasty and cardiac revascularization treatments and statistics* [Online]. Available: www.americanheart.org/Heart_and_Stroke_A_Z_Guide/angioc.html.

American Heart Association (AHA). (1999b). *Atherosclerosis* [Online]. Available: www.americanheart.org/Heart_and_Stroke_A_Z_Guide/athero.html.

American Heart Association (AHA). (1999c). *Cardiovascular disease statistics* [Online]. Available: www.americanheart.org/Heart_and_Stroke_A_Z_Guide/cvds.html.

American Heart Association (AHA). (1999d). *Cardiovascular rehabilitation* [Online]. Available: www.americanheart.org/Heart_and_Stroke_A_Z_Guide/cvdre.html.

American Heart Association (AHA). (1999e). *Cholesterol levels* [Online]. Available: www.americanheart.org/Heart_and_Stroke_A_Z_Guide/cholle v.html.

American Heart Association (AHA). (1999f). *Congenital cardiovascular disease* [Online]. Available: www.americanheart.org/Heart_and_Stroke_A_Z_Guide/conghd.html.

American Heart Association (AHA). (1999g). *Congenital heart defects statistics* [Online]. Available: http://americanheart.org/Heart_and_Stroke_A_Z_Guide/conghds.html.

American Heart Association (AHA). (1999h). *Congestive heart failure* [Online]. Available: www.americanheart.org/Heart_and_Stroke_A_Z_Guide/congest.html.

American Heart Association (AHA). (1999i). *Economic cost of cardiovascular diseases* [Online]. Available: www.americanheart.org/statistics/10econom.html.

American Heart Association (AHA). (1999j). *Heart attack and angina statistics* [Online]. Available: www.americanheart.org/Heart_and_Stroke_A_Z_Guide/has.html.

American Heart Association (AHA). (1999k). *Prevention, primary* [Online]. Available: www.americanheart.org/Heart_and_Stroke_A_Z_Guide/prevpri.html.

American Heart Association (AHA). (1999l). *Prevention, secondary* [Online]. Available: www.americanheart.org/Heart_and_Stroke_A_Z_Guide/prevsec.html.

American Heart Association (AHA). (1999m). *Risk factors and coronary heart disease* [Online]. Available: www.americanheart.org/Heart_and_Stroke_A_Z_Guide/riskfact.html.

American Heart Association (AHA). (1999n). *Target heart rate* [Online]. Available: www.americanheart.org/Heart_and_Stroke_A_Z_Guide/target.html.

American Lung Association (ALA). (1998a). *A1-AD related emphysema* [Online]. Available: www.lungusa.org.

American Lung Association (ALA). (1998b). *Asthma-ALA fact sheet-asthma in adults* [Online]. Available: www.lungusa.org/asthma/index.html.

American Lung Association (ALA). (1998c). *Chronic bronchitis* [Online]. Available: www.lungusa.org.

American Lung Association (ALA). (1998d). *Emphysema* [Online]. Available: www.lungusa.org.

American Lung Association (ALA). (1998e). *Emphysema* [Online]. Available: www.lungusa.org/diseases/luna1ad.html.

American Lung Association (ALA). (1998f). *Facts about lung cancer* [Online]. Available: www.lungusa.org.

American Lung Association (ALA). (1998g). *Facts about pulmonary fibrosis and interstitial lung disease* [Online]. Available: www.lungusa.org/diseases/pulmfibrosis.html.

American Lung Association (ALA). (1998h). *Lung disease in minorities: Chronic obstructive pulmonary disease—emphysema and chronic bronchitis* [Online]. Available: www.lungusa.org/pub/minority/copd.htm.

American Lung Association (ALA). (1998i). *Lung disease in minorities: Focus—asthma* [Online]. Available: www.lungusa.org/pub/minority/f-asthma.htm.

American Lung Association (ALA). (1998j). *Lung disease in minorities: Lung cancer* [Online]. Available: www.lungusa.org/pub/minority/lungcncr.htm.

American Lung Association (ALA). (1998k). *Sarcoidosis* [Online]. Available: www.lungusa.org/home2.html.

Canobbio, M. (1990). *Cardiovascular disorders*. St Louis: Mosby.

Carbone, L. (1999). An interdisciplinary approach to the rehabilitation of open-heart surgical patients. *Rehabilitation Nursing, 24*(2), 55-61.

Connors, G., & Hilling, L. (Ed.). (1998). *Guidelines for pulmonary rehabilitation programs: American Association of Cardiovascular and Pulmonary Rehabilitation—Promoting health and preventing disease* (2nd ed.). Champaign, IL: Human Kinetics.

Fischbach, F. (1988). *A manual of laboratory diagnostic tests* (3rd ed.). Philadelphia: J.B. Lippincott.

Glanze, W.D. (Ed.). (1987). *The Signet/Mosby medical encyclopedia*. New York: Mosby.

Huang, S., Kessler, C., McCulloch, C., & Dasher, L. (1989). Cardiac rehabilitation of the myocardial patient. In *Coronary care nursing*. Philadelphia: W.B. Saunders.

Loeb, S. (Ed.). (1992). Teaching patients with chronic conditions. Bethlehem Pike, PA: Springhouse Corp.

National Cancer Institute (NCI). (1998). *General information about lung cancer* [Online]. Available: www.healthtouch.com/level1/leaflets/nci/nci062.htm

National Heart, Lung and Blood Institute (NHLBI). (1998a). *Cholesterol and heart disease IQ quiz* [Online]. Available: www.healthtouch.com/level1/leaflets/nhlbi/nhlbi008.htm.

National Heart, Lung and Blood Institute (NHLBI). (1998b). *Lowering blood cholesterol levels: Diet, exercise and weight control* [Online]. Available: www.healthtouch.com/level1/leaflets/nhlbi/nhlbi014.htm.

North American Nursing Diagnosis Association (NANDA). (1999). *Nursing Diagnoses: Definitions and Classification 1999-2000*. Philadelphia: Author.

Saint Joseph's Regional Medical Center (SJRMC). (1996). *The beat goes on: Educational materials for the cardiac patient and family*. South Bend, IN: Author.

Tierney, L.M., McPhee, S.J., & Papadakis, M.A. (Ed.). (1994). *Current medical diagnosis and treatment* (33rd ed.). Norwalk, CT: Appleton & Lange.

Wilson, S.F., & Thompson, J.M. (1990). *Respiratory disorders*. St. Louis: Mosby.

Suggested resources

Allen, J.K., & Redman, B.K. (1996). Cardiac rehabilitation in the elderly: Improving effectiveness. *Rehabilitation Nursing, 21*(4), 182-186, 195.

Carpenito, L. (1989). *Nursing diagnosis: Application to clinical practice*. Philadelphia: Lippincott.

Dettenmeir, P. (1992). *Pulmonary nursing care*. St. Louis: Mosby.

Eakes, G.G., Mayo, C., & Whicker, S. (1997). Growth and development of a cardiac rehabilitation support group. *Rehabilitation Nursing, 22*(4), 173-176.

Goodwin, B.A. (1999). Home cardiac rehabilitation for congestive heart failure: A nursing case management approach. *Rehabilitation Nursing, 24*(4), 143-147.

Herbert, R., & Gregor, F. (1997). Quality of life and coping strategies of clients with COPD. *Rehabilitation Nursing, 22*(4), 182-187.

Jaffe, M.S., & Skidmore-Roth, L. (1993). *Home health nursing care plans* (2nd ed.). St. Louis: Mosby.

Kamwendo, K., Hansson, M., & Hjerpe, I. (1998). Relationships between adherence, sense of coherence, and knowledge in cardiac rehabilitation. *Rehabilitation Nursing, 23*(5), 240-245, 251.

King, K.M., & Teo, K.K. (1998). Cardiac rehabilitation referral and attendance: Not one in the same. *Rehabilitation Nursing, 23*(5), 246-251.

Milligan, N.P., Havey, J., & Dossa, A. (1997). Using a 6-minute walk test to predict outcomes in patients with left ventricular dysfunction. *Rehabilitation Nursing, 22*(4), 177-181.

Missik, E. (1999). Personal perceptions and women's participation in cardiac rehabilitation. *Rehabilitation Nursing, 24*(4), 158-165.

Romeo-Ashton, K.C., & Saccucci, M.S. (1996). A follow-up study of ethnic and gender differences in cardiac rehabilitation. *Rehabilitation Nursing, 21*(4), 187-191.

Scherer, Y.K., Schmieder, L.E., & Shimmel, S. (1998). The effects of education alone and in combination with pulmonary rehabilitation on self-efficacy in patients with COPD. *Rehabilitation Nursing, 23*(2), 71-77.

Scherer, Y.K., & Shimmel, S. (1996). Using self-efficacy theory to educate patients with chronic obstructive pulmonary disease. *Rehabilitation Nursing, 21*(5), 262-266.

Stanhope, M., & Knollmueller, R.N. (1992). *Handbook of community and home health nursing: Tolls for assessment, intervention, and education*. St. Louis: Mosby.

Steinke, E.E., & Patterson-Midgley, P.E. (1998). Perspectives of nurses and patients on the need for sexual counseling of MI patients. *Rehabilitation Nursing, 23*(2), 64-70.

Suter, P.M., Suter, W.N., Perkins, M.K., Bona, S.L., & Kendrick, P.A. (1996). Cardiac rehabilitation survey: Maintenance of lifestyle changes and perceptions of program value. *Rehabilitation Nursing, 21*(4), 192-195.

Wenger, N.K. (1994). Guidelines for exercise training of elderly patients with coronary artery disease. *Southern Medical Journal, 87*(5).

Zimmerman, B.W., Brown, S.T., & Bowman, J.M. (1996). A self-management program for chronic obstructive pulmonary disease: Relationship to dyspnea and self-efficacy. *Rehabilitation Nursing, 21*(5), 253-257.

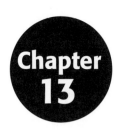

Understanding Acute and Chronic Pain

Judy A. Harris, MS RN CRRN CRC

"Pain is a part of life. Sometimes it is useful and can be a warning of danger, injury, or illness" (Association for the Care of Children's Health & McGrath, 1994, p. 1).

"Pain cannot be seen, palpated, imaged, or scientifically verified" (Steele-Rosomoff, 1996).

Pain is a subjective experience with marked differences in severity, quality, and impact in patients attempting to describe what appears to be the same phenomena (Turk, 1993). Pain is whatever the person experiencing it says it is, and it exists whenever he or she says it does (McCaffery, 1979). Reports of pain should be believed and taken seriously because "…there is no direct relationship between physical pathology and the intensity of pain" (Turk, 1993, p. 1). The person reporting the pain is the most knowledgeable about it.

"The goal of the pain management rehabilitation nurse is to improve the level of functioning and the quality of life for those affected by pain" (Association of Rehabilitation Nurses [ARN], 1994). A review of the literature indicates that effective pain management continues to be a challenge for nurses in all settings. Rehabilitation nurses must evaluate the patient's pain in its entirety, including the effects on the patient's personal, family, and community roles. Only by considering the global picture will nurses be able to achieve the excellent pain management outcomes anticipated by the patient.

I. Overview

A. Definitions of Pain

1. Acute pain

   a. "The state in which an individual experiences and reports the presence of severe discomfort or an uncomfortable sensation, lasting from 1 second to less than 6 months" (Carpenito, 1995, p. 217)

   b. Has an identifiable source and is accepted as a warning system for the body: "It signals when tissue damage may occur and thus alerts us to protect ourselves from injury or to care for an injury that already occurred" (Leo & Huether, 1998, p. 432).

2. Chronic pain

   a. "The state in which an individual experiences pain that is persistent or intermittent and lasts for more than 6 months" (Ellis & Nowlis, 1994, p. 227)

   b. Often has an unknown cause: If the cause is known, the pain does not respond to usual therapy (Leo & Huether, 1998).

3. Limited pain: Has an existing, known physical pathology (McCaffery, 1979)

4. Intermittent pain

   a. Has an existing, known, and understood physical pathology

   b. Involves periods during which the patient is free of pain (McCaffery, 1979)

5. Persistent pain

   a. Is also known as chronic nonmalignant or benign pain

   b. Has a known or unknown physical pathology that is resistant to treatment (McCaffery, 1979)

B. Epidemiology

1. Prevalence

a. The management of pain is becoming a higher priority in the United States as evidenced by health policy makers, health professionals, regulators, and the public becoming more knowledgeable about pain management (American Academy of Pain Medicine [AAPM] & American Pain Society [APS], 1997).

b. The National Institutes of Neurological Disorders and Stroke (NINDS) estimate chronic pain to be the third largest health problem in the United States. Pain accounts for 40 million visits per year to physicians for "new" pain (NINDS, 1998).

c. "According to the American Chronic Pain Association, 86 million Americans are affected by chronic pain to some degree—that's 1 out of 3 Americans" (Cooper, 1995, p. 1).

d. "Sixty-five million Americans suffer from painful disabilities each year" (Menard, 1999, p. 1).

2. Cultural considerations

a. "The face of American society is changing from white to multicolored, from European-American to African- and Asian-American, from one that is almost exclusively of the Judeo-Christian tradition to one that encompasses Islam, Hinduism, Buddhism, and other religious traditions" (Showalter, 1997, p. 1). This changing population has implications for how pain is assessed and managed.

b. All personal experiences are perceived through the culture from which one emerges. In other words, different cultures reinforce different behaviors (Swartz, 1998).

1) One person's heritage may promote "being strong" (stoic) as opposed to "expressing oneself" (emotive), which causes the person's response to pain to differ from a person of another heritage.

2) "Expressive patients often come from Hispanic, Middle Eastern, and Mediterranean backgrounds, while stoic patients often come from Northern European and Asian backgrounds" (Showalter, 1997).

3) Southeast Asian and Native American cultures frequently express their illness through altered states of consciousness (e.g., trances, hallucinations) (Swartz, 1998).

c. Rehabilitation nurses must have an understanding of the impact of culture on the patient's pain experience.

1) Through personal and professional experience
2) By reviewing research findings

d. Rehabilitation nurses collaborate with the patient to develop a care plan that strives to improve health status in a holistic and cost-effective manner.

3. Age: Pain disorders and the perception of pain cross all age ranges.

4. Gender

a. The expression of pain is readily acceptable by women in Western society; however, men are expected to be stoic.

b. There is a cultural bias in which women may not be taken seriously when reporting their level of pain and men who report pain may be given a greater level of credibility (Ellis & Nowlis, 1994).

C. Etiology

1. Acute pain: The result of trauma or injury (e.g., accidents, falls, burns), disease processes, medical treatments and diagnostics, postsurgical interventions, and disease processes

2. Chronic pain: Can be the result of everything noted in acute pain, however, the pain prevails despite healing. "The cause of chronic pain is often unknown, and if the cause is known, the pain does not respond to usual therapy" (Leo & Huether, 1998, p. 423).

D. Pathophysiology of Pain (Leo & Huether, 1998)

1. Origin of the stimulus: Nociceptors

a. Nociceptors are naked nerve endings found at the ends of small unmyelinated and lightly myelinated afferent neurons.

b. Unimodal nociceptors are mechanosensitive only. They are found in the skin, mucous membranes, and some wall linings of body cavities.

c. Polymodal nociceptors are mechanosensitive, thermosensitive, and chemosensitive. They are more common and are found in deep tissue and the skin.

2. Stimulus transmission

a. Stimulation of nociceptors produces impulses that are transmitted through Ad-fibers and C-fibers to the spinal cord where they form synapses with neurons in the dorsal horn.

  1) Most terminate ipsilaterally but some terminate contralaterally.
  2) Although the clinical significance of this is unclear, it may explain why pain returns after these fibers are surgically dissected.

b. Myelinated Ad-fibers transmit rapidly and are responsible for the initial pain response, whereas small, unmyelinated C-fibers produce a slower response and are believed to be felt several seconds after an injury (e.g., if you touch a hot stove, Ad-fibers cause you to withdraw your hand prior to C-fibers transmitting the burning pain sensation).

c. "Ad-fibers terminate in lamina I, the marginal zone, lamina II, the substantia gelatinosa, and lamina V of the spinal cord" (Leo & Huether, 1998, p. 426).

  1) Pain that returns after surgical resection of these fibers is most likely related to the crossing of these fibers.
  2) "Secondary neurons transmit the information from the substantia gelatinosa and laminae to the ventral and lateral horn, crossing, in the same or adjacent spinal segments, to the other side of the cord. From there the impulse is carried through the spinothalamic track to the brain" (Leo & Huether, 1998, p. 426).

d. Acute pain is noted in the neospinothalamic tract, whereas dull and burning pain is noted in the paleospinothalamic tract.

3. Termination of the stimulus

a. The neospinothalamic tract transmits information to the midbrain, postcentral gyrus, and the cortex.

b. The paleospinothalamic tract transmits information to the reticular formation, pons, limbic system, and the midbrain.

II. Pain Theories

A. Specificity Theory

1. Proposes cutaneous stimulation of touch, warmth, cold, and pain at specific skin receptor sites: "Stimulation of the pain receptor nerve endings precipitates transmission of the painful stimuli" (Leo & Huether, 1998, p. 426).

2. "Postulates a direct relationship between the stimulus and the perception of pain: It does not take into account the adaptation to pain or the psychosocial implications" (Leo & Huether, 1998, p. 426).

B. Intensity Theory

1. Suggests that pain is the result of excessive or intense stimulation of sensory receptors

2. Does not account for why some intense stimulation of sensory sites does not result in the perception of pain

C. Pattern Theory

1. Proposes that the perception of pain is directly related to the stimulus intensity (i.e., length of time and amount of tissue involved) and the summation of the impulses

2. Raises concerns due to the lack of agreement among theorists of where the summation is received (brain vs. spinal cord) and the lack of accountability for adaptation

D. Gate Control Theory

1. Is the most widely accepted theory of pain

2. Postulates a "gating mechanism" within the spinal cord ("The Gate Control Model Opens A New Era In Pain Research," 1998)

  a. Nociceptor impulses are transmitted from specific skin sites via large A- and small C-fibers to the spinal cord, terminating in the substantia gelatinosa.

  b. The cells of the substantia gelatinosa function as the gate: The large, fast conducting fibers "close the gate," and the small, slower cells "open the gate."

    1) The closed gate results in a decrease in the stimulation of trigger cells, a decrease in pain impulses, and a decrease in pain perception. If persistent stimulation of the large fibers occurs, it results in adaptation.

2) The opposite occurs with an open gate. Increased stimulation of trigger fibers, increased transmission of impulses, and increased pain perception occurs when the substantia gelatinosa opens the gate.

c. In addition to the substantia gelatinosa control of the gate, the central nervous system (CNS) may open, close, or partially close the gate ("The Gate Control Model Opens a New Era in Pain Research," 1998) (see Figure 13-1).

III. Clinical Manifestations of Pain

A. Acute Pain

1. Indicator: The individual promptly seeks attention to relieve the pain.

2. Types

a. Somatic pain

1) Refers to the skin or surface area of the body

2) Presents symptoms such as sharp and well-localized pain; dull, aching, poorly localized pain; and accompanying nausea and vomiting (Leo & Huether, 1998)

b. Visceral pain

1) Refers to internal organs, abdomen, or skeleton

2) Presents specific symptoms

a) Poorly localized pain due to the small number of mechanoreceptors involved

b) Nausea and vomiting

c) Hypotension

d) Restlessness

e) Shock (in some cases)

3) Is usually perceived at a different site of the body and radiates away from the actual site of the pain

c. Referred pain

1) Involves pain that is present in an area that is removed from the original site of pain

2) Involves both the same spinal segment that supplies the actual site of pain and the referred site: As the stimulation transpires, the brain center cannot distinguish between the two sites of pain.

3. Manifestations

a. Physiological responses (in response to a warning of or actual tissue damage)

1) Increased heart rate, respiratory rate, blood pressure, and blood sugar level

2) Decreased gastric acid secretion and motility and blood flow to the viscera and skin

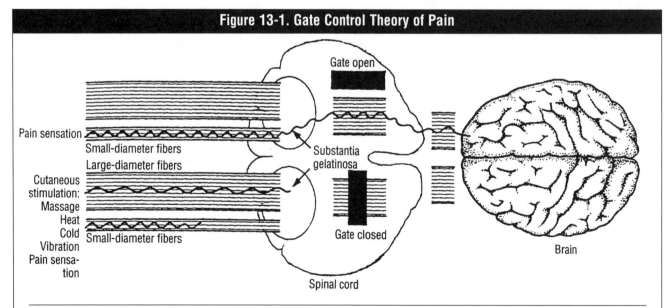

Figure 13-1. Gate Control Theory of Pain

Pain sensation
Small-diameter fibers
Large-diameter fibers
Cutaneous stimulation: Massage Heat Cold Vibration Pain sensation
Small-diameter fibers
Gate open
Substantia gelatinosa
Gate closed
Spinal cord
Brain

Reprinted with permission of W.B. Saunders Company and D.D. Ignatavicius from Ignatavicius, D.D., & Bayne, M.V. (1991). *Medical-surgical nursing: A nursing approach* (p. 109). Philadelphia: W.B. Saunders. (Modified by permission from Potter, P.A., & Perry, A.G. [1989]. *Fundamentals of nursing: Concepts, process, and practice.* St. Louis: Mosby.)

3) Pallor and flushing, dilated pupils, and diaphoresis
    b. Psychological responses: Fear, anxiety, and uneasiness while the person waits for information about the cause, treatment options, and prognosis of acute pain
    c. Behavioral response: Promptly seeks attention to relieve the pain
B. Chronic Pain
    1. Literature review: The accepted definition of chronic pain is pain that persists for longer than 6 months that is either persistent or intermittent.
    2. Suspected nervous system alterations
        a. A decreased level of endorphins
        b. A predominance of C neuron stimulation and neuron sensitivity change
        c. Spontaneous impulses arising from regenerating peripheral nerves
        d. Alterations in dorsal root ganglia as a resultant to a peripheral nerve injury
        e. A change in pain inhibition in the spinal cord
    3. Manifestations
        a. Physiological responses
            1) Intermittent pain mimics acute pain.
            2) Persistent pain allows the body to adapt, resulting in normal or near-normal physiologic presentation without accompanied pain relief.
        b. Psychological responses
            1) Depression
            2) Sleep disturbances (either too much or not enough)
            3) Appetite changes
            4) Potential for being fixated on the pain syndrome itself
        c. Behavioral responses
            1) In one extreme, the patient experiencing pain may be so overwhelmed with the pain that he or she pushes all other life experiences aside.
            2) On the other extreme, the patient experiencing pain may make all attempts possible to block the pain from taking over his or her life (e.g., the patient may decline to discuss the pain or may even participate in activities that place the patient at risk for harm).

IV. Variances in Pain Across the Life Span
A. The Role of the Rehabilitation Nurse
    1. Systematically assess the various dimensions of pain and their impact on the individual's quality of life
    2. Acknowledge that pain is a multidimensional problem that affects the individual's functioning level, psychological being, social interactions, and family and friends
    3. Give high priority to the patient's self-report, the family's report, observed behaviors (e.g., verbal, vocal, and body language), and physiological measures (McCaffery, 1997) (see Table 13-1)
    4. Recall that "unfortunately, in many infants, young children, or children with cognitive or physical impairments, self-report is not available, and behavioral or biological measures must be used" (McGrath, Unruh, & Finley, 1995, p. 1) [see *"Research Perspective"* in this chapter.]
    5. Remember that the perception of pain crosses all age ranges and special attention must be focused on young and elderly people.

B. Infants
    1. Infants experience pain but can't express where they hurt or the way they feel ("Assessment of Pain in Children," 1999).
    2. Parents are the advocates when an infant, child, or child with physical or cognitive impairments cannot communicate.
    3. Pain is generally recognized by a disturbance in infant behavior, such as a change in vocal or facial expression or body movement (McGrath et al., 1995).
        a. A cry that is not relieved by feeding, changing, or comforting
        b. A change in facial expression: Lowered and drawn-together eyebrows, a vertical bulge between the brows in the forehead, tightly closed eyes, an open squarish mouth, or chin quivers (Leo & Huether, 1998)
    4. It is essential to perform a thorough assessment to rule out any contributing physiological involvement.

  a. Elevated heart rate, blood pressure, and respiration (noted only with sharp, acute pain)

  b. Flushing, pallor, and diaphoresis (noted in acute, sharp pain episodes)

C. Toddlers

 1. Toddlers may express pain through crying, facial expressions (as in infants), agitation, aggression, rocking, and rubbing or guarding a body part with their hands.

 2. Delays in healing, as well as changes in the child's sleep, appetite, or play schedule may develop if pain is left untreated (O'Connor-Von, 1999).

D. Preschoolers

 1. May be able to indicate the presence of pain but not identify its location

 2. Identify pain through descriptors such as "hurt," "owie," or "boo-boo" (McGrath et al., 1995): Rehabilitation nurses must collaborate with parents to determine the language used at home to identify pain.

3. Can indirectly indicate their pain through parents' reports of the child not acting normally

4. Can express the amount of pain they are experiencing by using their hands: Putting the hands together (as if praying) indicates little or no pain, whereas holding the hands far apart indicates the most pain (O'Connor-Von, 1999).

5. Can begin to use formal instruments to indicate where they have pain (see Figures 13-2 and 13-3)

  a. Faces scale: A series of faces from happy (no pain) to very upset (the worst

---

Table 13-1. Pain Assessment Tool

Physiological	Pain History	Observed Behaviors	Family Involvement	Role Changes
Complete physical	Causal factor	Nonverbal behavior	Is there family support?	Home
Diagnostics	Onset	Facial expressions	Does the family reinforce pain behaviors?	School
Psychosocial history	Location	Body language	Is the family supportive of the patient's recovery?	Work
Past history	Intensity		What are the family's financial concerns?	Church
Family history	Variation over 24 hours			Community
Review of records	What aggravates it			
Collaboration with colleagues	What eliminates it			
	Current treatments			
	Medication regime			
	Adjunct therapies			
	Sleep patterns			
	Appetite changes			
	Coping patterns			
	Mood			
	Substance use			
	Activities and exercise			
	Family functioning			
	Cultural influences			
	Education of diagnosis			

Sources consulted

McCaffery, M. (1979). *Nursing management of the patient with pain* (2nd ed.). Philadelphia: Lippincott.

Swartz, M.H. (1998). Caring for patients in a culturally diverse society. In M.H. Swartz (Ed.), *Textbook of physical diagnosis: History and examination* (3rd ed., pp. 43-69). Philadelphia: W.B. Saunders.

pain possible) are shown to the child who is asked to point to the face that most resembles how he or she feels.

b. Number scales: The child is asked to rate the pain with 0 representing "no pain" and higher numbers representing "the worst pain." Scales of 0–5 or 0–10 are used.

c. Poker Chip Tool: Can be instrumental at this age because it is well validated and concrete.

1) Four poker chips are placed in front of the child. The chips are described as pieces of hurt.

2) The first chip is described as "just a little hurt," the second is "a little

---

Figure 13-2. Pain Diagram

Pain Diagram

Mark the areas on this body where you feel the described sensations.
Use the appropriate symbols.
Mark areas of radiation.
Include all affected areas.

Numbness	Pins & Needles	Burning	Aching	Stabbing
- - - - -	00000	xxxxx	*****	/ / / / /
- - - - -	00000	xxxxx	*****	/ / / / /
- - - - -	00000	xxxxx	*****	/ / / / /

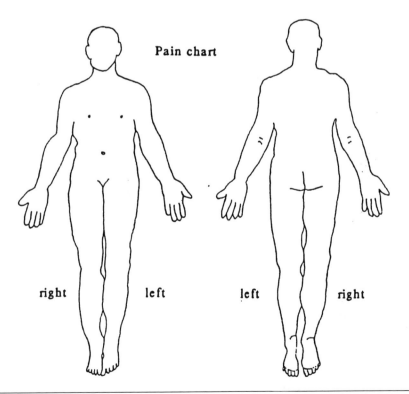

Pain chart

right   left   left   right

Reprinted with permission of Aspen from Skogsbergh, D.R., & Chapman, S.A. (1994). Dealing with the chronic patient. *Topics in Clinical Chiropractic, 1*(4).

---

more hurt," the third chip is "more hurt," and the fourth chip is "the most hurt you could have."

   3) The child is asked, "How many pieces of hurt do you have?" (McGrath et al., 1995).

   d. Body outlines: The child is asked to color on the picture to show where his or her pain is.

E. School-aged Children
   1. Can use some descriptors (e.g., shooting, stabbing, burning)
   2. Can use the faces and numbers scales

F. Adolescents and Adults
   1. Can provide a self-report of their pain using various instruments such as word descriptors and numerical scales
   2. Are able to participate in a full assessment

G. Elderly People
   1. Self-reports of pain are the most reliable.
   2. Rehabilitation nurses should incorporate several factors when assessing an elderly person's pain.
      a. Provide a quiet milieu
      b. Proceed at a slow pace
      c. Allow sufficient time for the person to respond
      d. Use direct and focused questioning
      e. Exchange information at a volume the person can hear
      f. Use enlarged written information
      g. Involve the family or caregiver to fill in details of the person's condition, especially if the person is fatigued or has cognitive deficits (e.g., deficits in memory, attention span, language [aphasia], visual-spatial skills, or fatigue) (Todd, 1997)
      h. Use questions that are age-appropriate
         1) Where do you hurt?
         2) Does the pain stay there or move around?
         3) Is the pain always there?
         4) Does the pain interrupt your sleep or prevent you from falling asleep?
         5) What are you unable to do because of the pain (e.g., activities of daily living [ADLs], shopping, housekeeping, visiting with friends, going to church)?
         6) What has worked in relieving your pain in the past?
         7) What has not worked in the past? (Kruse, 1999)
      i. Use assessment tools, including word scales with descriptors (e.g., mild, moderate, or severe), the 0–10 number scale, and the faces scale (see Figure 13–3). The faces scale may be most appropriate for individuals with dementia or aphasia (Todd, 1997).
   3. Several factors may inhibit appropriate pain management in elderly people.
      a. Fear of addiction to or side effects of pain medications
      b. A belief that pain is the inevitable consequence of aging and that reporting pain may indicate that something more serious is wrong (e.g., if the healthcare provider does not ask about the pain, the older patient may perceive that it should not exist)
      c. A tendency to be uncomfortable with medical technology and, if provided with unfamiliar equipment, a fear of using or breaking it
   4. Healthcare providers may not manage an elderly person's pain properly due to the inaccurate perception that elderly people experience less pain.
      a. Healthcare providers may believe that if the patient does not report pain, he or she is not experiencing it.
      b. Elderly people's sensitivity to the side effects of pain medications, especially narcotics, may indicate that these should be avoided.

V. The Effects of Pain on Family and Society
   A. Effects on Family Roles
      1. Pain affects the entire family.
      2. When an individual is sick, other members of the family often must carry out the sick person's responsibilities. In a short-term illness, this is usually not a problem; however, when the episode becomes chronic, the effects on the family become evident.

a. Adversely effects on relationships

b. Emotional liability

c. Health problems

3. Rehabilitation nurses should involve the family (with the patient's permission) whenever possible.

4. The family's support can reinforce the positive outcomes the patient has established (Lubkin & Jeffrey, 1998).

B. Effects on Society

1. AAPM (1996) reported that 65 million Americans suffer from painful disabilities each year and that nearly 90% of all diseases are identified because of pain.

2. Chronic pain is one of the most costly health problems in America according to the National Institute of Health (NIH) (University of Kentucky HealthCare Chandler Medical Center, 1999).

3. The effects of pain rapidly accumulate ("Peptides Implicated in Body's Response to Pain," 1998).

a. $65 billion lost in work productivity and 4 billion workdays

b. 90 million visits per year to physicians for "new" pain

c. $3 billion in sales of over-the-counter analgesics

4. These statistics do not take into account the

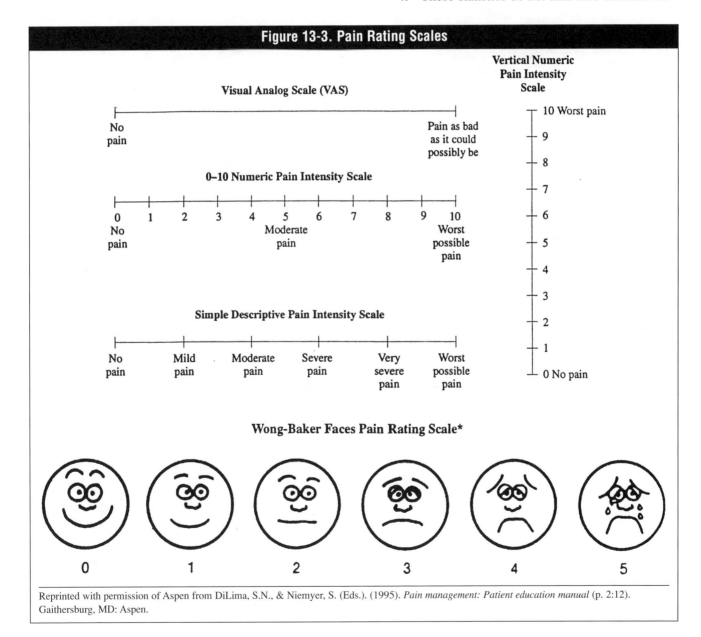

Figure 13-3. Pain Rating Scales

Reprinted with permission of Aspen from DiLima, S.N., & Niemyer, S. (Eds.). (1995). *Pain management: Patient education manual* (p. 2:12). Gaithersburg, MD: Aspen.

detrimental effects of pain and suffering by the patient and family.

VI. Pain Management

A. Overview
1. Pain management is a complex biological, psychological, social, spiritual, and cultural process.
2. Pain behaviors vary from individual to individual.
   a. Verbal indicators (i.e., what the patient reports) are considered the most useful.
   b. Nonverbal indicators (i.e., observable behaviors) often complement the picture and help design an individualized treatment plan.
3. Simon & McTier (1996) outlined a scale with 10 indicators that was developed and is in use at the University of Alabama at Birmingham (UAB) in which the healthcare professional observes the patient's pain.
   a. Verbal vocal complaints
   b. Nonverbal vocal complaints
   c. Down time (i.e., time spent lying down each day between 8 am and 8 pm because of pain)
   d. Facial grimaces
   e. Standing posture (e.g., stooped, favoring one side of the body)
   f. Mobility (e.g., limping, slow pace)
   g. Body language (e.g., clutching or rubbing site of pain)
   h. Use of visible supportive equipment (e.g., braces, crutches, cane)
   i. Stationary movement (e.g., squirming, restlessness)
   j. Use of medication
4. Frequent use of the healthcare system (e.g., scheduled office appointments, ER visits, "doctor shopping") are other behaviors to consider when working with patients (Simon & McTier, 1996).
5. Rehabilitation nurses work with the patient to teach him or her about the diagnosis and available treatment options (see Table 13-2) and help the patient establish realistic goals (ARN, 1994).
6. Because most chronic pain is not curable, the goal is to help the patient improve his or her quality of life and return to enjoyable activities.

B. Using an Outcomes Approach to Pain Management
1. Description: Inconsistent and ineffective pain management continues to be noted by patients, healthcare professionals, and the insurance industry (Barnason, Merboth, Pozehl, & Tietjen, 1998).
2. Roles of the rehabilitation nurse: The determination of the patient's pain status and the extent of its communication through nursing interventions are necessary steps toward achieving patient outcomes (Malek & Olivieri, 1996).
   a. Assess the patient
   b. Observe all cues (verbal, nonverbal, family report)
   c. Diagnose the patient's pain
   d. Coordinate and facilitate appropriate interventions for better pain management
   e. Establish rapport with the patient
   f. Educate the patient on the various resources available and advocate for their implementation
   g. Help the patient and other healthcare providers eliminate the myths that may have previously blocked pain management (see Figures 13-4 and 13-5)

C. Applying the Nursing Process to Pain Management
1. Assess the patient: Interview the patient, communicate, observe, and collect, verify, and organize the data
2. Diagnose: State the actual or potential healthcare problems
3. Plan: Set healthcare priorities based upon the patient's input and develop goals for nursing interventions
4. Implement the plan: Collect data on an ongoing basis and revise the plan as needed to help the patient reach the highest level of wellness
5. Evaluate the outcomes: Determine whether goals are achieved
6. Manage care: Build rapport with the patient

Table 13-2. Pharmacological and Nonpharmacological Pain Management

Type of Treatment	Interventions		Indicators	Action
Over-the-counter drugs	Acetaminophen	(APAP)	Inflammatory pain	Blocks pain impulses by inhibiting prostaglandin synthesis in the CNS
	Aspirin	(ASA)		
NSAIDs (not limited to those listed here)	Diclofenac sodium	(Voltaren)	Inflammatory pain and bone pain	Inhibits prostaglandin synthesis
	Ketoprofen	(Orudis)		
	Naproxen sodium	(Anaprox)		
Antidepressants	Nortriptyline hydrochloride	(Pamelor)	Neuropathic pain	Inhibits the reuptake of serotonin
	Imipramine hydrochloride	(Tofranil)		
	Sertraline hydrochloride	(Zoloft)		
	Paroxetine hydrochloride	(Paxil)		
	Fluoxetine hydrochloride	(Prozac)		
	Amitripyline pamoate	(Elavil)		
Anticonvulsants	Phenytonin sodium	(Dilantin)	Neuropathic pain, facial pain	Decreases abnormal impulses in the nervous system
	Gabapentin	(Neurotin)		
	Divalproex sodium	(Depakote)		
	Carbamazepine	(Tegretol)		
Benzodiazepines	Diazepam	(Valium)	Muscle spasms	Depresses the CNS at the limbic and subcortical levels of the brain
	Midazolam hydrochloride	(Versed)		
Muscle relaxants	Methocarbamol	(Robaxin)	Skeletal muscle pain and spastic pain	Reduces impulse transmission from the spinal cord to skeletal muscle
	Baclofen	(Lioresal)		
	Carisoprodol	(Soma)		
	Cyclobenzaprine hydrochloride	(Flexeril)		
Other (nonopioids)	Tramadol hydrochloride	(Ultram)	Moderate to severe pain	Uses synthetic mu agonist, inhibits reuptake of serotonin
Antiarrhythmics	Lidocaine hydrochloride	(Lidocaine)	Neuropathic pain	Interferes with transmission of nerve impulses
	Mexiletine hydrochloride	(Mexitil)		
Transdermal patch	Fentanyl transdermal	(Duragesic)	Moderate to severe pain	Binds with opiate receptors in the CNS, altering the perception and emotional response to pain
Opioids	Meperidene hydrochloride	(Demerol) ↑ conf.	Moderate to severe pain	Binds with opiate receptors in the CNS, altering the perception and emotional response to pain
	Morphine sulfate	(Morphine)		
	Codeine sulfate	(Codeine)		

Note. Avoid meperidene, which can be a cortical irritant ("Pain Disorders," 1999).

Type of Treatment	Interventions	Indicators	Action
Cutaneous stimulation	Cold	Decreased nerve conduction, inflammation, and muscle spasms	Reduces pain associated with acute sprains, strains, low back pain, and abdominal pain
	Heat	Vasodilation, increased oxygen and nutrients to damaged tissue, and increased metabolic rate	Reduces pain associated with chronic musculoskeletal injuries, tendonitis, and non-inflammatory arthritis
	Mechanical pressure: Massage	Decreased edema, increased blood flow, decreased muscle spasms, and break-up adhesions	Reduces edema of complex regional pain syndromes i.e., mastectomy, overused muscles, and contractures following burns
Electrical stimulation	Transcutaneous electrical nerve stimulation (TENS)	High frequency to block spine transmission; low frequency to increase the production of endorphins	Reduces pain associated with post-op, neuropathies, HIV, shingles, PVD, phantom pain, and nerve damage
Implantable therapies	Spinal cord stimulation	To block the pain signal to the brain	Reduces pain associated with nerve damage and moderate to severe pain
	Intrathecal pain therapy	To block the pain message to the brain by directing small doses of medicine (morphine) that bind to pain receptors in the spinal cord	Reduces unrelenting, intractable pain
Therapies	Independent exercise Physical therapy Occupational therapy	To prevent contractures and muscle atrophies	Reduces pain associated with all syndromes, unless contraindicated
Counseling	Psychotherapy Individual therapy Group therapy Support groups	To increase patient's coping skills and provide support to the patient and family	Alleviates chronic pain syndromes
Alternative therapies	Acupuncture	To provide a local analgesic effect (i.e., the "chi") and stimulate chemical modulators	Reduces musculoskeletal pain
	Art Biofeedback Distraction Meditation Music Prayer Slow rhythmic breathing	To decrease the focus on pain and redefine pain cognitively	Reduces muscle tension and works as an adjunct to pharmacological interventions

Table 13-2. Pharmacological and Nonpharmacological Pain Management (Continued)

Type of Treatment	Interventions	Indicators	Action
Cognitive therapies	Relaxation therapy Self-hypnosis Guided imagery Autogenic training	To decrease the focus on pain and redefine pain cognitively	Reduces muscle tension and works as an adjunct to pharmacological interventions
	Patient education	To provide education about medications, implications for various modalities, and developmental lifestyle changes	Alleviates chronic pain syndromes
	Guided imagary	To allow pleasant images to replace pain	
	Autogenic training	To use suggestions to move pain, substitute for pain, or change the meaning of pain	
Pain management	Multidisciplinary	To decrease pain, increase activity tolerance, decrease medication use, and decrease utilization of medical services	

Sources consulted

Harris, J. (1998). Protocols for an interdisciplinary rehabilitation approach to pain management. *Inside Case Management, 5*(2), 8-10.

Pasero, C.L., & McCaffery, M. (1996). Managing postoperative pain in the elderly. *American Journal of Nursing, 96*(10), 39-45.

Todd, C. (1997). *Pain in the elderly, Part 1: Assessing a complex population* [Online]. Available: http://www.nurse.ceu.com/geri.htm.

Figure 13-4. Myths About Pain

- Healthcare providers are the authority on the existence and extent of the patient's pain.

- The patient is not in pain if he or she does not report it.

- Pain is an unavoidable process of aging.

- As a person ages, his or her perception of pain decreases.

- For pain to be "real," it must have an associated physical cause.

- Everything that can be done for the pain is always done.

- Addiction is perceived when a person repeatedly requests something else for pain.

- When pain is reported, it automatically implies a progression of the disease or something else is wrong.

- By requesting additional medication or assistance, the person in pain is making a nuisance of himself or herself.

- The pain a person is experiencing is not worthy of being reported.

Sources consulted

Barnason, S., Merboth, M., Pozehl, B., & Tietjen, M.J. (1998). Utilizing an outcomes approach to improve pain management by nurses: A pilot study. *Clinical Nurse Specialist, 12*(1), 28-36.

Malek, C.J., & Olivieri, R.J. (1996). Pain management: Documenting the decision making process. *Nursing Case Management, 1*(2), 64-73.

Figure 13-5. Nursing Interventions for Pain

Establish a rapport with the patient so he or she can understand the nurse's role in pain management

Teach the patient that he or she is the most accurate reporter of the pain experience

Instruct the patient that all individuals experience pain and that pain is individualized

Educate the patient about pharmacological and adjunct interventions in the management of pain and determine the patient's preferences

Evaluate the patient's response to pharmacological interventions, determine whether an adjunct intervention or additional medication is indicated to potentiate positive outcomes, and facilitate the intervention

Collaborate with other healthcare professionals to advocate for the interventions necessary to help the patient manage his or her pain

Educate the patient on lifelong interventions and facilitate appropriate referrals in managing cost-effective and timely outcomes

---

and family, advocate for appropriate services, collaborate with colleagues, contain costs through early intervention of services and quality outcomes.

D. North American Nursing Diagnosis Association (NANDA) Diagnoses for Pain
   1. Exchanging: Risk for injury
   2. Relating: Social isolation
   3. Valuing: Spiritual distress
   4. Choosing: Ineffective individual coping, ineffective coping in the community, ineffective/compromised family coping, and ineffective management of therapeutic regimen
   5. Moving: Activity intolerance, impaired home maintenance management, and impaired physical mobility
   6. Perceiving hopelessness and powerlessness
   7. Knowing: Knowledge deficit
   8. Feeling: Anxiety and fear (Carpenito, 1995)

Research Perspective

Colwell, C., Clark, L., & Perkins, R. (1996). Postoperative use of pediatric pain scales: Children's self-report versus nurse assessment of pain intensity and affect. *Journal of Pediatric Nursing, 11(4), 375-381.*

The literature reveals that pain management is undertreated in all populations, including pediatrics. The authors specifically examined nurses' use of pediatric pain scales and compared their estimates of children's pain intensity and affect with children's self-reports. This quasiexperimental study examined a patient sample of 120 postoperative children between the ages of 5 and 17. The Analog Chromatic Continuous Scale (ACCS) was used to measure pain intensity, and the McGrath Affective Faces Scale (MAFS) was used to measure the affective pain dimension.

The data analysis found the following:

- Only 36% of the nurses used a pain scale specifically adapted for children.

- Nurses who used the ACCS found the tool better matched the child's self-report of pain intensity than their cohorts who made an estimate of the child's pain intensity.

- Nurses who used the MAFS tool showed an improved rating of the child's anxiety as opposed to those who did not use the tool.

Implications for practice

Effective pain management in all populations, including pediatrics, falls within the role responsibilities of rehabilitation nurses. Research has shown the validity and reliability of various instruments, including the ACCS and the MAFS. These tools helped direct the nurses to discriminate between pain and anxiety and provide the most appropriate pain management interventions. The authors recommended further research in the testing of the reliability and validity of pediatric scales, especially for older children.

Tools demonstrating reliability, validity, and ease of use should be used to supplement patients' self-reports of pain in all populations. As noted in this study, nurses should be educated in the value of these tools, the ease of their use, and their effectiveness in helping to better manage patients' pain. The U.S. healthcare system demands quality, cost-effective interventions that promote positive outcomes for both providers and consumers of services. It is the responsibility of every nurse to manage the patient's pain effectively. Rehabilitation nurses have a responsibility to validate their practice through current research and the nursing process. Advocating for the implementation of accepted research findings into practice and the measurement of outcomes is needed.

References

American Academy of Pain Medicine (AAPM). (1996). *A patient's guide to pain medicine* [Brochure]. Glenview, IL: Author.

American Academy of Pain Medicine (AAPM) & American Pain Society (APS). (1997). The use of opioids for the treatment of chronic pain: A consensus statement. *The Clinical Journal of Pain, 13*(1), 6-8.

Assessment of pain in children: Pediatric. (1999, March). [Online]. Available: http://pedspain.nursing.uiowa.edu/Assess/Assessme.htm

Association for the Care of Children's Health & McGrath, P. (1994). *Measuring pain in children* [Online]. Available: http://pedspain.nursing.uiowa.edu/Assess/Assessme.htm

Association of Rehabilitation Nurses (ARN). (1994). *The pain management rehabilitation nurse: Role description* [Brochure]. Skokie, IL: Author.

Barnason, S., Merboth, M., Pozehl, B., & Tietjen, M.J. (1998). Utilizing an outcomes approach to improve pain management by nurses: A pilot study. *Clinical Nurse Specialist, 12*(1), 28-36.

Carpenito, L.J. (1995). Comfort, altered: Acute pain, chronic pain. In D.L. Hilton (Ed.), *Nursing diagnosis: Application to clinical practice* (6th ed., pp. 205-235, 1138-1143). Philadelphia. J.B. Lippincott.

Colwell, C., Clark, L., & Perkins, R. (1996). Postoperative use of pediatric pain scales: Children's self-report versus nurse assessment of pain intensity and affect. *Journal of Pediatric Nursing, 11*, 375-381.

Cooper, J.R. (1995). *Many people must live with pain daily* [Online]. Available: http://www.coolware.com/health/medical_reported/pain.hlth

DiLima, S.N., & Niemyer, S. (Eds.). (1995). *Pain management: Patient education manual*. Gaithersburg, MD: Aspen.

Ellis, J.R., & Nowlis, E.A. (Eds.). (1994). *Nursing: A human needs approach* (5th ed.). Philadelphia: J.B. Lippincott.

The gate control model opens a new era in pain research. (1998). [Online]. Available: http://www.library.ucla.edu/libraries/biomed/his/PainExhibit

Harris, J. (1998). Protocols for an interdisciplinary rehabilitation approach to pain management. *Inside Case Management, 5*(2), 8-10.

Ignatavicius, D.D., & Bayne, M.V. (1991). *Medical-surgical nursing: A nursing approach*. Philadelphia: W.B. Saunders.

Kruse, L. (1999, May). *Gerontology assessment: Healthcare professional version* [Online]. Available: http://www.nursing.uiowa.edu/sites/Adultpain/GenePain/Geraas

Leo, J., & Huether, S.E. (1998). Pain, temperature regulation, sleep, and sensory function. In K. McCance & S.E. Huether (Eds.), *Pathophysiology: The biological basis for disease in adults and children* (3rd ed., pp. 422-459). St. Louis: Mosby.

Lubkin, I.M., & Jeffrey, J. (1998). In L.B. Ames (Ed.), *Chronic illness: Impact and interventions* (pp. 149-180). Toronto: Jones & Bartlett.

Malek, C.J., & Olivieri, R.J. (1996). Pain management: Documenting the decision making process. *Nursing Case Management, 1*(2), 64-73.

McCaffery, M. (1997). Pain management handbook. *Nursing 97, 27*(4), 42-45.

McCaffery, M. (1979). *Nursing management of the patient with pain* (2nd ed.). Philadelphia: Lippincott.

McGrath, P.J., Unruh, A.M., & Finley, G.A. (1995). Pain management in children. *Pain Clinical Updates, 3*(2) [Online]. Available: http://www.halcyon.com/iasp

Menard, R.G. (1999). *A patient's guide to pain management* [Brochure]. Glenview, IL: American Academy of Pain Medicine (AAPM).

National Institute of Neurological Disorders and Stroke (NINDS). (1998). *Peptides implicated in body's response to pain* [National Institutes of Health (NIH) news release, Online]. Available: http://www.ninds.htm.gov/whatsnew/PRESS WHN/1998/pain.htm

O'Connor-Von, S. (1999, March). *Pain assessment in children: Parent and family version* [Online]. Available: http://pedspain.nursing.uiowa.edu/Assess/Chiasst.htm

Pain disorders. (1999, April). [Online]. Available: http://www.neuropsychiatry.com/boland/pain.html

Pasero, C.L., & McCaffery, M. (1996). Managing postoperative pain in the elderly. *American Journal of Nursing, 96*(10), 39-45.

Peptides implicated in body's response to pain [NIH News Release]. (1998). [Online]. Available: www.ninds.nih.gov/whatsnew/presswhn/1998/pain.htm

Showalter, S. (1997). *Culture and pain: The face of society is changing...* [Online]. Available: http://www.nursing.uiowa.edu/sites/Adultpain/GenePain/Culture.htm

Simon, J.M., & McTier, C.L. (1996). Development of a chronic pain assessment tool. *Rehabilitation Nursing, 21*(1), 13-19.

Skogsbergh, D.R., & Chapman, S.A. (1994). Dealing with the chronic patient. *Topics in Clinical Chiropractic, 1*(4).

Steele-Rosomoff, R. (1996). The painful truth about pain management. *Rehabilitation Nursing, 21*(1), 6.

Swartz, M.H. (1998). Caring for patients in a culturally diverse society. In M.H. Swartz (Ed.), *Textbook of physical diagnosis: History and examination* (3rd ed., pp. 43-69). Philadelphia: W.B. Saunders.

Todd, C. (1997). *Pain in the elderly, Part 1: Assessing a complex population* [Online]. Available: http://www.nurse.ceu.com/geri.htm.

Turk, D. (1993). Assess the person, not just the pain. *Pain Clinical Updates, 1*(3) [Online]. Available: http://www.halcyon.com/tasp/PCU95c.html.

University of Kentucky HealthCare Chandler Medical Center. (1999). *Chronic pain: Statistics of chronic pain* [Online]. Available: www.uk.healthcare.uky.edu/disease/spine/

Suggested resources

Acute Pain Management Guideline Panel. (1992). *Acute pain management in infants, children, and adolescents: Operative and medical procedures—Quick reference guide for clinicians* (AHCPR Pub. No. 92-0020). Rockville, MD: Agency for Health Care Policy and Research (AHCPR), Public Health Service, U.S. Department of Health and Human Services.

Agency for Health Care Policy and Research (AHCPR). (1994). *Management of cancer pain: Clinical practice guidelines* (AHCPR Pub. No. 94-0592). Washington, DC: U.S. Department of Health and Human Services.

Carr, D.B., Jacox, A.K., Chapman, C.R., et al. (1992). *Acute pain management operative or medical procedures and trauma: Clinical practice guideline no. 1* (AHCPR Pub. No. 92-0032). Rockville, MD: Agency for Health Care Policy and Research (AHCPR), Public Health Service, U.S. Department of Health and Human Services.

Copp, L.A., Anderson, V.C., Brown, M.J., Dougherty, R.J., Greenfield, W., Hogan, C.M., Johnson, J.E., Kornfeld, D.S., et al., (1986). *The integrated approach to the management of pain.* [NIH Consensus statement Online]. Available: http://odp.od.nih.gov/consensus/cons/055/055_statement.htm.

Dellasegra, C., & Keiser, C.L. (1999, May). Pharmacologic approaches to chronic pain in the older adult. *The Nurse Practitioner* [Online]. Available: http://www.springnet.com/ce/j/05a.htm

International Association for the Study of Pain (IASP). (1995, July). Pain measurement in children. In *Pain Clinical Updates, 3*(2) [Online]. Available: http://weber.u.washington.edu/~CRC/IASP.html

Keck, J.F., Gerkensmeyer, J., Joyce, B., & Schade, J. (1999, April). *Reliability and validity of the faces and word descriptor scales to measure pain in verbal children* [Online]. Abstract available: http://www.mosby.com/mosby/open/hcom_wong.fm

Kruse, L. (1999, March). *Gerontology assessment: Patient and family version—Adult* [Online]. Available: http:www.nursing.uiowa.edu/sites/AdultPain/GenePain/Geroas

McCaffery, E. (1996). The impacts of pain: Assessing and managing its cost in the workplace. *Business and Health Special Edition, 14*(11A), 3-30.

McCaffery, M. (1996). The scientific method: Clinical practice guidelines facilitate better care of patients with chronic pain. *Continuing Care, 15*(3), 18-20.

McCaffery, M. (1998). How to make the most of non-opioid analgesics. *Nursing 98, 28*, 54-55.

National Institute of Neurological Disorders and Stroke (NINDS). (1989, November). *Chronic pain: Hope through research* (NIH Pub. No. 90-2406) [Online version prepared for Healthtouch (1997, September)]. Available: http://www.health touch.com

O'Connor, S. (1999, March). *Pain assessment in children: Healthcare professional version* [Online]. Available: http://pedspain.nursing.uiowa.edu/Assess/Chiasst.htm

Simon, J.M. (1996). Chronic pain syndrome: Nursing assessment and evaluation. *Rehabilitation Nursing, 21*(1), 6.

Todd, C. (1997). *Pain in the elderly, Part 2: Assessing a complex population* [Online]. Available: http://www.nurse.ceu.com/geri.htm.

Vines, S.W., Cox, A., Nicoll, L., & Garrett, S. (1996). Effects of a multimodal pain rehabilitation program: A pilot study. *Rehabilitation Nursing, 21*(1), 25-30.

Chapter 14

Specific Disease Processes Requiring Rehabilitation Interventions

Karen Cervizzi, MSN RN CRRN CNA

Patricia A. Haldi, MN RN CRRN CDE

Carol Ann Ottey, MSN RNC CRRN

Life with a chronic illness is still life.

Rehabilitation nurses play an important role in caring for people with a wide variety of chronic illnesses and disabilities. This chapter covers the following specific disease processes that require rehabilitation interventions:

- Diabetes mellitus
- Parkinson's disease
- Burns

- Multiple sclerosis
- HIV/AIDS
- Cancer

Coping with a chronic condition is very stressful, and rehabilitation nurses are the ideal practitioners to provide and coordinate the patient and family education and interventions to help the patient integrate the illness into daily life and become as independent as possible. It is very important for rehabilitation nurses to have current knowledge and the requisite skills to prevent complications and modify the effects of chronic conditions regardless of the practice setting.

I. Diabetes Mellitus (DM)

A. Overview

  1. A progressive, chronic, and potentially disabling disease

  2. Is rapidly becoming one of the major health concerns of the 21st century

  3. Involves an increasing number of individuals who require rehabilitation nursing care

    a. DM is a comorbidity condition commonly treated in rehabilitation (along with stroke, heart disease, amputation, renal failure) and is a major management issue: Optimal recovery from any of these conditions relies primarily on the control of acute and chronic hyperglycemia.

    b. DM complicates treatment and can challenge the rehabilitation nurse.

  4. Encompasses a group of genetically and clinically heterogeneous disorders characterized by glucose intolerance in which the body does not produce or properly respond to insulin (American Diabetes Association [ADA], 1998)

B. Types

  1. Type 1

    a. Previously known as insulin dependent diabetes mellitus (IDDM) or juvenile-onset diabetes

    b. Can develop at any age, but usually develops before age 30

    c. Composes 5%–10% of the total number of people with diabetes

  2. Type 2

    a. Previously known as noninsulin dependent diabetes mellitus (NIDDM), or adult-onset diabetes

    b. Composes 90%–95% of the total number of people with diabetes

3. Other types: Insulin resistance is seen in gestational diabetes and diseases such as polycystic ovary disease and acanthosis nigricans.

C. Epidemiology/Incidence (ADA, 1998; Lipsett & Geiss, 1993; National Diabetes Data Group, 1979)

1. In 1998, approximately 123 million people worldwide had diabetes (2.1% of the world's population). It occurs more commonly in minority groups than in the white population.

2. An estimated 10.3 million Americans have diabetes, and an additional 5.4 million are unaware that they have diabetes (this makes up 5.9% of the U.S. population). These numbers are expected to double by 2010.

3. Diabetes is the sixth most common cause of death in the United States and is the leading cause of adult blindness, chronic renal failure, and nontraumatic amputations.

4. Individuals with diabetes have two to four times the risk of atherosclerosis and are three times more likely to have a heart attack or stroke than those who do not have diabetes.

D. Etiology (ADA, 1998)

1. Type 1 diabetes is an autoimmune disorder involving B-cell destruction by islet cell antibodies (ICAs).

2. Type 2 is primarily caused by any one or a combination of the following: islet cell malfunction, diminished insulin release pre- and postinsulin receptor, cellular resistance to insulin in fat, liver, and muscle, loss of first-place insulin release (i.e., insulin released within 10 minutes of eating). Increased insulin production is needed to move glucose into cells. The need for exogenous insulin is variable.

3. Gestational diabetes applies to having glucose intolerance during pregnancy. After pregnancy the intolerance subsides or continues as Type 1 or Type 2. Even if the intolerance returns to normal, chances are high that it will reappear in the future.

4. Secondary diabetes is a result of other disorders or treatments that trigger the diabetes. Frequently, reversing the underlying disorder or stopping the offending agent is impossible

and results in the need for continued diabetes therapy.

5. Risk factors for diabetes
   a. Type 1
      1) Family history of diabetes
      2) Age: Younger than 25 years old
      3) Environmental factors
   b. Type 2
      1) Family history of diabetes
      2) Race: Minorities are at a higher risk than whites
      3) Age: Older than 35 years old
      4) Environmental factors
      5) Obesity: Body fat of more than 25% for men and more than 30% for women
      6) Physical inactivity

E. Pathophysiology

1. Release of insulin (which is a hormone) from the pancreas
   a. Two phases
      1) Phase 1: Stored insulin from beta cells is released within the first 5 minutes after glucose ingestion.
      2) Phase 2: Insulin is released and newly synthesized by beta cells.
   b. Release
      1) Type 1: Endogenous insulin release is deficient. Pathologic and biochemical changes occur in stages. It may take up to 9 years before clinical onset of symptoms occurs (ADA, 1998, p. 175).
      2) Type 2: Endogenous insulin release may be normal, inefficient, or deficient (Lipsett, & Geiss, 1993; Peragallo-Dittko, Godley, & Meyer, 1993; Ridkin, 1988).
   c. Insulin resistance by liver, fat, and muscle cells: Common in obese individuals with Type 2 diabetes
   d. Insulin deficiency: Common in thin individuals with Type 2 diabetes

2. Clinical manifestations (see Table 14-1)

3. Diagnostic criteria for diabetes: Results are confirmed on a subsequent day (The Expert Committee on the Diagnosis and Classification of Diabetes, 1998)

a. For DM (Type 1 or Type 2): Any one of the following tests, plus symptoms of diabetes (e.g., polyuria, polydipsia, polyphagia, unexplained weight loss)

  1) Casual plasma glucose (any time of day without consideration of last meal): More than 200 mg/dl

  2) Fasting plasma glucose (no food for at least 8 hours): More than 126 mg/dl

  3) 2-hour Oral Glucose Tolerance Test (OGTT)/75 gm glucose load test:

More than 200 mg/dl

b. For impaired fasting glucose (IFG): Fasting plasma glucose (i.e., no food for at least 8 hours) of more than 110 mg/dl, but less than 126 mg/dl

c. For impaired glucose tolerance (IGT): 2-hour OGTT of more than 140 mg/dl, but less than 200 mg/dl

F. Management Options

  1. Nutritional therapy

    a. Eliminate the sugar-restricted diet and the idea that only "diabetic" food can be

Table 14-1. Symptomatic Manifestations of Diabetes Mellitus

Primary Symptoms	Secondary Symptoms	Tertiary Symptoms
Poor wound healing	Infection, chronic ulceration, limb amputation	Dysfunctional denial
Skin and feet	Dryness and cracking, callous formation, ulceration, deformities (e.g., Charcot's foot)	Dysfunctional grief
		Body image crisis
		Social isolation
Peripheral neuropathy (e.g., numbness, tingling, pain, decreased sensation in extremities)	Cold intolerance, rest and sleep disturbance, inadequate hand and finger movement (e.g., carpal tunnel syndrome)	Ineffective coping with anxiety, reactive depression, anger
		Marital conflict/divorce
Gastroparesis (e.g., bowel, bladder, sexual dysfunction)	Constipation, urinary retention, UTIs, gastroparesis, vaginal dryness, declined libido, and orgasmic ability	Loss of job, financial stability, self-esteem, and self-worth
Blurred vision, cataracts, blindness, retinopathy	Errors with insulin drawing and mixing, declining ability to visual inspect skin and feet	Loss of ability to provide adequate self-care, causing loss of independence and control over life, living situation, location (i.e., often needing nursing home placement if unable to do self-insulin management)
Hypoglycemia	Mild symptoms (sweating, trembling, impaired concentration, dizziness), severe symptoms (mental confusion, lethargy, unconsciousness)	Falls, accidents
		Hypotension with exercise
		End-stage renal disease
Hyperglycemia	Specific symptoms (polyuria, polydipsia, blurred vision, polyphagia, weight loss), nonspecific symptoms (weakness, malaise, lethargy, headaches), gastrointestinal symptoms (nausea, vomiting, abdominal pain), respiratory symptoms (Kussmaul's, ketonuria, metabolic acidosis hyperventilation, coma)	Microvascular disease
		Macrovascular disease
Weight changes (i.e., more or less than ideal body weight)	Obesity with ideal body weight of more than 25% in women and more than 30% in men; central adipose tissue accumulation; inadequate nutrition	
Chronic systemic dysfunction	Orthostatic hypertension, cardiac denervation, hypoglycemia unaware, proteinuria	

consumed; focus on serving size, not carbohydrate choices

b. Eliminate predetermined nutrition prescriptions based on ADA caloric formulas and shift to individualized meal plans based on the patient's needs and preferences

c. Determine individualized dietary amounts of carbohydrates, fats, and protein according to height, weight, eating habits, food preferences, lipid profile, blood protein, and other medical conditions (e.g., end-stage renal disease)

d. Prescribe meal plans: This is done by the dietitian, who is an essential team member (American Association of Diabetes Educators [AADE], 1998).

   1) Exchange lists for meal planning

   2) Count carbohydrates on three levels

     a) Getting started (basic)

     b) Moving on (intermediate)

     c) Carbohydrate counting (advanced), using carbohydrate/insulin ratios

2. Exercise therapy

a. Exercise options and strategies for self-directed exercise: Identified by a physical therapist (AADE, 1998)

b. Benefits, effects, risks, and precautions: Vary depending on the individual

   1) Age and type of diabetes

   2) Physical conditioning and presence of other chronic diseases

   3) Presence of ketonuria

3. Medication therapy

a. Oral agents

   1) Categories of oral agents include sufonylureas, biguanide, alpha-glucosidase inhibitors, and thiazolidinediones.

   2) Modes of action of oral medications

     a) Stimulate pancreatic insulin production and secretion

     b) Decrease hepatic glucose production

     c) Decrease intestinal glucose absorption

     d) Increase insulin sensitivity (e.g.,

biguanide works in the liver, small instestine, and peripheral tissues to decrease hepatic glucose production and intestinal glucose absorption and improves insulin senstivity)

   3) Medication regimens can be simple or complex with options for monotherapy or polytherapy with dual-agent or triple-agent options.

   4) Complexity of regimen is enhanced with further addition of insulin therapy to oral therapy (e.g., BIDS, bedtime insulin and daytime sulfonylurea, are often used when oral therapy is not effective).

b. Insulin therapy options

   1) Conventional insulin therapy

     a) Daily routine dose(s) of long-lasting insulin (usually NPH or mixture of NPH and regular) either once or twice daily

     b) Factory premixtures of NPH and regular, which are prepared to simplify adminstration, facilitate correct dosing, and encourage compliance by eliminating mixing (e.g., 70/30, 50/50)

     c) Difficult to match typical insulin release pattern of a person without diabetes

   2) Intensive conventional therapy

     a) Daily routine dose(s) of long-lasting insulin (usually NPH or Lente) either once or twice daily, basal dose, with fast-acting insulin boluses: Uses carbohydrate/insulin ratios calculated according to future carbohydrate consumption (White, 1997)

     b) Less difficult to match insulin pattern of a person without diabetes

   3) Insulin pump therapy

     a) Requires high cognitive reasoning and motivation

     b) Provides ability to match typical insulin pattern of a person without diabetes

   c) Provides access to better blood glucose control and a more flexible lifestyle

4) Sliding scale treatment: Predetermined bolus dose of regular insulin, which is not determined by future carbohydrate consumption but rather on actual blood glucose level

5) Injection therapy

   a) Absorption rates differ between sites: The abdomen is the fastest, followed by the arms, thighs, and buttocks.

   b) Injections are routinely given subcutaneously, but are given intramuscularly in emergencies.

   c) Lipohypertrophy usually slows absorption.

   d) Exercise increases the rate of absorption by providing increased blood flow to the injection site.

G. Acute Problems Associated with Diabetes

  1. Hypoglycemia

    a. Causes: Not eating, too much insulin or oral diabetes medication, or extra exercise

    b. Symptoms

      1) Mild: Sweating, trembling, difficulty concentrating, lightheadedness, blurred vision

      2) Specific: Inability to self-treat, mental confusion, lethargy, unconsciousness

    c. Treatment options

      1) Begin with administration of 10–15 g of carbohydrate (5–10 g for children)

      2) Retest blood glucose level after 15 minutes

      3) Give an additional 15 g carbohydrate if blood glucose is still < 70 mg/dl (e.g., three glucose tablets, two tablespoons raisins, 8 oz low fat milk, half a can of regular soda)

      4) Consider preference, allergies, and food intolerance when making treatment choices (e.g., glucose gel for patients with dysphasia)

      5) Be careful not to overtreat and cause rebound hyperglycemia: Adding sugar to orange juice is not a standard of care.

      6) Follow the treatment with a snack or scheduled meal

  2. Hyperglycemia

    a. Causes: Eating too much food, not enough insulin or oral diabetes medication, stress, or illness

    b. Symptoms

      1) Specific: Polyuria, polydipsia, blurred vision, polyphagia, weight loss

      2) Nonspecific: Weakness, malaise, lethargy, headache

      3) Gastrointestinal: Nausea, vomiting, abdominal pain

      4) Respiratory: Kussmaul's breathing, metabolic acidosis, hyperventilation

    c. Treatment options: Insulin and fluids (refer to nursing standards)

H. Nursing Process

  1. Assessment

    a. Gather subjective data: Determine the patient's self-perceived compliance with medical and nutritional prescriptions for medication administration, blood glucose monitoring, meal planning, exercise, foot and skin care, sick-day management, and treatment and preventive methods for high and low glucose levels

    b. Determine the patient's acceptance of the disease, the effect on his or her lifestyle, and perceived social barriers for complying with treatment

    c. Observe the patient's functional ability and physical and psychological barriers (e.g., verbal and nonverbal communication, mobility, vision, cognition)

    d. Observe the patient's ability in self-glucose testing, self-insulin drawing and administration, and foot and skin care

  2. Plan of care

    a. Nursing diagnoses

      1) Ineffective individual coping related to denial and depression

2) Knowledge deficit related to disease cause, progression, and treatments
3) Self-care deficits related to the following:
   a) Physical, social, economical, and psychological barriers and limitations (e.g., medication administration, self-glucose testing)
   b) Neuropathy, limited mobility, and poor vision (e.g., foot and skin care)
   c) Lack of knowledge of target blood glucose levels
   d) Lack of financial and social support systems
   e) Lack of knowledge of follow-up needs and prevention of further complications related to the disease process
4) Altered nutritional intake (more or less than body requirements) related to lack of awareness about serving sizes, limited self-discipline, and compliance with dietary guidelines
5) Sensory-perceptual alterations related to neuropathy
6) Sexual dysfunction related to microvascular and macrovascular impairment

b. Goals
1) State barriers to and develop methods of effective coping
2) Increase level of independent self-administration of medication and glucose testing
3) Perform or direct daily foot checks and skin care
4) Identify adequate nutritional intake according to ADA guidelines
5) Practice selecting proper serving sizes of favorite foods
6) Identify ways to compensate for altered sensory-perceptual sensations
7) Identify individual concerns with and compensate for sexual dysfunction
8) Learn target levels of blood glucose (BG)
9) Identify variances of BG levels and corrective actions

10) Identify and obtain needed adaptive equipment (e.g., talking meters, insulin bottle holders, dose dialing insulin syringes, premixed syringes, magnifying guides)
11) Identify and obtain insurance and Medicare benefits for diabetes education and equipment (e.g., meters, strips, lancets, therapeutic shoes)

3. Interventions
   a. Teach coping strategies (e.g., stress management, breathing exercises)
   b. Provide opportunities for assisted practice with self-medication program (e.g., drawing, mixing, and injecting insulin)
   c. Direct daily self-foot checks and skin care (e.g., using skin cream)
   d. Promote identification and selection of proper food servings
   e. Suggest ways to compensate for altered sensory-perceptual sensations (e.g., wear diabetic socks at night to increase warmth, circulation, and comfort)
   f. Teach compensation for sexual dysfunction (e.g., cream for vaginal dryness)
   g. Teach problem-solving skills to treat and prevent blood glucose variances and to know how to get help
   h. Describe adaptive equipment (e.g., talking meters, insulin bottle holders)
   i. Discuss insurance and Medicare benefits for education, equipment, and continued assistance (e.g., nursing home or assisted living placement, support groups)
   j. Discuss yearly follow-up care (e.g., annual eye exam, HbA1c test, kidney function test)

II. Multiple Sclerosis (MS)

A. Overview
1. A chronic neuroimmunologic condition that affects the white matter of the central nervous system (CNS)
2. Primarily affects adults in the prime years of life
3. Characterized by numerous etiologic possibilities, an uncertain prognosis, and a course that consists of episodes of remission and relapse

4. An unpredictable disease that can result in diverse neurologic impairments and that necessitates a collaborative approach to care

5. A degenerative progressive disease with sites of inflammatory demyelination (loss of the myelin sheath that surrounds the nerve fiber tracts) in the CNS

6. Involves partial or complete destruction of the myelin sheath followed by sclerotic plaques or scar tissue formation

7. Is associated with various signs and symptoms due to the loss of myelin sheath integrity that interfere with the efficiency of nerve impulse conduction within the CNS

B. Epidemiology
1. Incidence
   a. Affects 400,000 Americans
   b. Approximately 8,000–10,000 new cases are diagnosed yearly
   c. A major cause of disability and economic hardship in young adults between the ages of 20 and 40
   d. Occurs more often in women than men, in people who live in colder northern latitudes, in Caucasians, and in people who have first-degree relatives with MS (Phipps, Sands, & Marek, 1999)

2. Disease patterns (Lublin & Reingold, 1996)
   a. Relapsing-remitting MS: The most typical pattern of the disease
      1) Defined by relapses followed by either complete, partial, or no recovery of previous function
      2) Involves no disease progression between relapses
   b. Secondary-progressive MS
      1) Can begin as a relapsing-remitting course followed by progression that is unpredictable
      2) Involves acute attacks that can result in a progressive worsening level of disability
   c. Primary-progressive MS: Identified by a continuous worsening of the patient's disability but with no actual relapses or remissions
   d. Progressive-relapsing MS
      1) Marked by disease progression from the onset with definite acute relapses
      2) Involves disease progression that continues to escalate between relapses

C. Etiology
1. The specific cause remains unknown.
2. Factors that may cause MS are viral, immunologic, and genetic.
   a. A latent viral infection may either cause inflammation of white matter or trigger an autoimmune reaction that precipitates the demyelination process.
   b. Although there is no specific genetic pattern of transmission for MS, researchers support a multigenic predisposition to the disease because specific genetic markers are found more frequently in patients with MS (Ignatavicius, Workman, & Mishler, 1998).

D. Pathophysiology
1. Overview
   a. Normally, an intact blood brain barrier protects the brain from immune cell activity. In MS, the protective barrier is breached as activated T cells, antibodies, and macrophages mistakenly attack the myelin sheath and destroy the oligodendrocytes that produce it (Phipps et al., 1999).
   b. Research suggests that an axonal transection occurs in MS patients (Trapp, Peterson, Ransohoff, Rudick, & Mork, 1998).
   c. Demyelination appears as diffuse and discrete lesions (plaques) throughout the brain and spinal cord.
      1) Although natural healing (remyelination) may restore some myelin function, the characteristic plaque formation or sclerosis interferes with normal nerve conduction.
      2) Nerve impulses slow down initially; eventually, the impulses are completely blocked.
      3) The wide variety of signs and symptoms reflect the anatomic location of the demyelination and plaque formation (Beare & Myers, 1998).

2. Clinical manifestations (see Table 14-2)
   a. Primary symptoms
      1) Occur as the result of the nerve conduction deficits caused by demyelination and plaque formation
      2) Reflect a specific area of dysfunction in the CNS (Beare & Myers, 1998)
   b. Secondary symptoms
      1) Occur as a consequence of primary symptoms
      2) Include problematic complications resulting from decreased neurologic function
   c. Tertiary symptoms
      1) Evolve as the cumulative and detrimental effects of the disease affect all aspects of the person's life
      2) Include psychosocial, vocational, financial, and emotional issues and problems
3. Diagnosis (Phipps et al., 1999)
   a. There is no specific laboratory or radiologic test to definitively diagnose MS.
   b. Because MS can mimic other diseases and the initial symptomatic presentation varies and fluctuates so greatly in severity, MS is difficult to accurately diagnose.

A diagnosis is often made only after more than one occurrence and subsequent relapses (Taggart, 1998).

   c. A diagnosis of MS is based on a history of episodic neurologic disability and actual signs of neurologic dysfunction on physical examination.
   d. Diagnostic tests that can support a suspected MS diagnosis include the following:
      1) Magnetic resonance imaging (MRI)
         a) Pinpoints demyelinated plaque in the CNS
         b) Is used in serial form to monitor disease progression (Halper & Holland, 1998)
      2) Cerebrospinal fluid analysis: Reveals the presence of oligoclonal (immunoglobulin G) bands and increased protein (Halper & Holland, 1998)
      3) Evoked potential studies (somatosensory, auditory, visual): Demonstrates a slowing or delay in electrical impulse conduction (Halper & Holland, 1998)

Table 14-2. Symptomatic Manifestations of Multiple Sclerosis		
Primary Symptoms	**Secondary Symptoms**	**Tertiary Symptoms**
Muscle weakness, paralysis, spasticity, and hyperreflexia	Falls, fractures, skin breakdown, contractures, and other injuries	Loss of job
Mild to disabling fatigue	Marked reduction in carrying out all aspects of self-care	Complete change in roles
Visual impairments (e.g., diplopia, scotoma, decreased acuity)	Decreased safety within the environment due to decreased visual input	Social isolation
Numbness, tingling, pain, and tremors	Interruption in adequate rest and disrupted sleep	Divorce
Bowel, bladder, and sexual dysfunction	UTIs, bowel and bladder incontinence or retention, and marked decline in libido and orgasmic ability	Ineffective coping with anxiety, denial, anger, reactive depression, and suicide
Ataxia, nystagmus, dysarthria (scanning speech), and dysphagia	Problems affecting a safe gait pattern, communication ability, and swallowing function	Loss of financial stability, self-esteem, and self-worth
Cognitive changes (e.g., memory loss, impaired judgment), emotional lability and depression	Marked decline in healthy and effective coping strategies that are implemented to cope with life's challenges	

E. Management Options
1. Goal: To decrease the number and frequency of relapses, alleviate symptoms, maintain independence, and ensure the highest quality of life (Costello & Cerreta, 1998)
2. Pharmacotherapy (see Figure 14-1)
    a. Involves the potential use of drugs from different classes, such as anti-inflammatory agents, immunomodulators, immunosuppressants, and others
    b. Is most often used to treat spasticity and tremor, urinary retention or frequency, chronic pain, fatigue, and depression

---

Figure 14-1. Pharmacotherapeutic Agents Used to Treat MS

Treatment of Acute Relapses
Short course of anti-inflammatory corticosteroids
- Methylprednisolone (Solu-Medrol)
- ACTH
- Prednisone

Treatment to Reduce the Frequency of Relapses
Parenteral injections of immunomodulators (effective for only one or two MS disease patterns)
- Interferon beta – 1b (Betaseron)
- Interferon beta – 1a (Avonex, Rebif)
- Glatiramer acetate (Copaxone)

Treatment of Disease Progression
Immunosuppressants that halt disease progression
- Azathioprine (Imuran)
- Methotrexate (Rheumatrex)

Treatment of Spasticity and Tremor
- Baclofen (Lioresal)
- Dantrolene (Dantrium)
- Tizanidine (Zanaflex)
- Diazepam (Valium)
- Clonazepam (Klonopin)
- Botulinum torin (Botox)

Treatment of Urinary Retention
- Bethanechol chloride (Urecholine)

Treatment of Urinary Frequency and Urgency
- Propantheline (Pro-Banthine)
- Oxybutynin (Ditropan)

Treatment of Chronic Pain Fatigue and Depression
- Carbamazepine (Tegretol)
- Pemoline (Cylert)
- Amitriptyline (Elavil)
- Imipramine (Tofranil)
- Fluoxetine (Prozac)

---

3. Alternative approaches (e.g., bee sting therapy, dietary modifications): Numerous investigational therapy trials are in progress.
4. Use of a collaborative team of professionals, including physicians, physical and occupational therapists, spiritual advisers, social workers, psychologists, vocational rehabilitation specialists, legal advisers, and nurses (Taggart, 1998)

F. Nursing Process
1. Assessment
    a. Obtain a complete health history and information about current symptoms, time of onset, and past history of relapses
    b. Pay particular attention to mental state and overt coping abilities
    c. Determine how the disease has affected the patient's lifestyle and family
    d. Observe the patient's overall appearance
    e. Investigate physical mobility, urinary elimination, self-care activities, and safety concerns
    f. Assess for spasticity, weakness, incontinence, and visual impairments
2. Plan of care
    a. Nursing diagnoses (Beare & Myers, 1998; Smeltzer & Bare, 1996)
        1) Impaired physical mobility related to weakness, spasticity, and tremor
        2) Fatigue related to the MS disease process
        3) Self-care deficits (e.g., bathing, dressing, feeding, toileting) related to weakness, spasticity, and tremor
        4) Alterations in urinary elimination (e.g., retention, frequency, urgency) related to spinal cord involvement and decreased functional ability
        5) Knowledge deficit related to the variable nature of symptoms and multifaceted treatment options
        6) Ineffective individual coping related to the variability of the disease course, cognitive impairments, decreased independence, and changes in family and vocational roles

b. Goals

   1) Improve mobility
   2) Conserve energy
   3) Achieve independence in activities of daily living (ADLs)
   4) Improve bladder function and prevent complications
   5) Improve knowledge about the disease and appropriate treatment options
   6) Develop effective coping strategies

3. Interventions

   a. Improve mobility

      1) Encourage progressive, resistive exercises according to the prescribed physical therapy program
      2) Gradually build up tolerance through a daily exercise program
      3) Use assistive devices (e.g., walker, cane, wheelchair, motorized scooter)
      4) Avoid physical and emotional stressors and exposure to extreme heat

   b. Conserve energy

      1) Avoid vigorous exercise
      2) Ensure the patient gets adequate sleep and takes frequent rests
      3) Space all activities and allow for rest periods

   c. Achieve independence in ADLs

      1) Encourage a balance between assisted and independent activities as necessary
      2) Encourage the use of self-help devices to make care easier
      3) Avoid extremes in body temperature and use air conditioning when needed

   d. Improve bladder function and prevent complications

      1) Avoid giving the patient caffeinated beverages
      2) Teach intermittent self-catheterization or external catheter procedures
      3) Instruct the patient to identify and prevent urinary tract infections (UTIs)

   e. Improve knowledge

      1) Provide information to help manage the disease on a continuous basis
      2) Encourage the patient to ask questions
      3) Review educational information with the patient and family

   f. Develop effective coping strategies

      1) Encourage the patient and family to verbalize feelings and concerns
      2) Refer the patient and family to support groups (e.g., Multiple Sclerosis Association of America, National Multiple Sclerosis Society)
      3) Make referrals for psychological counseling as necessary

III. Parkinson's Disease (PD)

A. Overview

   1. A slowly progressive neurodegenerative disease of the brain
   2. Involves manifestations that occur when there is significant damage to or destruction of dopamine-producing neurons in the substantia nigra within the basal ganglia of the brain
   3. Begins very insidiously and is characterized by a prolonged course of illness
   4. Leads to marked disability with the initiation and execution of smooth coordinated voluntary movements and balance
   5. Involves no known way to stop or cure the disease
   6. Is one of the more common chronic diseases of the nervous system

B. Types

   1. Primary PD

      a. A chronic debilitating disease caused by an idiopathic dopamine deficiency in the basal ganglia of the brain
      b. Characterized by tremor, rigidity, bradykinesia, and postural instability

   2. Parkinsonism syndrome: Refers to a group of symptoms (e.g., tremors, stiffness, slow movements) where there is an exact known cause of injury to the dopamine-producing cells

C. Epidemiology/Incidence

   1. 1.5 million Americans have PD: The disease shows no socioeconomic or cultural preferences.
   2. PD occurs in men slightly more often than women.
   3. PD most commonly occurs after age 50: With an aging population, the prevalence of PD is likely to increase.

The Specialty Practice of Rehabilitation Nursing: A Core Curriculum, 4th Ed.

4. Approximately 10% of people with PD are younger than age 40 (Henkel, 1998).

D. Etiology

1. Primary PD is idiopathic with no known cause.

2. PD may be caused by a combination of genetic and environmental factors (e.g., virus, toxins, free radical exposure) (Beare & Myers, 1998).

3. Secondary parkinsonism is caused by the use of neuroleptic agents in response to brain trauma, tumors, ischemia, encephalitis infections, and arteriosclerosis (Phipps et al., 1999).

E. Pathophysiology

1. Overview

   a. Normally, there is a balance between the neurotransmitters dopamine (DA) and acetylcholine (ACh), which are responsible for controlling and refining motor movements and have opposing effects.

   b. An increase in the excitatory effects of ACh due to depletion of DA causes the manifestations of PD.

   c. A shift in the balance of neurotransmitter activity is responsible for the patient's difficulty in controlling and initiating voluntary movements (Lewis, Collier, & Heitkenper, 1996).

2. Clinical features: Classic manifestations (Phipps et al., 1999)

   a. Tremor

      1) Occurs in the tongue, lips, jaw, chin, and limbs
      2) May involve a "pill rolling" movement of the thumb and finger
      3) Is present at rest and diminishes with active movement

   b. Rigidity or "cogwheeling": Resistance to movement caused by constant contraction of opposing muscle groups due to abnormal muscle stiffness and jerky movements with passive motion

   c. Bradykinesia: Abnormal slowness of movement that hinders the ability to initiate normally spontaneous movements

   d. Postural instability, which causes a stooped-over, flexed posture: Diminished postural reflexes lead to frequent falls that are associated with balance and coordination problems.

   e. Other symptoms: Masklike facial appearance; difficulty with chewing, swallowing, and voice changes; autonomic disturbances (e.g., orthostatic hypotension, constipation, excessive perspiration, oily skin); and numerous cognitive losses (e.g., memory, problem solving, depression)

3. Diagnosis (Phipps et al., 1999)

   a. Diagnosis is made clinically from the patient's history and presenting symptoms.

   b. No specific laboratory or radiologic

Table 14-3. Drugs Prescribed for Symptomatic Control of Parkinson's Disease

Drug Category and Name	Action
Monoamine oxidase B inhibitor: Selegiline (Eldepryl)	Used in the early stages of PD by delaying the breakdown of naturally occurring dopamine
Devodopa, carbidopa, levodopa (Sinemet)	Is the first-line, gold-standard therapy that restores deficient dopamine to the brain without causing extreme, uncomfortable peripheral side effects
Dopamine agonists: Bromocriptine (Parlodel), Pergolide (Permax), Pramipexole (Miropex), Ropinirole (ReQuip)	Directly stimulates the dopamine receptors in the brain to produce more dopamine
Antiviral: Amantadine (Symmetrel)	Acts by releasing dopamine from neuronal storage sites
Anticholinergic: Benzatropine (Cogentin), Trihexyphenidyl (Artane)	Counteracts the action of ACh in the CNS
Catechol-o-methyltransferase inhibitor: Tolcapone (Tasmar)	Used in combination with Sinemet to block the enzyme that metabolizes levodopa, thus allowing more levodopa to be available for conversion to dopamine

studies are available to support a positive diagnosis.

c. Definite diagnosis is made after assessing the patient's response to antiparkinson medications.

F. Management Options
   1. General notes
      a. Currently, there is no known treatment that halts neuronal degeneration.
      b. Current options provide symptom relief and improve the quality of life.
   2. Types of treatment
      a. Pharmacotherapy: Involves the use of drugs from various classes (e.g., monoamine oxidase B inhibitor; levodopa [carbidopa, levodopa]; dopamine agonist; antiviral; anticholinergic; and catechol-o-methyltransferase inhibitor) (Begany, 1997; Phipps et al., 1999; Segatore, 1998) (see Table 14-3)
      b. Surgical interventions: Offer selected patients diminution of some symptoms; however, cannot improve the disease course or guarantee long-lasting disease improvement (Henkel, 1998)
         1) Pallidotomy and thalamotomy: Destroys groups of brain cells that are responsible for some of the most distressing symptoms
         2) Neural transplantation of the adrenal medulla into the basal ganglia: Decreases symptoms
         3) A recently approved device that can be surgically implanted deep within the brain and is connected to a pulse generator: The patient can self-activate the device that blocks the brain signals that cause tremors.

G. Nursing Process
   1. Assessment
      a. Obtain a complete health history and information about current symptoms, time of onset, and progression
      b. Pay particular attention to mental status, ability to answer questions, and overt coping abilities
      c. Determine how the disease has affected the patient and family and ask about

what aspects of the disease are most troublesome

      d. Observe overall appearance, posture, and gait pattern
      e. Determine level of extremity stiffness, tremors, and ability to move
      f. Investigate safe mobility, self-care activities, nutritional intake, and verbal communication
   2. Plan of care
      a. Nursing diagnoses (Monahan & Neighbors, 1998; Smeltzer & Bare, 1996)
         1) Ineffective individual coping related to depression and increasingly severe physical limitations
         2) Knowledge deficit related to disease progression, treatment, ongoing adaptations, and availability of support systems
         3) Impaired physical mobility related to tremor, rigidity, bradykinesia, and postural instability
         4) Self-care deficits (e.g., bathing, dressing, feeding, toileting) related to tremor, rigidity, bradykinesia, and postural inability
         5) Altered nutritional intake (less than body requirements) related to difficulty with chewing, swallowing, and drooling
         6) Impaired verbal communication related to low pitch voice, slow speech, and difficulty moving facial muscles
      b. Goals
         1) Develop positive coping mechanisms
         2) Develop a sound knowledge base about the disease and treatments
         3) Improve mobility
         4) Achieve independence in ADLs
         5) Achieve a satisfactory nutritional status
         6) Improve verbal communication
   3. Interventions
      a. Develop positive coping mechanisms
         1) Allow the patient to freely verbalize feelings and concerns
         2) Encourage participation in support groups (e.g., Parkinson's Disease

Foundation, Parkinson's Support Groups of America, National Parkinson Foundation)

3) Encourage the patient to establish realistic, attainable goals

4) Support the use of prescribed psychotherapy and medication to combat depression

b. Develop a sound knowledge base about the disease and treatments

1) Teach the patient about the common signs, symptoms, and progression of PD

2) Discuss aspects of the disease that are unique to PD and the use of antiparkinson drugs (e.g., "on-off," "wearing off," and "freezing" phenomena)

3) Educate the patient and family about the desired effects and side effects of prescribed medications and surgical treatments

4) Offer suggestions to make living with PD easier

5) Inform the patient and his family of local and national support groups for assistance and education

c. Improve mobility

1) Encourage active and passive range of motion (ROM) exercises according to the prescribed physical therapy program

2) Allow time for rest after activity and avoid rushing

3) Administer medications as prescribed to avoid exacerbation of symptoms

4) Use warm baths and massage to help relax muscles

5) Teach the patient to concentrate on walking erect by consciously using a wide-based gait and deliberately swinging the arms

d. Achieve independence in ADLs

1) Encourage the use of devices to make self-care easier (e.g., raised toilet seats, trapeze bar, grab bars, long-handled shoehorns, elastic shoelaces)

2) Allow adequate time to accomplish self-care

3) Make environmental modifications to enhance safety and independence

e. Achieve satisfactory nutritional status

1) Encourage the patient to sit upright for all meals

2) Offer semisolid foods and thickened liquids if choking occurs

3) Use stabilized plates, plate guards, nonspill cups, and large-handle utensils

4) Augment caloric intake with supplementary feedings

5) Monitor weight weekly

f. Improve verbal communication

1) Reinforce exercises prescribed by the speech-language therapist

2) Inform family and friends to wait for the patient to answer questions

3) Encourage the patient to engage in conversation and read aloud

IV. Human Immunodeficiency Virus (HIV) and Acquired Immunodeficiency Syndrome (AIDS)

A. Overview

1. AIDS was first recognized in 1981 as a serious life-threatening illness and has since become a worldwide epidemic.

2. Although significant breakthroughs in prevention, treatment, and diagnosis have increased survival times, the long-term prognosis for people with HIV/AIDS remains poor.

3. Despite developments and considerable research, no cure or vaccine is available, and the infection rate has remained unchanged worldwide for a decade (Centers for Disease Control and Prevention [CDC], 1998c).

4. It is estimated that 14 million people have died of AIDS since the start of the epidemic (CDC, 1999).

5. Avoiding behaviors that put a person at risk of infection is the only way to prevent the infection.

6. Nurses play a vital role in caring for people with HIV/AIDS and are challenged to stay up-to-date on the most current research, as information in this area is constantly developing.

B. Types
1. AIDS: The most advanced stage of a progressive immune function disorder caused by the retrovirus HIV
2. HIV
   a. Attacks the immune system and leaves the body defenseless to numerous infections and health problems
   b. Involves two strains that cause AIDS but have differing geographic distributions
      1) HIV-1: Accounts for the majority of infections worldwide
      2) HIV-2: Appears to be prevalent in Western African countries but has only limited distribution in other areas
C. Epidemiology (Avert, 1998; CDC, 1998a, 1998c, 1999)
1. Globally, more than 33.4 million people are living with HIV/AIDS, and 1.1 million of them are younger than age 15.
2. 5.8 million new HIV infections were reported in 1998, which is equivalent to 16,000 new infections every day.
3. Women are the fastest growing group of people with HIV/AIDS.
4. HIV/AIDS is the second leading cause of death in people 25–44 years of age.
D. Etiology
1. Natural history: The result of the interaction between the immune system and HIV has been studied since 1981. Considerable progress has been made in understanding the disease.
2. A person with HIV may be asymptomatic for many years and not even know that he or she is infected; however, as the immune system weakens, the person will become ill more often.
3. HIV varies considerably from individual to individual, but once the virus enters the body and infects cells, the course of HIV infection is categorized according to signs, symptoms, and cell count (Bradley-Springer, 1995; Casey, Cohen, & Hughes, 1996).
   a. Primary infection: Period from infection with HIV to the development of HIV-specific antibodies
      1) Onset is 0–12 weeks from initial infection.
      2) Virus infects white blood cells called CD4+ T-cells, which are the master coordinators of the immune system.
      3) Immune system clears virus to lymphatic organs.
      4) The CD4+ T-cell count declines from 1,000/ul to 500/ul.
      5) Physical characteristics are similar to flu or mononucleosis (e.g., fever, arthralgias, myalgias, lymphadenopathy, pharyngitis, anorexia, weight loss).
   b. Clinical latency: Asymptotic period
      1) Onset is 12 weeks–8 years from initial infection.
      2) HIV destroys cells of the immune system.
      3) The virus is present primarily in lymphatic tissue and slowly spreads throughout the body.
      4) Clinical symptoms are usually absent or mild. Vague symptoms include fever, headache, and night sweats.
      5) CD4+ T-cell counts are 500-750/ul.
   c. Early symptomatic HIV disease
      1) Onset is 8–10 years from initial infection.
      2) Viral replication destroys the lymph nodes and allows a greater amount of the virus to be released in circulation.
      3) Signs and symptoms progress from mild to moderate (e.g., frequent fever, sweating, yeast infection, generalized lymphadenopathy, skin rashes, chronic diarrhea, fatigue, memory loss, oral candidiasis, tuberculosis, oral hairy leukoplakia, shingles, thrombocytopenia, increased persistent generalized lymphadenopathy [PGL], Kaposi's sarcoma [KS], developmental delays and failure to thrive [in children]).
      4) CD4+ T-cell counts are 200–500/ul.
   d. Advanced HIV disease/AIDS
      1) Onset is 10–11 years from initial infection.
      2) Immune system fails.
      3) One or more opportunistic infections (OIs) or diseases develop.

4) Clinical manifestations involve the loss of lean body mass and wasting syndrome.
5) CD4+ T-cell counts are 0–200/ul.
6) Death usually occurs from infection, cancer, or wasting syndrome.

E. Pathophysiology
1. Transmission
a. HIV is transmitted from human to human through exposure of infected body fluid (e.g., blood, semen, vaginal secretions, breast milk).
b. Common modes of transmission
1) Sexual contact (e.g., oral, vaginal, anal)
2) Sharing a needle or syringe (e.g., IV drug use, tattooing, body piercing)
3) Blood transfusion
4) Tissue or organ donation
5) Prenatal contact from mother to infant before or during birth or during breastfeeding
6) Occupational exposure (e.g., needle stick)
c. HIV is not spread through casual contact (e.g., touching, hugging, shaking hands, sharing eating utensils, eating food prepared by a person with HIV, coughing, sneezing, using restrooms, touching animals or insects, working or attending school with an HIV-infected person).
2. Clinical manifestations
a. Common signs and symptoms of HIV infection include fever, fatigue, weight loss, sore throat, rash, night sweats, shortness of breath, yeast infection, lymphadenopathy, gastrointestinal distress, pain, and dementia (InteliHealth, 1997; OnHealth, 1998a).
b. Individuals with AIDS are susceptible to OIs, which are life-threatening illnesses caused by organisms that are normally fought off by a healthy immune system (InteliHealth, 1997) (see Figure 14-2).
1) Diagnosis and treatment of OIs are essential to increase life span.
2) Children are susceptible to OIs as well as conjunctivitis, ear infection, and tonsillitis (InteliHealth, 1997).

3. Diagnosis
a. Early testing for HIV will enable appropriate treatment, prevent certain OIs, and alert the HIV-infected person to avoid high-risk behavior to prevent the spread of the infection (Bradley-Springer, 1995).
b. HIV testing should be accompanied by pre- and posttest counseling, education, and risk assessment.
1) Pretest counseling
a) Review test procedures
b) Explain the meaning of positive and negative test results
c) Provide information on HIV and AIDS
d) Set a plan for risk reduction
e) Describe the importance of follow-up care
f) Prepare the patient for potential psychological and emotional reactions to a positive test result
2) Posttest counseling
a) If the test is negative, provide advice on retesting (if the person engages in high-risk behavior) and preventing the spread of HIV
b) If the test is positive, evaluate the person's potential for suicide; provide crisis intervention

---

Figure 14-2. Opportunistic Infections (OIs) Associated with AIDS

Viral: Cytomegalovirus disease, herpes simplex, pneumonitis or esophagitis

Bacterial: Mycobacterium tuberculosis, recurrent pneumonia, recurrent Salmonella septicemia

Protozoal: Pneumocystis carinii pneumonia (PCP), toxoplasmosis of the brain

Fungal: Candidiasis of bronchi, trachea, lungs or esophagus

Neurological: Dementia, headaches

Neoplastic processes: Lymphoma, Kaposi's sarcoma (KS), cervical carcinoma

Wasting syndrome: Chronic diarrhea, weakness, weight loss, constant or intermittent fever for at least 30 days

---

if needed and information on symptoms of HIV/AIDS; teach health maintenance; refer for medical follow-up and tuberculosis (TB) screening, support groups, clinical trials, or experimental protocols; and discuss potential discrimination

 c. Confidentiality with HIV testing is very important, because disclosure may result in discrimination.

 d. Types of test available (CDC, 1998b)

  1) Antibody testing

   a) Detects the presence of antibodies to HIV

   b) Involves a delay of 3 weeks to 6 months before a detectable antibody is produced

  2) Antigen testing

   a) Detects the virus (HIV RNA) in the blood

   b) Is detectable 1 week earlier than antibody testing, but the test is labor intensive and costly (InteliHealth, 1997)

   c) May be performed if an antibody test is negative and the person is highly likely to be positive

F. Management Options

 1. Early intervention allows the individual to survive longer: Research has focused on antiretroviral agents to inhibit disease progression, prophylactic therapy to prevent OIs, therapy to restore the damaged immune system, and vaccine development (Bradley-Springer, 1995).

 2. The Food and Drug Administration (FDA) has approved a number of drugs for treating HIV infection.

  a. Nucleoside analog reverse transcriptase inhibitors: AZT (zidovudine), ddC (zalcitabine), ddI (didanosine), d4T (stavudine), and 3TC (lamivudine)

  b. Non-nucleoside reverse transcriptase inhibitors: Delvaridine (Rescriptor), and nevirapine (Viramune)

  c. Protease inhibitors: Ritonavir (Norvir), saquinivir (Invirase), indinavir (Crixivan), and nelfinavir (Viracept)

 3. The most effective treatment strategy is combination drug therapy because a combination of drugs can attack different stages of the HIV life cycle and produce a more sustained antiviral effect in a person with HIV.

 4. A number of treatments are available for some opportunistic diseases (e.g., radiation and chemotherapy for KS and other forms of cancer, pentamidine to treat pneumocystic carinii pneumonia [PCP]).

  a. Adults with HIV whose CD4+ T-cell counts drop below 200/ul are given prophylactic treatment to prevent the occurrence of PCP. Those that have survived an episode of PCP are given medications to prevent reoccurrence (InteliHealth, 1997).

  b. A study done by CDC and the Cote d'Ivoire Ministry of Public Heath found the first evidence that trimethoprim/sulfamethoxazole can significantly reduce the death rate among HIV-infected tuberculosis patients in Africa (CDC, 1998a).

 5. Alternative and complementary therapies include therapeutic touch, massage therapy, meditation, imagery, tai chi, and herbal medicine.

 6. Health promotion and disease prevention can be effective to prevent the spread of infection.

  a. Promote a lifestyle that prevents or decreases the risk of HIV infection

  1) Abstain from sexual activity or use a condom for all insertive sexual practices with a partner who has or may have HIV

  2) Stop using IV drugs; stop sharing needles and equipment; use a clean needle and syringe or disinfect them after each use; decrease the number of injections; and avoid engaging in risky sexual activity

  3) Screen all potential blood donors for high-risk behaviors and signs and symptoms of AIDS and test all human tissue for transplantation for HIV antibodies

4) Adhere to safety guidelines to prevent occupational exposure

b. Promote a healthy lifestyle in people who are already infected

1) Decrease high-risk behavior
2) Attend regular medical and psychiatric evaluations and follow-ups
3) Maintain proper nutrition and diet, which promote optimal immune functions
4) Maintain food safety by keeping food at the proper temperature, cooking food thoroughly, and avoiding contamination (because people with HIV infection are vulnerable to food-borne illness) (Kubic, 1997; Ungvarski & Flaskerud, 1999)
5) Reduce and control stress
6) Avoid or limit cigarettes, alcohol, and drugs
7) Exercise regularly
8) Attend counseling on birth control, pregnancy, and breast feeding: Collaborative research by CDC and the Thai Ministry of Public Health suggested that a course of ADT given late in pregnancy and during delivery reduced the rate of HIV transmission to infants of infected mothers by half (CDC, 1998).

G. Nursing Process

1. Assessment

a. Begin with a thorough history to evaluate the course of HIV infection

1) Immunization history
2) Dietary evaluation
3) Risky behaviors (e.g., sexual history, drug use, occupational exposure)
4) Signs and symptoms that may indicate presence of HIV infection and AIDS-related illness
5) Psychosocial evaluation (e.g., support systems, financial state, coping strategies)

b. A complete physical and functional assessment (because any body system can be affected)

2. Plan of care

a. Nursing diagnoses

1) Anxiety
2) Fear
3) Anticipatory grieving
4) Grieving
5) Ineffective individual coping
6) Social isolation
7) Parental role conflict
8) Altered nutrition (less than body requirements)
9) Pain
10) Activity intolerance

b. Goals (Bradley-Springer, 1995)

1) For asymptomatic stage

a) Promote health
b) Prevent further transmission of HIV
c) Promote adjustment to HIV infection
d) Provide support

2) For symptomatic stage

a) Prevent and treat OIs
b) Manage problems caused by HIV infection
c) Maintain and maximize quality of life

3) For terminal stage

a) Promote comfort
b) Maintain dignity

3. Interventions

a. Provide active support
b. Promote adequate intake of nutrients and calories
c. Provide health education
d. Manage skin integrity, pain, and other HIV/AIDS-related symptoms

4. Evaluation: Modify care according to the stage of HIV and the patient's response to nursing interventions

V. Burns

A. Overview

1. Burns

a. A burn is tissue damage resulting from exposure to flames or hot liquids, contact with an electrical current, or exposure to radiation, strong acids, or alkalis chemicals.

b. Rehabilitation of the patient with burns requires interdisciplinary teamwork to achieve restoration of function and reintegration into the community.

c. Rehabilitation nurses must be knowledgeable in wound management and healing, as well as the pathophysiology and psychological components associated with burn injuries.

2. Skin

   a. The skin is the largest organ of the body.

   b. The skin's major functions are to protect internal organs from infection and trauma, prevent the loss of fluid, and regulate body temperature.

   c. Exposure to heat above 120ºF will damage the skin, interfere with its primary functions, and cause burn injuries.

B. Epidemiology (Aronovitch, 1999; National Center for Prevention and Control, 1998)

   1. Approximately 2 million Americans sustain burns each year; 100,000 of them require hospitalization.

   2. Most burn injuries occur in children ages 1–5 years and men 17–30 years of age.

   3. A fire department responds to a fire approximately every 18 seconds.

   4. Most burn injuries occur in the home and are preventable.

      a. 3,360 deaths occurred in 1997 as a result of residential fires.

      b. The most common causes of fire were cooking and heating equipment.

   5. People younger than 1 year and people older than 65 years have higher mortality rates due to burns because their skin is thinner.

C. Etiology

   1. Thermal

      a. Flame (e.g., house fire, burning leaves)

      b. Hot liquid (e.g., boiling water)

      c. Steam

      d. Tar

   2. Chemical: Strong acids or alkalis compounds (e.g., common household cleaning agents) that are ingested or inhaled or come in contact with skin or mucous membranes. The amount of damage depends on the concentration and quantity of the agent, duration of skin contact, and the degree of penetration into the tissue (OnHealth, 1998b).

   3. Electrical: Exposure to electrical current.

The amount of damage depends on the type of circuit, voltage, amperage, the pathway of the current through the body, and the duration of contact.

   a. Exposed or faulty wiring

   b. High-voltage power lines

   c. Strikes of lightning

4. Radiation

   a. Sunburn

   b. Therapeutic radiation for cancer treatment

D. Pathophysiology

   1. Classifications of burn

      a. Severity of burn (see Figure 14-3)

      b. Extent of burn

         1) Total body surface area: Percentage of the burn injury compared to healthy tissue

         2) Rule of 9: A formula that divides the body into anatomical sections, each representing 9% or a multiple of 9% (the perineum = 1%)

Figure 14-3. Levels of Burn Severity

First Degree (partial thickness)

Does not extend below the epidermis

Is dry and very painful

Heals in a matter of days

Second Degree

Involves the epidermis and part of the dermis

May be superficial (e.g., moist, painful, blisters) or deep thickness (e.g., less painful); may have a white or red base

Superficial burns heal in 1-2 weeks; deep thickness burns heal in 3 weeks or more

Third Degree (full thickness)

Extends into dermis

Is dry and involves no pain, because sensory nerves are damaged; can be any color (e.g., white, black, yellow, brown)

Autograft is the usual form of treatment

Fourth Degree

Extends beyond fat and into the muscle and bone

Involves no pain and has variable color

Amputation of extremity is often necessary; autografting is the primary method for healing

---

The Specialty Practice of Rehabilitation Nursing: A Core Curriculum, 4th Ed.

c. Level of skin damage (OnHealth, 1998b)
  1) Minor burns: First-degree burns and some second-degree burns
  2) Major burns
    a) Widespread second-degree burns
    b) All third- and fourth-degree burns
    c) Electrical burns: Despite minimal skin damage, interior damage can be extensive and damage the heart.
    d) Burns of the eyes, face, feet, hands, and perineum (regardless of the estimated percentage) (Richard & Staley, 1994)
d. Age: Burn victims younger than 2 years of age and older than 60 years have a higher mortality rate than other age groups with similar burn injuries (Trofino, 1991). In both groups, the skin is thin and more prone to infection.
e. Preexisting conditions: Heart disease, diabetes, sickle-cell anemia, and lung disease complicates wound management (Trofino, 1991).

2. Clinical manifestations
  a. Systemic responses: A major burn can affect all body systems (see Figure 14-4)
  b. Complications from burn surface
    1) Pain related to exposed nerve endings in partial-thickness burns and donor sites
    2) Scars
      a) Hypertrophic scars are raised above the level of normal skin, but are within the boundaries of the burn wound and result from an imbalance between collagen synthesis and collagen lysis.
      b) Scar tissue affects thermal regulation. Shivering is not possible with full-thickness scar with extensive grating. A cool environment is preferred.
    3) Contractures: Tightening and shortening of the tendons and muscles resulting in immobility and decreased ROM. Prevention is the most

---

Figure 14-4. Systemic Responses to Burn Injury

Vascular Alterations

Vasoconstriction occurs from exposure to heat and from stress response, resulting in decreased blood flow.

Dilation of adjacent vessels and capillaries and increased capillary permeability occur after the initial vasoconstriction.

Sodium pump is disturbed.

Fluid shifts from the vascular space into the extracellular space resulting in edema. (If edema is not corrected, ischemia in the underlying tissues can occur.)

Cardiac output is decreased as a result of hypovolemia.

Fluid resuscitation must be initiated to prevent cell shock and to maintain cardiac output and renal and tissue perfusion. (Adults with burns of a total body surface area [TBSA] greater than 15% require fluid resuscitation.)

Pulmonary Alterations

Obstruction can occur when damage around the neck area becomes tight or when superheated air, steam, gases, flames, or smoke are inhaled.

Depending on the severity, treatment can range from humidified air to mechanical ventilation.

Hematologic Alterations

Destruction of red blood cells in the burned area results in anemia.

Hematocrit level and sluggish blood flow increases as the fluid shifts to the extravascular space, resulting in possible ischemia of underlying tissue and thrombosis.

Immune Response

Immune responses decrease due to damage of the protective skin layer, stress, protein and caloric malnutrition, and side effects of immunosuppressant medication and steroids.

The individual is highly susceptible to infection.

Gastrointestinal Alterations

Ileus is due to vasoconstriction.

Parenteral route is used if an ileus is present.

Nutritional Alterations

Metabolic rate increases, resulting in increased caloric need of about two times normal (Wilson, 1996).

The metabolic rate will slowly return to normal when the wound is healed (Wilson, 1996).

Blood glucose rises.

Nutritional support may include oral supplements, tube feeding, intravenous supplements, or total parental nutrition.

---

effective treatment (e.g., splinting, exercising, positioning, using pressure garments). Surgery may be required, depending on the severity and location of contractures.

4) Heterotopic ossification: Abnormal deposit of new bone in soft tissue surrounding a joint that does not normally ossify (Trofino, 1991)

5) Surgical interventions: May be required if mobility is limited

6) Altered sensation: Diminished or absent response to sharp/dull, hot/cold; caution is needed to avoid further injury.

7) Pruritus or itching as the wound heals

E. Management Options
1. Prevention
    a. House fires
        1) Use a smoke detector on each floor and replace and test batteries at least once a year
        2) Have a fire extinguisher in the kitchen
        3) Install a sprinkler system
        4) Place fire-fighting decals on the window of children's bedrooms
        5) Keep matches and lighters out of reach of children
        6) Have a fire escape plan and practice fire drills
    b. Hot water
        1) Do not exceed a maximum temperature of 120° F
        2) Turn handles of pots and pans inward while cooking
    c. Chemical: Lock out of reach from children all flammable and caustic substances
    d. Electrical
        1) Cover outlets with plastic protectors
        2) Do not use appliances with frayed or worn cords
    e. Ultraviolet rays of sun
        1) Avoid long exposure to sun
        2) Wear hats and sunscreen with a minimum sun protector factor (SPF) of 15

2. Management of burn surface
    a. Burn location and severity determines treatment: Wound care should focus on cleaning the wound and removing debris until healthy tissue is present.
    b. Wound management includes moist dressing, infection control, debridement of necrotic tissue (i.e., removal of dead tissue), or surgical care.
        1) Nonsurgical care
            a) Apply a topical antimicrobial agent (e.g., silver sulfadiazine) and leave the wound open to air or apply a sterile occlusive or semiocclusive dressing to cover the wound
            b) Expose the area to light and maintain a cool environment
            c) Use daily hydrotherapy, which promotes cleansing and removes bacteria
            d) Debride the wound to remove contaminated tissue and eschar
        2) Surgical care
            a) Surgical excision of damaged tissue
            b) Escharotomy: An incision into the dermal fascia of the chest or limbs; performed to relieve pressure and allow the skin to separate freely to restore normal function if edema below the burn has resulted in resisted movement or arterial circulation
            c) Grafting: To close deep partial-thickness or full-thickness wounds
                (1) Autograft: Uses the patient's own skin from another site
                    (a) The donor site is the harvested area of the patient's own skin.
                    (b) Partial-thickness wounds require an absorbent dressing due to excessive drainage (Wilson, 1996).
                (2) Cadaver skin: Obtained through a graft bank

3. Management of complications

   a. Begin positioning and splinting immediately on admission to maintain the functional position of joints and prevent contractures: After the graft is stable, the splint should be worn continuously for at least 3 months.

   b. Use pressure garments against the skin to reduce scar formation for 23 hours per day for 1–2 years until the scar is fully mature (Wilson, 1996)

   c. Use massage therapy to reduce scar formation

   d. Manage pain by administering narcotics and using diversional activities (e.g., music, imagery, relaxation techniques) during dressing changes

F. Nursing Process

1. Assessment

   a. Begin with a history

      1) Cause of burn and any contributing factors

      2) Pain (e.g., location, quality, duration, intensity)

      3) Dietary evaluation

      4) Psychosocial evaluation (e.g., support systems, coping strategies)

   b. Perform a complete physical and functional assessment, including the amount of burn area involved and the depth, severity, and any complications from the injury

   c. Use a body diagram to document the location and appearance of burns, grafted areas, and donor sites

2. Plan of care

   a. Nursing diagnoses

      1) Alteration in comfort

      2) Pain

      3) Self-care deficit

      4) Alteration of skin integrity

      5) Potential for infection

      6) Alteration in nutrition (less than body requirements)

      7) Impaired physical mobility

      8) Anxiety

      9) Fear

      10) Social isolation

      11) Ineffective family coping

      12) Body image disturbance

   b. Goals

      1) Promote health

      2) Promote comfort and pain relief

      3) Prevent and manage any complications caused by burn injuries

      4) Provide support for altered body image

      5) Prevent and control infection

3. Interventions

   a. Provide care for the wound and the development of healing tissue

   b. Position, splint, and maintain joint mobility

   c. Prevent infection

   d. Provide pain relief

   e. Ensure adequate nutrition and hydration

   f. Provide psychological support and health education regarding health status, treatments, nutritional needs, prevention of infections, and support groups

4. Evaluation: Modify care according to the patient's response to nursing interventions

VI. Cancer

A. Overview

1. Cancer encompasses a group of diseases characterized by the growth and spread of abnormal cells that result in death if not controlled.

2. Remarkable progress against cancer has been made. The cancer incidence and death rate dropped between 1990 and 1995 (OnHealth, 1998c).

3. There are four major types of cancer.

   a. Carcinoma: Originates in the skin, lungs, breast, pancreas, and other organs and glands

   b. Sarcoma: Arises in bone, muscle, fat, or cartilage

   c. Lymphoma: Affects the lymphatic system

   d. Leukemia: Affects the blood

B. Epidemiology (American Cancer Society [ACS], 1998, 1999; OnHealth, 1998c)

1. Approximately 8.2 million Americans who are alive today have a history of cancer.

2. Since 1990, approximately 12 million cancer cases have been diagnosed. In 1999, approximately 1,221,800 cancer cases were expected to be diagnosed.

3. Approximately 563,100 Americans are expected to die of cancer in 1999; this amounts to more than 1,500 people per day.

4. Cancer is the second leading cause of death in the United States; one of every four deaths is caused by cancer.

5. Between 1990 and 1999, approximately 5 million people died as a result of cancer.

C. Etiology/Risk Factors
   1. Habits, traits, or use of substances that increase a person's chance of developing cancer
   2. Age: The risk for nearly all cancers increases with age.
   3. Inherited or familial predisposition
   4. Environment: Smoking, sunlight, alcohol, diet, and occupational exposure to carcinogens

D. Pathophysiology
   1. Cancer cells
      a. Characteristics
         1) Variable size and shape
         2) Loss of capacity for specialized function
         3) Continued growth after division
            a) Normal cells usually die after 50–60 divisions; however, cancer cells continue in an uncontrolled growth pattern.
            b) Cancer cells continue to grow despite a diminished concentration of growth hormones.
      b. Tumor growth
         1) Cancer cells accumulate and form a mass of abnormal cells (or tumors) that may compress, invade, and destroy normal tissues.
         2) Most cancers form tumors, but not all tumors are cancerous.
            a) Benign: Noncancerous tumors that stop growing and do not spread to other parts of the body
            b) Malignant: Cancerous tumors

c. Carcinogenesis
   1) The process through which cancer develops and abnormal cells grow and proliferate out of control
   2) Change or mutation in the nucleus of a cell: Millions of cells in the human body die and are replaced every second. The body's immune system typically recognizes mutant cells and destroys them before they multiply, but some mutant cells survive and cause cancer (Otto, 1997).
   3) Involves carcinogens, which are substances that start or promote the process (e.g., various chemicals, gases, and other substances found in the air, water, foods, pesticides, and industrial settings; tobacco smoke; cleaning products; paints; certain viruses—HIV, hepatitis B, Epstein-Barr) (OnHealth, 1998c)

d. Metastasis
   1) Abnormal cells that multiply out of control
   2) The spread of a tumor from the original site to another site via the lymphatic system or blood vessels
   3) Note: Cancer is classified by the body part where it started

2. Symptoms that may signal the presence of cancer (OnHealth, 1998c)
   a. A change in the size, color, shape, thickness of a wart, mole, or mouth sore
   b. A sore that resists healing
   c. Persistent cough, hoarseness, or sore throat
   d. Thickening or lumps in the breasts, testicles, or elsewhere
   e. A change in bowel or bladder habits
   f. Any unusual bleeding or discharge
   g. Chronic indigestion or difficulty swallowing
   h. Persistent headaches
   i. Unexplained loss of weight or appetite
   j. Persistent fatigue, nausea, or vomiting
   k. Persistent low-grade fever, either constant or intermittent
   l. Repeated instances of infection

3. Diagnosis
   a. Noninvasive: Radiological studies, computed tomography (CT), MRI, ultrasonography, nuclear medicine studies, laboratory studies, and tumor markers (i.e., substances measurable in the blood that are not produced or are produced in a lesser amount in healthy people)
   b. Invasive procedures: Biopsy (ranges from needle biopsy to surgical procedure), endoscopy
   c. Staging
      1) The process used to describe the extent of the disease or the spread of cancer from the original site (McCorkle, Grant, Frank-Stromborg, & Baird, 1996; Otto, 1997)
      2) Tumor-Node-Metastasis (TNM) staging system: The most common system, which assesses tumors in three ways to determine a "stage" (i.e., I, II, III, IV) (McCorkle et al., 1996; Otto, 1997)
         a) T: Extent of the primary tumor
         b) N: Absence or presence of regional lymph node involvement
         c) M: Absence or presence of metastases
   d. Early detection and treatment: Offers better chances of the cancer being cured
   e. Screening examinations by healthcare professionals: Can help detect cancer of the breast, colon, rectum, cervix, prostate, testis, oral cavity, and skin
   f. Self-examination for breast and skin cancer: May result in early detection of tumors

E. Management Options
   1. Prevention measures
      a. Do not smoke or chew tobacco: ACS estimated that in 1999, approximately 173,000 cancer deaths would be caused by tobacco use (ACS, 1999).
      b. Limit alcohol intake: ACS estimated that in 1999, approximately 20,000 cancer deaths would be related to excessive alcohol use (ACS, 1999).
      c. Eat a well-balanced diet: Reduce the intake of fat, increase daily intake of natural fiber (e.g., fresh fruits, vegetables, whole grains), and avoid processed, smoked, cured, fried, or barbecued foods. Approximately one-third of the 563,100 cancer deaths expected to occur in 1999 were related to nutrition and could have been prevented (ACS, 1999).
      d. Protect skin from sun's rays
         1) Use sunscreen outdoors
         2) More than 1 million skin cancers that were expected to be diagnosed in 1999 could have been prevented (ACS, 1999).
      e. Exercise regularly
      f. Follow occupational hazard guidelines if exposed to carcinogens
         1) Limit exposure to carcinogens at home
         2) Avoid using aerosol cleaning products
         3) Wear gloves when using carcinogenic chemicals
         4) Follow safety warnings when using paint, solvents, pesticides, household cleaners, and other carcinogenic chemicals
   2. Cancer treatment modalities: Used to cure, control, or provide palliation; options depend on the stage of the tumor and the level of metastasis
      a. Surgery: The oldest form of treatment; offers the greatest chance for cure for many types of cancer
         1) Biopsy: Obtain specimens of suspected tissue
         2) Curative resection: Resect lesions
         3) Palliation: Relieve symptoms to improve quality of life
      b. Radiation: A stream of high-energy particles or waves used to destroy or damage cancer cells in a specific area
         1) Used before surgery to shrink a tumor so it can be removed more easily
         2) Used after surgery to stop the growth of cancer cells that remain
         3) Side effects: Irritation to the overlying skin, nausea, vomiting, anorexia,

bone marrow depression, anemia, thrombocytopenia, leukopenia

c.   Chemotherapy: The use of drugs to treat cancer by interfering with the stages of the dividing cell cycle

1)   Anticancer drugs are more powerful when used in combination: More than 50 anticancer drugs are currently in use.

a)   Drugs of different actions can work together to kill more cancer cells.

b)   Use of multiple drugs can reduce the chance of developing a resistance to one particular drug (ACS, 1999).

2)   Side effects: Nausea, vomiting, fatigue, temporary hair loss, mouth sores or dryness, difficulty swallowing, diarrhea, increased vulnerability to infection

d.   Bone marrow transplantation (BMT)

1)   Autologous BMT: Patient's own bone marrow is used.

2)   Allogenic BMT: Patient receives a donor's bone marrow.

a)   Syngenic: Donor is an identical twin.

b)   Related: Donor is a relative.

c)   Unrelated: Donor is not a relative.

e.   Hormone therapy: Drug treatment that interferes with hormone production or action to kill or slow the growth of cancer cells

f.   Immunotherapy: Treatment that promotes or supports the immune system's response to cancer

g.   Gene therapy: Manipulates genetic material inside cancerous cells to make them easier targets (OnHealth, 1998c)

h.   Alternative and complementary therapy: Unconventional therapies that have not been scientifically tested, but may complement conventional care and may help relieve certain symptoms and side effects

1)   Body work: Promotes relaxation (e.g., massage, reflexology)

2)   Exercise: Controls fatigue, muscle

tension, and anxiety

3)   Mind/body medicine: Improves quality of life through behavior modification (e.g., guided imagery, hypnotherapy, biofeedback, art or music therapy)

i.   Nutrition and diet: Can play a role in cancer prevention, but no diet can cure cancer. A proper diet with vitamins, minerals, and other nutrients may inhibit the development of cancer by neutralizing carcinogens, ensuring proper immune function, and preventing tissue and cell damage (OnHealth, 1998c).

3.   Treatment of side effects

a.   Pain: Goal of pain management is to relieve suffering and control pain.

1)   Medication

a)   Nonprescription: Aspirin, acetaminophen, ibuprofen

b)   Prescription: Codeine, morphine

2)   Other methods: Relaxation techniques, imagery, distraction, music, humor, biofeedback, hypnosis

3)   Invasive techniques: Surgery, nerve block, acupuncture

b.   Nausea: Eat light snacks throughout the day rather than heavy meals

c.   Increased risk for infection

1)   Arises from underlying disease, side effects of treatment (e.g., neutropenia, immune suppression), disruption of mucous membranes or skin, presence of long-term venous access device, impaired nutrition, and prolonged hospitalization

2)   Can be managed via prevention; prompt recognition of suspected infection; treatment of skin complications; administration of antibiotics, antifungals, or antiviral agents; fever management; platelet or blood transfusion for bleeding

d.   Fatigue

1)   Minimize symptoms that interfere with sleep

2)   Avoid stimulants

3)   Pace activities to save energy

4)   Exercise

e.   Weight loss

1) Can be a cause of treatment side effects that impair nutritional status, uncontrolled pain that impairs appetite, fatigue that affects the ability to obtain and eat food

2) Can be treated according to the cause of the weight loss and the overall goals

3) Can be treated with oral or parenteral nutritional supplementation

f. Arm care precautions for women following breast or axillary surgery

   1) Perform ROM exercises

      a) Ensures full use and flexibility of the arm to help alleviate damage to the nerves and muscles that accompanies breast cancer surgery (Baum, 1994)

      b) Reduces the risk and severity of lymphedema (i.e., the accumulation of lymph fluid in the tissues of the upper extremity after breast cancer surgery), which occurs most commonly in women with breast cancer who had axillary node dissection followed by radiation

   2) Avoid sunburn and burns while cooking, baking, or smoking

   3) Wear protective gloves while gardening

   4) Wear loose-fitting watches, jewelry, and clothing

   5) Treat cuts immediately and monitor for signs of infection

   6) Use the unaffected arm for intravenous access, blood draws, and blood pressure; avoid giving chemotherapy with the affected arm

   7) Avoid carrying heavy objects with the affected arm

g. Monitor for oncologic emergencies: Hypercalcemia, disseminated intravascular coagulation (DIC), alteration in blood-clotting mechanism, septic shock, pleural effusion, spinal cord compression, neoplastic cardiac tamponade

F. Clinical Management of Cancers Requiring Rehabilitation

1. Brain tumors

   a. Cancer of the CNS is the fourth leading cause of cancer death in people ages 15 to 34 years and accounts for less than 2% of all malignancies (Otto, 1997).

   b. Glioma is the most common CNS tumor.

   c. Brain tumors have better outcomes in children than in adults.

   d. Clinical manifestations vary according to the location and size of the tumor, but may include headache, seizure activity, nausea and vomiting, memory deficit, and changes in speech, motor skills, and vision.

   e. Diagnosis: Neurologic assessment, CT, MRI, biopsy

   f. Treatment

      1) Types: Surgery, radiation therapy, chemotherapy

      2) Complications of CNS surgery: Intracranial bleeding, cerebral edema, infection, neuromotor deficits, thrombosis, and hydrocephalus

2. Spinal cord tumors

   a. Schwannoma and meningioma are the most common types.

   b. Clinical manifestations: Related to the site and size of tumor and may include pain, weakness, sensory loss, muscle spasms, and loss of bowel and bladder control

   c. Diagnosis: Neurologic assessment, CT, MRI, biopsy

   d. Treatment: Surgery, radiation therapy, chemotherapy

3. Bone cancer

   a. Cancer that originates in the bone (primary bone cancer) is rare; however, cancer that spreads to the bones from other parts of the body is more common.

      1) Primary bone cancer generally attacks young people and is more likely to occur in bones that have been fractured or infected in the past.

      2) The likelihood of a cure for primary bone cancer depends on how early it is detected and how rapidly it spreads (OnHealth, 1998c).

b. Symptoms: A hard lump felt on the surface of the bone, pain (especially at night), swelling in bones and joint, spontaneous bone fracture, fever, weight loss, fatigue, and impaired mobility (Groenwald, Frogge, Goodman, & Yarbro, 1998)

c. Diagnosis: X rays, other imaging tests, biopsy

d. Treatment

1) Surgical removal when possible: If the cancer is in the arm or leg, amputation is usually avoided and the bone is reconstructed with a metal prosthesis.

2) Radiation and chemotherapy

a) May be given before surgery to reduce the size of the tumor

b) May be used after surgery to kill remaining cells

c) Used to treat inoperable bone cancer

3) Therapy: Should begin as soon as possible to avoid stiffness and improve mobility and, if amputation was unavoidable, to help the patient learn how to use the prosthesis

e. Common types

1) Osteosarcoma

a) Tends to affect teenagers whose bones are in a stage of rapid growth

b) Has an incidence rate that is twice as high in men as in women (Groenwald et al., 1998)

c) Most common sites: Knee (distal end of femur), proximal tibia, humerus (McCorkle et al., 1996)

2) Chondrosarcoma

a) Tends to attack middle-aged adults

b) Originates in the cartilage

c) Most common sites: Pelvic bone, long bones, scapula

3) Ewing's sarcoma

a) Tends to occur in children between the ages of 5 and 9 and in young adults between the ages of 20 and 30

b) Originates in the bone marrow and is commonly located in femoral diaphysis, skull, pelvis, ileum, humerus, fibula, or ribs (McCorkle et al., 1996)

G. Nursing Process

1. Assessment

a. History

1) Signs and symptoms of underlying disease and side effects of treatment

2) Pain: Quality, location, duration, intensity, relieving factors

3) Dietary evaluation with food preferences

4) Use of complementary therapies

5) Psychosocial evaluation (e.g., support systems, coping strategies)

b. Complete physical and functional assessment to determine the degree of loss of function

2. Plan of care

a. Nursing diagnoses

1) Impaired skin integrity

2) Pain

3) Activity intolerance

4) Impaired physical mobility

5) Altered nutrition (less than body requirements)

6) Anxiety

7) Coping, ineffective individual

8) Coping, ineffective family

9) Anticipatory grieving

10) Spiritual distress

b. Goals, according to phase of illness

1) Acute phase: To obtain remission status and prevent and control side effects of treatment

2) Intermittent or chronic phase: Rehabilitation for side effects of treatment and complications

3) Palliative phase: To provide comfort, emotional support, symptom management, and attain peaceful death

3. Interventions

a. Minimize infection, maximize comfort, decrease muscle wasting, minimize pain, manage nausea and vomiting, and provide emotional support by helping the patient and family express grief

b. Provide health education about side effects of therapy, risk of injury due to immunosuppression medication, health promotion, and support groups

c. Provide pain relief and comfort: It is important to accept the patient's report of pain and to use a consistent method or scale to evaluate pain. *[Refer to Chapter 13 for more information about pain management.]*

4. Evaluation: Modify care according to the patient's response to nursing interventions, focusing on quality of life

References

American Association of Diabetes Educators (AADE). (1998). *A core curriculum for diabetes education* (3rd ed.). Chicago: Author.

American Cancer Society (ACS). (1998, July). *Cancer: Treatment* [Online]. Available: http://www3.cancer.org/cancerinfo

American Cancer Society (ACS). (1999). *Cancer: Prevention and risk factors* [Online]. Available: http://www3.cancer.org/cancerinfo

American Diabetes Association (ADA). (1998). Report of the Expert Committee on the Diagnosis and Classification of Diabetes Mellitus. *Diabetes Care, 21*(Suppl. 1).

Aronovitch, S.A. (1999). *Burn care I: RTN continuing education* [Online]. Available; http://www.rtngroup.com/hc-ceulburn.html

Avert. (1998). *Worldwide HIV & AIDS estimates* [Online]. Available: http://www.avert.org/wwstatsg98.htm

Baum, M. (1994). *Breast cancer.* New York: Oxford University Press.

Beare, P.G., & Myers, J.L. (1998). *Adult health nursing* (3rd ed.). St. Louis: Mosby.

Begany, T. (1997). Update on Parkinson's disease. *Patient Care, 31*(10), 12-25.

Bradley-Springer, L. (1995). *HIV/AIDS: Nursing care plans.* El Paso, TX: Skidmore-Roth.

Casey, K.M., Cohen, F., & Hughes, A. (1996). *ANAC's core curriculum for HIV/AIDS nursing.* Philadelphia: Nursecom, Inc.

Centers for Disease Control and Prevention (CDC). (1998a, July 24). Addressing the global epidemic: CDC's international activities. *CDC Update* [Online]. Available: http://www.cdc.gov/nchstp/hiv-aids/pubs/facts/internat.htm

Centers for Disease Control and Prevention (CDC). (1998b, November 13). Are there other test available? *CDC Update* [Online]. Available: http://www.cdc.gov/nchstp/hiv-aids/pub/faq/faq8.htm

Centers for Disease Contro and Preventionl (CDC). (1998c, December 28). The HIV and AIDS epidemic in the United States, 1997-1998. *CDC Update* [Online]. Available: http://www.cdc.gov/nchstp/hiv-aids/pubs/facts/hivrefs.htm

Centers for Disease Control and Prevention (CDC). (1999, May 13). How many people have HIV & AIDS. *CDC Update* [Online]. Available: http://www.cdc.gov/nchstp/hiv-aids/pubs/faq/faq13.htm

Costello, K.M., & Cerreta, E. (1998). *Multiple sclerosis: Disease modification and disease management.* Luncheon symposium presented at the Association of Rehabilitation Nurses 24th Annual Educational Conference, Dallas, TX.

Groenwald, S.L., Frogge, M.H., Goodman, M., & Yarbro, C.H. (1998). *Clinical guide to cancer nursing* (4th ed.). Boston: Jones and Bartlett.

Halper, J., & Holland, N. (1998). New strategies, new hope: Meeting the challenge of multiple sclerosis, Part I. *American Journal of Nursing, 98*(10), 26-32.

Henkel, J. (1998). New treatments stow onslaught of symptoms: Parkinson's disease. *FDA Consumer, 32*(4), 13-18.

Ignatavicius, D.D., Workman, M.L., & Mishler, M.A. (1998). *Medical-surgical nursing across the health care continuum* (3rd ed.). Philadelphia: W.B. Saunders.

InteliHealth (Home to John Hopkins Health Information). (1997, May). *AIDS Fact Sheet: HIV infection and AIDS* [Online]. Available: http://www.ihtIH?t=7154&c=36380&p=br,AOL

Kubic, M. (1997, Jan/Feb). New ways to prevent and treat AIDS. *FDA Consumer.*

Lewis, S.N., Collier, I.C., & Heitkenper, M. (1996). *Medical-surgical nursing assessment and management of clinical problems* (4th ed.). St. Louis: Mosby.

Lipsett, L.F., & Geiss, L. (1993, April 9). Statistics: Prevalence, incidence, risk factors and complications of diabetes [Memorandum]. *AM Diabetes Association Bulletin.*

Lublin, F.D., & Reingold, S.C. (1996). Defining the clinical course of multiple sclerosis: Results of an international study. *Neurology, 46*, 907-911.

McCorkle, R., Grant, M., Frank-Stromborg, M., & Baird, S.B. (1996). *Cancer nursing: A comprehensive textbook* (2nd ed.). Philadelphia: W.B. Saunders.

Monahan, F.D., & Neighbors, M. (1998). *Medical-surgical nursing foundations for clinical practice* (2nd ed.). Philadelphia: W.B. Saunders.

National Center for Prevention and Control. (1998, October). Fact sheet on fire-related injuries and death among U.S. residents [Online]. Available: http://www.cdc.gov/ncipc/duip/fire2.htm

National Diabetes Data Group. (1979). Classification and diagnosis of DM and other categories of glucose intolerance. *Diabetes, 28*, 1039-1057.

OnHealth. (1998a, July). AIDS. *OnHealth Conditions A-Z* [Online]. Available: http://onhealth.com/ch1

OnHealth. (1998b, July). Burns. *OnHealth Conditions A-Z* [Online]. Available: http://onhealth.com/ch1/resource/conditions/items,246.asp

OnHealth. (1998c, July). Cancer. *OnHealth Conditions A-Z* [Online]. Available: http://onhealth.com/ch1/resource/conditions/items, 249.asp

Otto, S.E. (1997). *Oncology nursing* (3rd ed.). St. Louis: Mosby.

Peragallo-Dittko, V., Godley, K., & Meyer, J. (1993). *A core curriculum for diabetes education* (2nd ed.). Chicago: AADE & AADE Education and Research Foundation.

Phipps, W.J., Sands, J.D., & Marek, J.F. (1999). *Medical-surgical nursing: Concepts and clinical practice* (6th ed.). St Louis: Mosby.

Phipps, W.J., Sands, J.K., & Marek, J.F. (1999). *Medical-surgical nursing: Concepts and clinical practice* (6th ed.). St. Louis: Mosby.

Richard, R.L., & Staley, M.J. (1994). *Burn care and rehabilitation*. Philadelphia: F.A. Davis.

Ridkin, H. (Ed.). (1988). *Physician's guide to non-insulin dependent Type 2 diabetes: Diagnosis and treatment* (2nd ed.). Alexandria, VA: American Diabetes Association.

Segatore, M. (1998). Managing the surgical orthopedic patient with Parkinson's disease. *Orthopedic Nursing, 17*(1), 13-21.

Smeltzer, S.C., & Bare, B.G. (1996). *Brunner and Suddarth's textbook of medical-surgical nursing* (8th ed.). Philadelphia: Lippincott-Raven.

Smeltzer, S.C., & Bare, B.G. (1996). *Brunner and Suddarth's textbook of medical surgical nursing* (8th ed.). Philadelphia: Lippincott.

Taggart, H.M. (1998). Multiple sclerosis update. *Orthopedic Nursing, 17*(2), 23-26.

Trapp, B., Peterson, J., Ransohoff, R., Rudick, R., & Mork, S. (1998). Axonal transection in the lesions of multiple sclerosis. *New England Journal of Medicine, 338*(5), 278-285.

Trofino, R.B. (1991). *Nursing care of the burn-injured patient*. Salem, MA: F.A. Davis.

Ungvarski, P.J., & Flaskerud, J.H. (1999). *HIV/AIDS: A guide to primary management* (4th ed.). Philadelphia.: W.B. Saunders.

White, J.R. (1997). Combination oral agent/insulin therapy in patients with type 2 diabetes mellitus. *Clinical Diabetes, 15*(2), 103.

Wilson, R.E. (1996). Care of the burn patient. *Ostomy/Wound Management, 42*(8), 16-34.

Suggested resources

American Diabetes Association (ADA). (1998a). Diabetic nephropathy [Position statement]. *Diabetes Care, 21*(Suppl. 1), S50-S53.

American Diabetes Association (ADA). (1998b). Diabetic retinopathy [Position statement]. *Diabetes Care, 21*(Suppl. 1), S50-S53.

American Diabetes Association (ADA). (1998c). Foot care in patients with diabetes mellitus [Position statement]. *Diabetes Care, 21*(Suppl. 1), S47-S49.

American Diabetes Association (ADA). (1998d). Gestational diabetes mellitus [Position statement]. *Diabetes Care, 21*(Suppl. 1), S54-S55.

American Diabetes Association (ADA). (1998e). Nutrition recommendations and principles for people with diabetes mellitus [Position statement]. *Diabetes Care, 21*(Suppl. 1), S32-S35.

Cook, L.C. (1996, November). Diabetes update 1996. *Caring Magazine*, pp. 10-19.

DeFronzo, R.A. (1998). *Current therapy of diabetes mellitus*. St. Louis: Mosby.

Duffy, J.C., & Patout, C.A. (1990, December). Management of the insensitive foot in diabetes: Lessons learned from Hansen's disease. *Military Medicine, 155*.

Faugier, J., & Hicken, I. (1996). *AIDS and HIV: The nursing response*. London: Chapman & Hall.

Goldstein, B.J., Cotter, V.T., Morley, J.V., & Setter, S.M. (1998). *Type 2 diabetes in the long-term care environment: A practical approach to patient care—A multidisciplinary continuing education monography*. Jointly sponsored by Thomas Jefferson University, Jefferson Medical College, and Medical Education Systems, Inc. Midwest Office: 5840 N. Canton Center Road, Suite 270, Canton, MI 48187-2614, www.mesinc.com

Halper, J., & Holland, N. (1998). New strategies, now hope: Meeting the challenge of multiple sclerosis, Part II. *American Journal of Nursing, 98*(11), 39-45.

Hernendez, C.A., & Grinspun, D.R. (1955). The challenges of teaching clients with cerebrovascular accidents to manage their diabetes. *The Diabetes Educator, 20*(4), 311-316.

Jameson, D.L. (1994). *Perceived and actual level of knowledge of DM among staff nurses: A replication*. Unpublished master's thesis. Sacred Heart Medical Center, 101 West 8th Ave., PO Box 2555, Spokane, WA 99220-2255.

Jayne, R.L., & Rankin, S.H. (1993). Revisiting nurse knowledge about diabetes: An update and implications for practice. *The Diabetes Educator, 19*(6), 497-501.

Kahn, J.O., & Walker, B.D. (1998). *The AIDS knowledge base: Primary HIV infection—Guides to diagnosis, treatment, and management* [Online]. Available: http://hivinsite.ucsf.edu//akb/1997/04prihiv/index.html

Kelly, J.M. (1994). Implementing a patient self-medication program. *Rehabilitation Nursing, 19*(2), 87-90.

Leggett-Frazier, N., Turner, M.S., & Vincent, P.A. (1994). Measuring the diabetes knowledge of nurses in long-term care facilities. *The Diabetes Educator, 20*(4), 307-310.

Libman, H., & Witzburg, R.A. (1996). *A primary care manual for HIV infection* (3rd ed.). Boston: Little, Brown.

National Cancer Institute (NCI) Cancer Trials. (1999, May 17). *Chemotherapy side effects* [Online]. Available: http://cancertrials/nci.nih.gov/NCI-Cancer-Trials.

National Cancer Institute (NCI). (1999). *NCI's research programs* [Online]. Available: http://wwwosp.nci.nih.gov/newosp/spa/bypass2000

Ropka, M.E., & Williams, A.B. (1998). *HIV: Nursing and symptom management*. Sudbury, MA: Jones & Bartlett.

U.S. Department of Health and Human Services, Public Health Service, National Institutes of Health. (1994, September). *Diabetes control and complications trial* (DCCT). (NIH Publication No. 94-3874.) Bethesda, MD: Author.

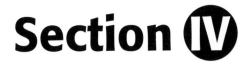

Section IV

Rehabilitation Nursing Across the Life Continuum

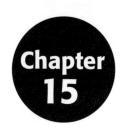

Developmental Theories and Tasks Across the Life Span: Individuals and Families

Linda L. Pierce, PhD RNC CRRN CNS

Developmental theories provide the backdrop for understanding the process of human development. Each theory provides a framework for relating life history and past circumstances to the individual's and/or family's tasks of functioning, engaging in healthy relationships, and developing ways to understand the world. Developmental theories propose that individuals and families grow and change and master the tasks of living across the life span through increasing levels of separation, mastery, and independence.

This chapter reviews two types of developmental theories:
- individual human development from intrapsychic, interpersonal, social learning, cognitive, behavioral, and interactionist perspectives
- family development and functioning

I. Individual Human Development Theories (see Table 15-1)

A. Overview
   1. Complex factors and forces foster the development of human beings.
   2. Human traits are built and exist as enduring behavioral patterns.
   3. Unique individual personal dispositions and preferences are demonstrated through behavioral patterns.
   4. Behavior patterns lead to successful or unsuccessful management of life and its circumstances.
   5. Nursing assessment, diagnosis, intervention, and resultant evaluation depends upon a firm understanding of individual human developmental theories (Whiting, 1997).

B. Theories
   1. Intrapsychic theory: Freud (1959), the early and long dominant theorist in the field of personality development
      a. Individuals experience conflict between their natural instincts and society's restrictions on them.

   b. Conflict experienced in childhood influences the individual's adult personality.
   c. Libidinal or instinctual drives influence behavior and are related to the individual's attempt to gain pleasure through the mouth, anus, or genitalia (Glod, 1998; Jarvis, 1996; Whiting, 1997).
      1) Oral phase
         a) Occurs in the first year of life
         b) Involves exploring the world through the mouth: Mouth, lips, and tongue are the center of existence for the infant.
         c) Begins development of the infant's personality, which depends on the mother's (or mothering person's or caretaker's) sense of personal security in self and satisfaction in the mother role
         d) Involves maternal experiences, which are taken on by the infant: The infant experiences whatever the mothering person feels.

e) Leads to the infant being vulnerable (e.g., if mother's anxiety is pervasive and infant begins life with a deficit in adaptive abilities)

2) Anal phase
   a) Occurs from about 18 months to 3 years of age
   b) Centers on buildup and release of tension in the orifices; involves experiencing pleasure in expelling urine and feces
   c) Is challenging for parents' coping ability in allowing child to move away, to seek freedom or a greater sense of self
   d) Brings psychological problems to the forefront due to toilet training and other issues related to rules of culture and custom
   e) Involves ambivalence
      (1) Complying through proper elimination on the part of the infant and interjecting the values of the parents
      (2) Complying through retention or inappropriate discharge of feces or urine by the infant, which brings retribution and further anxiety
      (3) Holding on and letting go responses by the infant lead to various behaviors known as anal characteristics
   f) Involves approaching the issue of toilet training by the parents as well as the infant's corresponding response, which can govern adult personality

3) Phallic phase
   a) Occurs from about 3 to 6 years of age
   b) Draws on the foundation that has been established in the previous two stages
   c) Involves becoming aware of individuals' separateness; learning gender or how males and females differ; sex-typing
      (1) Having a romantic attraction to the parent of the opposite sex (Oedipus complex)
      (2) Having a rivalry with the same-sex parent
      (3) Producing guilt and fear from attraction and rivalry
      (4) Resolving guilt and fear by identifying with the same-sex parent
      (5) Repressing sexual urges and imitating the sex-related behaviors, attitudes, and beliefs of the parent of the same sex
      (6) Sex-typing, which has a broader scope than just learning appropriate sex roles, in that children learn, assimilate, and internalize their parents' ideals and values
   d) Familiarizes the child with the standards of society (by the parents' words and deeds) and leads to the development of the conscience

4) Latent and genital phase
   a) Occurs from 6 to 12 years (latent) and from puberty (genital)
   b) Involves hiding sexuality, which happens in 6- to 12-year-olds as they engage in the larger world and are absorbed by its challenges; the libidinal drive seems to be less important and receives less attention
   c) Involves reawakened oedipal strivings during adolescence
   d) Rechannels energy toward peers of the opposite sex in an effort to rework the libidinal drive
   e) Involves individuals' responses during the preceding stages, which may cause serious adjustment problems if brought into adulthood
   f) Can involve feelings of constant jeopardy, in which the person is unable to turn energy away from

Table 15-1. Summary of Individual Human Development Theories

Theory and Theorist	Description	Infancy (0–12 months)	Birth–2 years old	Toddler (12–36 months)	2–7 years old
Intrapsychic (Freud, 1959)	Conflict between individuals' natural instincts and society's restrictions on them experienced in childhood influence individuals' adult personality; children are thought to progress through four stages of psychosexual development (Glod, 1998; Whiting, 1997)	Oral	N/A	Anal	N/A
Interpersonal (Sullivan, 1956, 1964)	Repeated experiences between parents/caretakers and children lead to development of a good self and a bad self, which is the basis for healthy development; six stages represent processes by which an individual's identity develops in the context of relationships (Glod, 1998; Whiting, 1997)	Infancy	N/A	Childhood	N/A
Social Learning (Erikson, 1963)	Interaction between parents/caretakers and child is essential to healthy psychological growth; each phase of normal development requires the individual to accomplish age-appropriate developmental tasks through eight phases of development from infancy to older adulthood (Glod, 1998)	Trust vs. mistrust	N/A	Autonomy vs. shame and doubt	N/A
Cognitive (Piaget, 1952)	Motor activity involving concrete objects results in the development of mental functioning; children move through four general periods of cognitive development in the same sequence although not according to the same timetable (Glod, 1998)	N/A	Sensorimotor	N/A	Preoperational
Behavioral (Pavlov, 1927; Skinner, 1953)	Individuals' development is influenced by stimulus-response interaction; individuals' behavior is shaped through the consistency of responding; two attributes of the human brain—flexibility and plasticity—allow for a developmentally significant variety of adaptive sequences (Glod, 1998)	N/A	N/A	N/A	N/A
Interactional (Schaie, 1981)	Development of individuals in a progressive direction occurs when goodness of fit (consonance) exists; poorness of fit (dissonance) involves discrepancies between individuals and their environment, which results in distorted development and maladaptive functioning; starting with dependency in infancy, interference with development of independence in adolescence is likely to inhibit the establishment of interdependence in adulthood (Schaie, 1981; Whiting, 1997)	Dependency	N/A	N/A	N/A

Major Points

- Human development is a complex, interactive, and multifaceted process that involves a variety of forces.
- Some older theories of development (Freud, 1959; Piaget, 1952) emphasize completion of development early in childhood.
- Other theories (Pavlov, 1927; Skinner, 1953) are not age-specific but allow for a developmentally significant diversity of adaptive sequences.

Periods of Development

Preschooler (3–5 years old)	School age 5–12 years old	7–11 years old	11–15 years old	Childhood (1–12 years old)	Adolescence (12–18 years old)	Early adulthood (18–25 years old)	Adulthood (26–65 years old)	Older adulthood (older than 65 years old)
Phallic, oedipal	Latent and genital	N/A	N/A	N/A	N/A	N/A	N/A	N/A
Childhood, juvenile	Juvenile, preadolescence	N/A	N/A	N/A	Early to late adolescence	Adulthood	Adulthood (continues)	Adulthood (continues)
Initiative vs. guilt	Industry vs. inferiority	N/A	N/A	N/A	Identity vs. role confusion	Intimacy vs. isolation	Generativity vs. stagnation	Integrity vs. despair
N/A	N/A	Concrete operational	Formal operational	N/A	N/A	N/A	N/A	N/A
N/A	N/A	N/A	N/A	N/A	N/A	N/A	N/A	N/A
N/A	N/A	N/A	N/A	Decreasing dependency	Dependency to independence	Inter-dependency (adulthood)	Inter-dependency (adulthood) (continues)	Inter-dependency (adulthood) (continues)

* Many theories (Erikson, 1963; Schaie, 1981; Sullivan, 1956, 1964) view individual development as a continuous process that unfolds throughout the life span rather than as a process that is limited to a few early years in relationships with limited numbers of people (Glod, 1998; Whiting, 1997).

the self to a more productive activity and may produce problems of a sexual nature

    g) Results in self-absorption and defensiveness to protect the self or ego

    h) Brings out defensive measures used in earlier phases of development (e.g., repression, introjection, projection, denial, isolation, ambivalence, regression, sublimation) (Freud, 1959; Glod, 1998; Jarvis, 1996; Whiting, 1997)

2. Interpersonal theory: Sullivan (1956, 1964), one of psychiatry's most influential thinkers

  a. Sullivan's theory departed from Freudian concepts.

  b. The term *integrating tendencies* describes behavior by which one person moves toward another person.

  c. Healthy development is based upon repeated experiences between parents and/or caretakers and children that lead to the development of a good self and a bad self (Glod, 1998; Whiting, 1997).

  d. Seven stages of development represent processes by which the person's identity develops in the context of relationships.

    1) Infancy

      a) Developing both good and bad self-representations

      b) Beginning to realize a sense of sequential time in which things are causally related

    2) Childhood: Beginning to develop interpersonal relationships with peers, language skills, and gender identity

    3) Juvenile: Expanding interactions to social, group, and societal relationships

    4) Preadolescence

      a) Forming peer relationships with individuals of the same sex

      b) Developing the ability to form a meaningful nondependent relationship

    5) Early adolescence: Developing sexuality and gender identity

    6) Late adolescence: Beginning to assume responsibility

    7) Adulthood: Containing these interpersonal themes that continue to emerge in new relationships

  e. Personality is shaped by previous relationships.

  f. Difficulties in development are viewed as manifestations of disordered interpersonal relationships (Glod, 1998; Sullivan, 1956, 1964; Whiting, 1997).

3. Social Learning Theory: Erikson (1963), one of the first developmental theorists to suggest that the interaction between parent or caretaker and child is essential to healthy psychological growth (i.e., parents raise the child, and the child influences the parents)

  a. Through satisfactory completion of the developmental task of each psychosocial stage (listed below), individuals become ready to move through the stages of development from infancy to adulthood (Glod, 1998; Luggen, 1998; Whiting, 1997).

  b. There are eight sequential psychosocial stages.

    1) Trust versus mistrust (infancy)

      a) Viewing the universe as reliable

      b) Seeing relationships as stable and available

    2) Autonomy versus shame and doubt (toddlerhood)

      a) Understanding control over one's body and thinking

      b) Understanding disappointment in self and others

    3) Initiative versus guilt (preschool years): Dealing with predominately genital issues

    4) Industry versus inferiority (school age): Dealing with latency, school, and relationships outside the family

    5) Identity versus role confusion (adolescence)

      a) Clarifying personal identity

      b) Depersonifying internal representations

    6) Intimacy versus isolation (young adulthood)

a) Rediscovering attachment

b) Developing mature bonding

7) Generativity versus stagnation (middle adulthood)

    a) Being creative and productive

    b) Carrying out parental responsibilities (Erikson, 1963; Glod, 1998; Whiting, 1997)

8) Integrity versus despair (older adulthood): Feeling a sense of completeness, based on an integrated philosophy of one's unique life (Erikson, 1963; Glod, 1998; Luggen, 1998; Whiting, 1997)

4. Cognitive theory: Piaget (1952)

   a. The major focus of this theory is to understand how children evolve ways of knowing and how they develop right and wrong answers (Glod, 1998).

   b. Every child passes through stages of cognitive development in the same sequence, although not according to a given timetable.

   c. Every child develops strategies for interacting with the environment and knowing the environment's properties.

   d. A gradual progression takes place from one period of cognitive development to another; acquisition of each new operation builds on existing ones.

   e. Differentiation and complexity occur and are matched by increasing integration and coordination of schemata in this process of development (Drucker, 1979; Ricci-Balich & Behm, 1996).

   f. Infants possess both fixed and flexible reflexes that enable them to develop abstract intelligent behavior (Glod, 1998).

   g. Children move through four general periods of cognitive development.

1) Sensorimotor

    a) Occurs from 0 to 2 years of age

    b) Development proceeds from reflex activity to representation and sensorimotor learning.

      (1) Feeling and actions are inseparable.

      (2) Sucking and touching actions by infants are innate at first.

      (3) Individuals begin to understand how personal behavior affects the world and become involved in trial-and-error actions.

2) Preoperational

    a) Occurs from 2 to 7 years of age

    b) Development proceeds from sensorimotor representation to prelogical thought.

      (1) By maintaining stable and consistent images, children are able to create a representational world.

      (2) Children begin to fantasize and usc symbols to represent objects and feelings.

3) Concrete operational

    a) Occurs from 7 to 11 years of age

    b) Development proceeds from prelogical thought to logical, concrete thought.

      (1) Rules are devised to govern behavior.

      (2) Trial-and-error is replaced by the ability to problem solve.

4) Formal operational

    a) Occurs from 11 to 15 years of age

    b) Development proceeds from logical, concrete thought to logical solutions to all kinds or categories of problems.

      (1) Reasoning and abstract conceptualizations are used to help guide future actions.

      (2) The ability to "walk in another's shoes" is gained.

      (3) Deductive logic is used (Glod, 1998; Piaget, 1952; Whiting, 1997).

5. Behavioral theories: Pavlov (1927) and Skinner (1953)

   a. Overview

1) Behavior is developed through the stimulus-response interaction.

2) Behavior is shaped through consistency of responding.

3) Two attributes of the human brain—flexibility and plasticity—allow for a developmentally significant variety of adaptive sequences (Glod, 1998).

4) Human behavior is derived from behavioral principles and aversive childhood experiences (Glod, 1998; Whiting, 1997).

b. Classical conditioning theory (Pavlov, 1927)

1) Conditioning occurs when a once-neutral stimulus becomes analogous with a response, after the two have been associated with each other (Glod, 1998; Pavlov, 1927).

2) Derived in part from Pavlov's work with dogs, behavioral theory suggests that internal responses can be changed by modifying behavior.

c. Environmental consequences of behavior theory (Skinner, 1953)

1) Skinner's theory extends Pavlovian theory to human beings.

2) Learning is influenced by the effect of individuals' behaviors.

3) During development, actions are weakened or strengthened.

4) Shaping behavior occurs with positive and negative reinforcers, which are events that increase or decrease the likelihood that a given action will result; these action responses also reflect learning (Glod, 1998; Skinner, 1953).

6. Interactional model: Schaie (1981)

a. Development focuses on the concept of goodness of fit and the related ideas of consonance and dissonance.

b. Many outcomes may be influenced by the development that occurs during childhood and adolescence (Whiting, 1997).

1) Development occurs when consonance (or goodness of fit) exists.

a) Involves having environmental demands and expectations in accord with the individual's capacity to respond

b) Results in a sense of comfort or consonance, which makes progressive, optimal development possible

(1) The progression from dependence to interdependence occurs through each developmental stage.

(2) Adaptation results in and corresponds with the demands of the child's chronological age and particular interests.

(a) Developing dependency in infancy (0–1 year of age)

(b) Developing decreasing dependency in childhood (1–12 years of age)

(c) Experiencing conflict in dependency in early adolescence; struggling toward independence in middle adolescence; and attaining independence in late adolescence (older than 13 years of age)

(d) Achieving interdependency in adulthood (older than 21 years of age)

2) Development of dissonance (or poorness of fit) involves discrepancies between the individual and the environment.

a) Results in distorted development from the discrepancies

b) Results in maladaptive functioning from the discrepancies (Schaie, 1981; Whiting, 1997)

C. Critique

1. Older theories of development emphasize completion of development early in childhood.

2. Today, theories assert that individual human development is complex and cannot be classified and categorized.

3. Two attributes of the human brain—flexibility and plasticity—allow for a developmentally significant variety of adaptive sequences.

4. Although early life experiences and influences are significant, they are not the only producers of healthy or negative outcomes (Whiting, 1997).

II. Family Development and Function Theories (see Table 15-2)

A. Overview
   1. The family is a group of people in varying stages of development.
   2. There is a family group stage of development.
   3. Family life stages of development can be useful to rehabilitation nurses who are assessing and intervening with families across the life span.
   4. The needs of the family can be anticipated, depending upon the family's developmental stage (Hogarth & Weeks, 1997).

B. Theories
   1. Family Life Cycle: Duvall (1977)
      a. Basic tasks of families
         1) Keeping the family together: Physical maintenance
         2) Allocating resources: Meeting the family's needs and allocating goods, facilities, space, and authority
         3) Dividing the work within the family: Division of labor
         4) Teaching family members active participation in society: Socialization of family members
         5) Providing for reproduction: Recruitment and release of family members
         6) Maintaining order: Keeping structure and organization within the family
         7) Placing family members into society
         8) Maintaining motivation and morale: Giving encouragement and affection, meeting personal and family crises, refining a philosophy of life and a sense of family loyalty through use of rituals (Hogarth & Weeks, 1997; Youngblood, 1999)
      b. Stages of family development
         1) Marriage and the joining of families
            a) Establishing an identity as a couple
            b) Establishing relationships with extended families
            c) Making decisions about parenthood
         2) Families with infants
            a) Maintaining the couple's relationship while bonding with and integrating the infant into the family
            b) Maintaining the couple's relationship while assuming the parenting role
         3) Families with preschool children
            a) Teaching socialization to children
            b) Learning to adjust to the children being with babysitters or other adults
         4) Families with schoolchildren
            a) Helping the children develop peer relationships
            b) Adjusting to longer periods of separation by both parents and children
         5) Families with teenagers
            a) Adjusting to increased autonomy, which the children are developing
            b) Focusing on midlife issues
         6) Families as launching centers
            a) Adjusting to the children leaving home and becoming independent adults
            b) Adjusting the couple's relationship as they are required to do less parenting
         7) Families of middle years (empty nesters)
            a) Adjusting to living alone again as a couple as the last child leaves home
            b) Beginning to prepare for retirement
            c) Developing new relationships with adult children and grandchildren
         8) Families in retirement (retirement to death)
            a) Beginning to prepare for death of spouse

b) Adjusting to loss of family members and friends (Duvall, 1977; Hogarth & Weeks, 1997)
2. Family Life Cycle: Stevenson (1977) based the stages of family development on the length of the couple's relationship.
   a. The emerging family (years 1–10 of the relationship)

1) Initiating work and career paths by the couple
2) Deciding to and having children by the couple
   b. The crystallizing family (years 11–25 of cohabitation)
      1) Dealing with adolescent children; a two-way relationship between parents

---

Table 15-2. Summary of Family Development and Function Theories

Theory	Description	*Stage 1*	*1–10 years*	*Stage 2*	*Stage 3*
Duvall's (1977) Family Life Cycle	Family development is an eight-stage division that allows for differentiation of the family's changes over time and an analysis of the relationship between the family and the individual's developmental tasks. These cycles begin with the establishment of the marital relationship and are primarily based upon the age or school placement of the eldest child. Successful accomplishment of the tasks in each stage promotes growth and provides a basis for success in the next developmental stage. On the other hand, failure to successfully complete each stage's developmental tasks may result in unhappiness, societal disapproval, and difficulties in accomplishing the tasks within the next stage (Hogarth & Weeks, 1997; Youngblood, 1999)	Marriage and the joining of families	N/A	Families with infants	Families with preschool children
Stevenson's (1977) Family Life Cycle	Four stages of family development are identified that are based on the couple's relationship over time. Success or failure of the family is dependent upon the developmental tasks accomplished in each stage beginning in the first year of the relationship. The last stage ends with the death of one partner and the remaining partner grieving and continuing to grow (Hogarth & Weeks, 1997; Stevenson, 1977)	N/A	The emerging family	N/A	N/A

Major Points
- Family life cycle is defined as the existence of a nuclear family unit (i.e., mother, father, child) from its inception to its dissolution.
- Family life cycle stages are viewed as the amount of time needed to complete each stage of family development.
- The family is a task-performance group that also has specific stage-related behaviors.
- A family evolves over time. The life history of a family is divided into expected stages of development.
- Each stage of development is characterized by relevant tasks and predictable crises associated with the achievement or nonachievement of specific developmental tasks.

and children
2) Launching children into independent status
3) Continuing to grow as a couple
4) Beginning participation in community life by the couple
c. The integrating family (years 26–40 of the relationship)

1) Renewing and enhancing the couple's relationship
2) Continuing work roles by the couple
3) Developing leisure activities by the couple
4) Making adjustments on the part of the children to aging parents
d. The actualizing family (more than 40 years of living together)

Periods

Stage 4	Stage 5	Stage 6	11–25 years	Stage 7	26–40 years	Stage 8	More than 40 years
Families with schoolchildren	Families with teenagers	Families as launching centers	N/A	Families of middle years (empty nesters)	N/A	Families in retirement (retirement to death)	N/A
N/A	N/A	N/A	The crystallizing family	N/A	The integrating family	N/A	The actualizing family

- The life cycles defined by Duvall (1977) and Stevenson (1977) are based on a traditional nuclear family form. Neither theory reflects today's lifestyle changes and various types of families (e.g., divorce, alternative marriage, single parenting).
- Duvall's theory assumes that an intact family (i.e., marriage and children) has universal tasks as well as specific developmental tasks that must be accomplished by the family at eight different stages.
- Stevenson's four stages of family development are based on the length of the couple's relationship and specific developmental task completion throughout the relationship (Carter & McGoldrick, 1989; Youngblood, 1999).

1) Continuing development by the couple
2) Dealing with aging, chronic illness and disease, dying spouse or parents, and death
3) Grieving and continuing to grow if one partner dies (Hogarth & Weeks, 1997; Stevenson, 1977)

C. Critique
   1. Theories such as Duvall's (1977) and Stevenson's (1977) that describe family life stages can be useful for studying families and for practicing rehabilitation nurses because the needs of the family can be anticipated depending on the stage of the family.

2. Because the life cycles defined by both Duvall and Stevenson are based on the traditional nuclear family form, caution is needed when rehabilitation nurses assess nontraditional families.

3. Duvall's and Stevenson's work cannot be used to describe many of the families in today's society that reflect varying lifestyles and forms (e.g., divorce, alternative marriage, single parenting) (Carter & McGoldrick, 1989; Youngblood, 1999).

References

Carter, B., & McGoldrick, M. (1989). *The changing family life cycle: A framework for family therapy.* Needham Heights, MA: Allyn & Bacon.

Drucker, J. (1979). Development from one to two years: Ego development. In J. Noshpitz (Ed.), *Basic handbook of child psychiatry* (Vol.1, pp. 157-165). New York: Basic Books.

Duvall, E. (1977). *Marriage and family development* (5th ed.). Philadelphia: Lippincott.

Erikson, E. (1963). *Childhood and society* (2nd ed.). New York: Norton.

Freud, S. (1959). Inhibitions, symptoms, and anxiety. In J. Strachey (Ed.), *The standard edition of the complete psychological works of Sigmund Freud* (Vol. 18, pp. 1-64). London: Hogarth Press.

Glod, C. (1998). Developmental and psychological theories of mental illness. In C. Glod (Ed.), *Contemporary psychiatric-mental health nursing* (pp. 64-72). Philadelphia: F.A. Davis.

Hogarth, C., & Weeks, S. (1997). Families and family therapy. In B. Johnson (Ed.), *Psychiatric-mental health nursing: Adaptation and growth* (4th ed., pp. 277-298). Philadelphia: Lippincott.

Jarvis, C. (1996). Assessment of the whole person. In C. Jarvis (Ed.), *Physical examination and health assessment* (pp. 1-46). Philadelphia: W.B. Saunders.

Luggen, A. (1998). Developmental theories. In A. Luggen, S. Travis, & S. Meiner (Eds.), *NGNA core curriculum for gerontological advanced practice nurses* (pp. 7-9). Thousand Oaks, CA: Sage.

Pavlov, I. (1927). *Conditioned reflexes: An investigation of the physiological activity of the cerebral cortex.* New York: Oxford University Press.

Piaget, J. (1952). *Origins of intelligence in children.* New York: International Universities Press.

Ricci-Balich, J., & Behm, J. (1996). Pediatric rehabilitation. In S. Hoeman (Ed.), *Rehabilitation nursing: Process and application* (2nd ed., pp. 660-682). St. Louis: Mosby.

Schaie, K. (1981). Psychological changes from midlife to early old age: Implications for the maintenance of mental health. *American Journal of Orthopsychiatry, 51*(4), 199-218.

Skinner, B.F. (1953). *Science and human behavior.* New York: Macmillan.

Stevenson, J. (1977). *Issues and crises during middlescence.* New York: Appleton-Century-Crofts.

Sullivan, H. (1956). *Clinical studies in psychiatry.* New York: Norton.

Sullivan, H. (1964). *The fusion of psychiatry and social science.* New York: Norton.

Whiting, S. (1997). Development of the person. In B. Johnson (Ed.), *Psychiatric-mental health nursing: Adaptation and growth* (4th ed., pp. 357-373). Philadelphia: Lippincott.

Youngblood, N. (1999). Family-centered care. In P. Edwards, D. Hertzberg, S. Hays, & N. Youngblood (Eds.), *Pediatric rehabilitation* (pp. 129-143). Philadelphia: W.B. Saunders.

Suggested resources

Armour, M. (1995). Family life cycle stages: A context for individual life stages. *Journal of Family Social Work, 1*(2), 27-42.

Cronau, H., & Brown, R. (1998). Growth and development: Physical, mental, and social aspects. *Primary Care: Clinics in Office Practice, 25*(1), 23-47.

Litchfield, R. (1999, April). *Developmental perspectives on human growth* [On-line]. Available: www.rglitch.bibl.anderson.edu/

Quinn, A. (1993). Commentary on Erik Erikson: Ages, stages, and stories [Original article by S. Weiland]. *AWHONN's Women's Health Nursing Scan, 7*(6), 4.

Weiland, S. (1993). Erik Erikson: Ages, stages, and stories. *Generations, 17*(2), 17-23.

Chapter 16

Pediatric Rehabilitation Nursing

Penny A. Adsit, MHSA BSN RN CRRN

Dalice Hertzberg, MSN RN CRRN

Increasing numbers of children are surviving congenital, traumatic, or acquired diagnoses. As a result, more children with rehabilitation needs are being served throughout the country. Many general rehabilitation hospitals are finding themselves serving pediatric populations; however, very little literature exists to assist those who serve this specialized population.

Nurses and other rehabilitation providers must work with schools, community, and other healthcare facilities when working with children with rehabilitation needs and their families. Special attention is required so that these children remain a part of their families and community while developing the independence to transition into the community as adults.

I. Overview

A. Definitions
1. Pediatric rehabilitation nursing: "Pediatric rehabilitation nursing is the specialty practice committed to improving the quality of life for children and adolescents with disabilities and for their families as well. The goal of the rehabilitation process is for children, regardless of their disability or chronic illness, to function at their maximum potential and become contributing members of both their families and society" (Association of Rehabilitation Nurses [ARN], 1992, pp. 1–2) (see Figure 16-1).
2. Habilitation: Needing new skills and abilities to meet maximum potential (i.e., children usually have not learned some skills as they continue to progress through the developmental levels)
3. Rehabilitation: Relearning skills and abilities or adjusting existing function to meet age-related developmental expectations

B. Practice Settings
1. Pediatric rehabilitation hospitals (inpatient and outpatient)
2. Pediatric rehabilitation units in rehabilitation hospitals
3. Subacute rehabilitation units (inpatient)
4. Day treatment programs
5. Health department outpatient services
6. State children's rehabilitation services
7. School or day care centers
8. Home health agencies
9. Family homes

C. General Principles
1. Family-centered care: A philosophy of care that recognizes the role of the family in the lives of children
   a. All children are part of a family even if the family is not considered "traditional" in American culture.
   b. Including the family in care ensures that family members and the child receive support in coping with the child's disability or chronic illness.
2. Community-based delivery systems: Services that are delivered in the child's environment (e.g., early intervention center, school, day care, home)
3. Developmental issues
   a. Pediatric rehabilitation nurses should have a basic knowledge of developmental levels and how they affect children who are unable to meet these milestones. *[Refer to Chapter 15 for more information about developmental levels.]*
   b. The child's developmental level should

be considered when determining the rehabilitation plan and interventions.

    c. Interventions should incorporate appropriate recreational activities, toys, and fun, as well as therapeutic interventions.

4. Developmental levels

    a. Infant/toddler (1–3 years old)

    b. Preschooler (3–5 years old)

    c. School-age child (6–12 years old)

    d. Adolescent (12–21 years old)

5. Assessment: Each child should be assessed for the following items, regardless of his or her disability or illness.

    a. Current developmental level

    b. Delays related to developmental level for child's age

    c. The impact of the child's disability on his or her developmental level

    d. Plans for transition into adult services

6. Interventions

    a. Focus on helping the child meet his or her developmental milestones as much as possible

    b. Investigate alternative ways to achieve tasks if developmental milestones cannot be met through therapy or assistive devices

    c. Attempt to map the future by being proactive rather than reactive

    d. Facilitate adaptation to the disability and treatment

    e. Promote community integration

    f. Provide resources and referrals to meet transitional needs when the child is no longer eligible for pediatric services

II. Specific Pediatric Diagnoses

A. Acquired Accidents and Trauma

  1. Brain injury

    a. Definition: A major or minor injury to the brain that results in physical, emotional, or cognitive changes

    b. Assessment components

      1) Developmental level

      2) Glasgow Coma Scale (Edwards, 1999)

      3) Rancho Los Amigos Scale (Edwards, 1999)

      4) WeeFIM® instrument (Edwards, 1999)

      5) Disability Rating Scale (Edwards, 1999)

      6) Hearing and vision studies

      7) Functional and cognitive level

  c. Rehabilitation issues that must be addressed

      1) Independence level appropriate for developmental level

---

Figure 16-1. Roles of Pediatric Rehabilitation Nurses

Advocate
- Functions as a child and family advocate
- Facilitates the entire family's transition from hospital to home and community
- Promotes community and governmental knowledge of pediatric rehabilitation issues

Coordinator
- Works as a valued member of the healthcare team
- Brings together the expertise of health professionals and integrates that knowledge into a comprehensive continuum of care
- Facilitates the design and implementation of the child and family's individual plan of care

Leader
- Demonstrates leadership through clinical expertise
- Acts as an agent of change
- Consults with other health professionals
- Delegates responsibilities to other members of the team

Primary Care Provider
- Implements nursing care based on sound knowledge base, scientific principles, and a documented therapeutic plan

Teacher
- Shares knowledge and skills
- Offers counseling and support to families about the special needs of their children and adolescents with disabilities
- Teaches other individuals (both in the healthcare field and in the community) about the special aspects of children's and adolescents' rehabilitation needs

Team Member
- Works as part of an innovative and creative unit
- Collaborates in the development of new service delivery models that best meet the needs of young clients and their families

Reprinted with permission of the Association of Rehabilitation Nurses from ARN. (1992). *Pediatric rehabilitation nursing role description* [Brochure]. Skokie, IL: Author.

---

2) Need for cognitive rehabilitation
3) Prevention of further injury and complications
4) Family involvement
5) Behavior modification techniques
6) Plans for return to home, school, and community

d. Patient education topics

1) Developmental levels and techniques to help the child reach developmental milestones (this is especially helpful for parents)
2) Use and care of equipment and assistive devices
3) Community reintegration strategies
4) Prevention of further injury and use of protective equipment
5) Behavior modification techniques

2. Spinal cord injury (SCI)

a. Definition: A traumatic injury to the spinal cord and roots (Edwards, 1999) that could be caused by accidents, sports, violence, falls, and other injuries

b. Assessment components

1) Health history
2) Functional and cognitive levels
3) Developmental levels
4) Skin integrity
5) Bladder and bowel function
6) Psychosocial issues
7) Family history

c. Rehabilitation issues that must be addressed

1) Bladder and bowel management
2) Skin care
3) Mobility
4) Pulmonary function
5) Risk for heterotrophic ossification
6) Risk for autonomic dysreflexia
7) Risk for spasticity and contractures
8) Risk for sexual dysfunction
9) Risk for osteopenia

d. Patient education topics

1) Bladder and bowel program
2) Skin care
3) Autonomic dysreflexia (if injury is at T6 or above)
4) Medications
5) Community reintegration strategies

3. Burns

a. Definitions

1) The loss of any of the three layers of skin by thermal, electrical, chemical, or irradiation burns
2) Classified as first-, second-, or third-degree burns
3) Based on the depth (thickness) of skin affected (e.g., superficial, partial thickness, full thickness)

b. Assessment components

1) Skin integrity
2) Respiratory condition
3) Mobility and functional levels (using WeeFIM, Pediatric Evaluation of Disability Inventory [PEDI], Scale of Independent Behavior) (Himes & Kuntz, 1999)
4) Pain
5) Nutrition
6) Self-image (using Vinland Adaptive Behavior Scale) (Himes & Kuntz, 1999)
7) Developmental level (using Battelle Developmental Inventory)
8) Family history and coping

c. Rehabilitation issues that must be addressed

1) Potential for infection (e.g., skin, respiratory)
2) Location of burns that may affect functional ability
3) Comfort level
4) Nutrition
5) Pressure-relief garments
6) Restoration of self-image
7) Elimination pattern

d. Patient education topics

1) Prevention of complications, contractures, and loss of function
2) Care and use of pressure-relief garments
3) Signs and symptoms of infection
4) Wound care
5) Social reintegration strategies
6) School and community reintegration strategies
7) Psychosocial and behavioral interventions
8) Personal care
9) Nutrition

4. Limb deficiency
   a. Definition: The absence of one or more limbs, caused by accidents, diseases, malignancies, or congenital conditions
   b. Assessment components
      1) Developmental level
      2) Musculoskeletal system
      3) Mobility
      4) Skin integrity and/or residual limb care and condition
   c. Rehabilitation issues that must be addressed
      1) Independence level
      2) Function of limb
      3) Prosthetic management
      4) Skin and/or residual limb management
      5) Pain management
      6) Self-esteem and self-concept
   d. Patient education topics
      1) Use and care of equipment and/or prosthesis
      2) Residual limb wrapping
      3) Skin care
      4) Pain management
      5) Community reintegration strategies

B. Acquired Diseases
   1. Human immunodeficiency virus (HIV)
      a. Definition: A virus that causes multior-gan systemic illness due to suppression of the immune system; the course of the disease is variable but inevitably fatal
      b. Assessment components
         1) Multisystem analysis
         2) Disease progression
         3) Developmental level
         4) Central nervous system (CNS) impairment
         5) Community resources
      c. Rehabilitation issues that must be addressed
         1) Prevention of infection
         2) Neurologic involvement
         3) Independence level
         4) Coping
      d. Patient education topics
         1) Medication regimen
         2) Pain management techniques
         3) Prevention of complications

      4) Confidentiality and stigma
      5) Use and care of equipment and assistive devices
      6) Community reintegration strategies
   2. Cancer
      a. Definition: Abnormal cell growth and/or mutation that can invade vessels and transport mutated cells to other sites in the body; the most common pediatric cancers are leukemia, lymphoma, and sarcomas
      b. Assessment components
         1) Developmental level
         2) Family assessment
         3) Community resources
         4) Functional ability related to disease progression
      c. Rehabilitation issues that must be addressed
         1) Pain management
         2) Independence level related to developmental level
         3) Disease progression
         4) Coping
      d. Patient education topics
         1) Use and care of equipment and assistive devices
         2) Medication regimen
         3) Pain management techniques
         4) Community reintegration strategies

C. Congenital Diseases and Birth Defects
   1. Myelodysplasia or spina bifida
      a. Definition: A defect in which the neural tube fails to close during the first 3–4 weeks of fetal development, resulting in the spinal cord developing outside the body and enclosed in a small sac
      b. Assessment components
         1) Developmental level
         2) Hydrocephalus (shunts are common)
         3) Bladder and bowel function
         4) Skin integrity
         5) Scoliosis and kyphosis
         6) Orthopedic disorders (e.g., clubfoot, hip dysplasia)
         7) Cognition
         8) Location and severity of lesion
         9) Latex allergies
         10) Visual perceptual deficits

11) Cardiopulmonary function
12) Ability to perform activities of daily living (ADLs)
13) Family history and genetics

c. Rehabilitation issues that must be addressed

1) Developmental level
2) Functional and cognitive abilities
3) Ability to perform ADLs
4) Independence level related to growth and developmental level
5) Seizures and potential for shunt malfunction
6) Nutrition
7) Bowel and bladder management
8) Skin care
9) Self-concept and self-esteem

d. Patient education topics

1) Bladder and bowel program
2) Skin care and pressure-relief techniques
3) Use and care of equipment and/or orthoses
4) ADLs
5) Independence
6) Transfers and ambulation (if appropriate to level of lesion)
7) Community integration strategies

2. Joint and orthopedic conditions

a. Types and definitions

1) Legg-Calve-Perthes disease: A condition most frequently occurring in males in which the femoral capital epiphysis develops avascular necrosis when the child is 4–8 years old
2) Osteogenesis imperfecta: A genetic condition that results in brittle bones; commonly associated with fractures that can occur with normal movement and care of the child with this condition
3) Blount's disease (Tibia Vara): A condition resulting from an abnormality of the proximal medial tibial epiphysis and metaphysis in which the child has severe bowing of one or both legs
4) Leg length discrepancy: A disorder that can be the result of congenital malformations of the fibula,

infections, trauma that affects the epiphyses, or neurologic disorders such as poliomyelitis
5) Juvenile rheumatoid arthritis: A chronic inflammation that involves the connective tissue, joints, and viscera, which begins before the age of 16
6) Sickle-cell disease: A genetic disease that can cause osteopenia
7) Achondroplasia: A genetic condition, which is visible at birth, that involves atypical head and limb growth

b. Assessment components

1) Developmental level
2) Level of disability related to diagnosis
3) Mobility
4) Ability to perform ADLs
5) Use and care of equipment and assistive devices
6) Family history and genetics
7) Medications

c. Rehabilitation issues that must be addressed

1) Joint protection
2) Maximum independence level based on the severity of diagnosis
3) Mobility
4) ADL modification
5) Safety
6) Pain management

d. Patient education topics

1) Medication regimen
2) ADLs
3) Safety
4) Mobility vs. joint protection
5) Pain management
6) Use and care of equipment and assistive devices
7) Community reintegration strategies

3. Cerebral palsy (see Figure 16-2)

a. Definition: A mild to severe condition that results from damage to the developing brain that produces a permanent but not unchanging disorder of movement and posture

b. Assessment components

1) Developmental level
2) Cognitive level

3) Communication
4) Ability to perform ADLs
5) Feeding pattern
6) Toileting
7) Muscle tone
8) Ambulation
9) History of seizure disorder and other associated conditions
10) Musculoskeletal system
11) Skin integrity

c. Rehabilitation issues that must be addressed

1) Neurodevelopmental and sensory therapies
2) Independent living skills
3) Positioning (depending on severity)
4) Feeding problems
5) Communication
6) Seizure management
7) Spasticity management

d. Patient education topics

1) Skin care
2) Home exercise program
3) Medications
4) Spasticity management techniques
5) Self-care and feeding techniques
6) Community integration strategies

D. Chronic Illnesses
1. Cystic fibrosis

a. Definition: An autosomal recessive genetic defect that primarily affects the respiratory and digestive systems; a fatal, genetic disease that results from parents who both have the cystic fibrosis gene

b. Assessment components

1) Developmental level
2) Respiratory function
3) Gastrointestinal function
4) Pancreatic function
5) History of respiratory problems and infections
6) Symptom progression
7) Coping skills
8) Family history and genetics

c. Rehabilitation issues that must be addressed

1) Independence level
2) Pulmonary function
3) Nutritional status

d. Patient education topics

Figure 16-2. Types of Cerebral Palsy

Spastic
- Hyperactive reflexes, increased muscle tone, muscle clonus/spasms, persistent infantile reflexes, motor weakness
- *Hemiplegia:* Most frequent type, involves one side of the body, usually arm is weaker and leg is more spastic, affected side is smaller, fine motor movement of the hand has mild to severe involvement with posturing of the hand and flexion of the elbow and wrist, child can walk but has gait changes with knee flexion and plantar flexion of the foot, sensory deficits or cortical neglects of affected side; often seen from early head trauma or stroke
- *Diplegia:* Involvement of all four extremities, lower more involved than upper, with weakness and varying levels of increased tone, upper extremities more mildly involved; often seen with prematurity
- *Quadriplegia:* Involvement of total body, increased muscle tone, rigid in flexion and extension of all four extremities, usually severe impairment of postural and motor control, hip adductor spasticity causing "scissoring" of the legs, plantar flexion of the feet, hands fisted with thumb inside, feeding and speech difficulty with oral motor involvement, exaggerated startle reflex, highest incidence of associated conditions and severe impairments; impairment of cognitive functioning often caused by some type of anoxia

Athetoid
- Characterized by abnormal involuntary movements of all extremities that disappear during sleep, resulting in "worm-like" writhing and flailing of extremities and trunk, facial grimacing, dystonic movements of the tongue and mouth, poorly articulated speech, forced movements of hand and feet, distorted posturing; often caused by newborn kernicterus

Ataxic
- Hypotonia, "floppy" muscle tone with balance and coordination impairment; walk with wide-based, unsteady gait; uncoordinated upper extremity function; least common type

Mixed
- Combination of several types of cerebral palsy; severe delayed cognitive ability and other conditions common with this type

Sources consulted

Logigian, M.K., & Ward, J.D. (Eds.). *Pediatric rehabilitation: A team approach for therapists.* Boston: Little, Brown.
Gold, J. (1993). Pediatric disorders: Cerebral palsy and spina bifida. In M.S. Eisenberg, R.L. Glueckauf, & H.H. Zaretsky (Eds.), *Medical aspects of disability* (pp. 281-306). Philadelphia: W.B. Saunders.
Reprinted with permission of W.B. Saunders from Hays, S.R. (1999). Management of central nervous system impairment. In P.A. Edwards, D.L. Hertzberg, S.R. Hays, & N.M. Youngblood (Eds.), *Pediatric rehabilitation nursing* (p. 328). Philadelphia: W.B. Saunders.

1) Medication regimen
2) Prevention of complications
3) Management of emergencies
4) Community integration strategies

2. Asthma

   a. Definition: A lung disease characterized by reversible airway obstruction, inflammation of the airways, and increased airway responsiveness to internal and external stimuli; also typically involves childhood immunity problems

   b. Assessment components

     1) Developmental level
     2) Family history and coping
     3) Environmental allergies
     4) Onset and exacerbation of symptoms
     5) Cardiorespiratory system
     6) Functional limitations

   c. Rehabilitation issues that must be addressed

     1) Independence level related to developmental level
     2) Medication management
     3) Environmental modification
     4) Physical therapy

   d. Patient education topics

     1) Self-administration and self-management of medications
     2) Avoidance of triggers for asthma attack
     3) Environmental modifications to remove allergens

3. Bronchopulmonary dysplasia

   a. Definition: Chronic obstructive lung disease, which develops in premature infants as a result of medical interventions for life-threatening conditions such as respiratory distress syndrome, meconium aspiration, and persistent pulmonary hypertension

   b. Assessment components

     1) Developmental level
     2) Respiratory condition
     3) Current and past treatments, including mechanical ventilation, tracheostomy, and medications
     4) Cardiac assessment for symptoms of right-side heart failure
     5) Feeding patterns

6) Family coping

   c. Rehabilitation issues that must be addressed

     1) Developmental interventions
     2) Respiratory support (e.g., oxygen, tracheostomy, mechanical ventilation)
     3) Chest physiotherapy
     4) Medication therapy
     5) Nutritional management

   d. Patient education topics

     1) Management and administration of technology in the home and community
     2) Medication management
     3) Development of independence
     4) Community integration
     5) Family coping skills

4. Technology dependence

   a. Definition: A dependence on technology for a range of functions, including communication, environmental control, mobility, and basic survival

   b. Assessment components

     1) Developmental level
     2) Ability to perform ADLs
     3) Respiratory system
     4) Feeding patterns
     5) Toileting
     6) Ambulation
     7) Musculoskeletal system

   c. Rehabilitation issues that must be addressed

     1) Independence level appropriate for developmental level
     2) Prevention of further injury and complications
     3) Family involvement
     4) Operation and maintenance of assistive technology
     5) Personal care and assistance
     6) Cost of care and reimbursement
     7) Return to home, school, community

   d. Patient education topics

     1) Operation and maintenance of assistive technology
     2) Community integration
     3) Training of community service providers

III. Long-Term Planning

A. Community Services
1. Community services promote normality for children because they can continue to live with their families.
2. Some communities do not have the services that children need, so families are forced to make compromises.
   a. To find services that are available for the child
   b. To remove the child from the home to obtain needed services

B. The Philosophy of Inclusion
1. Inclusion is a philosophical viewpoint that purports that children with disabilities are an integral part of the community and should participate with their peers in typical activities.
2. Inclusion activities include playgroups, school, recreation, social activities, and work.

C. Home Health Care
1. Home health care is available in most communities, but its high cost prohibits some families from taking full advantage of it.
2. Families must make decisions about providing services themselves or letting the child go without home care if the services are unaffordable.
3. Many of the child's physical needs can be met by the family.
4. Living at home is usually considered better for the child's psychological and social well-being than living in an institution.

D. School Programs
1. The Individuals with Disabilities Education Act (IDEA) ensures that all children and young adults ages 3–21 years receive a free, appropriate public education.
2. Education and special education services should be delivered in the least restrictive environment (LRE) that is very similar to educational settings for nondisabled children.
3. Children who require special education are entitled to receive an Individualized Education Plan (IEP) that is reviewed yearly to best meet the individual child's educational needs.

4. Children with disabilities may also receive related services (e.g., physical therapy, occupational therapy, speech therapy, nutrition, other health-related services) as mandated by IDEA.
5. Child Find is a system that each school district must have in place to identify and evaluate children who are eligible for special education services.

E. Early Intervention Programs
1. IDEA provides for early educational services for young children from birth to 3 years of age.
2. Eligible children may have a congenital disability, may exhibit developmental delays, or may be at risk for delays.
3. Eligible children and their families receive an Individualized Family Service Plan (IFSP) that plans interventions to eliminate or reduce the developmental delay or disability and offers family support.

F. Health Promotion and Preventive Measures
1. Immunizations
2. Screening (identification of children who need in-depth assessment particularly related to developmental delays or other health problems)
3. Preventive health education for the child and family
4. Health education for legislators and community leaders
5. Positive health education for the community

G. Transition to Adulthood and Independent Living Situations
1. Functional independence assessment
2. Primary factors in successful psychosocial and independent living models (Blomquist, Brown, Peersen, & Presler, 1998)
   a. Attitude
   b. Adjustment
   c. Control
   d. Environmental accessibility
   e. Availability of independent living support services
3. Areas of assessment for helping plan the transition to independent living (Blomquist et al., 1998)

a. Ability to perform ADLs

b. Level of mobility

c. Transportation needs

d. Healthcare needs

e. Living arrangements (e.g., where, with whom, community options, housekeeping skills)

f. Housing (e.g., adaptations needed, ability to maintain a home)

g. Recreation and leisure activities

h. Personal awareness and desire for companionship

i. Community participation

j. Educational level and needs

k. Existing employment opportunities and job support systems

l. Financial management strategies

m. Legal issues

H. Vocational Rehabilitation and Higher Education
1. Consideration should be provided early as to the child's future potential in the workforce.

   a. Developmental level

   b. Progress toward independence

   c. Cognitive learning abilities

2. While not all children have the potential to be working members of society, many are overlooked simply because they are not aware of available resources for gaining more independence by participating in vocational training and higher education as a result of the Vocational Rehabilitation Act.

3. Vocational rehabilitation programs will sometimes help clients obtain higher education.

I. Legislation That Affects Children with Disabilities
1. Individuals with Disabilities Education Act (IDEA)

2. Rehabilitation Act

3. Americans with Disabilities Act (ADA) of 1990

4. Vocational Rehabilitation Act

5. Title V Legislation (Maternal and Child Health Bureau)

6. Child Protection Legislation

IV. The Future of Pediatric Rehabilitation
A. In Health Care
1. Additional medical developments will result in more children surviving congenital, traumatic, and acquired disabilities and conditions.

2. Debates will continue and become more prevalent regarding the inadequate amount of funding that goes to a small percentage of the healthcare population (e.g., children with disabilities and chronic conditions).

3. More sophisticated technology will be available to preserve and improve life, but this will come at an increasing expense, making it accessible only to those with private insurance or substantial income.

4. The population of adults with disabilities who have survived childhood disabilities and chronic diseases will increase and affect the healthcare system as a whole.

5. There will be a greater emphasis on the use of healthcare outcomes to legitimize services.

6. There will be increased use of genetic history of disease to deny potentially costly insurance benefits.

7. Pediatric rehabilitation will continue to develop as a recognized specialty.

B. In the Community at Large
1. There will be an increased need for home care education and for training caregivers in various settings.

2. There will be an increased need for accommodations for children who are technology-dependent in schools and in the community.

3. There will be less hospital-based care and more community- and home-based care.

4. Legislation and litigation will continue to be a means to provide services to pediatric population at both the state and federal levels.

References

Association of Rehabilitation Nurses (ARN). (1992). *Pediatric rehabilitation nursing role description* [Brochure]. Skokie, IL: Author.

Blomquist, K.B., Brown, G., Peersen, A., & Presler, E.P. (1998). Transition to independence: Challenges for young people with disabilities and their caregivers. *Orthopaedic Nursing, 17*(3), 27-35.

Edwards, P.A. (1999). Traumatic injuries. In P.A. Edwards, D.L. Hertzberg, S.R. Hays, & N.M. Youngblood (Eds.), *Pediatric rehabilitation nursing* (pp. 509-524). Philadelphia: W.B. Saunders.

Hays, S.R. (1999). Management of central nervous system impairment. In P.A. Edwards, D.L. Hertzberg, S.R. Hays, & N.M. Youngblood (Eds.), *Pediatric rehabilitation nursing* (pp. 317-336). Philadelphia: W.B. Saunders.

Himes, C.H., & Kuntz, K.R. (1999). Pediatric burn rehabilitation. In P.A. Edwards, D.L. Hertzberg, S.R. Hays, & N.M. Youngblood (Eds.), *Pediatric rehabilitation nursing* (pp. 494-508). Philadelphia: W.B. Saunders.

Suggested resources

Allen, K., Wilcyzynsky, S., & Evans, J. (1997). Pediatric rehabilitation: Defining a field, a focus and a future. *International Journal of Rehabilitation & Health, 3*(1), 25-40.

Anonymous. (1997). Helping parents cope…their child has a severe disability. *Pediatric Mental Health, 16*(2), 3.

Arango, P. (1997). Family voices: Building voices for our children with special health care needs. *Pediatric Nursing, 23*(4), 400-402.

Batshaw, M., & Perrett, Y. (1998). *Children with disabilities.* Baltimore: Paul H. Brookes Publishing.

Deaton, A. (1996). Ethical issues in pediatric rehabilitation: Exploring an uneven terrain. *Rehabilitation Psychology, 41*(1), 33-32.

Dorman, S. (1998). Technology briefs: Assistive technology benefits for students with disabilities. *Journal of School Health, 68*(3), 120-123.

Fowler, F. (1996). The challenges of pediatric rehab. *Rehab Management: The Interdisciplinary Journal of Rehabilitation, 9*(1), 78, 81.

Gormley, M., Jr., & Krach, L. (1997). Pediatric functional assessment. *Rehab Management: The Interdisciplinary Journal of Rehabilitation, 19*(6), 32, 34-35, 103.

Guillett, S. (1998). Assessing the child with disabilities. *Home Healthcare Nurse, 16*(6), 402-409.

Kaye, H. (1997). *Education of children with disabilities.* Washington, DC: U.S. Department of Education, National Institute of Disability and Rehabilitation Research.

McCabe, M. (1996). Pediatric functional independence measure: Clinical trials with disabled and nondisabled children. *Applied Nursing Research, 9*(3), 136-138.

Molnar, G. (1992). *Pediatric rehabilitation.* Baltimore: Williams and Wilkins.

Schaaf, R., Sherwen, L., & Youngblood, N. (1997). An interdisciplinary, environmentally-based model of care for children with HIV infection and their caregivers. (1997). *Physical and Occupational Therapy in Pediatrics, 17*(3), 63-85.

Selekman, J. (1991). Pediatric rehabilitation: From concepts to practice. *Pediatric Nursing, 17*(1), 11-14, 33.

Wallace, H., MacQueen, J., Biehl, R., & Blackman, J. (1997). *Mosby's resource guide to children with disabilities and chronic illness.* St. Louis: Mosby.

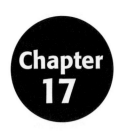

Chapter 17

Gerontological Rehabilitation Nursing

Kristen L. Easton, MS RN CRRN-A CS

It is no secret that the rapid growth in the elderly population will have a major impact on the healthcare delivery system. In 1990, people older than 65 years accounted for 12.7% of the United States population, or 38 million people (Fowles, 1994). By the year 2050, it is projected that nearly 20% of the U.S. population will be at least 65 years old, and the oldest-old—or frail elderly people—will be the fastest growing age group in the country. As a person's age increases, so does the likelihood of experiencing chronic illness and functional limitations. In light of these statistics, rehabilitation nurses must be prepared to meet the demands of an aging society. This can only be accomplished through special knowledge and training in the areas of gerontology and rehabilitation.

I. Overview of the Aging Process

A. Theories of Aging

1. Genetics/DNA: Each person has a genetic program that helps predetermine life expectancy.

2. Wear and tear: The length of life is inversely related to the rate of living (i.e., the more wear and tear placed upon the body, the faster one ages).

3. Lipofuscin: This lipoprotein byproduct of metabolism increases with age, resulting in visible signs of aging.

4. Radiation: Stressors related to radiation in the environment cause signs of aging.

5. Stress: Aging is related to or influenced by life stress.

6. Gene mutation: Over time, genes mutate and cause the body to age.

7. Autoimmune: The body perceives old, irregular cells as hostile agents and begins to attack itself.

8. Nutritional: Length of life and age-related changes can be either positively or negatively influenced by nutritional intake.

9. Environmental: Pollutants in one's life surroundings, such as air and noise pollution, adversely affect health and cause signs of aging.

B. Physiological Effects of Normal Aging and the Possible Effects of Aging on Functional Ability and Rehabilitation Potential

1. Cardiac/circulatory system

a. Decreased cardiac output

b. Valvular changes that may result in heart murmurs

c. Decreased ability to adapt to increased demands

d. Decreased contractility

e. Increased incidence of varicose veins

f. Increase in thickness of capillary walls (Miller, 1995)

g. Increase in systolic blood pressure (Eliopoulos, 1999)

2. Respiratory system

a. Less elasticity of the lungs

b. Increase in carbon dioxide retention due to a less efficient system

c. Less useful oxygen with each breath

d. Reduced vital capacity

e. Decrease in blood oxygen level (Ebersole & Hess, 1998)

3. Musculoskeletal system

a. Decreased muscle mass

b. Changes in range of motion (ROM) in joints

c. Decrease in overall height due to compression of vertebra over time

d. Decreased bone density leading to increased risk for fractures

e. Decrease in cartilage surface of joints leading to possible limitations in ROM

4. Genitourinary system

   a. In women

     1) Decrease in estrogen with perimenopause and menopause

     2) Decrease in vaginal lubrication often leading to pain during sexual intercourse

     3) Stress incontinence (common but treatable)

     4) Other types of incontinence (common but not a normal part of aging)

   b. In men

     1) No significant changes in sexual libido or previous patterns of behavior

     2) Longer refractory times during phases of sexual intercourse

     3) Less complete erections and less frequent orgasms

     4) Enlarged prostate, resulting in poor urinary stream

   c. In both men and women

     1) Decreased bladder capacity

     2) Increase in urinary frequency and nocturia

5. Nervous system

   a. Slower voluntary reflexes

   b. Deep tendon reflexes still responsive

   c. More difficulty responding to multiple stimuli

   d. Decreased kinesthetic sense

   e. Complaints of feeling tired (even if staying in bed longer) due to sleep pattern changes such as a decrease in Stage IV, rapid-eye-movement (REM) sleep

   f. Decreased dopamine levels, which may contribute to Parkinsonian features such as abnormal gait

6. Sensory system

   a. Vision

     1) Presbyopia: Farsightedness or trouble focusing on near objects due to age-related changes in the shape of the eye

     2) Decreased peripheral vision

     3) Cataracts (extremely common but highly treatable with surgery and intraocular lens implants)

     4) Decreased tear production, which leads to increased susceptibility to infections

     5) Changes in depth perception

   b. Hearing

     1) Presbycusis: Decrease in hearing acuity, especially the ability to detect high frequency tones

     2) Impacted wax

     3) Need for hearing aids, which may amplify extraneous noises

   c. Smell: General decrease in acuity

   d. Taste: Atrophied taste buds, which can cause a person to use more seasoning on food

   e. Pain

     1) Increased tolerance for pain

     2) General decreased sensitivity to light touch

     3) Increased pain threshold

7. Neurological system

   a. Cognition

     1) Some memory loss is common but should be distinguished from abnormalities such as those that occur with Alzheimer's disease.

     2) Intelligence and ability to learn are not affected.

   b. Proprioception (awareness of body position in space): May decrease with age, which can result in less coordination and balance that could lead to falls

8. Endocrine system

   a. Changes in sex hormones

   b. Decreased efficiency of the entire system

   c. Changes in thyroid hormone production and glucose tolerance, which may require treatment (e.g., thyroid changes may lower the metabolic rate)

9. Hematological system

   a. Anemia, particularly iron deficiency and pernicious types

   b. Hypoalbuminemia

     1) Serum albumin has been shown to be a predictor of geriatric rehabilitation outcomes.

2) Albumin of less than 3.0 g/dl may place a person at risk for poor outcomes, including pressure ulcers.

10. Immune system

   a. Generally less efficient

   b. Possibly less resistant to infections

   c. Possible absence of "typical" symptoms of illness (e.g., elevated temperature with pneumonia)

11. Integumentary system

   a. Skin

     1) Becomes more wrinkled, thinner
     2) Loses elasticity
     3) Is dry, which may lead to itching
     4) Has an increased potential for skin tears and bruising

   b. Hair

     1) Pigment loss, resulting in what appears as gray or white hair
     2) Development of facial hair (in women)
     3) Balding (in men)

   c. Nails: More brittle

   d. Fat: Distributed more on the trunk and less on the arms and legs

12. Gastrointestinal system

   a. Slowed absorption in intestines

   b. Decreased digestive enzymes

   c. Decreased saliva production

   d. Decreased esophageal and intestinal peristalsis

   e. Constipation

   f. Weaker gag reflex and/or delayed swallowing, which can increase the risk of aspiration

13. Renal system

   a. Potential loss of up to half of the functioning nephrons

   b. Decreased glomerular filtration rate

II. The Combination of the Effects of Aging and Chronic Illness and Disability

A. General Considerations

1. The aging process affects all living things; however, with the presence of a disability or chronic illness, the effects of aging are often compounded.

2. As more people live to old age with disabilities and functional limitations (especially those that occurred when they were younger), more research will be needed on the effects of aging with a disability.

3. Certain factors are common among many disease processes.

   a. Fatigue

   b. Decreased endurance

   c. Higher incidence of skin breakdown

B. Aging and Specific Diseases and Disabilities

1. Stroke

   a. Hemiparesis or hemiplegia, combined with changes in sensory perception, balance, and coordination, increase the risk for falls.

   b. Neurogenic bowel compounds problems with constipation.

   c. Neurogenic bladder increases the risk of incontinence.

   d. Impaired swallowing is complicated by normal aging changes, such as decreased esophageal peristalsis and decreased salivary secretions.

   e. Adequate nutritional intake may be difficult when impaired swallowing is present; tube feedings may be necessary to prevent aspiration.

   f. Impaired physical mobility may be complicated by preexisting arthritis or other limiting factors.

   g. Immobility increases the risk of pressure ulcers on already fragile skin.

2. Spinal cord injury (SCI)

   a. General: Aging with SCI affects all body systems due to the hazards of prolonged immobility.

   b. Skin: The aging, fragile dermis is more susceptible to pressure ulcers as a result of immobility and paralysis.

   c. Temperature: Less perspiration and less tolerance to temperature extremes are associated with aging; with SCI, heat intolerance is also common.

   d. Muscles and bones: ROM decreases with age; active ROM is absent with complete SCI; muscle mass and muscle atrophy decreases with age and disuse after SCI.

e. Bowel and bladder: Incontinence increases with age (but it is not a normal part of aging) and is complicated by neurogenic bowel and bladder after SCI.

f. Cardiopulmonary function

1) Less useful oxygen is available with each breath with aging.

2) Respiratory status is compromised after all cervical and most thoracic SCIs: Many clients do not have a strong cough and are prone to respiratory infections.

3) Incidence of deep vein thrombosis (DVT) increases after SCI.

g. Nutrition and metabolism

1) Metabolism slows with age and the need for calories decreases.

2) With SCI, less activity decreases caloric need.

3) All elderly clients need a diet high in protein, roughage, vitamins, and minerals.

h. Renal system

1) Glomerular filtration rates decrease with age.

2) Clients with SCI need routine renal studies because they are at an increased risk for reflux and kidney damage due to complications of neurogenic bladder.

i. Sexuality

1) Changes in physical function with normal aging may adversely affect self-esteem.

2) Obvious body image changes occur with paralysis after SCI.

3) Older clients must deal with self-esteem and self-concept issues as well as role changes.

j. Sensory perception: Clients may experience changes related to decreased touch sensation, but some sensory perception may be absent or diminished after SCI, depending on the level and completeness of the injury.

3. Multiple sclerosis (MS)

a. Fatigue associated with MS is complicated by decreased endurance with advanced age as well as exacerbations over time.

b. New medications that decrease the number of plaques and the number of annual exacerbations present new challenges for those who may be living a long life with MS.

c. It becomes more challenging to manage medications (especially frequent subcutaneous injections) with advanced age and to deal with functional limitations that may affect fine motor coordination.

4. Traumatic brain injury (TBI), which involves long-term consequences associated with aging

a. Increased caregiver burden when constant supervision is needed

b. Life changes among the family members of the older adult with TBI

c. Decisions regarding long-term care placement when the family or caregiver is unable to manage at home

5. Amputation

a. The use of upper extremities may place undue stress on nonweight-bearing joints (especially shoulders), which can lead to early complications

b. The cost of maintaining adaptive equipment (e.g., wheelchairs, prostheses) is high if the injury occurred in younger years; the client can expect to use several different chairs and prostheses throughout his or her lifetime.

6. Other neurological and musculoskeletal disorders

a. Parkinson's disease (PD)

1) The three cardinal signs of PD may be complicated with changes occurring with advanced age.

a) Bradykinesia

b) Rigidity

c) Tremors

2) Joints become less mobile with normal aging; clients with PD are especially dependent upon medication management to maintain mobility.

3) Swallowing is often impaired and complicated by the normal aging

processes of decreased esophageal peristalsis and salivary secretions.

4) Altered sleep patterns are commonly associated with PD and normal aging.

b. Postpolio syndrome: Fatigue resurfaces years after the initial incidence of polio and presents a major concern.

c. Lupus: This disease affects all body systems; the signs and symptoms of fatigue, sensitivity to sunlight, pain, and potential for infection are complicated and compounded by the aging process.

d. Joint replacements, which are often needed for mobility and pain management with osteoarthritis

1) There is a limited life span of the prosthetics used for replacement.

2) Improper rehabilitation can place undue stress on other joints.

3) Hip pinning may be an alternative to hip replacement after fracture.

7. Other chronic problems

a. Diabetes

1) Foot care: This is important for all elderly people, but it is particularly crucial for older adults with diabetes. The following instructions are especially important.

a) Do not trim corns, bunions, or calluses

b) See a podiatrist about ingrown toenails

c) Do not go barefoot

d) Keep feet clean by washing regularly with warm water and soap

e) Avoid putting lotion between the toes

f) See a healthcare professional promptly about any type of foot sore

g) Do not use home remedies in lieu of being treated by a physician

2) Medications: It is important to keep blood sugar under control with a balance of exercise, diet, and medications to prevent complications.

3) Selected complications that are compounded with aging

a) Visual disturbances

(1) Diabetic retinopathy can result in blindness.

(2) Cataracts and decreased peripheral vision are common with normal aging.

(3) Surgery for cataracts or other visual problems may be complicated by longer healing times and the higher risk of infection with diabetes.

b) Wound healing

(1) Wounds heal more slowly as a person ages and even more slowly if the person has diabetes.

(2) Elderly clients have a higher risk of infections.

c) Peripheral vascular disease (PVD) or diabetic neuropathy

(1) Diabetes is a primary cause of PVD.

(2) Decreased sensation in the extremities is compounded by diabetes.

b. Burns

1) Skin is more fragile and less elastic with age, and the risk of infection and healing time increases.

2) The potential for complications related to fluid volume changes and electrolyte imbalances increases.

c. Multiple trauma: Elderly clients have slower healing times and increased risk of infection as well as less reserve in other body systems to recover from extreme trauma.

d. Cardiac and respiratory disease

1) Elderly clients have less of a cardiac reserve to meet the increased demands of normal aging.

2) Carbon dioxide retention increases with age and is further complicated if chronic obstructive pulmonary disease (COPD) is present.

3) Impaired gas exchange is a common problem in elderly people with COPD.

4) Smoking greatly increases the risk of respiratory disease.

III. Special Considerations for Older Adults Participating in Rehabilitation

A. Fall Prevention and Safety Promotion

1. Background and statistics

   a. Falls account for a substantial number of accidental deaths in elderly people (Ross, 1991).

   b. Mortality from falls rises with increased age (Liddle & Gilleard, 1995; Ross, 1991).

   c. More than half of nursing home clients fall more than once (Steinmetz & Hobson, 1994).

2. Risk assessment for falls

   a. Risk factors for falls (Easton, 1999)

      1) Age: Older than 60 years old; elderly people

      2) Diagnosis: Increased risk with stroke and brain injury

      3) Altered physical capabilities: Impaired mobility, weakness, hemiplegia, impaired balance, decreased endurance

      4) Altered mental state: Confusion, restlessness, sedation, altered consciousness, history of seizures, dementia

      5) Altered elimination: Bowel and bladder incontinence, urgency, frequency, nocturia

      6) Cognitive and sensory impairments: Impaired memory or judgment, aphasia, neglect, impaired hearing or vision

      7) Altered proprioception

      8) Time of hospitalization: Falls are more likely to occur when the client first changes settings (due to unfamiliarity with surroundings) and again as discharge approaches (due to gaining confidence and being encouraged to increase independence).

      9) Medication that affects fluid balance or sensorium: Diuretics, laxatives, sedatives, hypnotics, tranquilizers, antidepressants, antihypertensives, drug and alcohol abuse

      10) Psychological factors: Denying that a fall occurred, impulsivity, history of removing safety devices, hesitancy in calling for help

   b. Tools: Preexisting tools are available, but it may be most efficient to analyze the factors related to falls in the specific institution or workplace.

3. Goals of safety or fall prevention programs

   a. Decrease incidence of falls, including the physical and emotional consequences of falls (Liddle & Gilleard, 1995)

   b. Promote safety among clients

4. Interventions

   a. Develop and implement a safety promotion or fall prevention plan

   b. Promote strength and endurance training for older adults

   c. Make the home and hospital setting safe

      1) Keep walkways clear

      2) Remove clutter

      3) Remove throw rugs

      4) Teach the client and family about risk factors for falls (see Figure 17-1)

      5) Be careful around stairs, pets, and small children

      6) Use adaptive devices correctly

5. Evaluation

   a. Evaluation should be done in terms of long- and short-term goals.

   b. Documentation of falls should include

Figure 17-1. Potential Environmental Risk Factors for Falls

- Flooring, such as throw rugs, high-pile carpeting, slippery or wet tile
- Outdoor walkways that are wet or have leaves, snow, or ice on them
- Small children and pets
- Stairs and steps (especially those without handrails and those not clearly marked)
- Clutter in walkways and around the bedroom and bathroom areas
- Lack of handrails in the bathroom
- Adaptive equipment such as rolling walkers, canes, splints
- Poor lighting in rooms or walkways
- Lack of a system to call for help (e.g., whistle, bell)
- Long cords such as those for phones or supplemental oxygen tanks
- Poor arrangement of living space, which requires a person to reach or move in ways that offset balance

the person's condition, vital signs, cause of fall, time of day, location, treatment rendered, and other relevant factors.

    c. Data collected should be used to formulate specific safety interventions for each individual.

B. Teaching and Learning Strategies

    1. Principles of adult learning

        a. Adults need a motivation to learn.

        b. Adults build on past learning experiences.

        c. Adults are independent learners.

    2. Components of the nursing assessment

        a. Readiness to learn

        b. Motivation to learn

    3. Specific strategies for teaching older adults (see Figure 17-2)

C. Medication Management

    1. Polypharmacy: Older adults commonly take many medications, which can result in an increased risk of adverse reactions because of many factors.

        a. Drugs are excreted more slowly by the kidneys.

        b. Absorption in the intestines is slower.

        c. The above factors cause the drugs to remain present in the body for a longer time.

        d. Older adults may use over-the-counter medications and/or herbal therapies that they do not consider "drugs."

    2. Use of medication boxes

        a. Organizes the client's medications

        b. Provides a system for management to decrease the risk of making medication errors at home

        c. Allows family members to help monitor or set up the client's medications

    3. Family and client education

        a. Include the client and the family or caregiver

        b. Follow the principles of teaching and learning with family members as well as with the client

        c. Allow time for demonstration and return demonstration

        d. Teach more than one family member whenever possible

D. The Nurse's Role in Preparation for Placement in a Long-Term Care Facility

    1. Address cultural influences

        a. Realize that people with some cultural backgrounds consider placement in a nursing home to be unacceptable and that other resources must be explored.

        b. Explore cultural norms and influences with the family and client

    2. Help select a facility

        a. Know the options available in the community

        b. Obtain information through industry organizations such as the American Health Care Association (AHCA)

        c. Access facilities' survey histories from the Health Care Financing Administration (HCFA) Web site (www.hcfa.gov) or from state health departments

    3. Assist family members with placement decisions

        a. Provide the family with viable options and lists of community resources

        b. Use mutual goal-setting techniques

        c. Consult with the client's case manager or social worker for specific information on area facilities

        d. Refer the family to information checklists available in the facility or through agencies such as the American Association of Retired Persons (AARP) or the United Way

IV. **Psychosocial, Ethical, and Legal Issues Associated with Aging**

A. Psychosocial Issues

    1. Grief and loss

        a. Life changes with age

            1) Retirement

            2) Death of a spouse, children, friends

            3) Possible decline in health including chronic illness and disability

            4) Menopause

            5) Possible change in economic status

            6) Possible social isolation

7) Possible change in living arrangements
b. Role changes with age
   1) Widowhood
   2) Caregiver role reversal (i.e., the person who traditionally has provided care becomes the person who is being cared for)
2. Stress and coping

a. Assess coping strategies in relation to the amount of stress the person is experiencing
b. Promote the use of positive coping strategies
3. Death and dying
   a. Older adults may be undertaking an end-of-life review.

Figure 17-2. Suggestions for Teaching Elderly Adults

Visual
Use bright, direct lighting, unless contraindicated due to visual disturbances (such as recent cataract surgery)
Do not stand by a window; avoid glare
When using visual aids, use large, well-spaced letters (black on white is best)
Keep clients close to the speaker, or if in a large room, be certain that the audience can see and hear the speaker
For individual teaching, make sure that the client's glasses are clean

Auditory
Limit distractions: Eliminate extraneous noise, close doors, turn off television or radio, limit interruptions
Face the audience; speak directly to the individual in a one-to-one setting
Never cover your mouth when speaking (many elderly people rely on lip reading to compensate for hearing deficits)
Speak slowly and clearly
If appropriate, wear bright lipstick to help elderly people who lip read
Before proceeding, ask if the client can hear you
Utilize assistive devices as needed (make certain that hearing aids and microphones are turned on and that batteries are working)

TEACHING TOPICS

General Teaching and Learning Suggestions
Keep teaching sessions short and to the point
Design handouts to be simple and clear
Relate the relevance of the topic to adult experiences within the group
Employ the principles of adult learning when planning an educational session
Pace the presentation to reflect the unique needs and understanding of the group or individual
Avoid the temptation to overload with too much information
Remember that adults need a motivation to learn
Provide immediate feedback to questions and comments
Give an overview of the material to be covered and explain its relevance
Keep information simple and specific; avoid technical jargon
Use a variety of teaching modalities such as videotapes, hands-on experiences, samples of products, group discussion, overheads, pamphlets, handouts
Emphasize the client's learning responsibility
Be enthusiastic about the subject; if the teacher isn't, the learner will not be
Summarize important points
Teach a procedure close to the time it will take place
When teaching skills, allow time for practice, return demonstrations, questions, and review sessions
Stick to the essentials needed to maintain life and prevent complications, but be prepared to address additional questions
Keep the environment conducive to learning; for group sessions, the room temperature should be comfortable for the majority, potentially noxious stimuli (such as cigarette smoke) should be avoided, seats must be easily accessible
Use a large enough room to accommodate those with wheelchairs, walkers, and other assistive devices, make certain exits are not blocked, have additional nursing personnel available should needs arise (such as toileting)
Be thoroughly familiar with resources available within the community and the individual facility

Reprinted with permission of W.B. Saunders Company from Easton, K.L. (1999). *Gerontological rehabilitation nursing* (p. 176). Philadelphia: W.B. Saunders.

b. They may experience anticipatory grieving.

c. They enter Erikson's development stage for older age: Ego integrity vs. despair. *[Refer to Chapter 15 for more information on developmental stages.]*

B. Ethical and Legal Issues and Moral Dilemmas
[Refer to Chapter 3 for more information.]

1. Withholding treatment: To withhold treatment rather than beginning treatment and then withdrawing it (advance directives make the client's wishes explicit)

2. Withdrawing treatment: To remove life-sustaining interventions after they have been implemented (e.g., disconnecting a ventilator from a person who is unable to breathe independently, discontinuing nutritional interventions for a person who cannot otherwise eat or drink independently)

3. Advance directives

   a. Living will
      1) Is used in cases of terminal illness
      2) Makes the client's wishes known in advance when death is imminent as certified by a physician

   b. Declaration document of life-prolonging procedures
      1) Describes steps to take to prolong life
      2) Is determined by the client

   c. Durable power of attorney for health care
      1) Allows another person to make decisions on behalf of the client
      2) Can encompass health, financial, property, and other issues

   d. Healthcare representative: Allows a healthcare professional to make decisions at the client's behest regarding health-related issues

4. Use of physical and chemical restraints

   a. The use of physical restraints must be justified and documented.

   b. Physical restraints should only be used when the person is a danger to himself or herself or others.

   c. Chemical restraints are inappropriate except in the most extreme circumstances for client safety.

d. Good alternatives to restraints exist and should be explored.

e. Restraint use can actually increase the likelihood of injury in many instances.

f. A physician order is required for restraint use and must include documentation of the medical condition requiring restraint, the type of restraint, the length of time for use, and guidelines for release and repositioning (according to OBRA 1987 guidelines)

5. Rehabilitation of clients who are terminally ill

   a. Nurses should explore their own feelings about the rehabilitation of those who are at the end of life.

   b. There are many potential examples of situations that involve rehabilitating elderly people with terminal illnesses.
      1) Late-stage cancer, including melanoma
      2) Rapidly growing, inoperable tumors
      3) End-stage renal disease
      4) Last stages of AIDS
      5) Other incurable diseases

6. Abuse or mistreatment of older adults: May take many forms, including neglect or financial, passive or active physical, and sexual abuse

   a. Characteristics of abusers
      1) May have been victims of abuse themselves
      2) Can be men or women
      3) May be family members or caregivers
      4) May have social and emotional problems or a history of psychological problems
      5) May abuse drugs or alcohol
      6) May have a high level of stress or frustration, minimal coping abilities, and lack of knowledge

   b. Characteristics of victims (DeCalmer & Glendenning, 1993; Pritchard, 1995, 1996): Many rehabilitation clients are at risk because of the following factors.
      1) Are socially isolated
      2) Are elderly
      3) Are in poor health

4) Are widowed
5) Have significant physical limitations
6) Can be men or women (although women are victims more frequently)
7) Are dependent on others
8) Have a history of family violence

c. Possible signs and symptoms of abuse or mistreatment
1) Poor physical hygiene
2) Dehydration or malnutrition
3) Multiple bruises of different colors (indicating different stages of healing)
4) A withdrawn, cowering, fearful, anxious, depressed, or hopeless demeanor
5) Presence of burns, skin tears, broken bones, or severe rashes that, when explained, do not fit the injury or trauma

d. Nursing interventions (see Figure 17-3)
1) Perform a complete history and physical assessment
2) Make certain the explanation fits the injury, realizing that rehabilitating elderly people may experience falls as they increase their level of independence
3) Be alert to possible signs and symptoms of abuse or neglect
4) Interview the suspected abuser and the victim separately
5) Consult with available resources as needed (e.g., psychologist, social worker)
6) Report any suspected case of abuse: This can be done anonymously to an office of Adult Protective Services.
7) Do not alienate the suspected perpetrator
8) Take necessary steps to protect the client

7. Suicide among elderly people
a. Elderly white men are at highest risk for suicide.
b. Elderly people tend to use more lethal means of suicide (e.g., firearms, hanging)
c. Suicide is associated with alcoholism, diagnosis of a terminal disease, depression, presence of a chronic disease, those who are unmarried and live alone, those with few support systems, drug abuse, bereavement, intractable pain, and social isolation.
d. The risk can be lessened by strengthening social supports, treating depression, increasing involvement in social activities, and taking definitive action when suicidal ideations are expressed.

Figure 17-3. Nursing Indications for the Prevention of Elder Abuse

- Establish a trusting relationship with the elderly person
- Be able to refer families to resources available in the community
- Strengthen social supports
- Encourage regular respite for the caregiver
- Identify caregivers who are at the highest risk of being abusers and target interventions to prevent stress from caregiver burden
- Be aware of risk factors and contributing factors
- Perform thorough physical assessments and carefully document findings, including the client's appearance, nutritional state, skin condition, mental attitude and awareness, need for aids to enhance sensory perception
- If abuse is suspected, interview the caregiver and other possible informants to confirm or refute suspicions
- Know the laws governing the reporting of abuse

Reprinted with permission of W.B. Saunders Company from Easton, K.L. (1999). *Gerontological rehabilitation nursing* (p. 336). Philadelphia: W.B. Saunders.

References

DeCalmer, P., & Glendenning, F. (Eds.). (1993). *The mistreatment of the elderly people*. London: Sage.

Easton, K.L. (1999). *Gerontological rehabilitation nursing*. Philadelphia: W.B. Saunders.

Ebersole, P., & Hess, E. (1998). *Toward health aging: Human needs and nursing response*. St. Louis: Mosby.

Eliopoulos, C. (1999). *Manual of gerontological nursing*. St. Louis: Mosby.

Fowles, D.G. (1994). *A profile of older Americans*. Washington, DC: American Association of Retired Persons and Administration on Aging, U.S. Department of Health and Human Services.

Liddle, J., & Gilleard, C. (1995). The emotional consequences of falls for older people and their families. *Clinical Rehabilitation, 9*(2), 110-114.

Miller, C. (1995). *Nursing care of older adults: Theory and practice*. Philadelphia: J.B. Lippincott.

Pritchard, J. (1995). *The abuse of older people: A training manual for detection and prevention*. London: Jessica Kingsley Publishers.

Pritchard, J. (1996). Darkness visible…elder abuse. *Nursing Times, 92*(42), 26-31.

Ross, J.E.R. (1991). Iatrogenesis in the elderly: Contributors to falls. *Journal of Gerontological Nursing, 17*(9), 19-23.

Steinmetz, H.M., & Hobson, S.J.G. (1994). Prevention of falls among the community-dwelling elderly: An overview. *Physical and Occupational Therapy in Geriatrics, 12*(4), 13-29.

Suggested resources

Ashely, M.J., Gryfe, C.I., & Arnies, A. (1977). A longitudinal study of falls in an elderly population II: Some circumstances of falling. *Age and Ageing, 6*, 211-220.

Atwood, S.M., Holm, M.B., & James, A. (1994). Activities of daily living capabilities and values of long-term-care facility residents. *The American Journal of Occupational Therapy, 48*(8), 710-716.

Berry, G., Fisher, R., & Lang, S. (1981). Detrimental incidents including falls in an elderly institutional population. *Journal of the American Geriatric Society, 29*(7), 322-324.

Campbell, J., & Humphreys, J. (1993). *Nursing care of survivors of family violence*. St. Louis: Mosby.

Commodore, D.I.B. (1995). Falls in the elderly population: A look at incidence, risks, healthcare costs, and preventive strategies. *Rehabilitation Nursing, 20*(2), 84-89.

Evans, L.K., & Strumpf, N.W. (1990). Myths about elder restraint. *IMAGE: Journal of Nursing Scholarship, 22*(2), 124-127.

Fagier, J., & Greenwood, M. (1993). Outside risk. *Nursing Times, 89*(40), 56-58.

Frost, M.H., & Wilette, K. (1994). Risk for abuse/neglect: Documentation of assessment data and diagnoses. *Journal of Gerontological Nursing, 29*(8), 37-45.

Janelli, L.M., Kansi, G.W., & Neary, M.A. (1994). Physical restraints: Has OBRA made a difference? *Journal of Gerontological Nursing, 20*(6), 17-21.

Koroknay, V.J., Werner, P., Cohen-Mansfield, J., & Braun, J.V. (1995). Maintaining ambulation in the frail nursing home resident: A nursing administered walking program. *Journal of Gerontological Nursing, 21*(11), 18-24.

McIntosh, J.L. (1992). Epidemiology of suicide in the elderly. *Suicide Life Threatening Behavior, 22*(1), 15-35.

Meehan, P., Saltzman, L., & Sattin, R. (1991). Suicides among the older United States residents: Epidemiologic characteristics and trends. *American Journal of Public Health, 81*, 1198-1200.

Mellick, E., Buckwalter, K., & Stolley, J. (1992). Suicide among elderly white men: Development of a profile. *Journal of Psychosocial Nursing, 30*(2), 29-34.

Roberts, B.L., & Wykle, M.L. (1993). Pilot study results: Falls among institutionalized elderly. *Journal of Gerontological Nursing, 19*(5), 13-20.

Section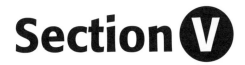

The Delivery and Evaluation of Rehabilitation Services

● ●

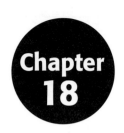

Environment of Care and Service Delivery

Patricia A. Quigley, PhD ARNP CRRN

Scientific and technological advances, the aging population, duration and quality of life, and cost-conscious healthcare systems have influenced the delivery of rehabilitation services, the environments in which rehabilitation services are provided, and the role of rehabilitation nurses in all healthcare settings. Additionally, models of care delivery have been redesigned to maximize continuity and coordination of client care in settings with diminishing lengths of stay and changes in skill mix. The delivery and evaluation of rehabilitation services requires oversight by expert rehabilitation nurses who serve as client advocates to maximize client care services without jeopardizing quality outcomes and client safety throughout the continuum of care.

This chapter describes and contrasts rehabilitation environments throughout the continuum of care and demonstrates how the nursing and rehabilitation process is applied in the delivery of rehabilitation services. Rehabilitation nurses must become familiar with ethical principles, decision-making models, and alternatives to deal with the many challenges of healthcare reorganization and service redesign.

Rehabilitation should be practiced in all healthcare settings and rehabilitation nursing care should be an integral component of care delivery. The role of the rehabilitation nurse is paramount to ensure that basic rehabilitation techniques are performed and that specialized rehabilitation care is provided in the appropriate setting based on the client's medical stability and tolerance for rehabilitation efforts.

I. Practice Settings in Which Rehabilitation Occurs

A. Critical Care
1. Description: Intensive medical/surgical care settings within hospitals
2. Severity of clients' medical stability
   a. Critically ill, life-threatening illnesses or conditions
      1) Require 1:1 or 1:2 nurse/client staffing
      2) Require physiological assessment more frequently than every 4 hours
   b. Unable to tolerate intensive rehabilitation
3. Models of nursing care delivery
   a. Primary care nursing
      1) One nurse is assigned and responsible for the total care of a client during the shift of care.
         a) Ensures that the client and other providers know who is accountable for the specific client's care

      b) Provides 24-hour accountability for the client's care
      2) For successful primary nursing, extensive communication and collaboration is required with all members of the healthcare team, client, and family (Lyon, 1993).
   b. Primary nurse for a shift of care
      1) Financial constraints, the decreased availability of RNs, and the shift of acute nursing care to outpatient care settings (so that length of stay on medical/surgical units is less than 72 hours) have caused many acute care settings to adopt this model.
      2) One RN is assigned as a primary nurse for a client for the shift, rather than for the client's length of stay.
   c. Case managers
      1) Background
         a) Although case management

began in the 1950s, nurses have only recently accepted the importance for professional nurses to accept this role.

b) Case management is one of the most recent care delivery models for RNs to embrace (McBride, 1992).

c) This model of care delivery is comprehensive, client-centered, and allows continuous care across the continuum.

2) Roles of nurse case managers

a) Coordinate care and service delivery, improve continuity of care, monitor outcomes

b) Function as client advocates

c) Direct, coordinate, and supervise care

d) Maximize positive financial outcomes and use continuous quality improvement and utilization review (Johnson & Schubring, 1999)

d. Nurse liaisons: Evaluate clients and help them gain access to services at freestanding rehabilitation facilities

e. Minimum Data Set (MDS) coordinators

1) Initiate and instruct the care team in completing MDS assessment forms and resource utilization group (RUG) codes

2) Serve as a resource for team members about the prospective payment system (PPS) process in subacute and long-term care settings

f. Advanced practice nurses (APNs) (e.g., clinical nurse specialist, advanced registered nurse practitioner): Provide clinical leadership and expertise as direct and indirect care providers

4. Aspects of rehabilitation nursing care

a. Prevent medical and functional complications (e.g., positioning, passive range of motion) and readmission

b. Maintain function: Engage clients to participate in care (e.g., eating, bathing, dressing) within medically indicated restrictions and precautions

c. Promote independence: Engage clients in increasing self-care actions and monitor progress toward goal achievement

d. Delegate and supervise aspects of rehabilitation and restorative care provided by licensed practical nurses (LPNs) and technicians

5. Documentation: Centers on medical management

a. Systems review: Assess and manage physiological systems

b. Systems outcomes: Stabilize physiological status

c. Critical pathways: Use process standards as adjuncts to a client's plan of care that define when and by whom critical care interventions must be done

6. Client and family education

a. Medical management

b. Self-care management

c. Exercise and health promotion

7. Discharge planning: Focuses on the transition to the next clinical setting

B. Acute Care

1. Description: 25% of rehabilitation nurses practice in acute care facilities.

a. Episodic care settings (in hospitals and acute rehabilitation units) for acute illness

b. Acute rehabilitation settings (the traditional setting for rehabilitation care)

c. Rehabilitation units in general hospitals

d. Freestanding rehabilitation centers

e. Comprehensive integrated inpatient rehabilitation programs: "Coordinated and integrated medical and rehabilitation services that are provided 24 hours per day and endorse the active participation and choice of the persons served throughout the entire program" (CARF, 1998, p. 101)

2. Severity of clients' medical stability: Require medical management by physicians or APNs

a. Medically stable: Medical management is secondary to or concurrent with rehabilitation needs.

1) Require ongoing medical management

2) Require 24-hour nursing care, 7 days per week

b. Ability to tolerate intensive rehabilitation

1) Require 1–3 hours of therapy per day
2) Require rehabilitation nursing skills and care

3. Models of nursing care delivery

a. Team nursing: Task-oriented client care delivery

b. Modified primary nursing: Uses a primary nurse (RN) and associate nurses (RNs or licensed practice nurses [LPNs])

c. Interdisciplinary team care

1) Shared accountability among team members to meet client and family rehabilitation needs
2) Shared goals that cross discipline-specific boundaries
3) "Characterized by a variety of disciplines that participate in the assessment, planning, and/or implementation of a person's program: There must be close interactions and integration among the disciplines so that all members of the team interact to achieve team goals" (CARF, 1998, p. 310).

d. Transdisciplinary team care: Boundary-free plans of care that focus on client and family goals

4. Aspects of rehabilitation nursing care

a. Prevent complications

b. Restore abilities

5. Documentation

a. Focuses on clinical pathways: Combines aspects of critical pathways to focus on client needs or problems. Outcomes are achieved according to predetermined goals at predetermined intervals (James A. Haley VAMC, 1995).

b. Centers on client needs: Clinical pathways address the client's individualized needs and plan of care through teamwork among various team members.

6. Client and family education: Provides outcome-directed teaching and learning

7. Discharge planning

a. "A major challenge faced today by nurses is the increased complexity of patients' discharge needs caused by decreased length of stay in the hospital" (Closson, Mattingly, Finne, & Larson, 1994, p. 287).

b. The period immediately after rehabilitation is the most critical to clients; many gains may be lost within the first 3 months of discharge from an acute rehabilitation program (Mor, Granger, & Sherwood, 1983).

c. Follow-up interventions can help increase clients' functional outcomes and reduce healthcare utilization following discharge from rehabilitation.

1) Deterioration was found to be related to the client's or the caregiver's failure to understand or sustain the rehabilitation program (Moskowitz, Lightbody, & Frietag, 1972).
2) Frequent follow-up after discharge (e.g., by telephone) may reduce healthcare utilization and enhance functional outcomes (Evans et al., 1990).

C. Subacute Care

1. Description

a. Postacute care setting for clients whose medical treatment precludes participation in an acute rehabilitation program or who are classified as slow to progress and would not qualify for a regular rehabilitation program (Mayer, Buckley, & White, 1990)

b. A service area available since the mid-1980s for people who are not quite ready for intensive, acute rehabilitation therapy

c. "A comprehensive and cost-effective inpatient program for patients who have had an acute event as a result of an illness, injury, or exacerbation of a disease process; have a determined course of treatment; and do not require intensive diagnostic and/or invasive procedures" (International Subacute Healthcare Association [ISHA], as cited in Griffin, 1995, p. 4).

d. A care option that serves as an alternative to an acute care hospital admission or as an alternative to continued hospitalization: The client receives less acute nursing care and less intense rehabilitation (CARF, 1998) than in a freestanding or hospital-based setting.

    e. Categories of subacute care (Griffin, 1995)

      1) Transitional

        a) Short stay (5–30 days)

        b) For clients who need medical care and monitoring

        c) Requires highly skilled nursing care, pharmacological management, and rehabilitation services

      2) General

        a) Short stay (10–40 days)

        b) Requires rehabilitation and nursing services

      3) Chronic

        a) Longer length of stay (60–90 days)

        b) For clients with long-term medical diseases (e.g., progressive neurological disease)

      4) Long-term care: Average length of stay can be 25 days or longer

2. Severity of clients' medical stability: Varied acuity levels and problems

    a. Medically complex but stable (e.g., cardiovascular clients with congestive heart failure, clients with septicemia or osteomyelitis)

      1) Require skilled nursing care

      2) Require medical monitoring and specialized care

      3) Require assistance with activities of daily living (ADLs)

    b. Medically unable to tolerate an intensive rehabilitation program (e.g., clients recovering from surgery, oncology clients, wound care clients)

      1) Need less than 1 hour of therapy daily

      2) Need at least 3 hours of therapy weekly

    c. Clients needing respiratory care

      1) Require ventilator care or weaning

      2) Require nursing care

    d. Clients recuperating from surgery

      1) Require skilled nursing care

      2) Require rehabilitation services

    e. Clients with chronic wounds: Require skilled nursing care

3. Models of nursing care delivery

    a. Team nursing: One RN is the designated team leader for staff members who provide care to a group of clients (this model was created to advance nursing care in functional nursing models).

    b. Functional nursing: Client care is divided by tasks.

    c. Case management: 1:1 care is usually provided by a live-in nurse (this was a form of nursing care practiced in the early 20th century).

    d. Multidisciplinary team care: Discipline-specific care is directed to client needs, but not integrated across disciplines or services; boundaries and turf issues exist between disciplines.

4. Aspects of rehabilitation nursing care

    a. Prevent complications

    b. Maintain functional status and capabilities

    c. Restore self-care skills in functional ADLs

5. Client and family education: Provides outcome-directed teaching and learning

D. Long-Term Care

1. Description

    a. Long-term acute care (LTAC)

      1) Posthospital settings with an average length of stay of 30 days, combining services for clients in need of intensive medical and extended skilled nursing care as well as rehabilitation and respiratory management

      2) Highly specialized centers of care: Some acute rehabilitation facilities are licensed as LTAC facilities.

      3) Geropsychiatric care and some mental health centers that also provide rehabilitation services

    b. Long-term care (LTC)

      1) Posthospital centers for clients in need of extended skilled nursing care

and attendant care due to the inability to live alone

2) Inpatient settings that provide long-term rehabilitation due to chronic disability
   a) Skilled nursing facilities
   b) Residential facilities
   c) Transitional living centers
   d) Long-term care hospitals

2. Severity of clients' medical stability
   a. Medically stable: Clients at low potential for medical instability
   b. Unable to tolerate intensive rehabilitation programs but have regular, direct individual contact with rehabilitation physicians as determined by medical and rehabilitation needs
   c. Require routine rehabilitation nursing and have a low risk of needing high medical-acuity skilled nursing
   d. Receive a minimum of 1–3 hours of services 5 days per week from interdisciplinary team members
   e. Receive client and family education and training opportunities on an ongoing basis (CARF, 1998).

3. Models of nursing care delivery
   a. Functional nursing
      1) Nursing care is divided by labor (i.e., assembly-line nursing); this model dates back to the 1920s.
      2) The division of labor determines the technical aspects of the job to be performed.
      3) Each job is broken down to its simplest component to increase attention on quantity, not quality.
      4) Nurses' aides provide care.
   b. Partners in care: Cross-trained staff, which often includes teams of professional licensed nurses and technical support personnel, assist with specific tasks.

4. Documentation
   a. Minimum Data Set-Post Acute Care (MDS-PAC) assessment
      1) Medicare's payment system for medical rehabilitation facilities, which takes effect October 1, 2000, will include standard assessment data as well as disability and outcome data.
      2) The MDS-PAC assessment will include as much of the Functional Independence Measure (FIM™) instrument as possible.
   b. Clinical pathways
      1) Monitor client outcomes at predetermined intervals to provide a framework for interdisciplinary team members to plan, monitor, revise, and evaluate client responses to care throughout the rehabilitation process
      2) Determine trend variances in outcomes for clinical cohorts (Quigley, Smith, & Strugar, 1998)
   c. Nursing Intervention Classification (NIC) (Moorehead, McCloskey, & Bulechek, 1993) and Nursing Outcomes Classification (NOC) systems
      1) Designed to standardize nursing intervention and outcome terms and link them with North American Nursing Diagnosis Association (NANDA) classification for nursing diagnoses
      2) Contain six domains (physiological [basic], physiological [complex], behavioral, safety, family, health system), 26 classes, and more than 400 interventions that are also compatible with ICD codes and DRG classification systems
      3) Have been tested for use in LTC settings
      4) Have a comprehensive coding structure for all of nursing practice (Iowa Intervention Project, 1995)
   d. Omaha Classification System (OCS) (Martin & Scheet, 1992)
      1) Serves as a guide for nursing practice and nursing documentation in home health care and nurse-managed care centers
      2) Has three components
         a) Problem Classification Scheme, which contains 44 actual or potential nursing diagnoses that affect the client or family
         b) Problem Rating Scale for

Outcomes, which was designed by community health nurses to help nurses systematically measure client changes and responses

c) The Intervention Scheme, which delineates four categories of interventions: health teaching, guidance, and counseling; treatments and procedures; case management; and surveillance

e. FIM instrument: Measures client outcomes in terms of functional status gains from admission to discharge throughout the continuum of care and is developed and updated by the Uniform Data System for Medical Rehabilitation (UDSMR)

5. Client and family education: Promotes self-care actions to prevent complications, maintain functional status, and increase functional gains

E. Community-Based Care
   1. Description
      a. Care is based in the communities in which people with rehabilitation needs manage their care and daily activities independently, with assistance, or with supervision.
      b. Clients and family members work as partners with healthcare providers to attain mutually established goals (Hoeman, 1996).
      c. Rehabilitation is provided in settings that are within community or residential settings.
      d. According to CARF (1998), when a residence is provided by the organization, it is "designed, constructed, furnished, and maintained in ways similar to others in the neighborhood consistent with the needs and preferences of the person served" (p. 296).
   2. Types of community-based care
      a. Day treatment care or programs: Provide supervised care and therapeutic recreational activities

b. Independent living centers and congregate living facilities: Provide daily supervision and skilled nursing care
c. Community reentry programs and assisted care living facilities
d. Rural outreach programs
e. Home healthcare services: Neal (1999) reported the results of a study examining the congruence between rehabilitation principles and home health nursing practice. Data from 30 home health nurses suggested congruence between rehabilitation and home health nursing principles.
f. Hospice services
g. Nursing centers (e.g., Pine Street Inn [Boston]): Healthcare clinics run by nurses
h. Outpatient clinics
i. Senior citizen centers

3. Documentation
   a. Home Healthcare Classification (HHC)
      1) Generated from a study funded by the Health Care Financing Administration (HCFA) to develop a method to assess and classify home health Medicare clients, predict resource requirements, and measure outcomes (Bowles & Naylor, 1996)
      2) Bases cohort models on four types of provider visits for 30 days or for the episode of care (30–120 days or more)
      3) Includes measures of socioeconomic and functional status, medical diagnosis, surgical procedures, as well as nursing components of diagnoses, interventions, and discharge status (Saba, 1992)
   b. HomeFIM™ instrument
      1) Designed to measure the functional status of individuals receiving home care rehabilitative services
      2) Provides documentation of functional gains for insurance effectiveness and efficiency for third-party payers
      3) Offers the critical link in the continuum of care between the comprehensive inpatient rehabilitation program,

outpatient, and home health services (Kedron, 1998)

    4. Client and family education: Provides information regarding continuous life planning

II. Care Delivery Across the Life Span

A. Young Children

    1. Heery (1992) described pediatric rehabilitation as the process of restoring childhood.

    2. Interactions between parent and child are critical.

B. Adolescents

    1. Critical development needs include developing a sense of independence, socialization, and sexuality education.

    2. The major focus is on helping the adolescent with a disability to adapt to educational settings.

C. Adults

    1. Programs focus on the individual's unique social, psychological, and vocational needs.

    2. Healthcare professionals should consider how working partners effect the care of family members.

D. Older Adults

    1. Due to the increasing aging population in general (aging-related services) and the increase in people aging with disabilities (disability-related services), rehabilitation nurses must focus on this population.

    2. Healthcare professionals should consider how long-distance care effects the family.

III. Continuum of Care: Longitudinal Outcomes and Documentation

A. Overview

    1. Clients, families, and other providers (e.g., visiting nurses associations) participate in mutual goal setting and monitoring goal achievement.

    2. Outcomes are setting-oriented and cumulative throughout the continuum of care.

    3. Long-term outcomes can be achieved only after short-term, integrated outcomes are met.

    4. Outcomes must be monitored in relation to expected outcomes within a time frame and across settings.

    5. Family meetings are critical to reaching

consensus about future hospitalizations, planning for healthcare needs, and insurance coverage.

B. ARN Standards

    1. Rehabilitation nurses provide services designed to prevent complications of physical disability, restore optimal functioning, and help the individual adapt to an altered lifestyle (ARN, 1994).

    2. Rehabilitation nursing is practiced in rehabilitation settings, defined as any environment in which nurse-patient interactions are grounded in the philosophy and concepts of rehabilitation nursing practice (ARN, 1994).

C. Documentation: Environment of Care and Service Delivery System

    1. Each environment of care has specific requirements for documentation defined by standards of nursing care and practice, accreditation bodies, third-party payers, and regulatory and institutional policies.

    2. Rehabilitation nurses must develop or select a standardized language for use with computerized, integrated team documentation systems that links to all points on the continuum of care (Cervizzi & Edwards, 1999).

    3. Documentation systems must promote quality, cost-effective client care, customer satisfaction, and outcomes.

D. Client and Family Education: Social Structure of Care

    1. Educate families regarding 24-hour responsibilities and requirements for care

    2. Discuss issues of coordination of services and increased responsibility of care providers

    3. Provide access to support groups

E. Discharge Planning: Preparing for Transitions

    1. "Discharge preparation: Hospital-based activities to anticipate a safe, smooth transition from that setting" (Steele & Sterling, 1992, p. 80)

    2. "Discharge readiness: A multifaceted, multistaged concept that provides an estimate of a client's ability to leave an acute care facility" (Steele & Sterling, 1992, p. 80)

    3. Rehabilitation team meetings: Include the client and family and enable all participants

to reach consensus regarding the ongoing needs and plans for rehabilitation throughout the continuum of care and a method to evaluate the effectiveness of that care

IV. Changes in Health Care

A. In the Healthcare Environment
   1. Managed care and Medicare PPS are affecting care delivery and client access to rehabilitation services.
   2. Rehabilitation services are moving to specialty centers, home care, and outpatient care.

B. In the Roles of Rehabilitation Nurses
   1. Managed care and Medicare PPS necessitate rehabilitation nurses' leadership as client advocates and care managers.
   2. Rehabilitation nurses must ensure that clients receive timely, quality, comprehensive, cost-effective care with appropriate providers in the appropriate setting.
   3. Rehabilitation nurses must practice within and across a variety of settings as case managers and clinical practitioners.

References

Association of Rehabilitation Nurses (ARN). (1994). *Standards and scope of rehabilitation nursing practice* (3rd ed.). Skokie, IL: Author.

Bowles, K., & Naylor, M. (1996). Nursing intervention classification systems. *Image: The Journal of Nursing Scholarship, 28*(4), 303-308.

CARF...The Rehabilitation Accreditation Commission. (1998). *Standards manual and interpretive guidelines for medical rehabilitation.* Tucson, AZ: Author.

Cervizzi, K., & Edwards, P. (1999). Where is rehabilitation nursing documentation going? *Rehabilitation Nursing, 24*(3), 92.

Closson, B., Mattingly, L., Finne, K., & Larson, J. (1994). Telephone follow-up program evaluation: Application of Orem's Self-Care Model. *Rehabilitation Nursing, 19*(5), 287-292.

Evans, R., Hendricks, R., Bishop, D., Lawrence-Umlau, D., Kirk, C., & Halar, E. (1990). Prospective payment for rehabilitation: Effects on hospital readmission, home care, and placement. *Archives of Physical Medicine and Rehabilitation, 71*, 291-294.

Griffin, K. (1995). *Handbook of subacute health care.* Gaithersburg, MD: Aspen.

Heery, K. (1992). Restoring childhood through rehabilitation. *Rehabilitation Nursing, 17*, 193-195.

Hoeman, S. (Ed.). (1996). *Rehabilitation nursing: Process and application* (2nd ed.). St. Louis: Mosby.

Iowa Intervention Project. (1995). Validation and coding of the NIC taxonomy structure. *IMAGE: The Journal of Nursing Scholarship, 27*(1), 43-49.

James A. Haley VAMC. (1995). *Clinical pathways for in-patient rehabilitation programs.* Tampa, FL: Author.

Johnson, K., & Schubring, L. (1999). The evolution of a hospital based decentralized case management model. *Nursing Economics, 17*(1), 29-48.

Kedron, M. (1998). Introducing HomeFIM™ Instrument. *The FIM System^{SM} Update, 2*(3), 1.

Lyon, J.C. (1993). Models of nursing care delivery and case management: Clarification of terms. *Nursing Economics, 11*, 163-169.

Martin, K., & Scheet, N. (1992). *The Omaha System: Application for community health nursing.* Philadelphia: W.B. Saunders.

Mayer, G.G., Buckley, R.F., & White, T.L. (1990). Direct nursing care given to patients in a subacute rehabilitation center. *Rehabilitation Nursing, 15*, 86-88.

McBride, S.M. (1992). Rehabilitation case managers: Ahead of their time. *Holistic Nursing Practice, 6*, 67-75.

Moorehead, S., McCloskey, J., & Bulechek, G. (1993). Nursing intervention classifications: A comparison with the Omaha and the Home Healthcare Classification. *Journal of Nursing Administration, 23*(10), 23-29.

Mor, V., Granger, C., & Sherwood, C. (1983). Discharged rehabilitation patients: Impact of follow-up surveillance by a friendly visitor. *Archives of Physical Medicine and Rehabilitation, 64*, 346-353.

Moskowitz, E., Lightbody, F., & Frietag, N. (1972). Long-term follow-up of poststroke patients. *Archives of Physical Medicine and Rehabilitation, 59*, 167-172.

Neal, L. (1999). Research supporting the congruence between rehabilitation principles and home health nursing practice. *Rehabilitation Nursing, 24*(3), 115-121.

Quigley, P., Smith, S., & Strugar, J. (1998). Successful experiences with clinical pathways in rehabilitation. *Journal of Rehabilitation, 64*(2), 29-32.

Saba, V. (1992). Home health care classification. *Caring, 11*(5), 58-60.

Steele, N., & Sterling, Y. (1992). Application of the case study design: Nursing interventions for discharge readiness. *Clinical Nurse Specialist, 6*(2), 80-84.

Suggested resources

Bower, K. (1995). Case management designed for the care continuum. In K. Zander (Ed.), *Managing outcomes through collaborative care: The application of care mapping and case management* (pp. 20, 167). Chicago: American Hospital Publishing.

Clinton, B. (1992). The Clinton health care plan. *New England Journal of Medicine, 327*(11), 804-806.

Crummer, M., & Carter, V. (1993). Clinical pathways: The pivotal tool. *Journal of Cardiovascular Nursing, 7*, 30-37.

Erkel, E. (1993). The impact of case management in preventative services. *Journal of Nursing Administration, 23*(1), 27-32.

Hampton, D. (1993). Implementing a managed care framework through care maps. *Journal of Nursing Administration, 23*, 21-27.

Tahan, H. (1993). The nurse case manager in acute care settings: job description and function. *Journal of Nursing Administration, 23*(10), 53-61.

Wood, R., Bailey, N., & Tilkemeier, D. (1992). Managed care, the missing link in quality improvement. *Journal of Nursing Care Quality, 6*, 55-65.

Chapter 19

Outcome Measurement and Performance Improvement

Terrie Black, MBA BSN RNC CRRN

Accountability and validation of value have become essential components of the healthcare delivery process. Today, outcomes of care are emphasized like never before (Black, 1999). Outcomes focus on the effectiveness of care or the results of services delivered by a clinician or team of clinicians. Monitoring outcomes can help do the following:

- track efficiency and effectiveness

- identify trends

- facilitate communication among the patient, family, treatment team, payers, referral source, and other stakeholders

- assess follow-up measures to determine if progress is continuing after discharge

- identify areas for improvement

Internal stakeholders interested in outcomes may include a rehabilitation program's case managers, administrators (e.g., managers, members of the board of directors), or clinicians (e.g., rehabilitation nurses, therapists, physicians, quality improvement managers, researchers). Externally, other groups who may ask for outcomes include case managers, payers, referral sources (e.g., community physicians, the general public, patients and families, other interested stakeholders).

Outcomes can be benchmarked according to past trends within an organization or corporation, against national and regional standards or norms, and against best practice standards. Corporations can identify outcomes and use various sites or regions as a basis for comparison. Measuring and monitoring rehabilitation outcomes can be used to market an individual program or organization, meet accreditation standards, and identify areas for performance improvement (Wilkerson, 1997a). Outcomes can also be used to improve rehabilitation nursing care and as the basis for research. This chapter examines outcomes of care in rehabilitation, describes the tools used by rehabilitation clinicians to collect information about outcomes, and profiles the agencies that accredit rehabilitation programs.

I. Overview

A. Primary Accreditation Agencies for Rehabilitation Providers
   1. Joint Commission on Accreditation of Healthcare Organizations (JCAHO)
   2. CARF...The Rehabilitation Accreditation Commission

B. Benefits of Accreditation
   1. Helps with the business, management, and quality strategies that organizations should have in place to meet consumer needs and maintain operations
   2. Demonstrates evidence to stakeholders that certain standards of excellence have been met, systems are in place to deliver quality services, results are expected based on the "norm," and processes thought to be of expert consensus are followed
   3. Offers confidence to consumers that an independent review process focuses on improving the quality of services
   4. Provides organizations with a template for efficient and effective operations
   5. Establishes a common level of program expectations and performance
   6. Focuses on meeting the needs of people with disabilities and others who need rehabilitation

7. Offers a mechanism for purchasers, providers, and consumers to interact

8. Identifies organizations or programs that have met standards and reinforces and supports those organizations

9. Affects reimbursement (CARF, 1998)

II. Accrediting Agencies

A. Joint Commission on Accreditation of Healthcare Organizations (JCAHO)

1. General

   a. Mission: To improve the quality of care provided to the public through the provision of healthcare accreditation and related services that support performance improvement in healthcare organizations (JCAHO, 1999)

   b. "Compliance": JCAHO's term for referring to standards

   c. Organizational structure: Governed by the Board of Commissioners

2. Historical perspective

   a. 1910: Dr. Ernest Codman proposed a system of "hospital standardization" in which hospitals track every patient to determine if treatment is effective.

   b. 1918: The American College of Surgeons (ACS) began on-site inspections of hospitals.

   c. 1926: The first 18-page standards manual was published.

   d. 1950: More than 3,200 hospitals achieved approval under the new program; as a result, the standard of care gradually improved.

   e. 1951: The American College of Physicians, the American Hospital Association, the American Medical Association, and the Canadian Medical Association joined to create the Joint Commission on Accreditation of Hospitals, whose primary purpose was to provide voluntary accreditation.

   f. 1964: The Joint Commission began charging for surveys.

   g. 1966: Long-term care accreditation began.

   h. 1970: RNs joined physicians in conducting surveys.

   i. 1982: The first public member began serving on the JCAHO Board of Commissioners.

   j. 1988: Accreditation for home care organizations began.

   k. 1989: Accreditation for managed care began.

   l. 1993

      1) The number and nature of Type 1 recommendations against an organization became public information.

      2) JCAHO began making random, unannounced surveys of accredited organizations.

   m. 1996: The Home Care Accreditation Program became JCAHO's largest accreditation program based on number of accredited organizations.

   n. 1997

      1) The ORYX initiative was launched to integrate outcomes and other performance measures into the accreditation process.

      2) JCAHO established cooperative agreements with CARF…The Rehabilitation Accreditation Commission for freestanding rehabilitation hospitals and rehabilitation units in hospitals.

   o. 1998: JCAHO announced its intent to begin offering international accreditation services.

3. Accreditation process

   a. An organization submits an application to JCAHO.

   b. The survey date is given to the organization.

   c. An initial conference with the organization's leaders is held on the first day of survey to finalize the survey schedule.

   d. The survey includes a tour of the facility, reviews of medical records and documentation, observation of staff, and interviews with patients and staff.

4. Accreditation decision(s) or outcomes

   a. Accreditation with commendation

   b. Accreditation without Type I recommendations

c. Accreditation with Type I recommendations

d. Provisional accreditation

e. Conditional accreditation

f. Preliminary nonaccreditation

g. Not accredited

5. The ORYX initiative

a. Introduced in 1997

b. Designed to help organizations strengthen their quality improvement efforts and to identify issues that require attention

c. Uses data from organizations to monitor performance between on-site survey visits

d. Supports JCAHO's mission and is a critical link between accreditation and patient care outcomes

e. Affects various rehabilitation settings, including hospitals, rehabilitation, long-term care, and home care (Dobrzykowski, 1997)

B. CARF...The Rehabilitation Accreditation Commission

1. General

a. Mission: To promote the quality, value, and optimal outcomes of services through a consultative accreditation process that centers on enhancing the lives of the people served (CARF, 1998)

b. "Conformance": CARF's term for referring to standards

c. Organizational structure

1) Four divisions

a) Medical rehabilitation: Accredits programs such as comprehensive integrated inpatient rehabilitation, brain injury, spinal cord injury systems of care, pain programs, outpatient, health enhancement, occupational rehabilitation, case management, home and community-based rehabilitation programs

b) Adult day services: Accredits community-based group programs designed to meet the needs of adults with impairments through individual plans of care to ensure that the program is structured, nonresidential, and provides a vast array of social support, as well as health and other services, in a protected setting

c) Behavioral health: Accredits providers of behavioral health programs (e.g., alcohol and drugs, mental health, psychosocial rehabilitation, integrated behavioral health)

d) Employment and community services: Accredits organizations that provide employment services, community services, and psychosocial rehabilitation programs

2) Membership: Includes associate members and sponsoring members (see Figure 19-1)

3) Board of Trustees

a) Composed of one person from each sponsoring organizations, as well as at-large trustees

b) Approves standards, awards accreditation, and oversees policies and financial matters (CARF, 1999)

2. Historical perspective

a. 1966: Founded as a nonprofit organization

b. 1973: Published a new program evaluation section of its standards manual for rehabilitation facilities

c. 1993: Accredited its first program in Canada

d. 1995: Enacted new standards for occupational rehabilitation and comprehensive pain management programs in the medical rehabilitation division

e. 1996: Accredited its first program in Sweden

f. 1997

1) Signed an agreement to accredit all Veterans Affairs rehabilitation programs over a 5-year period.

2) Began to offer a combined survey process with JCAHO to freestanding rehabilitation hospitals

g. 1998: Rewrote standards to be unidimensional as a result of the Standards Conformance Rating Scale (SCoRS) initiative

h. 1998: Accredited medical rehabilitation programs that are part of a larger entity, are recognized by JCAHO, and do not have to undergo JCAHO surveys for larger organizations

i. 1999: Published standards for adult day services

3. Development and creation of standards

a. National Advisory Committees (NACs): Each year, NACs are formed to review existing standards and create new standards. This is usually the starting point in the development of new standards. In years when there are no NACs, CARF solicits informal feedback from surveyors, consumers, other purchasers, and interested stakeholders.

b. Field review: Proposed standards are sent to the rehabilitation field for review by national professional groups, third-party purchasers, consumers, surveyors, and advocacy groups. Feedback, suggestions, and requests are evaluated by CARF.

c. Vote by Board of Trustees: New or revised standards are approved by the Board before they go into effect (CARF, 1999).

Figure 19-1. Members of CARF

Sponsoring Members

American Academy of Neurology
American Academy of Orthopaedic Surgeons
American Academy of Orthotists and Prosthetists
American Academy of Pain Medicine
American Academy of Physical Medicine and Rehabilitation
American Hospital Association
American Network of Community Options and Resources
American Occupational Therapy Association, Inc.
American Pain Society
American Physical Therapy Association
American Psychological Association
American Rehabilitation Association
American Speech-Language-Hearing Association
American Spinal Injury Association
American Therapeutic Recreation Association
Association of Rehabilitation Nurses
Brain Injury Association, Inc.
Department of Veterans Affairs
Federation of American Health Systems
Goodwill Industries International, Inc.
International Association of Jewish Vocational Services
International Association of Psychosocial Rehabilitation Services
Mental Health Corporations of America, Inc.
National Adult Day Services Association: A unit of The National Council on the Aging
National Association of Alcoholism and Drug Abuse Counselors
National Council for Community Behavioral Healthcare
Paralyzed Veterans of America
United Cerebral Palsy Associations

Associate Members

American Association of Spinal Cord Injury Psychologists and Social Workers
American Association on Mental Retardation
American Congress of Rehabilitation Medicine
American Horticultural Therapy Association
American Music Therapy Association, Inc.
American Osteopathic College of Rehabilitation Medicine
American Society of Neurorehabilitation
Association for Ambulatory Behavioral Healthcare
Commission on Rehabilitation Counselor Certification
Dietetics in Physical Medicine and Rehabilitation
National Alliance for the Mentally Ill
National Association of Children's Hospitals and Related Institutions
National Association of Psychiatric Treatment Centers for Children
National Association of Rehabilitation Professionals in the Private Sector
National Association of Social Workers
National Coalition of Art Therapies Associations
National Easter Seal Society
National Rehabilitation Association
National Therapeutic Recreation Society]
RESNA: The Rehabilitation Engineering and Assistive Technology Society of North America
Therapeutic Communities Association of New York, Inc.
Washington Business Group on Health

4. Accreditation process
    a. Contact CARF office to verify which standards manual to use: Standards manual year runs from July 1 to June 30.
    b. Perform a self-study: A facility may opt to complete a self-study and evaluation prior to and in preparation for the actual survey. CARF publishes numerous resources to help organizations in this process.
    c. Submit application at least 3 months prior to requested survey
    d. Schedule the survey date: Surveyors are selected based on their expertise and knowledge of the programs that are being surveyed. Generally, there will be an administrative surveyor and at least one program surveyor for medical rehabilitation programs.
    e. Have an orientation conference: Done the first day of the survey to allow surveyors to give an overview of the survey process and the organization to describe itself to the survey team
    f. Have an exit conference: Provides immediate feedback to the organization regarding strengths, areas for improvement, suggestions, and any recommendations made by the survey team
    g. Submit a quality improvement plan that addresses any recommendations in the survey report (CARF, 1999)
5. Key terminology related to CARF's survey process
    a. Recommendations: Statements reflecting nonconformance to specific standards. An organization must take action on each recommendation to come into conformance with the standards.
    b. Commendations: Statements of approval or praise offered to an organization for areas well implemented
    c. Suggestions: Ideas from the survey team for improving services within the organization based on experience in the rehabilitation field. Suggestions are not linked to conformance to the standards in that an organization is not required to implement or act upon them (CARF, 1999).

6. Accreditation decisions: Ultimately made by the Board of Trustees
    a. 3-year accreditation: Demonstrates substantial fulfillment of the standards
    b. 1-year accreditation: Evidence exists that the program is committed and capable; however, deficiencies also exist.
    c. Provisional accreditation: Deficiencies exist; however, the organization is committed to correct them (this decision can be given only once)
    d. Nonaccreditation: Major deficits exist in meeting standards and concerns exist about whether the organization meets the needs of the people it serves (CARF, 1999)

C. JCAHO/CARF Integrated Survey
    1. Integrated surveys apply only to the medical rehabilitation division.
    2. A crosswalk of JCAHO/CARF standards is available to freestanding rehabilitation organizations after an application has been completed to undergo an integrated survey.
        a. Minimal integration: Involves two survey teams, two standards manuals, two survey processes, two outcome decisions, and one survey time frame
        b. Moderate integration: Began in February 1999 and involves two survey teams, two manuals, two outcome decisions, one survey process, and one survey time frame
        c. Full integration: Anticipated to begin by the end of 2000 and will involve one survey process, one survey time frame, one survey team, and two separate outcome decisions

D. National Council on Quality Assurance (NCQA)
    1. Oversees managed care companies
    2. Uses the Health Employment Data Information Set (HEDIS) as its data set

III. Key Concepts in Rehabilitation

A. World Health Organization (WHO) Model (1980)
    1. Impairment: An abnormality of body structure, appearance, and organ or system function resulting from any cause. Impairments occur at the organ level (e.g., dysphagia, hemiparesis).

2. Disability: The consequences of impairment in terms of an individual's functional performance and activity. Disabilities represent disturbances at the level of the person (e.g., bathing, dressing, communication, walking, grooming).

3. Handicap: The disadvantages in work, family, and social roles experienced by an individual as a result of impairments and disabilities. Handicaps reflect interaction with and adaptation to the individual's surroundings.

B. Proposed International Classification of Impairments, Activities, and Participation (Wilkerson, 1997b; WHO, 1997)

1. Impairment: Abnormality of body structure, appearance, and organ or system function resulting from any cause

2. Activity: The nature and extent of function at the individual or person level

3. Social participation: The nature and extent of a person's involvement in life and various activities

IV. Tools for Monitoring Rehabilitation Outcomes

A. Global Adult Scales (which measure motor, physical, and cognitive elements)

1. Functional Independence Measure (FIM™) instrument (see Figure 19-2)

   a. Looks at severity of disability and need for assistance (burden of care)

   b. Designed to promote a uniform language among the rehabilitation team and to describe the severity of disability

   c. Is included in the Uniform Data Set for Medical Rehabilitation (UDSMR), which includes demographic, diagnostic, financial, and functional information about rehabilitation patients: UDSMR maintains databases for acute rehabilitation, subacute and skilled nursing facilities, and long-term hospitals.

   d. Includes 18 items (13 motor, 5 cognitive)

   e. Involves a hierarchy of motor items that progress from eating (easiest) to using stairs (most difficult)

   f. Uses a 7-level scale in which 1 = total assistance (patient performs less than 25% of an activity) and 7 = total independence (patient performs an activity without an assistive device or a helper in a safe and timely manner)

   g. Is used internationally and considered to be the "gold standard" in assessing functional status

   h. Is easy to use by members of any discipline

   i. Provides the basis for predicting outcomes for various patient populations (Black, Soltis, & Bartlett, 1999)

   j. Is the foundation for establishing Function-Related Groups (FRGs)

   k. Can be used to estimate the burden of care for activities of daily living (ADLs) (based on the FIM "Rule of Thumb Burden of Care" chart) (Deutsch, Braun, & Granger, 1997; UDSMR, 1996).

2. Patient Evaluation and Conference System (PECS) (see Figure 19-3)

   a. Comprehensive, lengthy interdisciplinary tool that examines 76 distinct functional areas

   b. Uses a 7-level scale in which 1 = most dependent and 7 = independent; 0 = a functional area that is either not tested or unmeasurable

3. PULSES: Represents the initial letters of the categories it measures

   a. P: Physical condition

   b. U: Upper extremities

   c. L: Lower extremities

   d. S: Sensory components

   e. E: Excretory function

   f. S: Social and mental status

4. Functional Assessment Measure (FAM) (Hall, 1997)

   a. Developed to serve as an adjunct to the FIM instrument to address some functional items that are essential to brain injury rehabilitation

   b. Measures 12 items, including cognitive, behavioral, communication, and community functioning

   c. Uses a 7-level scoring similar to the FIM instrument

Figure 19-2. Functional Independence Measure (FIM™) Instrument

FIM™ instrument

LEVELS		
	7 Complete Independence (Timely, Safely) 6 Modified Independence (Device)	**NO HELPER**
	Modified Dependence 5 Supervision (Subject = 100%+) 4 Minimal Assist (Subject = 75%+) 3 Moderate Assist (Subject = 50%+) **Complete Dependence** 2 Maximal Assist (Subject =25%+) 1 Total Assist (Subject = less than 25%)	**HELPER**

	ADMISSION	**DISCHARGE**	**FOLLOW-UP**
Self-Care A. Eating B Grooming C. Bathing D. Dressing - Upper Body E. Dressing - Lower Body F. Toileting			
Sphincter Control G. Bladder Management H. Bowel Management			
Transfers I. Bed, Chair, Wheelchair J. Toilet K. Tub, Shower			
Locomotion L. Walk/Wheelchair M. Stairs	W Walk C Wheelchair B Both	W Walk C Wheelchair B Both	W Walk C Wheelchair B Both
Motor Subtotal Score			
Communication N. Comprehension O. Expression	A Auditory V Visual B Both V Vocal N Nonvocal B Both	A Auditory V Visual B Both V Vocal N Nonvocal B Both	A Auditory V Visual B Both V Vocal N Nonvocal B Both
Social Cognition P. Social Interaction Q. Problem Solving R. Memory			
Cognitive Subtotal Score			
TOTAL FIM Score			

NOTE: Leave no blanks. Enter 1 if patient not testable due to risk

Figure 19-3. Listing of Patient Evaluation and Conference System (PECS) Items and Item Groupings

I. Rehabilitation Medicine (MED)
1. Motor Loss
2. Spasticity/Involuntary Movement
3. Joint Limitations
4. Autonomic Disturbance
5. Sensory Deficiency
6. Perceptual & Cognitive Deficits
7. Associated Medical Problems
8. Postural Deviations

II. Rehabilitation Nursing (NSG)
1. Performance of Bowel Program
2. Performance of Urinary Program
3. Performance of Skin Care Program
4. Assumes Responsibility for Self-care
5. Performs Assigned Interdisciplinary Activities
6. Patient Education
7. Safety Awareness

III. Physical Mobility (PHY)
1. Performance of Transfers
2. Performance of Ambulation
3. Performance of Wheelchair Mobility
4. Ability to Handle Environmental Barriers (e.g., stairs, rugs, elevators)
5. Performance of Car Transfer
6. Driving Mobility
7. Assumes Responsibility for Mobility
8. Position Changes
9. Endurance
10. Balance

IV. Activities of Daily Living (ADL)
1. Performance in Feeding
2. Performance in Hygiene/Grooming
3. Performance in Dressing
4. Performance in Home Management
5. Performance of Mobility in the Home Environment (including utilization of environmental adaptations for communication)
6. Bathroom Transfers

V. Communication (COM)
1. Ability to Comprehend Spoken Language
2. Ability to Produce Language
3. Ability to Read
4. Ability to Produce Written Language
5. Ability to Hear
6. Ability to Comprehend and Use Gesture
7. Ability to Produce Speech
8. Ability to Swallow
12. Impairment in Thought (Verbal Linguistic) Processing (NP4)

VI. Medications (DRG)
1. Knowledge of Medications

VII. Nutrition (NUT)
1. Nutritional Status—Body Weight
2. Nutritional Status—Lab Values
3. Knowledge of Nutrition and/or Modified Diet
4. Skill with Nutrition & Diet (Adherence to Nutritional Plan)
5. Utilization of Nutrition & Diet (Nutritional Health)

VIII. Assistive Devices (DEV)
1. Knowledge of Assistive Mobility Devices
2. Skill with Assuming Operating Position of Assistive Mobility Devices
3. Utilization of Assistive Mobility Devices

IX. Psychology (PSY)
1. Distress/comfort
2. Helplessness/self-efficacy
3. Self-directed Learning Skills
4. Skill in Self-management of Behavior and Emotions
5. Skill in Interpersonal Relations
6. Ability to Participate in the Rehabilitation Program
7. Acceptance/understanding of Disability

X. Neuropsychology (NP)
1. Impairment of Short-term Memory
2. Impairment of Long-term Memory
3. Impairment in Attention-concentration Skills
4. Impairment in Verbal Linguistic Processing
5. Impairment in Visual Spatial Processing
6. Impairment in Basic Intellectual Skills
7. Orientation
8. Alertness/Coma State

XI. Social Issues (SOC)
1. Ability to Problem Solve and Utilizc Resources
2. Family: Communication/Resources
3. Family: Understanding of Disability
4. Economic Resources
5. Ability to Live Independently
6. Living Arrangements

XII. Vocational/Educational Activity (V/E)
1. Active Participation in realistic Voc/Ed Planning
2. Realistic Perception of Work-related activity
3. Ability to Tolerate Planned Number of Hours of Voc/Ed
4. Vocational/Educational Placement
5. Physical Capacity for Work

XIII. Therapeutic Recreation (REC)
1. Participation in Group Activities
2. Participation in Community Activities
3. Interaction with Others
4. Participation and Satisfaction with Individual Leisure Activities
5. Active Participation in Sports

XIV. Pain (PAI)
1. Pain Behavior
2. Physical Activity
3. Social Interaction
4. Pacing
5. Sitting Tolerance
6. Standing Tolerance
7. Walking Tolerance
8. Use of Body Mechanics
9. Use of Relaxation Techniques
10. Performance of Medication Program

XVI. Pastoral Care (PC)
1. Awareness of Spiritual Dimensions of Illness/Disability
2. Knowledge of Spiritual Resources
3. Skill in Self-management of Spirituality
4. Utilization of Spiritual Resources

Reprinted with permission of Marianjoy Rehabilitation Hospital and Clinics and PECS, Inc., from Patient Evaluation and Conference System, Inc. (PECS). (Available from Marianjoy Rehabilitation Hospital and Clinics, PO Box 795, Wheaton, IL 60189)

B. Activity of Daily Living (ADL) Scales (which measure motor and physical elements) (Dittmar & Gresham, 1997) (see Figure 19-4)

1. Barthel Index

    a. Uses a 0–100 scoring system (100 = total independence, 0 = dependence) that assesses 10 domains

    b. Is popular in European rehabilitation facilities

2. Kenny Self-Care Evaluation

    a. Examines six domains: Transfers, bed activity, feeding, personal hygiene, dressing, and locomotion

    b. Uses a 4-level scale in which 0 = completely dependent and 4 = independent

3. Katz Index of Independence in Activities of Daily Living: Uses letters (e.g., A = independent, G = dependent) to score various functional areas

4. Klein-Bell Activity of Daily Living Scale

    a. Designed to help determine the patient's current level of function

    b. Includes 170 items in six functional areas: dressing, elimination, mobility, eating, bathing and hygiene, and emergency telephone communication

5. Quadriplegia Index Function (QIF)

    a. Is specific to people with quadriplegia

    b. Involves the domains of transfers, grooming, bathing, feeding, dressing, wheelchair mobility, bed activity, bladder program, bowel program, and understanding of personal care

    c. Uses a 4-level scale in which 4 = independent and 0 = dependent; 9 = areas that are not applicable

C. Instrumental Activities of Daily Living (IADLs) Scale (Dittmar & Gresham, 1997)

1. Encompasses activities that go beyond basic ADLs

2. Examples of IADLs: Doing laundry, shopping, preparing meals, using a phone, managing finances

D. Scales That Measure the Effects of Primary and Secondary Handicaps

1. Community Integration Questionnaire (CIQ): A 15-item tool that assesses home integration, social integration, and productive activity (Willer, Ottenbacher, & Coad, 1994)

2. Craig Handicap Assessment Reporting Technique (CHART) (Hall, Dukers, Whiteneck, Brooks, & Krause, 1998)

    a. Designed to assess the reintegration of people with spinal cord injury

    b. Includes 27 items categorized into five dimensions (e.g., physical independence, mobility, occupation, social integration, economic self-sufficiency)

    c. Has a maximum score for each dimension of 100

E. Pediatric Tools

1. WeeFIM® instrument (see Figure 19-5) (Braun, 1998)

Figure 19-4. Characteristics of Selected Activity of Daily Living (ADL) Scales

Scale	Items Included	Type of Scale	Evaluation
Katz Index of ADL	Bathing, dressing, toileting, transferring, continence, feeding; order of items reflects natural progression in loss and acquisition of function	Dichotomous rating of independence or dependence on each item; forms a six-level Guttman Scale	By professional raters
Kenny Self-Care Evaluation	Seventeen activities in six categories: bed activities, transfers, locomotion, personal hygiene, dressing, and feeding	Each activity rated on a four-point scale (0= complete dependence, 4= complete independence); an average score is created for each of six categories, allowing a possible total score of 24	By rehabilitation staff; scores constructed on the basis of observations
Barthel Index	Feeding, transferring, grooming, toileting, bathing, walking, or propelling a wheelchair; climbing stairs, bladder control, bowel control	Partial scores for performing ADLs with help, full score for independent performance; items weighted; full score of 100 signifies ability to do all tasks independently	By rehabilitation staff

Sources consulted

Jacelon, C.S. (1986). The Barthel Index: A review of the literature. *Rehabilitation Nursing, 11*(4), 9-11.

Katz, S., Lord, A.B., Moskowitz, R.W., Jackson, B.A., & Jaffe, M.W. (1963). Studies of illness in the aged. The index of ADL: A standardized measure of biological and psychological function. *Journal of the American Medical Association, 185*, 914-919.

a. Designed for children aged 6 months to 7 years and older

b. Derived from the FIM instrument

c. Can be used by members of any discipline

d. Measures actual performance across various settings

2. Pediatric Evaluation of Disability Inventory (PEDI) (Haley, 1999)

a. Provides an assessment of key functional areas in children between the ages of 6 months and 7 years

b. Examines performance in three domains: self-care, mobility, and social

3. Home Observation for Measurement of the Environment (HOME) (Molnar & Alexander, 1999)

a. Consists of 45 items

b. Identifies risk of developmental delay due to lack of environmental support for a child in the home

c. Assesses quality of child care

d. Bases data collection on actual observation

4. Functional Evaluation of Sensori-Neurologic Outcomes (FRESNO) (Roberts et al., 1999)

a. Includes 196 items in 45 key functional areas

Figure 19-5. WeeFIM® Instrument

WeeFIM® instrument

L E V E L S	7 Complete Independence (Timely, Safely) 6 Modified Independence (Device)	**No Assistance**
	Modified Dependence 5 Supervision (Subject = 100%) 4 Minimal Assist (Subject = 75%+) 3 Moderate Assist (Subject = 50%+) **Complete Dependence** 2 Maximal Assist (Subject = 25%+) 1 Total Assist (Subject = less than 25%)	**Assistance**

ASSESSMENT   GOAL

Self-Care
.1 Eating
.2 Grooming
.3 Bathing
.4 Dressing - Upper
.5 Dressing - Lower
.6 Toileting
.7 Bladder
.8 Bowel
Self-Care Total   *Quotient*

Mobility
.9 Chair, Wheelchair
.10 Toilet
.11 Tub, Shower
.12 Walk/Wheelchair
.13 Stairs
Mobility Total   *Quotient*

W Walk
C wheelChair
L crawL
B comBination

Cognition
.14 Comprehension
.15 Expression
.16 Social Interaction
.17 Problem Solving
.18 Memory
Cognitive Total   *Quotient*

A Auditory
V Visual
B Both

V Vocal
N Nonvocal
B Both

WeeFIM Total   *Quotient*

NOTE: Leave no blanks. Enter 1 if patient not testable due to risk

b. Encompasses five domains: self-care, motor, communication, cognition, and socialization

F. Outpatient Tools
1. LifeWare® assessment tools (Granger, 1999)
    a. Designed for outpatient medical rehabilitation programs
    b. Examines physical function, pain, affective well-being, and cognitive functioning
    c. Customized for various patient populations
        1) Musculoskeletal (two versions, one of which is abbreviated)
        2) Neurological
        3) Pulmonary
        4) Comprehensive
        5) Multiple sclerosis
2. Focus on Therapeutic Outcomes (FOTO) (Dobrzykowski & Nance, 1997)
    a. Created in 1992 as an outcomes measurement system for outpatient orthopedic rehabilitation
    b. Monitors the efficiency and effectiveness in the outpatient orthopedic population
3. Short form 36 (SF-36): Developed to assess a patient's well-being and perception of overall health (Ware & Sherbourne, 1992)

G. Home Environment Tools: Outcome and Assessment Information Set (OASIS)
1. Mandated by the Health Care Financing Administration (HCFA) for use in home care
2. Has 100 questions covering 14 categories of care (e.g., ambulation, management of medication, psychological and emotional behavior, living arrangements)
3. Involves data information being sent to state agencies
4. Is a standardized measurement for monitoring outcomes of adults in the home setting

H. Other Tools
1. Minimum Data Set (MDS) assessment
    a. Mandated by HCFA for use in long-term care and subacute settings
    b. Serves as the data collection instrument for prospective payment system (PPS)
    c. Utilizes Resource Utilization Groups,

Version III (RUGs-III), a 44-group patient classification system in which periodic assessments are done
    d. Involves patient information being sent to the fiscal intermediary for reimbursement and MDS information being sent to state survey and certification agencies (Medicare Payment Advisory Commission [MedPac], 1999)
2. Minimum Data Set-Post Acute Care (MDS-PAC)
    a. Mandated by HCFA to be the data collection instrument by which patients are placed into FRGs
    b. Will be the basis for reimbursement
    c. Becomes effective for rehabilitation programs in October 2000
    d. Is expected to be implemented in skilled nursing facilities and long-term care hospitals over the next several years

V. Program Evaluation
A. Overview
1. Performance indicators play a key role in the development of a successful outcomes system.
2. Performance indicators are quantitative values that can be collected by providers and reported to stakeholders.

B. General Considerations
1. When assessing for efficiency, effectiveness, and other critical outcomes of rehabilitation, an organization must use a system that has demonstrated reliability and validity.
    a. Reliability: Reproducibility of an instrument's findings
    b. Validity: Ability of the tool to measure what it was designed or intended to measure
2. Data collection instruments and systems used by rehabilitation programs should be valid and reliable.
3. Development of a successful program evaluation and outcomes system with an emphasis on rehabilitation nursing interventions should include specific critical design elements.
    a. Functional status: Documents the rehabilitation gains of physical function

b. Destination: Determines whether discharge to the community or to the least restrictive environment has been achieved

c. Efficiency: The extent to which a specific intervention, procedure, regimen, or service, when applied in routine circumstances, does what it is intended to do for a specific population (Last, 1995)

d. Patient perception: Satisfaction of the patient, family, and other various stakeholders

e. Effectiveness: The end results achieved in relation to the effort expended in terms of resources (e.g., money, time) (Last, 1995)

f. Follow-up: Determines whether progress was made or maintained after discharge from a rehabilitation program

VI. Quality and Performance Improvement in Health Care

A. Overview

1. Definition of quality improvement: "A management process or approach to continuous study and improvement of the processes of providing health care services to meet the needs of individuals and others" (JCAHO, 1999)

2. Historical figures in the development of quality improvement

a. Walter Shewhart (1920s): Created the quality cycle of Plan, Do, Check, Act (PDCA)

b. Armand Feigenbaum (1940s to present): Developed phrases of "total quality control" and "cost of quality"

c. W. Edwards Deming (1930s to present): Developed a 14-point plan that serves as the basis for total quality management (TQM). Although Deming's model was originally designed for the manufacturing industry, the concepts and philosophy have been adopted by the healthcare industry.

d. Joseph Juran (1950s): An engineer and attorney whose philosophy was to build upon quality improvement, quality control, and quality planning (i.e., the quality trilogy). Juran's philosophy supports the frameworks of CARF and JCAHO.

e. Philip Crosby (1960s to present): Identified zero defects as a performance standard with an emphasis on preventing errors

B. Tools for Quality Improvement (Brassard & Ritter, 1994)

1. Brainstorming: Allows team members to create as many creative ideas and solutions as possible; all suggestions are recorded to be evaluated at a later time.

2. Cause-and-effect diagram (Fishbone diagram): Allows team members to visually and graphically explore the relationship between the effects and possible causes to identified problems

3. Affinity diagram: Gathers large amounts of data and helps organize the information into groupings based on the relationships between the items

4. Check sheet: Allows team members to record and collect data from various sources so that patterns and trends may be identified

5. Run chart: Used to visually display data and to identify any changes that occur

6. Histogram: Displays the distribution of data and reveals the amount of variation within a process

7. Scatter diagram: Used to study the possible cause and effect between two variables

8. Control chart: Used to monitor, control, and improve variances in performance by identifying the source; is similar to a run chart, but with statistical upper and lower limits

9. Flowchart: A pictorial representation of various steps within a process that allows team members to easily identify the flow of events

10. Force field analysis: Identifies the forces in place that affect an issue or problem; ideally, it reinforces positives and eliminates negatives

11. Pareto chart: A display of bar graphs that can help focus on and determine which problems to solve and in which order so that efforts are directed to the problems that have the greatest improvement potential

C. Models for Performance Improvement

1. American Nurses Association (ANA) and Association of Rehabilitation Nurses (ARN) standards of care

a. 1973: ANA established generic standards of nursing practice for determining the quality of nursing care.

b. 1977: ANA published standards of rehabilitation nursing practice

c. 1986: ARN and ANA collaborated to revise the standards of rehabilitation nursing practice (McCourt, 1993).

c. 1994: ARN published revised standards for rehabilitation nursing practice.

2. JCAHO's Plan, Do, Check, Act (PDCA) approach

a. Plan what you want to accomplish

b. Do what you planned to do

c. Check the results

d. Act on the information

3. CARF's Quality and Accountability Initiative

a. Goals: To enhance the value of accreditation, conduct accreditation program research, and direct attention to outcomes measurement and management

b. Includes the 4-level Standards Conformance Rating Scale (SCoRS)

1) 0 = Nonconformance (does not meet standard)

2) 1 = Partial conformance (has substantial room for improvement)

3) 2 = Conformance (fully meets standard)

4) 3 = Exemplary conformance (significantly exceeds expectation for conformance)

VII. The Future of Outcomes Management

A. The Increasing Importance of Outcomes

1. Outcomes across the continuum will continue to have greater importance.

2. Some systems (e.g., WeeFIM, FIM instrument, LifeWare) are starting to support measurement across the continuum of care.

3. The emphasis of satisfaction will transition from provider to payer to patient or consumer (Jones & Evans, 1998).

a. Satisfaction is evidenced by disclosure statements that have a great influence in rehabilitation.

b. Example: CARF's medical rehabilitation division maintains a public disclosure policy in which an individual may request an organization's survey summary, and CARF provides the summary to the individual at no charge. This meets the "need to know" element for various stakeholders (e.g., consumers).

B. Greater Accountability to Stakeholders

1. Rehabilitation providers are experiencing an increase in accountability to demonstrate positive outcomes.

2. Rehabilitation providers are increasingly expected to share information about programs and outcomes.

C. Integrated CARF/JCAHO Surveys in Long-Term and Subacute Settings

D. Increased Focus on Measuring and Monitoring Outcomes

1. Measuring and monitoring outcomes and the quality and durability of outcomes will become an even larger component of rehabilitation nursing practice.

2. Management of patients' needs across the continuum will be critical for successful chronic disease management.

3. Rehabilitation nurses have the skills and knowledge to positively affect outcomes for patients.

References

Black, T.M. (1999). Outcomes: What's all the fuss about? *Rehabilitation Nursing, 24*(5), 188–189, 191.

Black, T.M., Soltis, T., & Bartlett, C. (1999). Using the Functional Independence Measure (FIM) instrument to predict stroke rehabilitation outcomes. *Rehabilitation Nursing, 24*(3), 109–114, 121.

Brassard, M., & Ritter, D. (1994). *The Memory Jogger II™: A pocket guide of tools for continuous improvement and effective planning.* Methuen, MA: Goal/QPC.

Braun, S. (1998). The Functional Independence Measure for children (WeeFIM instrument): Gateway to the WeeFIM system. *Journal of Rehabilitation Outcomes Measurement, 2*(4), 63–68.

CARF...The Rehabilitation Commission (CARF). (1998). *Performance indicators for rehabilitation programs, version 1.1.* Tucson, AZ: Author.

CARF...The Rehabilitation Commission (CARF). (1999). *Standards manual for medical rehabilitation.* Tucson, AZ: Author.

Deutsch, A., Braun, S., & Granger, C.V. (1997). The Functional Independence Measure (FIM^SM) instrument. *Journal of Rehabilitation Outcomes, 1*(2), 67–71.

Dittmar, S., & Gresham, G. (1997). Appendix A: Description and display of selected functional assessment and outcome measures in physical rehabilitation. In *Functional assessment and outcome measurement for the rehabilitation healthcare professional* (pp. 90–138). Gaithersburg, MD: Aspen.

Dobrzykowski, E. (1997). ORYX: The next evolution in accreditation. *Journal of Rehabilitation Outcomes, 1*(6), 22–23.

Dobrzykowski, E., & Nance, T. (1997). The focus on therapeutic outcomes (FOTO) outpatient orthopedic rehabilitation database: Results of 1994-1996. *Journal of Rehabilitation Outcomes Measurement, 1*(1), 56–60.

Granger, C. (1999). The LifeWare System. *Journal of Rehabilitation Outcomes Measurement, 3*(2), 63–69.

Haley, S. (1997). The Pediatric Evaluation of Disability Inventory (PEDI). *Journal of Rehabilitation Outcomes, 1*(1), 61–69.

Hall, K. (1997). The Functional Assessment Measure (FAM). *Journal of Rehabilitation Outcomes Measurement, 1*(3), 63–65.

Hall, K., Dukers, M., Whiteneck, G., Brooks, C.A., & Krause, J. (1998). The Craig Handicap Assessment and Reporting Technique (CHART): Metric properties and scoring. *Journal of Rehabilitation Outcomes Measurement, 2*(5), 39–49.

Jacelon, C.S. (1986). The Barthel Index: A review of the literature. *Rehabilitation Nursing, 11*(4), 9–11.

Joint Commission on Accreditation of Healthcare Organizations (JCAHO). (1999). *1999 accreditation manual for hospitals.* Oakbrook Terrace, IL: Author.

Jones, M., & Evans, R. (1998). Outcomes in a managed care environment. *Topics in Spinal Cord Injury Rehabilitation, 3*(4), 61–73.

Katz, S., Lord, A.B., Moskowitz, R.W., Jackson, B.A., & Jaffe, M.W. (1963). Studies of illness in the aged. The index of ADL: A standardized measure of biological and psychological function. *Journal of the American Medical Association, 185*, 914–919.

Last, J.M. (1995). *Dictionary of epidemiology* (3rd ed.). New York: Oxford University Press.

Medicare Payment Advisory Commission (MedPac). (1999, March). "Post Acute Care Providers: Moving toward prospective payment" in *Report to Congress: Medicare Payment Policy*, pp. 81–98.

Molnar, G., & Alexander, M. (Eds.). (1999). *Psychological assessment in pediatric rehabilitation in pediatric rehabilitation* (pp. 29–56). Philadelphia: Hanley and Belfus.

McCourt, A.E. (Ed.). (1993). *The specialty practice of rehabilitation nursing: A core curriculum* (3rd ed.). Skokie, IL: Rehabilitation Nursing Foundation of the Association of Rehabilitation Nurses.

Roberts, S., Wells, R., Brown, I., Bryant, J., Hutchinson, H.T., Kurushima, C., Garbarino, W., Dahl, B., & Vander Plaats, S. (1999). The FRESNO: A pediatric functional outcome measurement system. *Journal of Rehabilitation Outcomes, 3*(1), 11–19.

Uniform Data System for Medical Rehabilitation (UDSMR). (1996). *Guide for the Uniform Data Set for Medical Rehabilitation.* Buffalo, NY: State University of New York, Buffalo.

Ware, J.E., & Sherbourne, C.D. (1992). The MOS 36-item short health survey (SF-36): Conceptual framework and item selection. *Medical Care, 30*, 472–480.

Wilkerson, D. (1997a, August/September). Outcomes and accreditation. *Rehab Management*, pp. 112, 114–115, 124.

Wilkerson, D. (1997b, Winter). On the language and classification of disablement and a new ICIDH. *American Congress of Rehabilitation Medicine Newsletter*, pp. 5–7.

Willer, B., Ottenbacher, K., & Coad, M.L. (1994). The Community Integration Questionnaire. *American Journal of Physical Medicine and Rehabilitation, 73*(2), 103–111.

World Health Organization (WHO). (1980). *International classification of impairments, disabilities and handicaps.* Geneva: Author.

World Health Organization (WHO). (1997). *International classification of impairments, activities and participation (ICIDH-2): Beta-I draft for field trials.* Geneva: Author.

Suggested resource

Hoeman, S. (Ed.). (1996). *Rehabilitation nursing: Process and application* (2nd ed.). St. Louis: Mosby.

Chapter 20

The Impact of Information Technology and Computer Applications on Rehabilitation Nursing

Mary Ann Sawalski, MSEd BSN RN CRRN

"When the PC [personal computer] was born, the lives of countless persons with disabilities changed forever, and a new technology sprang into being" (Lazzaro, 1996, p. ix).

"The work of redefining human potential and creating a world of access to opportunity through technology has only just begun. It must continue until technology is a regular part of the lives of all individuals with disabilities who can benefit from it" (Alliance for Technology Access, 1996, p. ix).

Information technology and computer applications have developed and expanded beyond expectations in the last 10 years. This "electronic revolution" has changed the way business is done, regardless of whether it is banking, advertising, industry, art, or health care. The rapid transfer of information touches our daily lives personally, professionally, and socially.

Health care today is more effective, efficient, and reliable because of computer technologies and information systems. In fact, the specialty fields of nursing informatics and rehabilitation engineering developed in response to computerization. Diagnosis, care, treatment, education, and research related to individuals who need rehabilitation, who are living with disabilities, or who are delivering care are greatly affected by the use of computers. As a result, rehabilitation nurses must be knowledgeable about computer applications and their potential. Rehabilitation nurses can contribute to and enhance the potential benefits of computerization by appropriately using computer applications. The input of knowledgeable, experienced rehabilitation healthcare workers expands the benefits of the computer.

The expertise of nurses and other professionals in rehabilitation settings, including acute care, subacute, rehabilitation hospitals, home health, case management, and outpatient facilities, can range from using a computer as a glorified typewriter to using state-of-the-art, sophisticated programming networks. If there is no "cheerleader" or "salesman" of computerization in the nursing department, the rate of progress is usually slow at best. Nurses' lack of computer experience, heavy work schedules, and limited scheduled time for training and practice also are factors for the poor acceptance of computer use in some facilities. Facilities that are successful in computerized documentation will address these barriers.

Health care can be more effective, efficient, and reliable because of computer technology and information systems. "The Association of Rehabilitation Nurses (ARN) projects that in this increasingly complex environment, we will need to increase the number of nurses with advanced skills and practice responsibilities to continue to achieve optimal client outcomes" (ARN, 1995). The quality of client care and the integrity of the nursing profession will be directly affected by the way the nurses of the new millennium approach and embrace these new and powerful tools of information processing and rapid communication brought about by use of the computer, now and in the future.

This chapter reviews the range of computer applications used in health care. Due to the amount of information available and the rapid changes in computer technology, this information is designed to introduce the reader to computer technology, resources, and the Internet. It is not a comprehensive study of the numerous areas of computer applications and technology.

I. Precipitating Factors of Computerization in Rehabilitation

A. Changes in the Client's Home and Work Environment

1. Expectations of independence have increased.

   a. Shorter hospital and treatment stays require accelerated self-help.

   b. Independence expectations are greater with the shrinking of the nuclear family.

2. Public policy supports and encourages various levels of independence at home and in the workforce (Flippo, Inge, & Barcus, 1995).

3. Computerized assistive devices allow people with disabilities to produce the same or similar outcomes as the general population in the following areas:

   a. Activities of daily living (ADLs)

   b. Driving

   c. Work output

   d. Communication

4. Environmental assistive devices enhance the home, community resources, and the workplace.

   a. Adaptive lighting

   b. Access to vans, public transportation, toilets, and stairways

   c. Ergonomics applications that allow longer and easier sitting times

5. Employers are required (by legislation) to make reasonable adjustments in the work environment. These adjustments have expanded job opportunities for people with disabilities.

B. Reforms in Health Care

1. Decreased length of stay at rehabilitation hospitals

2. Case management focus

   a. Is outcomes oriented

   b. Identifies financial priorities and parameters

   c. Sets short- and long-range plans for the highest quality of services within parameters

3. Consolidation of resources

   a. Prevents overlap of services

   b. Compares choices for appropriate equipment and treatment within identified constraints

C. The Need for Refined Communication

1. Society is acclimating to the speed of information. Clients and their families expect to be more informed within a shorter time.

2. The continuum of care blends services as the client moves from hospital to rehabilitation to home.

3. Comprehensive healthcare records across the continuum are necessary.

   a. To facilitate diagnosis

   b. To determine plans of care

   c. To identify problems and untoward reactions

   d. To track positive and negative outcomes

4. Pertinent information concerning client status, customized educational information, and changes in diet, medication, and therapies can be available immediately.

5. Data management is increasingly important.

   a. Computerized data management systems facilitate physical, time, and financial management of large amounts of information.

   b. Requirements for an increase in data are evident by client, family, and healthcare industry demands in the following areas:

      1) Tracking costs of health care

      2) Clinical outcomes in general (e.g., case management)

      3) Clinical outcomes with a specific focus (e.g., therapy outcomes, medical reasons for Medicare coverage)

      4) Research to study trends

      5) Financial planning for clients, insurance companies, and healthcare providers

      6) Prospective payment systems (PPS) for long-term care and home health

II. Contributions of Computer Technology to Rehabilitation

A. Technological Advances

1. Adaptive equipment and assistive devices

   a. For clients with physical disabilities

      1) Speech input devices: The computer interacts with a human voice instead

of physical input devices such as a keyboard or a mouse (e.g., Via Voice™, Simply Speaking™) (IBM Corporation, 1999)

2) An eye-controlled keyboard for people with motor or speech difficulties but who have sight and eye control (e.g., VisionKey™); can be used with a variety of computers (e.g., Mac Access Passport, 1996b)

3) Adaptations such as switches, matrix keyboards, communication aids, joysticks, and video game controllers that allow clients with a variety of disabilities to use the keyboard or to prevent repetitive stress (Alliance for Technology Access, 1996; IBM Corporation, 1999) (see Figure 20-1)

4) One-handed keyboards and software (Flippo et al., 1995)

5) Computer controls using head movement or puffing instead of arm and hand movements (e.g., HeadMaster Plus™) (Mac Access Passport, 1999a)

b. For clients with visual disabilities

1) Screen magnifiers
   a) Enlarge text and images
   b) Reverse colors on screen to enhance clarity

2) Speech synthesizers (e.g., Screen Reader™): Convert information on screen into voice output

3) Refreshable braille displays
   a) Can display all typed information and screen formatting in braille
   b) Convert printed pages (via scanners) into speech or braille

4) Notetakers: Take class notes in braille or on a standard keyboard and store them in computerized files for later editing and reading in braille or via synthesized speech; also, braille labels are available for keyboard keys

5) Sip and puff switches: Are wireless and use the client's breath to click a switch

c. For clients with speech and hearing disabilities: How the client communicates depends not only on his or her tools and abilities but also on his or her personal

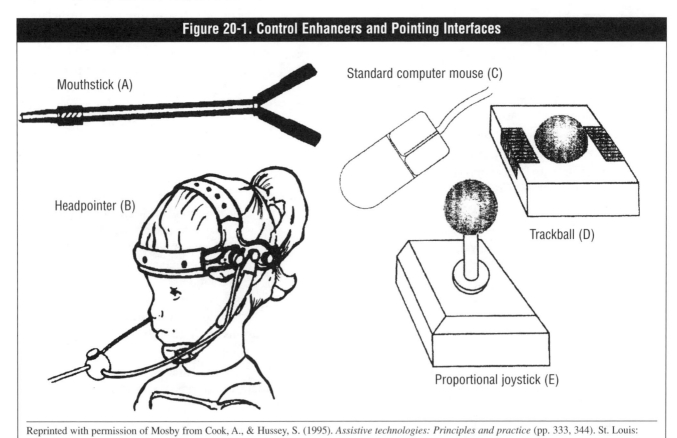

Figure 20-1. Control Enhancers and Pointing Interfaces

Mouthstick (A)

Headpointer (B)

Standard computer mouse (C)

Trackball (D)

Proportional joystick (E)

Reprinted with permission of Mosby from Cook, A., & Hussey, S. (1995). *Assistive technologies: Principles and practice* (pp. 333, 344). St. Louis: Mosby.

choice (e.g., some clients prefer to use the written word rather than robotic voice synthesizer sounds).

1) Visual voice tools: Basic tools for developing voice control
2) Speech viewer III™, a speech therapy tool for Windows™: Used as a tool for therapists and clients or as part of prescribed exercises for the client
3) Communication: A desktop or laptop computer can be used for communication between the person with a speech disability and the people with whom he or she interacts. Examples of communication enhancement include the following:
   a) Using small portable devices in transit or in the wheelchair as a computer (Note: These devices may be unwieldy).
   b) Using short messages, phrases, or sentences instead of spelling out individual words
   c) Converting representative pictures or objects into phrases or sentences if the client has problems comprehending the written word
   d) Interacting dynamically with message content, including synthesized speech with keyboard or mouse devices (e.g., Touch Talker™) that activate typed words or pictures into speech

d. For clients with cognitive disabilities

1) Computerized speech output (i.e., reading aloud) and using study tools for people with dyslexia and comprehension challenges
2) Speech synthesizers with screen readers (e.g., Screen Reader™): Convert screen information into voice output for use in letter-sound recognition
3) Intelligent word prediction programs that enhance the quality of written communication in clients with cognitive difficulties by presenting choices of "whole words" when a phonetic or partial word is given

2. Software and assistive technology
   a. For clients with physical disabilities
      1) Software for control of assistive computer devices (e.g., switches, matrix keyboards, communication aids, head-controlled mouse, joysticks, video game controllers)
      2) Virtual keyboards: Use image of keyboard on screen and the appropriate cursor controller to fit the disability in the same way virtual reality computer games are played
   b. For clients with visual disabilities: Home Page Reader™, a self-voicing Web browser that audibly communicates everything (including graphics) on the Web page
   c. For clients with speech and hearing disabilities: Programs are available that can help clients with the following skills:
      1) Cause-and-effect interactions
      2) Taking turns
      3) Early vocabulary
      4) Syntax
      5) Cognitive concepts
      6) Auditory processing
      7) Reading
   d. For clients with cognitive disabilities
      1) Software configurations that replace letters on the keyboard with common words or letter pairs
      2) Programmable software that can customize the keyboard to the client's needs
      3) Speech Solutions™: Available in nine languages with IBM's Via Voice™
      4) Software designed especially for children with special needs and exceptional learning (e.g., Edmark) (Edmark Corporation, 1999)

3. Environmental controls
   a. For clients with physical disabilities (Cook & Hussey, 1995)
      1) Adjustable workstations that meet the specific needs of clients with quadriplegia
      2) Padded arm, wrist, leg supports
      3) Customized furniture
      4) Flat overlays to prevent the person from accidentally pressing keys

b. For clients with visual disabilities
   1) Screen magnifiers
   2) Larger keys for keyboard
c. For clients with speech and hearing disabilities: Volume adjustment and control of voice input and output devices
d. For clients with disabilities: Environmental control, computerized control of lights, telephones, appliances, and intercoms that allow the client to have independent control of the surroundings

B. Diagnosis Augmentation
1. Provides early and accurate diagnoses
2. Allows the selection of appropriate treatment tracks
3. Decreases trial-and-error time, money, and client discomfort
4. Allows for noninvasive procedures (e.g., computerized tomography [CT] scan, magnetic resonance imaging [MRI], some lab tests) and rapid analysis or computation of data
5. Allows for a larger turnover of clients due to less time spent per test
6. Facilitates the dissemination of information to the testing department, nursing unit, or institution, as well as to the client
7. Enables differential diagnosis, which is essential in cases in which opposing treatment plans could increase the problem, as in the case of high-lumbar radiculopathy (Nader, Campagnolo, Tomaio, & Stitik, 1998).
8. Provides rapid and accurate identification of underlying pathophysiology, which allows for implementation of improved rehabilitation nursing and therapy practices
9. Promotes ease of comparison of symptoms to disease entities in large databases and narrows the field in difficult diagnostic situations
10. Broadens the knowledge of physiology and pathology in neurological and muscle systems by the use of electrodiagnostic equipment and computer analysis

C. Cognitive Rehabilitation Treatment
1. Diagnostic equipment advances

a. Provide potentially cost-effective and efficient clinical tools for diagnosing and tracking the progress of people with cognitive disabilities
b. Allow ongoing expansion of knowledge of physiology and pathologies of the brain, due to computerized enhancements (e.g., CT scan)
c. Enable computerized national data analysis of progress and problems in areas such as stroke and traumatic brain injuries

2. Educational therapeutic software: Available in limited areas of need. As positive outcome research increases, the data for validity and reliability of therapeutic and remediation outcomes will support the expansion of programs.
   a. Cognitive benefits of educational therapy software
      1) Enjoyment of tasks is enhanced due to the self-paced, nonjudgmental interaction, the "game" atmosphere, and active participation.
      2) Motivation increases because of success, enjoyment, instant accomplishment, and feedback.
      3) Self-esteem grows when success occurs. "Attention and receptive factors can affect cognitive performance," (Smith, 1996, p. 2) and computers facilitate this function.
   b. Precautions associated with educational therapy software
      1) Reliability and validity of the software must be determined.
      2) Standards and guidelines are being developed.
      3) Research that focuses on the variety of software programs and their outcomes will be necessary to fine-tune the software to achieve the desired results.
      4) Software must be matched to client's needs, and outcomes must be assessed.
      5) Computerized therapies must be part of a coordinated, monitored therapy and not used as an isolated therapy.
3. Methods of delivery of therapeutic tools: The

following studies showed positive results:

a. Adults who were moderately impaired with chronic aphasia used CATS, a Computerized Aphasia Treatment System (Katz & Nagy, 1984), which is a cost-effective and efficient therapy program (see Research Perspective in this chapter)

b. A 12-year-old client with a head injury and a 32-year-old stroke client showed significant gains on the Wechsler Intelligence and Memory Tests after using computer-assisted cognitive rehabilitation therapy (Bracy, 1983).

c. Clients at Palo Alto Veterans Administration Medical Center used computerized tasks and games as part of cognitive rehabilitation (Lynch, 1983).

d. Clients with head injuries performed computerized memory retraining with promising results (Kerner & Acker, 1985).

e. Noninstitutionalized elderly clients used video games in a training program designed to increase activity and perceptual motor functioning. After 2 months, the participants' showed significant improvement in skill levels as well as intellectual and perceptual motor functioning (Drew & Waters, 1986).

f. Clients with head trauma were studied for initial and long-term effects and gains after participating in computer-based cognitive rehabilitation. Clients showed significant increases in memory function, the gains were retained at discharge, and the rehabilitation program produced a lasting improvement that was not attributed to the passage of time (Marks, Parenté, & Anderson, 1986).

D. On-Line Access to Information
1. Internet: A rapid, worldwide communication system that can be accessed by using a computer, a phone line, and specific software

   a. The Internet allows access for any user who wishes to advance his or her opinions, theories, products, inventions, or other creative activities.

   b. A search (using a commercial vendor) can access information about millions of topics from around the world. Searches can be completed in seconds or minutes.

   1) Search engines and directories for rehabilitation-related information include the following:
      a) Yahoo
      b) Lycos
      c) HotBot
      d) Infoseek
      e) Alta Vista
   2) Searches can be targeted to a scope of topics (e.g., type of injury, case management, equipment development).

   c. The power of the Internet depends on the efficient use of databases.

   1) Databases serve as information banks or vast storage centers in the computer's internal or external memory system. The computer has the ability to use the same information in many ways.
   2) All necessary, available information in regard to a certain focus, subject, or client is identified and put into a database.
   3) All or portions of information can be captured for specific reports.

2. Intranet: A local network using an Internet-type structure, usually set up at a place of employment, which can bring workplace resources to individuals' personal computer screens in seconds. To have a functioning Intranet, the computers within the institution or facility must be interconnected, use the same software, and share data. Benefits include the following:

   a. The cost of purchasing and/or replacing multiple reference books as well as the misplacement of policy and procedure manuals can be decreased or eliminated by having the information stored on an Intranet system.

   b. An Intranet can facilitate computerized education within the facility for both providers and clients.

3. On-line nursing resources

   a. Interagency Council on Information Resources for Nursing (ICIRN): Presents nursing information in a variety of formats (e.g., print, electronic). The information is appropriate for all levels of nursing interests (ICIRN, 1998).

   b. Abstracts, bibliographies, and book lists

   c. Educational programs

   d. Grants and writers' manuals

   e. Audiovisuals and Internet resources

4. Precautions for using on-line information

   a. Accuracy and validity may be compromised.

     1) There is no government regulation of information in terms of accuracy. Some sponsors of Web sites may self-regulate their sites. The integrity, reliability, and validity of claims, techniques, tools, theories, and other information should be scrutinized to the level of veracity the nurse will need.

     2) Standards do exist for evaluating criteria. One plan includes addressing the following areas (McGonigle, 1998):

       a) Authority

       b) Timeliness and continuity

       c) Purpose

       d) Accuracy and objectivity

       e) Access

   b. False claims may cause a client and family to have unfounded hope, which can result in an increase in stress.

   c. Support groups and chat rooms are open to the lay public as well as organized or recognized health organizations. This mix can provide valid as well as speculative information.

   d. The sources for medications, "innovative" assistive devices, and other equipment should be scrutinized.

E. Electronic Documentation (see Figure 20-2)

1. Types of computerized documentation: Vary with available software programs; the range of implementation and appropriate use of computerized documentation is extensive.

   a. Computerized charting: The Rehabilitation Institute of Chicago (RIC) uses a state-of-the-art system that uses on-line care plans derived from the North American Nursing Diagnosis Association (NANDA) and the Nursing Intervention Classification (NIC) systems. RIC's system correlates these languages with care plan interventions (Cervizzi & Edwards, 1999). Benefits include the following:

     1) The clarity and organization of data make it easy to read and retrieve information.

     2) Documentation can easily be audited for consistency and accuracy.

     3) The same information can be accessed in multiple documents (e.g., vital statistics, lists).

     4) Relevant educational and community resources can be accessed rapidly to respond to client or family requests.

     5) Updated long-term treatment plans (or portions of plans) can be printed daily or even per shift.

     6) Clients' progress can be tracked in a timely manner.

       a) Progress toward client goals

       b) Effects of therapeutic efforts and outcomes

Figure 20-2. Computer Documentation Software Categories

Barcoding
Case management
Disease management
Education and training programs for health care
Financial information
Healthcare cards
Home health systems
Human resource systems
Internet and Intranet applications
JCAHO and OSHA annual in-service interactive training
Licensure requirements and government regulations
Managed care
Master client indexes
Materials management
On-line care plans
Outcomes management
Client record keeping
Client education systems
Pharmacy information systems
Physical assessments
Policy and procedure manuals
Scheduling
Therapy information systems

c) Progress in multidisciplinary and interdisciplinary areas

7) Standardized forms can be used to gather information: For example, assessments can cover predetermined areas of concern; physicians' orders can include date, directions, prespecified requirements; lists of assistive devices, Functional Independence Measure (FIM) instrument scores, and other required admission data can be monitored for completion in a timely manner.

8) Healthcare professionals can be alerted immediately when the client has an unusual weight loss, a need for fall prevention interventions, or shows depression symptoms.

9) Care plans can be easily updated or automatically marked as "needing to be updated" (depending on the program) and printed for daily use or client information.

b. Pharmacy modules

1) Provide physician order sheets
2) Outline the pharmacy order process
3) Provide client information
4) Track medication administration and inventory

c. Therapy modules

1) Use assessment tools with standard forms
2) Track time-sensitive data
3) Track and analyze progress
4) Create automatic reports for insurance, government, and other necessary parties

d. Nursing care charts

1) Can feed into other reports, Minimum Data Set (MDS) assessments, and care plans
2) Cue assessment needs
3) Flag unusual situations (e.g., medication reactions, lab test results, exaggerated blood pressure, weight differences)

e. Minimum Data Set (MDS) assessment software programs

1) Feed information into and receive information from the chart

2) Identify areas that require care planning
3) Offer care plan suggestions in pull-down menus
4) Identify time-driven data sets (as needed for next assessment)
5) Manage data for transmission to required government offices

2. Variety of data input devices

a. Stationary computers at the nurses' station or specified areas

b. Bedside terminals (e.g., computer monitors at the client's bedside)

1) Bedside charting system is usually menu-driven and clinically oriented.
2) Bedside charting is done at point of delivery, instead of making notations and then charting.
3) Information retrieved from a bedside chart is timely and convenient.

c. Portable terminals, or small handheld devices with a keypad or light wand

1) Provide instant clinical updates by charting a variety of information on-site or nearby
2) Decrease multiplication of effort due to the one-time entry system, instead of transcribing handwritten notes at the nurses' station
3) Are menu-driven and allow for more efficient time management in locating clinical information or a workspace for documentation
4) Can be costly: The high cost of providing and replacing equipment due to damage, loss, or theft are chief deterrents to this type of implementation.

3. Accuracy

a. Accurate data entries reduce duplication of effort, increase efficiency, and decrease cost.

b. Information can be as current as possible regarding the client's condition, therapies, medication administration, and lab tests.

c. Inaccurate data entries rapidly replicate mistakes on many records and can cause negative effects.

4. Security safeguards

a. Nurses, administrators, and physicians

act as client advocates to ensure security measures.

b. Confidentiality of information of any kind can be threatened with easy access.

 1) Paperless chart systems allow access to information by simply pressing a key.

 2) Security issues related to Internet or network systems must be addressed; healthcare administrators and supervisors should be required to do the following:

   a) Be cognizant of security measures in place in the facility

   b) Ascertain the adequacy of these security measures when conveying information from facility databases to outside agencies

c. Security measures with multiusers of a database system in an institution can be implemented.

 1) Administrators should define access levels according to clinical, management, privacy, and financial needs.

 2) Access to security code should be limited.

 3) Computer monitors should not be placed in easy view of the general public.

F. Employment Opportunities

 1. Main advantages to on-line employment services

  a. Reach a large audience

  b. Are less expensive to place than other classified ads

  c. Have the potential of rapid responses to questions, résumé submission, and application solicitation

 2. Factors for on-line job postings

  a. Organizations for people with specific disabilities may support or sponsor employment sites for people with specific disabilities.

  b. On-line job postings usually include any training, counseling, or other needs that will be addressed in the employment process.

  c. Some organizations maintain a job-finding database and offer to search for

employment opportunities to help people with disabilities find positions. By providing this service, the organizations can help job hunters match their abilities with potential jobs or counsel them to seek training in specific areas (America's Jobline, 1999).

 3. Exploration of new job types and titles evolving from changes in health care.

  a. Searches can be tailored to locate specific job requirements or responsibilities.

  b. General searches can be made to see what new jobs are available.

G. Research Enhancement

 1. Computerization enables data to be managed effectively, thus producing more accurate representations and research conclusions.

 2. Research information can be accessed rapidly and with little effort.

 3. Time and resources can be directed at actually doing research and not shuffling papers.

 4. By having efficient access to comparable research projects in a timely, organized manner, researchers can decrease time lost in duplicating existing research or in reviewing other studies.

H. Educational Developments

 1. New dimensions in education

  a. Advanced technologies decrease cost and labor-intensive factors of education.

  b. Advanced technologies can use animation, sound, or repetitive material, can control choice (limited or full), and can control the rate of material being presented to those with learning impairments.

  c. Innovative equipment and computer applications expand the educational environment and learning experiences.

  d. Educators must recognize and understand that the computer is a learning tool, not a process in itself, that should be used as an adjunct to a well-developed educational process.

 2. Types of educational processes

  a. Interactive education: The computer provides instant interaction, feedback, and nonjudgmental analysis of attempts at learning.

b. Virtual reality simulation via an interactive computerized system
1) Uses three-dimensional and other sensory stimuli to create a situation that will "feel" like reality. Examples of rehabilitation simulation situations include the following:
a) Retraining in driving a car: Allows clients to steer or brake in a realistic environment without encountering actual safety hazards until their skills are appropriate; after successful virtual training, the client can begin road training.
b) Reaching for objects: The client can see a variety of simulated situations and reach for or react to appropriate objects without the facility providing a large inventory of equipment.
c) Walking and using judgment concerning safety situations (e.g., stopping for traffic, avoiding obstacles)
d) Playing a game with others
e) Throwing a ball at a moving target
2) Has limitations due to the availability of virtual reality programming
3) Can be used in recreational, physical, and occupational therapy
c. Audiovisual presentations: These popular video-type presentations can be reproduced on the computer with the added advantage of having instant interaction and feedback.
1) A situation that needs logical input can be presented. At strategic segments, the student can offer logical solutions.
2) Feedback can be instantaneous.
3) The instructor and student can track correct and incorrect answers and use this information as a stepping stone to improvement.
4) Audiovisual presentations work well in the following areas:
a) Vocabulary improvement

b) Clinical simulations for professional or lay caregivers
c) Conflict management situations
d. Distance learning
1) Allows educational offerings to be experienced by those who are unable to attend on-site sessions
2) Can be effectively used when the learner faces the following obstacles:
a) Extensive distance or travel to site
b) Expensive transportation
c) Difficulty for people with certain disabilities to travel
d) Difficulty for a caregiver or family member to accompany the client due to time or other constraints
3. Teleconferences: Audio- and teleconferences were the pioneers in this area.
a. Education is delivered at one site with an audiovisual hookup at one or more remote sites.
b. The computer is used for visual displays, demonstrations, and interaction.
4. Libraries Without Walls and Universities and Colleges Without Walls projects: The Internet is a vital part of this new concept.
a. Universities and colleges offer college credit and continuing education classes via the Internet.
b. At specific times, course material is given on the Internet. The student can read the material on-line or download it.
c. Exams and assignments are most commonly transmitted to and from the student by e-mail, although faxing is also used.
d. Chat rooms or discussion times are available. Students can discuss topics "live" via the computer, while the instructor monitors the on-line session.
5. Categories of resources (see Figure 20-3)
a. Sources of information access for Libraries Without Walls: Comprehensive information on a variety of areas dealing with the libraries and not just book lists.
1) Equal Access to Software and

Figure 20-3. Internet Resources/Client Resources

General resources for people who are blind
www.blind.state.ia.us/vocrehab/default.htm
Resources, services, educational opportunities, guide dog schools; updated regularly

Braille
www.blind.state.ia.us/vocrehab
NFBTRANS, Grade II braille translation software package; can be downloaded

EASI/Libraries Without Walls
gophersite@sjuvm.stjohns.edu (click on Disability and rehabilitation resources, then EASI)
National program that focuses on students and professionals with disabilities; promotes "Libraries without Walls" program

Library of Neuropsychological Information (LONI) and Libraries Without Walls
http://www.neuroscience.cnter.com/lonimain.htm
Includes information on anatomy and physiology, differential diagnosis, grand rounds, diseases, guest lectures, software, and more

Nursing Resources
Books of interest to nurses
www.medbookstore.com
Wide variety of interest specific topics not easily found in other on-line bookstores

Cumulative Index to Nursing and Allied Health (CINAHL)
www.cinahl.com/library/library.htm
Literature search for nursing topics; available in CD-ROM; includes CINAHL news, journal lists, and directories

Nursing informatics
www.mrc.twsu.edu/informatic/resources/resources/.html
Information on specialized classes, curricula with degrees, informatics resources, and conferences

Nursing Information and Data Set Evaluation Center (NIDSEC)
www.nursingworld.org/pressrel/1998/nidsec.htm
Develops standards for information systems; recognizes Pathways Care Manager software program; evaluates care guides and critical paths

Nursing information resources
http://www.nln.org/journal/prod-journal_toc598_ess.htm#computerized
Interagency Council on Information Resources for Nursing (ICIRN); contains information on databases, abstracts, grants, internet resources, drugs, dictionaries, audiovisuals, and more

Rehabilitation nursing position statements
http://rehabnurse.org/resources/position/
Association of Rehabilitation Nurses (ARN) position statements on a variety of nursing interests such as advanced practice rehabilitation nursing, ethics, staffing, and others

General Rehabilitation Professional Resources
Clinical pharmacology guide to common drugs
http://www.cponline.gsm.com
Descriptions, mechanisms of action, adverse reactions, dosage and other pertinent clinical information

HealthStar: Healthcare Administration, Policies, and Planning
http://www.index.nlm.nih.gov.cgi/htsearch
Produced by the National Library of Medicine and the American Hospital Association; includes database leasing information; topics relate to healthcare administration

Medical topics
www.helix.com
Medical education, drug listings, daily medical news, Medline database of abstracts from 3,700 biomedical journals

Medical Literature Analysis & Retrieval System (MEDLARS)
http://www.nlm.nih.gov/pubs/factsheets/online_databases.htm#bioethics
Factual or literature search on health topics; has a database and file collection that contains more than 40 on-line databases.

National Rehabilitation Information Center (NARIC)
www.naric.com
Collection of rehabilitation literature, collects and disseminates information on federally funded research, has databases on 46 rehabilitation-related topics

Rehabilitation resources and miscellaneous information
www.nursingwebsearch.com
Search for "rehabilitation" and access more than 1,300 sites or narrow search; offers a broad scope of rehabilitation topics

Project DO-IT (Disabilities, Opportunities, Internetworking, Technology)
hawking.u.washington.edu or
http://weber.u.washington.edu/~doit/
Nationwide program that disseminates information about adaptive technology, workshops, presentations, brochures, presentation material, and videotapes

Social Security Administration
www.ssa.gov
Variety of general and specific information on social security benefits

Search Engines (If one search engine does not provide enough information, retry the search on another engine.)
Alta Vista (www.altavista.digital.com)
Excite (www.excite.com)
HotBot (www.hotbot.com)
Infoseek (www.infoseek.com)
Lycos (www.lycos.com)
Yahoo (www.yahoo.com)

Information (EASI)

    2) Library of Neurophysiological Information (LONI)

  b. Logistical information dissemination

    1) Universities and Colleges Without Walls and other organizations

      a) Sponsor in-service sessions, family and client classes, and conferences

      b) Offer posteducational sessions

      c) Allow on-line registration (which tells the student immediately if a class is filled or cancelled)

      d) Give immediate updates on schedule changes

  c. Updated sources of educational offerings

    1) An increasing number of educational institutions, professional organizations, and healthcare organizations post educational schedules on their Web sites.

    2) Using Internet search functions, a person can find out what class is available, where the class is held, and how to register.

  d. Educational data profiles

    1) Word processing tools, spreadsheets, databases, and commercial software allow easier tracking of client education, staff development, and continuing education activities.

    2) Records can be updated and retrieved easily and used as comprehensive documentation for evaluations or state inspections.

III. Challenges for Rehabilitation Nurses

A. Preparation of Registered Nurses to Use Computer Technology

  1. Reasons why rehabilitation nurses should educate themselves to use computers

    a. Computer technology plays an extensive role in rehabilitation practice.

    b. Nurses must understand and be able to work with the technology.

    c. Computer applications make the nurse's role manageable.

      1) By meeting documentation demands

      2) By using and understanding computerized equipment and devices

      3) By using time effectively in education and research

      4) By tracking and controlling clinical standards and outcome regulations

  2. How nurses can obtain specialized computer-related education

    a. Standardized computer knowledge requirements in nursing education are still evolving. (The American Nurses Association [ANA] has published standards and scope of practice for nursing informatics.) The nurse needs to know the content of the computer course. Many nursing schools still have little or no true computerized training. Sometimes, "computerization" consists of merely showing an interactive video or offering a word processing class.

    b. Have a basic understanding of computer function, which will help bring basic nursing settings in line with other services and businesses: For example, use current word processing programs and spreadsheets to generate reports, memos, in-service flyers, and client education information and to gather data. These computer applications can literally do in seconds what may take a novice computer user an hour or a day to do in an outdated system (e.g., sorting client information, typing reports on a typewriter, reading through numerous reports for abnormal lab tests).

    c. Take advantage of specialized orientation or training in the workplace: Computer software and hardware vary with each institution, so it is important for nurses to learn their facility's system.

    d. Take continuing education or college credit course in areas of special interest or special workplace needs

    e. Keep up-to-date with basic information on advancements in rehabilitation and assistive devices

      1) To become familiar with the assistive technology advances and their application to clients

      2) To be involved in client education and supervise the daily use of devices

      3) To contribute to possible improvements

3. Nursing informatics: A relatively new field for nurses in computer applications and information systems (McHugh, 1999)

    a. This field developed in response to the increased demand and pace of computerization in health care.

    b. Specialized classes—and even curriculums with degrees—are being offered.

    c. Informatics resources and educational conferences are available to nurses interested in this area.

B. Client Care

1. Every client is touched in some way by the many advances in technology brought about by computerization.

2. Rehabilitation nurses serve as catalysts, blending new technological advances with the care delivery process in positive and progressive paths.

3. Rehabilitation advanced practice nurses have many responsibilities in this area.

    a. Adhere to the areas identified in the ANA's *Nursing's Social Policy Statement* (1995)

      1) Provide comprehensive assessments

      2) Display expert skill in diagnosis and treatment of complex responses of individuals and groups

      3) Synthesize complex data to formulate appropriate decisions and plans

    b. Develop a wider knowledge base of medical/surgical rehabilitation diagnoses and be able to use easy-access reference tools, simulations, and three-dimensional models in computer reference programs: Software source books (e.g., *Health Care Software Sourcebook* [Aspen Reference Group, 1998]) are available from vendors, organizations, publishers, and others.

    c. Simplify the use of nursing diagnosis codes by referring to them in a computerized format

    d. Promote the use of computerized assessments

C. Computerized Applications

1. Rehabilitation care maps or pathways

    a. Case management: Computerized modules can be beneficial for the case management process.

      1) Allow checklisting to determine if an event has or has not occurred

      2) Enable note-taking and following detours

      3) Streamline tracking pathway compliance, type, and number of detours for summarization

      4) Analyze outcomes for a specific client and for a client group

    b. Software

      1) Care maps lend themselves to computer documentation very well.

      2) Many systems are being developed.

        a) At the 1998 Association of Rehabilitation Nurses (ARN) Annual Educational Conference, several software systems were presented (Cervizzi & Edwards, 1999).

        b) In November 1998, the ANA recognized a software program called Pathways Care Manager that addresses components of the nursing process in documentation as well as in care guides or critical paths (ANA, 1998).

        c) A multifacility hospital system in North Carolina developed a program called WakeMED that integrates clinical pathways throughout the continuum (Cervizzi & Edwards, 1999).

        d) The Ohio State University Medical Center has developed computerized clinical pathways that have three categories: transition, return to home and community (Cervizzi & Edwards, 1999).

2. Assistive technology awareness: Rehabilitation nurses, as the coordinating and supportive factors in the holistic approach to client care, should take advantage of staff development activities in these areas:

    a. New technologies that can support, educate, or evaluate holistic progress, and/or prevent complications: Rehabilitation nurses may be the first to observe an area that could be improved with another assistive device or pinpoint the reason why a specific device is not appropriate.

b. Environmental control devices: The degree of the client's environmental comfort affects the time that the client can stay with a task. These control devices can help eliminate or decrease physical complications (e.g., spasms, pressure areas).

c. Laws that support accessibility to computerization for people with disabilities: Knowing the potential for accessibility of computerization can open up areas of education, employment, and independence to clients with disabilities. Public Law 100-407, Technology-Related Assistance for Individuals with Disabilities Act (August 19, 1988), is a good resource to review.

3. Computerized tracking systems that monitor the client through the continuum

a. Allow data from previous care settings to be obtained and reviewed: Time-consuming retrieval can be streamlined with computerized systems.

1) Many software vendors have developed managed care information systems that can track and store information for retrieval, record keeping, clinical and financial analysis, and insurance information.

2) Software can monitor clinic or physician visits, generate reports, analyze outcomes, and transfer electronic data (Aspen Reference Group, 1998).

3) Information that has been accessed from a previous care setting can prevent ordering the same test twice or giving a medication that proved to be ineffective. It also allows the new staff to review and compare the client's and family's reactions to counseling or community resources.

b. Assess the progress of the plan of care, evaluate results, and obtain pertinent information for interested parties with current, easily accessible information

c. Simplify the documentation of services and outcomes

4. Computerized outcomes management: Outcomes analysis and management have become priority issues due to healthcare reform, managed care, health maintenance organizations (HMOs), prospective payment systems (PPS), and diagnosis-related groups (DRGs).

a. Measurement: Outcomes in individual health settings are measured against similar outcomes locally and nationally.

1) Use of the MDS assessment in long-term care settings

2) Use of the FIM instrument's computerized database by researchers (Black, Slotis, & Bartlett, 1999)

b. Application

1) Reports on comparison, analysis, and quality initiatives

2) Monitors care and identifies trouble areas and research into improved, cost-efficient methods of care delivery

3) Used by many types of healthcare organizations

a) Regulatory agencies and accrediting organizations (compliance and standardization)

b) Managed care companies and insurance companies (critical business decisions)

c) Individual institutions or healthcare settings (quality improvement)

c. Software programs

1) Use the required data-gathering tool (e.g., MDS assessment for long-term care facilities, mandated by the federal government)

2) Use the computerized documentation system in place at the facility

D. Research Applications

1. Rehabilitation and clinical research

a. Due to positive clinical outcomes verification and documentation of new effective techniques from research studies in medical rehabilitation, facilities are calling for "rapid incorporation...into clinical practice" (Fuhrer, 1998, p. 441).

b. Advancements through new technology include the following:

1) Methods of measuring clinical results

2) Data gathering and analysis methods
3) Objective measurements, which replace many subjective areas: Time and money can be saved by training a technician to manage advanced instrumentation, while the researcher can supervise and analyze. Examples of research using objective measures follow:
   a) The amount of pressure on a certain body area and the degree of muscle activity in movement in different situations (Doering et al., 1998; Visser, Pauwels, Duysens, Mulder, & Veth, 1998)
   b) How equipment such as electro-diagnosis and MRI can enhance nerve roots data and investigate neuronopathy (Bang, Han, & Lim, 1998; Liaw, You, Cheng, Kao, & Wong, 1998)
4) Decreased or eliminated need for tedious, time-consuming investigations of other similar studies through the use of sophisticated databases (Chae & Zorowitz, 1998; Fiedler, Granger, & Russel, 1998)

2. Nursing practice research: New paradigms arise with the advent of new technologies that can aid the advancement of rehabilitation nursing.
   a. Nursing research projects
      1) Omaha system: Describes and quantifies the practice of nurses and other health professionals (Martin & Bowles, 1997)
      2) The Nightingale Tracker Project: An electronic "point of care" communication system between instructors and students. It enhances teaching effectiveness through immediate teacher-student contact as needed (Connolly, Huynh, & Gornery-Moreno, 1999)
   b. Relevance of outcomes
      1) Information updates contain more data from a wide range of sources.
      2) Reviewing the analysis can be accomplished easily.
      3) Sources are available directly or

through the Internet.
   a) Abstract sources
   b) Computerized databases
   c) Grant resources
   d) Writers' manuals (ICIRN, 1998)

IV. **Benefits of Computer Technology**
   A. For Rehabilitation Clients and Their Families
      1. Requests for information can be easily accessed in an accurate, timely manner.
         a. Documentation of condition, test results
         b. Financial accounting
         c. Educational printouts or resources
      2. Community resources, self-help groups, and commercial products can be accessed in an inexpensive and easy manner.
      3. Client and family caregivers can receive education.
         a. Client education, a vital component of rehabilitative success, can be effectively achieved through one-on-one interaction by using a computer and minimal supervision.
            1) Reduces stress (e.g., loss of dignity, stigma of being "dumb") in retrying a certain task (e.g., learning to add again)
            2) Eliminates the barrier of excess competition in certain situations
               a) When working with peers who are more advanced
               b) When a client has not adapted to or is embarrassed by his or her disability
            3) Decreases negative outcomes by eliminating interactions with an instructor who may appear judgmental in word or body language
            4) Allows better student participation through reinforcement and limitless practice
            5) Decreases or eliminates embarrassment for reviewing the material before trying the task or understanding the concept
            6) In distance learning, eliminates the logistics of transporting a person with severe physical disabilities or of obtaining specialized equipment for a client with sensory impairments by

being able to use the computer and Internet at home

    7) Allows Internet use

      a) On-line registration for classes, job opportunities, government services

      b) Buying power at an extensive variety of stores

      c) Communication with others (e.g., e-mail, chat rooms)

      d) Easy access to unlimited information

  b. Caregiver education, which is necessary for compliance and support of the rehabilitative client, can be facilitated through computer use.

    1) The quantity of education time can be flexibly distributed without maintaining a continuous or rigid schedule for one-on-one time.

    2) The same information can be shared with other members of the client's family at different times if necessary or convenient.

    3) The family caregiver can supervise the client's practice sessions more accurately and needs less training to do so.

B. For Rehabilitation Nurses

  1. Increases educational opportunities and improves time, money, educational staff, and resources issues

    a. Nurses can take the time to participate in continuing education programs because of the increased availability of options.

    b. Nurses can choose the most convenient time for a class, eliminating unnecessary rushing, fatigue, or concern about work. Being in control of time improves the efficacy of the educational offering.

    c. All staff may receive education and still maintain adequate coverage on unit.

  2. Allows access to support group and chat rooms: Dealing with high-stress jobs, sharing frustrations about new legislation, or using a particular assistive device are some areas that may be discussed with on-line chat groups.

  3. Decreases repetitive, time-consuming documentation

  4. Decreases errors that result from multiple transcriptions of the same material

  5. Allows access to workplace information from one location (e.g., eliminates need to find charts, nursing records, manuals, call lab for results, library)

C. For Healthcare Providers

  1. Uses computerized financial packages

    a. Effective cost containment and cost management allows the maximum benefit from budgeted dollars.

    b. Computer applications are available for monitoring the cost and inventory of medical supplies, medications, linens, specialty beds, wheelchairs, assistive devices, food, and durable soft goods.

      1) Tracks immediate inventory use, inventory on hand, and inventory charged

      2) Tracks cost per case, per diagnosis, or per unit

  2. Monitors usage and purchasing decisions

    a. Tracks cost of specific types of supplies (e.g., for wound care, tube feedings)

    b. Tracks cost of client stay versus diagnosis

    c. Tracks specific care delivery and caps on services or money availability

    d. Matches client criteria with Medicare and insurance benefits

  3. Allows easy access to facility and organizational policy and procedure manuals

    a. Ready-made generic manuals (e.g., infection control, nursing procedures, disaster plans) on CD-ROM or computer disks can be purchased and customized for the facility.

    b. Internally developed manuals have some advantages over generic manuals.

      1) The manual is entered via the internal word processing system, which simplifies data entry, error correction, and the ability to update.

      2) The manual can be accessed easily; searching for an in-house policy is more efficient.

      3) An internal computerized manual eliminates the need for hard copies,

which saves space at the nursing station and eliminates the problem of lost or misplaced manuals.

4. Allows efficient cost management for educational and in-service sessions

   a. Reduces need for expensive instructors, speakers, or experts

   b. Reduces need to book multiple sessions to increase attendance: All staff may not be able to attend a mandatory in-service session at one time, but they can independently use computers to view the necessary information on-line.

   c. Allows unlimited access to self-directed or interactive education with one software purchase for the facility

   d. Increases resource efficiency by including reference material on a CD-ROM, a network, or even a single disk drive

      1) Prevents loss or theft of references, books, or policy and procedure manuals that can be difficult to replace

      2) Reduces loss of money and resources, which can be a critical consideration if no money is budgeted for replacement

D. For the Healthcare System

1. Increases public awareness and demand for available advances in technology and care through information on the Internet: For example, Public Law 100-407, Technology-Related Assistance for Individuals with Disabilities, acknowledges the advances made in modern technology and cites that many are important and even necessary tools for individuals with disabilities.

2. Encompasses financial, legislative, and clinical healthcare sectors in the quality monitoring processes

   a. Benchmarking and outcomes monitoring have expanded and increased in validity.

   b. Medicare requirements (e.g., MDS, PPS) in long-term care facilities has put high priorities and quality standards on rehabilitation and restorative care.

   c. JCAHO's and CARF's accreditation processes can be viewed by consumers.

3. Addresses certification requirements for the expanding assistive technology field to maintain and improve quality

   a. Practitioners, programs, suppliers, and equipment are included (Cook & Hussey, 1995).

   b. "Quality assurance is closely tied to reimbursement, and as the number of devices and practitioners increase, third-party payers are requiring some indication that the services and devices are necessary, safe, and effective" (Cook & Hussey, 1995, pp. 36–37).

4. Streamlines litigation of traumatic injury and types of data

   a. Businesses exist that act as clearinghouses for information concerning workers' compensation and other litigation cases.

   b. Databases are developed and maintained in which appropriate parties (e.g., lawyers, physicians, case managers, field nurses, insurance companies) may contribute or view information pertinent to a specific case.

V. Computer Resources

A. For Providers and Clients

1. Alliance for Technology Access

   a. A worldwide organization that provides information, support, and access regarding rehabilitation technology

   b. Target audience: Individuals with disabilities, their families, community groups, educators, technology developers, medical professionals, and advocates (Alliance for Technology Access, 1996; Apple Computer, Inc., 1999a)

2. Mac Access Passport

   a. A database for Macintosh computers containing descriptions of products for individuals with disabilities

   b. Provides telephone numbers to contact relevant organizations and learn about products (Apple Computer Inc., 1999b; Mac Access Passport, 1999b)

3. IBM Special Needs Systems: Independence Series products

   a. Help users in the areas of mobility, vision, education, dyslexia, and speech and hearing

   b. Include innovations such as a talking Web browser for people who are visually impaired or blind

c. Offer guidelines for software developers to make Web sites more accessible for all users (IBM Corporation, 1999)

4. EASI (Equal Access to Software and Information)

    a. A national program that focuses on students and professionals with disabilities

    b. Promotes the Libraries Without Walls trend in the educational community

    c. Publishes a journal, *Information Technology and Disabilities*

    d. Disseminates new assistive technology information to students, educators, professional organization staff, counseling staff, and businesses

5. Project DO-IT (Disabilities, Opportunities, Internetworking, and Technology)

    a. A national program for information dissemination about adaptive technology

    b. Promotes participation by people with disabilities in the sciences, mathematics programs, and other careers

    c. Assists university support groups, mentoring programs, and summer study activities

    d. Offers workshops and presentations for faculty, students, parents, and service providers

    e. Provides brochures, presentation materials, and videotapes (Lazzaro, 1996)

6. Resources for blind people

    a. Information on the Internet (see Figure 20-3)

        1) Offers resources, services, educational opportunities

        2) Lists guide dog schools

        3) Provides links to Federal Student Aid Application, the American Council for the Blind, and the National Federation for the Blind

        4) Includes information on aids and appliances

    b. Braille: Braille translation software packages (e.g., NFBTRAN) can be downloaded from the Internet.

    c. Other services

        1) Offer help with projects

        2) Provide information from committees around the world

        3) Provide support group information, such as IN-Touch (a Braille literacy group)

        4) Help users to use Windows more efficiently

        5) Offers information about independent living

B. For Rehabilitation Nurses and Other Professionals (see Figure 20-4)

1. On Yahoo search engine

    a. Traumatic Brain Injury Model System of Rehabilitation Care: Describes nature of injury and treatment

    b. CARE computer systems: Offers financial information management systems for rehabilitation as well as other settings

    c. Northwest Regional Spinal Cord Injury System: Provides state-of-the-art care, research, and information dissemination

    d. Software Rehabilitation Services: Analyzes, remediates, and tests software (COBOL source) for Y2K accuracy

    e. Rehabilitation Learning Center: Provides a computer-based rehabilitation environment that educates and trains individuals with acute or chronic spinal cord injuries

    f. Darci Institute of Rehabilitation Engineering: Describes assistive devices

    g. Minneapolis Rehabilitation Center (MRC): Provides vocational evaluations, computer training, job placement and training, among other services

2. Alta Vista sites: More than 1 million Web pages can be found in a general search for rehabilitation

    a. National Clearing House of Rehabilitation Training Materials (1999): Categorizes different needs and provides links to areas such as rehabilitation recruitment, counselors, associations, disability resources, educational resources, state agencies for vocational rehabilitation, assistive technology

    b. Redwood Disability Web Resources: Contains assistive technology information

    c. KneeGuru: Provides information on knee injuries, treatments, and physiology

d. Rehabilitation Engineering Research (at Cambridge University)

e. International Spinal Injuries and Rehabilitation Center

f. Tactile virtual screen

Figure 20-4. Web Sites of Rehabilitation-Related Organizations

Agency for Healthcare Policy and Research
www.ahcpr.gov

American Council for the Blind
www.acb.org

American Health Information Management
www.ahima.org

American Hospital Association
www.aha.org

American Nurses Association
www.nursingworld.org

American Society for Clinical Nutrition
www.faseb.org/ascn

American Society of Neuroscience Nurses
www..aann.org

Arthritis Foundation
www.arthritis.org

Association for the Advancement of Wound Care
www.medexpo.com/hmp/AAWC.html

Association of Rehabilitation Nurses
www.rehabnurse.org

Federal student aid application
www.fafsa.ed.gov

Health Care Financing Administration
www.hcfa.gov/

Health Informatics Standards Board (ANSI)
www.ansi.org.rooms/room_41

Joint Commission on Accreditation of Healthcare Organizations
www.jcaho.org

Microsoft Healthcare Users Group
www.mshug.org

National Association for Home Care
www.nahc.org

National Federation for the Blind
www.nfb.org

National Institutes of Health, Department of Nursing
www.nih.gov/ninr

U.S. Department of Health and Human Services
www.dhhs.gov

Wound Care Institute
www.woundcare.org

---

g. Iowa Department for the Blind (1999)

h. Salvation Army Thrift Stores

i. Research and welfare policies regarding computers and rehabilitation

j. Intelligent Wheelchair Resources

k. Able Home Aides Shop: A commercial site that showcases computers and specialized adaptive devices

3. Nursing literature on CD-ROMs and computer disks

a. Basic nursing textbooks, anatomy and physiology texts, pathology texts, and drug information guides are popular CD-ROMs.

b. A broad scope of information can be found in a small area of storage.

c. Hard copies of sections of or entire articles can be printed out easily and shared at the nursing station, with the client and family, in the classroom, or in the nurse's own resource collection.

4. On-line nursing journals: The number of nursing journals that are available on-line is increasing.

a. Lists are located at on-line library sites, as part of the services of some organizations, or from publishers.

b. Some nursing journals include the *American Journal of Nursing, Nursing Research*, and *Nursing Management.*

c. One of the most comprehensive lists of on-line journals can be found in the libraries of North Dakota State University at Fargo, where they offer access to 49 different nursing journals (NDSU Libraries—Nursing Journals, 1998).

d. Rehabilitation journals are available and cover a broad spectrum of services. The *American Journal of Physical Medicine and Rehabilitation* is one of the most well-known on-line rehabilitation resources.

e. The availability of on-line material varies with the journal or the Web site.

   1) Some abstracts are available free on-line.

2) Some journals can be viewed freely, but others require a subscription fee.

3) Most require registration on the site.

4) Some of the more technical sites require proof of licensure.

5) Many sites allow users to scan the archives for subject matter at no cost.

   f. Searching for material in this way is convenient and can save space previously used for copies of magazines.

5. On-line bookstores

   a. Allow convenient searches for books by topic, author, or title

   b. Can receive orders on-line and provide prompt service

   c. Examples of general on-line bookstores dealing with medical-related books: Amazon, Logan Brothers, Follett, Nursing Spectrum, and Barnes and Noble.

   d. Allow book access and topic searches to organizations for people with specific disabilities

6. Nursing Spectrum Career Fitness Online (1999)

   a. Covers a broad area of interests for nurses

   b. Includes support groups, chat groups, and resources

Research Perspective

Katz, R.C., & Wertz, R.T. (1997). The efficacy of computer-provided reading treatment of chronic aphasic adults. *Journal of Speech, Language and Hearing Research, 40*(3), 493-507.

This research studied the effectiveness of computerized reading treatment, computer stimulation through cognitive tasks and passage of time with no treatment on 55 adults with chronic aphasia who were randomly assigned to one of the three groups for 26 weeks. The participants were tested at the start of the study and again 3 and 6 months later using language measures from the Porch Index of Communicative Ability (PICA) "Overall" and "Verbal" modalities and the Western Aphasia Battery (WAB) "Quotient" and "Repetition" subtest.

The results at the end of 6 months showed significant improvement in the reading treatment group in five language measures. The computer stimulation group had significant improvement in one area, and the control group showed no improvement. Other promising positive effects included administration of this computerized treatment with minimal therapist assistance and carryover improvement in noncomputerized language. Use of appropriate software content was instrumental in positive results, not the use of the computer alone.

Implications for practice

The essence of rehabilitation practice is to enable people with disabilities to function at their highest possible level. Technology today has enhanced the survival rates of people who have a variety of disabilities. At the same time, healthcare reforms limit the financial and time allotments for rehabilitation.

Research into more efficient tools and methods for enhancing rehabilitation are crucial to the progress of this field. Studies such as this one can identify means of delivery of rehabilitation that can improve the quality of life of the people with disabilities and meet the demands of healthcare reform. Rehabilitation nurses who are aware of, promote, and encourage new and effective methods of care can make a difference in the ultimate outcome of their clients' rehabilitation.

References

Alliance for Technology Access. (1996). *Computer resources for people with disabilities: A guide to exploring today's assistive technology* (2nd ed.). Alameda, CA: Hunter House Publishing.

America's Jobline. (1999). *A public access job search network* [On-line]. Available: http://www.nfb.org/jobline.htm.

American Nurses Association (ANA). (1998, November 18). *ANA nursing information and data set evaluation center recognizes first product* [On-line, press release]. Available: http://www.nursingworld.org/pressrel/1998/nidsec.htm.

American Nurses Association (ANA). (1995). *Nursing's social policy statement*. Washington, DC: Author.

Apple Computer, Inc. (1999a). *Apple disability resources* [On-line]. Available: http://www.apple.com/education/k12/disability/message.html

Apple Computer, Inc. (1999b). *Mac Access Passport* [On-line]. Available: http://www.apple.com/education/k12/disability/message.html

Aspen Reference Group. (1998). *Health care software sourcebook 1998*. Gaithersburg, MD: Aspen.

Association of Rehabilitation Nurses (ARN). (1995). *ARN Web site* [On-line]. Available: http://www.rehabnurse.org/resources/position/padvance.htm

Bang, M., Han, T., & Lim, J. (1998). Acute sensory neuronopathy. *American Journal of Physical Medicine & Rehabilitation, 77*, 494-497.

Black, T., Slotis, T., & Bartlett, C. (1999). Using the Functional Independence Measure instrument to predict stroke rehabilitation outcomes. *Rehabilitation Nursing, 24*, 109-114.

Bracy, O. (1983). Computer based cognitive rehabilitation. *Journal of Cognitive Rehabilitation, 1*(1), 7-8.

Cervizzi, K., & Edwards, P. (1999). Where is rehabilitation nursing documentation going? *Rehabilitation Nursing, 24*, 92.

Chae, J., & Zorowitz, R. (1998). Functional status of cortical and subcortical nonhemorrhagic stroke survivors and the effect of lesion laterality. *American Journal of Physical Medicine & Rehabilitation, 77*, 415–420.

Connolly, P., Huynh, M., & Gornery-Moreno, M. (1999). On the cutting edge or over the edge? Implementing the Nightingale Tracker. *On-Line Journal of Nursing Informatics, 3*, 1.

Cook, A., & Hussey, S. (1995). *Assistive technologies: Principles and practice*. St. Louis: Mosby.

Doering, T., Resch, K., Steuernagel, B., Brix, J,. Schneider, B., & Fischer, G. (1998). Passive and active exercises increase cerebral blood flow velocity in young healthy individuals. *American Journal of Physical Medicine & Rehabilitation, 77*, 490–493.

Drew, B., & Waters, J. (1986). Video games: Utilization of a novel strategy to improve perceptual motor skills and cognitive functioning in the non-institutionalized elderly. *Journal of Cognitive Rehabilitation, 4*(2), 26–31.

Edmark Corporation. (1999). School versions. *Using Edmark software with children with special needs* [On-line]. Available http://www.edmark,com/prod/school/specialneeds.html

Fiedler, R., Granger, C., & Russel, C. (1998). Uniform data system for medical rehabilitation. *American Journal of Physical Medicine & Rehabilitation, 77*, 444-450.

Flippo, K., Inge, K., & Barcus, M. (Eds.). (1995). *Assistive technology*. Baltimore, MD: Paul H. Brookes Publishing.

Fuhrer, M., (1998). The National Center for Medical Rehabilitation Research: Beyond infancy, looking toward maturity. *American Journal of Physical Medicine and Rehabilitation, 77*, 368–375.

IBM Corporation. (1999, February). *Special needs systems* [On-line]. Available: http://www.austin.ibm.com/sns/index.html.

Interagency Council on Information Resources for Nursing (ICIRN). (1998). *Essential nursing references* [On-line]. Available: http://www.nln.org/journal/prod-journal_toc598_ess.htm#computerized.

Iowa Department for the Blind. (1999, April 30). *Vocational rehabilitation* [On-line]. Available: http://www.blind.state.ia.us/vocrehab/default.htm.

Katz, R., & Nagy, V. (1984). CATS: Computerized Aphasia Treatment System. *Journal of Cognitive Rehabilitation, 2*(4), 8–9.

Katz, R.C., & Wertz, R.T. (1997). The efficacy of computer-provided reading treatment of chronic aphasic adults. *Journal of Speech, Language and Hearing Research, 40*(3), 493-507.

Kerner, M., & Acker, M. (1985). Computer delivery of memory retraining with head injured patients. *Journal of Cognitive Rehabilitation, 3*(6), 10–23.

Laureate Learning Systems, Inc. (1999, January). *Special needs and language development software* [On-line]. Available: http://www.llsys.com/

Lazzaro, J. (1996). *Adapting PCs for disabilities*. New York: Addison Wesley.

Liaw, M., You, D., Cheng, P., Kao, P., & Wong, A. (1998). Central representation of phantom limb phenomenon in amputees studied with single photon emission computerized tomography. *American Journal of Physical Medicine and Rehabilitation, 77*, 368–375.

Lynch, W. (1983). Cognitive retraining using microcomputer games and commercially available software. *Journal of Cognitive Rehabilitation, 1*, 19–22.

Mac Access Passport. (1999a). *HeadMaster Plus* [On-line]. Available: http://www.apple.com/education/k12/disability/map.html

Mac Access Passport. (1999b). *Vision Key* [On-line]. Available: http://www.access.apple.com/FMPro

Marks, C., Parenté, F., & Anderson, J. (1986). Retention of gains in outpatient cognitive rehabilitation therapy. *Journal of Cognitive Rehabilitation, 4*(3), 20–23.

Martin, K., & Bowles, K. (1997). Omaha system report for the national committee on vital and health statistics [On-line]. Available: http://aspe.os.dhhs.gov/ncvhs/97041618.htm

McGonigle, D. (1998). How to evaluate web site [On-line]. Available: http://cac.psu.edu/~dxm12/siteval.html

McHugh, M. (1999). *Informatics—Resources and Links: Wichita State University* [On-line]. Available: http://www.mrc.twsu.edu/informatic/resources/resources.html

Nader, S.F., Campagnolo, D.I., Tomaio, A.C., & Stitik, T.P. (1998). High lumbar disc dilemma. *American Journal of Physical Medicine Rehabilitation, 77*, 539–543.

National Clearing House of Rehabilitation Training Materials. (1999, April). *Home page* [On-line]. Available: http://www.nchrtm.okstate.edu/index_3.html

NDSU Libraries—Nursing Journals. (1998, September). *Home page* [On-line]. Available: http://www.lib.ndsu.nodak.edu/subjects/lifesci/nursjnls.html

Nursing Spectrum Career Fitness Online. (1999). *Home page* [On-line]. Available: www.nusingspectrum.com

Public Law 100–407. (August 19, 1988). Technology-Related Assistance for Individuals with Disabilities Act.

Smith, G. (April, 1996). Computer and cognitive rehabilitation. *Ability Newsletter* [On-line]. Available: http://www.spin.net.au/~abilitycorp/cognitive_rehab.htm

Visser, E., Pauwels, J., Duysens, J., Mulder, T., & Veth, R. (1998). Gait adaptations during walking under visual and cognitive constraints: A study of patients recovering from limb-saving surgery of the lower limb. *American Journal of Physical Medicine Rehabilitation, 77*, 503–509.

Suggested resources

Anson, D. (1997). *Alternative computer access: A guide to selection*. Philadelphia: F.A. Davis.

Glaxo Wellcome Healthcare Education. (1997, February). *Helix* [On-line, advertisement]. Available: www.Helix.com.

Saver, C. (1999). The three faces of the internet. *Nursing Spectrum, 12*(13), 3.

Section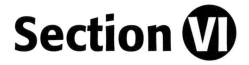

Rehabilitation Nursing in the 21st Century

· ·

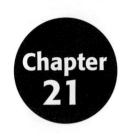

Chapter 21

Changes in American Health Care and the Implications for Rehabilitation Nurses

Teresa L. Thompson, PhD RN CRRN-A

Now that the field of rehabilitation has moved into the 21st century, rehabilitation professionals find themselves grappling with a decade filled with significant changes. Among these changes are the American with Disabilities Act (ADA), the move away from the acute setting, the recognition of diversity, the shift from the multidisciplinary model to an integrated transdisciplinary model of care, and the impact of the Balanced Budget Act of 1997 (Hartmann, 1998; Neal, 1999; Zollar, 1999). Professional rehabilitation nurses are required to know and use change theory in patient care as well as to become personally change-resilient to effectively provide and advocate for the services needed. Understanding the need for transformational change requires knowledge of the change process and the driving forces in the industry as well as having the professional grounding that can help determine what is nice to know and what is necessary to know (Burgess, 1996). By understanding the realities of change, rehabilitation nurses are more prepared to move across settings and meet the needs of individuals with disabilities and chronic illness.

I. Major Milestones Creating a Change Environment

A. The Americans with Disabilities Act (ADA) of 1990 (Glantz, 1997; U.S. Department of Justice, 1999)

1. Provisions of the ADA

   a. Title I

   1) Prohibits private employers, state and local governments, employment agencies, and labor unions from discriminating against qualified individuals with disabilities in job application procedures, hiring, firing, advancement, compensation, job training, and other terms, conditions, and privileges of employment

   2) Describes the traits of an individual with a disability

      a) A physical or mental impairment that substantially limits one or more major life activity

      b) A record of such an impairment

      c) Regarded as having such an impairment

   b. Title II

   1) Provides comprehensive civil rights for qualified individuals with disabilities

   2) Addresses public entities and requires that all activities, services, and programs of public entities be covered by the ADA, including activities of state legislatures and courts, town meetings, police and fire departments, motor vehicle licensing, and employment

   3) Directly influences access, program integration, communication, construction, and alterations

   c. Title III

   1) Addresses the public sector

   2) Defines those private entities that are required to meet ADA requirements

2. The impact of the ADA

   a. Allows people with disabilities to have equal opportunities, accessibility, and accommodations in employment, transportation, and public access

b. Has spawned ongoing litigation and clarification to further define the actual implementation and application of the ADA (Walter, 1997)

c. Has made rehabilitation nurses serve as advocates and use their knowledge of the ADA to inform patients and obtain needed resources and opportunities

B. Managed Care

1. Managed care has changed the emphasis in health care to one that looks at cost and the health of populations.

2. Fowler (1997) proposed three stages of managed care that emphasize the movement of the managed care process into the market.

   a. Stage 1
      1) Moves care to the ambulatory setting
      2) Allows insurers to purchase discounted services
      3) Marks the beginning of access control through prior authorization for services for managed care patients

   b. Stage 2
      1) Moves delivery of care to a postacute continuum as soon as the acute episode is stabilized
      2) Requires continuity across settings
      3) Forces payers and providers to look for new strategies for disease state management that address problems up-front to avoid or limit acute episodes of care

   c. Stage 3
      1) Is the most advanced stage of a managed care market
      2) Provides pre-illness care to avoid the costly and health-reducing effects of disease, chronic illnesses, and disabilities

3. Rehabilitation nurses are needed in each of these stages to advocate for access to managed care for individuals with disabilities and chronic illnesses.

C. Changes in the Rehabilitation Market

1. The influence of diagnosis-related groups (DRGs)

   a. In the mid-1980s, there was an increase in rehabilitation acute units.

   b. In the early 1990s, the overall census in all inpatient settings decreased.

   c. In the 1990s, competition for rehabilitation patients began and the growth of acute rehabilitation subsided.

   d. Internal and external case management of all patients has increased.

   e. Home health care has increased and has moved many rehabilitation nurses into the home care setting.

2. The growth of subacute rehabilitation

   a. In the early 1990s, the venue of subacute care arose out of the skilled nursing facility (SNF) sector. Some subacute programs were hospital-based; however, most were affiliated with SNFs.

   b. The growth of subacute programs created a definitional problem in rehabilitation between acute and subacute programs.

   c. Subacute programs have proved to be a real competitor for patients and staff. In general, subacute rehabilitation can offer services at a slower pace to patients who may not tolerate a full regime of therapy (DeJong & Sutton, 1997).

3. Developments by national rehabilitation companies in the for-profit market

   a. Companies provided inpatient, outpatient, and SNF subacute programs.

   b. Companies offered acute, subacute/SNF, long-term hospitals, and outpatient services.

   c. Companies drew on economies of scale in contracting for rehabilitation patient care with insurers.

4. A focus on marketing outcomes, which began in the late 1970s

   a. Outcomes, especially as they relate to function, are the most common measures across all levels of rehabilitation programs.

   b. Outcomes are used to communicate with consumers of rehabilitation services to describe the following:
      1) Comparison
      2) Contracting
      3) Selection of a rehabilitation setting
      4) Marketing and competition for the rehabilitation patient

5. A shift in care settings: Rehabilitation nurses have moved into all sectors of rehabilitation and chronic illness.

D. Recognition of a Transcultural Environment
 1. Acknowledges the rapidly changing demographics and increased awareness of cultural expectations
 2. Promotes cultural competence (Erlen, 1998; Taylor, 1998)
    a. Includes cultural self-awareness of values and beliefs
    b. Encompasses cultural knowledge, or the understanding of others' values, meanings, customs, and expressions
    c. Confronts prejudices, biases, judgments, and generalizations
    d. Improves communication
 3. Promotes culturally sensitive care, which provides for the preservation and maintenance, accommodation and negotiation, and the repatterning and restructuring of care to meet patients' cultural and healthcare needs (Leininger, 1997)
 4. Blends well with rehabilitation nursing philosophy, which is based on a holistic approach to the individual and ensures equal opportunity to care

E. Major Shifts in the Delivery, Environment, and Expectations of Health Care (Issel & Anderson, 1996)
 1. Customer orientation: This shift involved moving from viewing the person as the customer to viewing the population as the customer.
 2. Wellness orientation: With the movement to a focus on patient populations, the emphasis became health promotion, which redefined the health services that were provided and prioritized.
 3. Cost versus revenue: The emphasis is on managed care and capitation, and the responsibility lies with the provider to control costs.
 4. Approach to care: This shift involved moving from a departmental or an individual professional approach to an integrated, interdependent approach to care.
 5. Shift for patients: Patients are now viewed as consumers of cost and quality, which allows them to identify the types and cost of services needed to maintain wellness.

6. Continuity of information: Information is now brought to the patient across time and discipline boundaries.

F. The Balanced Budget Act of 1997
 1. Called for Medicare spending cuts that affect rehabilitation (Blecher, Haugh, Hudson, & Serb, 1998; Hartmann, 1998; Knapp, 1999; Neal, 1999; Zollar, 1999)
 2. Required a prospective payment system (PPS) to be applied in SNFs. The PPS has a fixed per-diem reimbursement. Implementation began in 1999, and the rate will be blended annually. The phase-in plan used an accelerating percent of the national fixed rate (e.g., 25%, 50%, 75%, 100%) combined with a proportionately declining institutional rate based on the facility's 1995 Medicare cost report (Stahl, 1998).
 3. Required the use of Resource Utilization Groups (RUGs) as the basis for rehabilitation PPS: RUGs-III are based on the Minimum Data Set (MDS) assessment's Resident Assessment Instrument (RAI) and Resident Assessment Protocols (RAPs), which must be done for each patient. RUGs categorize patients into four major categories (Knapp, 1999; Nathenson, 1999).
    a. Rehabilitation
    b. Extensive services
    c. Special care
    d. Clinically complex
 4. Required consolidated billing: SNFs must bill all Medicare Part B services with the Medicare Part A billing for all services provided to a resident in a nursing facility.
 5. Capped Medicare Part B payment: Rehabilitation therapy for postacute delivery services has a $1,500 cap (Fronheiser, 1998; Muse, 1999).
 6. Implemented the transfer rule: Patient transfers were expanded to include patients with specific diagnoses that move from the acute care hospital to the postacute setting (Esser, 1998; Zollar, 1999).

G. Disease State Management
 1. Disease state management is "a comprehensive, integrated approach to care and reimbursement based on a disease's natural course" (Todd & Nash, 1997, p. 4).

2. Disease management is population focused.

3. The managed care model of crib-to-grave enrollment motivates healthcare professionals to perform disease management. The use of services is disproportionate for patients with complicated medical problems.

4. Best practice guidelines to standardize approaches to care are expanding across healthcare settings.

5. Healthy People 2010 (Office of Disease Prevention and Health Promotion, 1999) seeks to improve systems for personal and public health.

   a. By increasing quality and years of healthy life

   b. By eliminating health disparities

   c. By promoting healthy behaviors

   d. By preventing and reducing diseases and disorders

   e. By promoting health communities

H. Alternative and Complementary Therapies

   1. The use of alternative and complementary therapies has increased. These therapies are now often incorporated into what is perceived as mainstream care.

   2. Alternative medicine practices are used by 42% of Americans, and $21.2 billion are spent on visits to alternative medicine practitioners (Snow, 1998, p. 65).

   3. There are many types of alternative and complementary therapies.

      a. Acupuncture: The Chinese practice of inserting needle points into specific body sites for symptom and/or pain relief. Acupuncture is thought to enable the body to release endorphins (Elliott, 1998; Morey, 1998; Sherwin, 1992).

      b. Acupressure, or therapeutic Chinese massage: "The palpitating, rubbing, and kneading of the flesh along meridian lines," which is used to relieve muscular tension (Hoeman, 1996, p. 213; Sherwin, 1992, p. 254)

      c. Biofeedback: "A method of autonomic nervous system control via self-regulation" (Hoeman, 1996, p. 213)

      d. Herbals and teas: Botanical products used in the treatment of disease (O'Neil,

Avila, & Fetrow, 1999)

      e. QiGong: The Chinese concept of life energy that "integrates breathing, meditation, and movement to strengthen, unblock, and balance the flow of vital energy within the person's body and spirit" (Elliott, 1998, p. 164). Tai chi is one form of QiGong (Sherwin, 1992).

      f. Reiki: The Japanese practice of transmitting energy to the body's *chakras* or energy points. Reiki blends the Japanese words *rei*, which means "universal" or "spiritual wisdom," and *ki*, which means "life energy" (Northrup, 1998; Sherwin, 1992).

      g. Therapeutic touch: Using the concept of energy transfer or exchange in the healing process (Hoeman, 1996; Sherwin, 1992)

   3. The National Center for Complementary and Alternative Medicine (NCCAM) was established in the National Institutes of Health in 1998 (Marwick, 1998).

   4. NCCAM identified seven categories of complementary and alternative medicine (NCCAM, 1998).

      a. Mind-body medicine: Behavioral, psychological, social, and spiritual approaches to health

      b. Alternative medical systems: Complete systems of theory and practice developed outside of the Western biomedical approach

      c. Lifestyle and disease prevention: Theories and practices designed to prevent the development of illness, identify and treat risk factors, or support the healing and recovery process

      d. Biologically based therapies: Natural and biologically based practices, interventions, and products

      e. Manipulative and body-based systems: Manipulation and/or movement of the body

      f. Biofield: Use of subtle energy fields in and around the body

      g. Bioelectromagnetics: Unconventional use of electromagnetic fields

5. Rehabilitation nurses should be aware of the cultural meanings of health and wellness and various alternatives that patients may use. This information should be gathered during the patient assessment. Incorporation of techniques requires additional education and review of the science and related research.

II. Change in an Ever-Changing Time

A. Descriptions of Change
   1. Previously known situation, process, or adaptation that is now new or altered
   2. Clear delineation of beginning and end
   3. "Resisting change is like holding your breath…do it long enough and you will die" (Te Tao Ching, in Scott & Rantz, 1994, p. 7).

B. Lewin's Change Theory
   1. Historical perspective: Social scientist Kurt Lewin (1947) is credited as the classical theorist of change theory; much of his work was done in the 1940s.
   2. Change theory concepts
      a. Behavior is a function of both personality and the environment, and the interaction between the two is dynamic.
      b. There are three stages of change.
         1) Unfreezing: Movement from a steady state to a state that is unsteady and amenable to change
            a) Discomfort with the present situation is induced or emerges.
            b) Status quo is questioned.
            c) Change relationship is established.
         2) Movement: Movement to higher level of behavior
            a) Problem is assessed and diagnosed.
            b) Options and alternatives are identified.
            c) Goals are established.
            d) Action is taken.
            e) Evaluation is made.
         3) Refreezing: Integration and stabilization of new learning
            a) New responses are integrated into lifestyle and relationships.
            b) Change is complete.

C. Types of Change
   1. Profound change: A phrase used to describe organizational change that combines inner shifts in people's values, aspirations, and behaviors with outer shifts in processes, strategies, practices, and systems (Senge et al., 1999). Nothing can change without personal transformation.
      a. The beginning and end of change is no longer clearly defined. Profound change builds on ongoing data gathering and adaptation (Porter-O'Grady, 1992).
      b. Change is often multidimensional and requires a more fluid approach.
      c. Senge (1994) described the "learning organization" as an approach to transition that is needed today. Learning organizations are those that seek to create their own future. Senge's model includes five disciplines (Birkner & Birkner, 1998; Senge, 1994).
         1) "Mental models: The personal biases and assumptions we use to make decisions that drive our behavior
         2) Personal mastery: Clarifying what is important and striving to see reality more clearly
         3) Shared vision: Building a common sense of purpose and commitment by developing shared images of the future we seek to create
         4) Team learning: Reflecting on action as a team and transforming collective thinking skills so that the team can develop intelligence and ability greater than the sum of individual members' talents
         5) Systems thinking: The language of interrelationships that shape the behavior of the systems in which we exist" (Birkner & Birkner, p. 157)
      d. Senge et al. (1999) noted that companies that fail to sustain significant change end up facing crises.
         1) Organizations (and professionals) must change their basic ways of thinking to initiate and sustain change.
         2) There must be a "commitment to" change versus a simple "compliance with" change.

e. External forces for change include technology, customers, competitors, market structure, and the social and political environment.

f. Internal realities of change depend on how the environment adapts.

g. "The timeless concern is whether these internal changes—in practices, views, and strategies—will keep pace with the external change" (Senge et al., 1999, p. 14).

2. Marshak's (1993) three types of change

a. Developmental change, which improves performance and is built on the past

b. Transitional change, which moves from one state to another

c. Transformational change, which "implies the transfiguration from one state of being to a fundamentally different state of being" (p. 47)

D. Managing Complex Change

1. Requires a multistep approach

2. Requires transformational leadership

3. Requires identification of the present state, transition state, and future state (Beckhard & Harris, 1987) (see Figure 21-1)

4. Involves communication of the demands requiring the change

5. Involves transformational leadership, including change, innovation, growth, and empowerment (Koerner & Bunkers, 1992)

E. The Rehabilitation Nurse as a Change Agent in Today's Healthcare Environment

1. Change is a central concern for nursing (DeFeo, 1990).

a. "Change in the rehabilitation setting can involve change in knowledge, attitude, behavior, or group organization or functioning" (Chin, Finocchiaro, & Rosebrough, 1998, p. 71).

b. As a change agent, the rehabilitation nurse proactively helps the patient or is involved in the change process within the organization.

c. Change parallels the nursing process.

1) Identify the problem to be addressed

2) Define changes needed

3) Identify the purpose of the change

4) Gather and use the elements required to accomplish the change

5) Implement actions to accomplish the change

6) Evaluate the change

d. Change requires a positive growth approach by the practitioner as well as the patient. The emphasis is on the knowledge, skill, and abilities that will be gained through change (Potter, Dawson, Barton, & Nitz, 1998).

2. The current demands of health care create an environment of profound change.

3. Rehabilitation nurses must have knowledge of change barriers, identify internal and external barriers to openness to change, and make a commitment to change.

a. Internal demands

1) Reorganization

2) Redesign

3) Reengineering

4) Continuous quality improvement

5) Redeployment

b. External demands

1) Managed care

2) New knowledge

3) Competition

4) Regulations

Figure 21-1. Changes and the Rehabilitation Corollary

Changes in the environment: Move from the acute to subacute, outpatient, and home health care

Changes in organizational priorities: Consolidation, restructuring, and internal development of subacute venues

Changes in structures: Move to transdisciplinary care

Changes in the ways work is done: Care maps, integrated assessments, and documentation by exception

Changes in roles: Increased case management, prior authorizations, and care by contract

Changes in culture: Cultural competence to address diversity; organizational cultural changes in response to managed care

Source consulted

Beckhard, R., & Harris, R.T. (1987). *Organizational transitions: Managing complex change.* Reading, MA: Addison Wesley.

---

4. The change process involves knowledge of classic information as well as making way for profound change.

5. Rehabilitation nurses must understand the external forces requiring change.
    a. Venue of care
    b. Expanded knowledge
    c. Upgrade of clinical knowledge and skills
    d. Fiscal accountability

6. Rehabilitation nurses must recognize their own attitudes or personality traits related to change. They must know the role that best describes their own positions and learn how to work with people who fall into the other groups.

7. Rogers (1995) described six types of behavioral groups.
    a. Innovators: Adventuresome
    b. Early adopters: Respected leader-type individuals in the organization
    c. Early majority: Deliberate
    d. Late majority: Skeptical
    e. Laggards: Hang on to traditional ways and ideas
    f. Rejecters

F. Major Hurdles to Change-Ready Thinking (Kreigel & Brandt, 1996)
    1. Fear
    2. Fatigue
    3. Comfort

G. Reasons for Taking a Proactive Approach to Change and Seeking Out Opportunities for Change

1. To improve the quality of care
2. To improve the cost-effectiveness of the delivery of care
3. To make the adaptations needed to maintain change

H. Resilience in Facing Change
    1. Attributes and traits that are characteristic to change-resilient people (Conner, 1996; Giordono, 1997; Jacelon, 1997)
        a. Positive thinkers
        b. Sense of being in control
        c. Resourceful
        d. Focused
        e. Self-disciplined
        f. Flexible
        g. Organized
        h. Proactive
    2. Traits that pose barriers to resilience to change (Giordono, 1997)
        a. Cynicism
        b. Distancing
        c. Avoidance

III. Conclusion

Rehabilitation nurses are driven to change both internally (as providers of care) and externally (as a part of healthcare organizations). Rehabilitation nurses who are aware of the various changes in health care and are open to new strategies are able to stay in the forefront of change. Rehabilitation nurses can develop the traits of resilience to change, which can then be translated to actual patient situations in which the individual is facing monumental change within his or her life.

References

Beckhard, R., & Harris, R.T. (1987). *Organizational transitions: Managing complex change.* Reading, MA: Addison Wesley.

Birkner, L.R., & Birkner, R.K. (1998). Learning organization update: Safety and health pros must prepare for careers as knowledge workers. *Occupational Hazards, 60*(10), 157.

Blecher, M.B., Haugh, R., Hudson, T., & Serb, C. (1998, December 5). The year that was: What it means for 1999. *Hospitals & Health Networks, 26*(1), 26–28, 30–34.

Burgess, C. (1996). Straight talk: Hitting the wall. *Rehab Management: The Interdisciplinary Journal of Rehabilitation, 9*(2), 25, 27.

Chin, P.A., Finocchiaro, D.N., & Rosebrough, A. (1998). *Rehabilitation nursing practice.* New York: McGraw Hill.

Conner, D.R. (1996). How can you survive continuous change? *Medical Economics, 73*(8), 109–114.

DeFeo, D.J. (1990). Change: A central concern of nursing. *Nursing Science Quarterly, 3*(2), 88–94.

DeJong, G., & Sutton, J.P. (1997). Rapid growth of postacute care services leads policy makers to reconsider bundling Medicare postacute services. *Rehabilitation Outlook, 5*(6), 84–85.

Elliott, L. (1998). Understanding natural therapies. *Washingtonian, 34*(2), 162–164.

Erlen, J.A. (1998). Culture, ethics, and respect: The bottom line is understanding. *Orthopaedic Nursing, 17*(6), 79–82.

Esser, C. (1998). Sorting out the Balanced Budget Act of 1997. *ARN Network, 14*(3), 1–2.

Fowler, F.J. (1997). Pricing and managed care. *Rehab Economics, 5*(1), 88–89.

Fronheiser, L.P. (1998). PPS's $1,500 cap: Hope for the best...plan for the worst. *Nursing Homes, 47*(4), 22–25.

Giordono, B.P. (1997). Resilience: A survival tool for the nineties. *AORN Journal, 65*(6), 1032–1034.

Glantz, L. (1997, February 27). Facts about the Americans with Disabilities Act [On-line]. Available: http://www.muskie.usm.maine.edu/research/disability/fact.htm

Hartmann, J. (1998). The Balanced Budget Act of 1997: How the prospective payment system affects providers of rehabilitation services. *Rehabilitation Nursing, 23*(5), 263–264.

Hoeman, S. (Ed.). (1996). *Rehabilitation nursing: Process and application* (2nd ed.). St. Louis: Mosby.

Issel, L.M., & Anderson, R.A. (1996). Take charge: Managing six transformations in health care delivery. *Nursing Economics, 14*(2), 78–85.

Jacelon, C.S. (1997). The trait and process of resilience. *Journal of Advanced Nursing, 25,* 123–139.

Knapp, M.T. (1999). Nurse's basic guide to understanding the Medicare PPS. *Nursing Management, 30*(5), 14–15.

Koerner, J.G., & Bunkers, S.S. (1992). Transformational leadership: The power of symbol. *Nursing Administrative Quarterly, 17*(1), 1–9.

Kreigel, R., & Brandt, D. (1996). *Sacred cows make the best burghers.* New York: Warner Books.

Leininger, M. (1997). Overview of the theory of culture care with the ethnonursing research method. *Transcultural Nursing, 8*(2), 32–52.

Lewin, K. (1947). Frontiers in group dynamics: Concepts, methods, and reality in social science. *Human Relations, 5*(1), 5–42.

Marshak, R.J. (1993). Managing the metaphors of change. *Organizational Dynamics, 22*(1), 44–56.

Marwick, C. (1998). Alterations are ahead at the OAM. *Medical News and Perspectives, 280*(18), 1553–1554.

Morey, S.S. (1998). NIH issues consensus statement on acupuncture. *American Family Physician, 57*(10), 2545–2546.

Muse, D. (1999). The rehab cap: An exercise in futility? *Nursing Homes, 48*(2), 46–50.

Nathenson, P. (Ed.). (1999). *Integrating rehabilitation and restorative nursing concepts into the MDS.* Glenview, IL: Association of Rehabilitation Nurses.

National Center for Complementary and Alternative Medicine (NCCAM). (1998). NCCAM Home Page [On-line]. Available: http://nccam.nih.gov/

Neal, L.J. (1999). Current issues: Important changes in home health care. *Rehabilitation Nursing, 24*(1), 4–6.

Northrup, C. (1998). *Women's bodies, women's wisdom.* New York: Bantam Press.

Office of Disease Prevention and Health Promotion, U.S. Department of Health and Human Services. (1999). Healthy People 2010 Home Page [On-line]. Available: http://www.odphp.osophs.dhhs.gov/pubs/HP2000/2010.htm

O'Neil, C.K., Avila, J.R., & Fetrow, C.W. (1999). Herbal medicines: Getting beyond the hype. *Nursing 99, 29*(5), 58–61.

Porter-O'Grady, T. (1992). Transformational leadership in an age of chaos. *Nursing Administrative Quarterly, 17*(1), 17–24.

Potter, M.L., Dawson, A.M., Barton, M.M., & Nitz, R.E. (1998). Change...ouch! *Nursing Management, 29*(11), 27–30.

Rogers, E. (1995). *Diffusion of innovation* (4th ed.). New York: Free Press.

Scott, J., & Rantz, M. (1994). Change champions at the grassroots level: Practice innovation using team process. *Nursing Administrative Quarterly, 18*(3), 7–17.

Senge, P. (1994). *The fifth discipline fieldbook.* New York: Currency Doubleday.

Senge, P., Kleiner, A., Roberts, C., Ross, R., Roth, G., & Smith, B. (1999). *The dance of change.* New York: Currency Doubleday.

Sherwin, D.C. (1992). Traditional Chinese medicine in rehabilitation nursing practice. *Rehabilitation Nursing, 17*(5), 253–255.

Snow, B. (1998). Internet sources of information on alternative medicine. *Database, 21*(4), 65–66.

Stahl, D.A. (1998). The nuts and bolts of prospective payment. *Nursing Management, 29*(7), 20–23.

Taylor, R. (1998). Check your cultural competence. *Nursing Management, 29*(8), 30–32.

Todd, W., & Nash, D. (Eds.). (1997). *Disease management: A systems approach to improving patient outcomes.* Chicago. American Hospital Association.

U.S. Department of Justice. (1999). Americans with Disabilities Act (ADA) Home Page [On-line]. Available: http://www.usdoj.gov/crt/ada/adahom1.htm

Walter, O. (1997, May 5). Disabling America. *National Review, 49,* 40–42.

Zollar, C. (1999). Transfer rule: Boon or bane for rehabilitation providers? *Rehabilitation Nursing, 24*(2), 48–50.

Suggested resources

Andrews, M.M. (1998). A model for cultural change. *Nursing Management, 29*(10), 62, 63, 66.

Bartol, G., & Richardson, L. (1998) Using literature to create cultural competence. *Image: Journal of Nursing Scholarship, 30*(1), 75–79.

Bonalumi, N., & Fisher, K. (1999). Health care change: Challenge for nurse administrators. *Nursing Administrative Quarterly, 23*(2), 69–3.

Disability Information Resources' Americans with Disabilities Act Information. (1997, December 19). [On-line]. Available: http://www.jsrd.or.jp/dinf_us/ada-home.html

Fadiman, A. (1997). *The spirit catches you and you fall down.* New York: Noonday Press.

Fetrow, C.W., & Avila, J.R. (1999). *Complementary and alternative medicines.* Springhouse, PA: Springhouse.

Flowers, C.R., Edwards, D., & Pusch, B. (1996). Rehabilitation cultural diversity initiative: A regional survey of cultural diversity within CILs. *The Journal of Rehabilitation, 62*(3), 22–29.

Gillett, D. (1997). Is your rehab unit managed care-ready? How to build on advantages SNFs already have. *Nursing Homes, 46*(8), 47–49.

Glantz, L. (1997, February 25). ADA Title II highlights [On-line]. Available: http://www.muskie.usm.maine.edu/research/disability/2high.htm

Glantz, L. (1997, February 27). ADA Title III fact sheet [On-line]. Available: http://www.muskie.usm.maine.edu/research/disability/fact3.htm

Grimaldi, P.L. (1998). Managed care glossary: Update II. *Nursing Management, 29*(10), 8–11.

Health Care Financing Administration (HCFA). (1997, December 23). HCFA Legislative Summary [On-line]. Available: http://www.hcfa.gov/regs/budget97.htm

Kerfoot, K. (1999). Creating a forgetting organization. *Nursing Economics, 17*(1), 64–65.

King, W.R. (1997). Organizational transformation. *Information Systems Management, 14*, 63–65.

Kirkham, S.R. (1998). Nurses' descriptions of caring for culturally diverse clients. *Clinical Nursing Research, 7*(2), 125–146.

Manion, J. (1993). Chaos or transformation. *Journal of Nursing Administration, 23*(5), 41–48.

Sampson, W. (1999). The braid of the "alternative medicine" movement. *Scientific Review of Alternative Medicine, 2*(2), 4–11.

Stahl, D.A. (1998). PPS challenges in postacute care. *Nursing Management, 29*(8), 10–12.

Strebel, P. (1996). Why do employees resist change? *Harvard Business Review, 74*(3), 86–92.

Sunoo, B.P. (1999). Alternative medicine: The arrival of new age health care. *Workforce, 78*(6), 88–90.

Sweeney, T., & Whitaker, C. (1994). Successful change: Renaissance without revolution. *Seminars for Nurse Managers, 2*(1), 196–202.

Tonges, M.C. (1997). The white water of change: A survivor's guide. *Nursing Management, 28*(11), 64, 66–67, 72.

Chapter 22

Rehabilitation Nursing: Past, Present, and Future

Patricia A. Edwards, EdD RN CNAA

The history of rehabilitation nursing is inexorably linked to the history of medicine, nursing, and rehabilitation. The timelines in this chapter provide a historical overview of rehabilitation and the major events, people, and factors that shaped the healthcare specialty known as rehabilitation nursing.

The initial change in attitude toward people with disabilities came with an interest in crippled children, particularly those affected by the outbreak of polio, at the turn of the 19th century. During the first decade of the 20th century, society began to focus on the needs of individuals with disabilities by providing a therapeutic environment for the treatment of specific disabilities and by beginning to address these individuals' educational and vocational needs. Many changes were stimulated as a result of society entering or recovering from war, enjoying the creativity and prosperity of peacetime, and attempting to treat and cure disease and its sequelae. In the second half of the 20th century, people with physical disabilities, composing a minority of approximately 45 million people in America, began to receive national support for their right to lead normal, high-quality lives despite their physical disabilities.

Rehabilitation was first practiced by nurses in the convalescent and sanitarium units of the early 1900s. The specialty practice of rehabilitation nursing began in the 1940s as World War II veterans returned home with spinal cord injuries and the aftermath of the polio epidemic left many people with disabilities with unmet needs. Both groups of patients required hospitalization over a long period of time.

The change, growth, creativity, and technological advances that characterized the 20th century have challenged rehabilitation nurses to expand their knowledge base and practice across the continuum of care. This chapter concludes with a number of possibilities for the future practice of rehabilitation nursing in the 21st century.

I. Past: A Historical Overview of Rehabilitation

A. Rehabilitation from Ancient Egypt Through the 18th Century

1. From ancient to modern times, mankind has been adapting and coping with physical disability

2. More than 5,000 years ago: An Egyptian physician recorded an assessment of a client

3. 2380 BC: Earliest record of crutches, discovered in hieroglyphics on an Egyptian tomb

4. Pre-Christian era: Many biblical references concern the crippled, lame, blind, and afflicted

5. 400–300 BC: Hippocrates, the father of medicine, recorded the use of artificial limbs as an attempt to replace amputated limbs and the basic principle that "exercise strengthens and inactivity wastes"

6. 200–100 BC: Galen, a Greek physician and writer, described the muscles and bones of the body

7. 30 AD: Celsius advocated the use of exercise after a fracture had healed to prevent the loss of function

8. 1601: The Poor Relief Act, the first show of responsibility and concern for people with disabilities, was passed in England

9. 1633: Vincent dePaul founded institutions for crippled children in France

10. 1750: John Hunter, a British physician, focused on the importance of the relationship between the client's will, range of motion, and muscle reeducation

11. 1798: Philippe Pinel began practicing psychiatric rehabilitation as well as occupational and recreational therapies as treatment methods in England (McCourt, 1993).

B. Rehabilitation in the 19th Century
1. 1829: The Perkins Institute, the first sheltered workshop for people with disabilities in the United States, was founded by Samuel Gridley Howe. The goal was to train blind people so they could work in the community
2. 1854: Florence Nightingale organized professional nursing in England
3. 1873: The first U.S. school of nursing was founded in New York at Bellevue Hospital
4. 1877: Clara Barton established the American Red Cross
5. 1889–1893: Interest in crippled children grew. The Cleveland Rehabilitation Center began offering services for children, and the first U.S. schools for children with physical disabilities were established (see Figure 22–1)
6. Advances in science and medicine increased the potential for the survival and physical restoration of people with disabilities
7. End of 19th century: Public health departments were established in major cities

C. Rehabilitation in the 20th Century
1. 1900-1919
   a. Society began to focus on the needs of individuals with disabilities.
      1) By providing a therapeutic environment for the treatment of specific disabilities
      2) By addressing educational and vocational needs
   b. Individuals promoted occupational and vocational training
      1) Susan Tracy, a nurse, teacher, and author who pioneered the discipline of occupational therapy
      2) Eleanor Slagle, a social worker
      3) George Barton, an architect recovering from tuberculosis
   c. The Home for Crippled Children was established in Pittsburgh in 1902 to care for children with disabilities
   d. Electrotherapy was used as a therapeutic modality, and physical therapy modalities were instituted at Massachusetts General Hospital
   e. The need for licensure and definition of the specialty of rehabilitation was identified

f. The Institute for Crippled and Disabled (est. 1917) and the Curative Workshop of Milwaukee (est. 1919) were pioneering ventures in the area of rehabilitation
g. World War I had a great impact on physical medicine
   1) The federal division of specialty hospitals and physical reconstruction at Massachusetts General Hospital (MGH) was developed in 1917 to treat wounded soldiers and others requiring rehabilitation
   2) Education and vocational rehabilitation was provided through the American Red Cross Institute for Disabled Men
   3) The first spinal centers incorporated concepts of functional reeducation.
   4) The U.S. Veterans' Administration (VA) was created

Figure 22-1. Early Pediatric Rehabilitation Facilities in the United States

1883	The Hospital for Sick Children, Washington, DC
1889	The Cleveland Rehabilitation Center, Cleveland, OH
1892	The Children's Country Home, Westfield, NJ, and The Blythedale Children's Hospital, Valhalia, NY
1893	The Boston Institute School for Crippled and Deformed Children
1895	Health Hill Hospital in Cleveland
1902	The Home for Crippled Children (now The Rehabilitation Institute), Pittsburgh, PA
1919	The Curative Workshop of Milwaukee
1922	Happy Hills Convalescent Center (now Mt. Washington Pediatric Hospital), Baltimore, MD
1930	Elizabethtown Hospital and Rehabilitation Center (now University Hospital Rehabilitation Center for Children and Adults), Elizabethtown, PA
1937	Children's Rehabilitation Institute (now the Kennedy Institute), Baltimore, MD
1940	Alfred I. DuPont Institute, Wilmington, DE (as a hospital for crippled children)
1949	Kennedy Memorial Hospital (now Franciscan Children's Hospital and Rehabilitation Center), Boston, MA
1950	Children's Orthopedic Hospital (now Cardinal Hill Rehabilitation Hospital), Lexington, KY

Source consulted

Edwards, P.A. (1992). The evolution of rehabilitation facilities for children. *Rehabilitation Nursing, 17*, 191-192.

2. 1920–1943
   a. 1920
      1) The Vocational Rehabilitation law provided for federal control of vocational rehabilitation
      2) The first Rehabilitation Act passed by Congress set in motion a focus on the emerging specialty of rehabilitation
   b. 1921: The Division of Physical Reconstruction and the Federal Board for Vocational Education were established
   c. Associations for physical and occupational therapists were developed. These organizations began to determine the role, placement, and governance of therapies, which became focus points of the emerging specialty of rehabilitation
   d. 1935: The Social Security Act defined rehabilitation as a process that helped a person with a disability become capable of engaging in a remunerative occupation. The government began providing rehabilitation services beyond the needs of the military and outside hospital walls
   e. 1938: The American Academy of Physical Medicine and Rehabilitation (AAPMR) was founded to set standards and requirements for the practice of rehabilitation medicine
   f. 1938–1941: In 1938, Dr. Frank Krusen established the hallmarks of physical medicine as controlling disease, relieving suffering, and shortening the period of disability. In 1941, Krusen wrote *Physical Medicine*, the first comprehensive book about treatment methods
   g. 1943
      1) The Sister Kenny Institute was established. Sister Kenny, a nurse, used muscular manipulation, which led to the theory of muscle reeducation. Her techniques pioneered the discipline of physical therapy, and her success with treatment of polio patients boosted the medical specialty of physiatry (McCourt, 1993).
      2) The Vocational Rehabilitation Act was enacted.

      a) Made funds available for professional training and research
      b) Broadened the scope of rehabilitation
      c) Provided a catalyst for the growth of the practice
   h. World War II played a tremendous role in the further development of rehabilitation programs
      1) Dr. Howard A. Rusk dramatically demonstrated the possibilities of rehabilitation when he showed how it could improve the lives of men who had been hospitalized since WWI
      2) New methods of handling shock and treating infection, as well as increasingly sophisticated trauma care, meant more people would survive

3. 1944–1960
   a. The number of industrial-related injuries increased, as did motor vehicle-related accidents and injuries.
   b. 1945
      1) Liberty Mutual hired the first rehabilitation nurse in the insurance industry, thus recognizing the importance of nurses in a rehabilitation role
      2) The American Paraplegia Association was founded
   c. 1946
      1) Rehabilitation programs began in U.S. VA hospitals.
      2) The term *physiatrist* began to be used to describe a physician specialized training in rehabilitation medicine
   d. 1947: Dr. Rusk established the first medical rehabilitation services in a U.S. civilian hospital
   e. Late 1940s: The first board certification exams in physiatry were conducted
   f. 1951: Alice Morrissey, BS RN, wrote the first textbook (*Rehabilitation Nursing*) in the field of rehabilitation nursing
      1) Principle contributions of nurses in rehabilitative care identified by Morrissey
         a) Basic bedside nursing
         b) Clinical teaching and rehabilitation nursing service management

c) An emphasis on the importance of nutrition and activities of daily living

2) Principle message of Morrissey's textbook: "Each sick person is regarded not as a patient with a disease but as a person with a future"

g. 1956-1969: Lena Plaisted, MS RN, founded the first graduate rehabilitation nursing program at Boston University in 1956. Plaisted wrote *The Clinical Specialist in Rehabilitation*, the first publication to describe this role, in 1969

h. During the 1950s: Barbara Madden, MA RN, contributed significantly to the development of nursing programs for acute and postpolio patients and helped establish regional respiratory centers

i. Increased strides were made in technology and a greater emphasis was placed on the needs of those with disabilities and on rehabilitation

j. The realm of rehabilitation was expanded to include treatment for people with stroke, cardiac conditions, arthritis, orthopedic injuries, and brain injuries

k. Mary Ann Mikulic was one of the first rehabilitation nursing clinical specialists appointed by the VA

4. 1960–1989

a. These 3 decades marked a period of increased recognition for the specialty practice of rehabilitation nursing. As one nurse said, "When starting my rehabilitation career in the '60s, I was frustrated that no one else in other specialty areas seemed to understand what we did in rehabilitation. My mentor acknowledged my frustration and said, 'Barbara, our day will come.' The day did come when I found others calling me about patient education, measuring outcomes, and discharge planning. Nurses in critical care wanted to know about autonomic hyperreflexia and how to talk to patients about sexuality. Finally I felt that what we did and what we knew were acknowledged and appreciated" (B. Warner, personal communication, July 7, 1999)

b. The Korean and Vietnam wars influenced continued progress in rehabilitation, due, in part, to the ability to treat wounded people more effectively on the battlefield and the availability of improved transport to medical treatment services, which led to a decrease in mortality rate (McCourt, 1993)

c. Increased medical technology, institution-based trauma care, and paramedics led to an increased survival rate from injury and focused on the further need for rehabilitation programs and services (McCourt, 1993)

d. The scope of rehabilitation broadened to include and meet needs of the following groups:

1) People with chronic diseases
2) An increasing elderly population
3) People reentering the workforce after traumatic injury, disease, or condition

e. 1962: Medicare legislation stimulated an increased demand for rehabilitation, and more rehabilitation nurses were hired by insurance companies (McCourt, 1993)

f. 1965

1) The Workers' Compensation and Rehabilitation law passed, placing an emphasis on the workplace
2) The American Nurses Association (ANA) published *Guidelines for the Practice of Nursing on the Rehabilitation Team: An Answer to a Growing Need*

g. 1966: The Commission on Accreditation of Rehabilitation Facilities (CARF) was established to serve as a consultative accrediting process in the rehabilitation industry. (Its current name is CARF...The Rehabilitation Accreditation Commission)

h. 1967: Amendments were passed to the Vocational Rehabilitation Act that focused on improving reentry for individuals with disabilities

i. Early 1970s: Regional health care became a focal point in rehabilitation services

j. 1973: The Rehabilitation Act was passed,

demonstrating increased public awareness of the needs of people with disabilities. The act included guidelines for nondiscrimination in employment and promoted community access through reducing and eliminating physical barriers

k. 1974: The Association of Rehabilitation Nurses (ARN) was established under the leadership of Susan Novak. In 1975, four chapters, representing the states of California, Illinois, and New York, were chartered

l. 1975: *ARN Journal* was developed with Dagny Engle serving as the editor. The introduction of the journal was a professional milestone for ARN and its members. In 1981, the journal's name was changed to *Rehabilitation Nursing*

m. 1976
   1) ARN was recognized by the nursing profession as a specialty organization, and the Rehabilitation Nursing Institute (RNI) was established
   2) ARN developed and published the standards and scope of rehabilitation nursing practice

n. 1978: Independent living programs helped change societal views of the dependency of people with catastrophic injuries (McCourt, 1993)

o. 1981: The International Year of the Disabled Person
   1) The needs of people with disabilities became more prominent as a social issue.
   2) The first edition of ARN's core curriculum for rehabilitation nursing was published under the title, *Rehabilitation Nursing: Concepts and Practice—A Core Curriculum*

p. 1984
   1) ARN developed a formal definition, philosophy, and conceptual framework of rehabilitation nursing and the association
   2) The first certification examination for the Certified Rehabilitation Registered Nurse (CRRN) credential was held

q. 1986

   1) RNI changed its name to the Rehabilitation Nursing Foundation (RNF), which more clearly represented the entity's goals and purpose to the outside world
   2) ARN revised and updated the standards and scope of rehabilitation nursing practice

r. 1987
   1) ARN revised its core curriculum and identified the following areas as future challenges (see Table 22-1):
      a) Insurance issues
      b) Increased impact and influence of rehabilitation
         (1) Increased knowledge and education
         (2) Medicine, drugs, and technological advances
         (3) Decreased social isolation and involvement
         (4) Continued independent living movement
         (5) Increased awareness of cost-effectiveness of rehabilitation
         (6) Clearly defined and available levels of rehabilitation care
   2) ARN formally implemented Special Interest Councils (currently called Special Interest Groups [SIGs]) in nine areas

s. 1989: RNF funded its first research grant

t. Rehabilitation techniques became more widely used in a variety of settings.
   1) Nursing homes
   2) Extended care facilities
   3) Inpatient rehabilitation units
   4) Home care programs
   5) Outpatient programs
   6) Private practice

II. Present–1990s: A Decade of Healthcare Reform and Rehabilitation Nursing Initiatives

A. Healthcare Reform
   1. The 1990s were marked by increasing survival and life expectancy rates, which consequently increased the need for rehabilitation services.
   2. 1990: The Americans with Disabilities Act (ADA) provided enhanced accessibility

options and opportunities for individuals with disabilities in community, employment, education, and healthcare arenas

3. Geriatric rehabilitation demanded greater attention, calling for an increased need for rehabilitation nurses and an increased emphasis on restorative care and prevention of disability

4. The decline in deaths from traumatic injuries and previously life-threatening diseases increased the need for rehabilitation nurses

    a. In critical and acute care settings

    b. As case managers for complex, multifaceted problems

5. The intensity of care increased at all points in the continuum, and care delivery expanded to outpatient and home care.

6. Early interventions and intense technological treatment increased

7. Lifelong care planning issues arose because individuals began living longer with chronic illness and disease

8. New roles, including working as case managers, emerged for nurses

9. Rehabilitation nurses influenced the standards set for rehabilitation facilities and participated in quality improvement and program evaluation activities

B. Rehabilitation Nursing Initiatives by ARN

1. 1990: The first role description for case managers was written by an ARN SIG

2. 1992–1996: ARN published the journal *Rehabilitation Nursing Research*

3. ARN initiated research to determine interventions and outcomes of specific nursing diagnoses

4. 1993: ARN published the third edition of its core curriculum with a new title, *The Specialty Practice of Rehabilitation Nursing: A Core Curriculum* (3rd ed.). It included the following areas of future challenges (see Table 22-1):

    a. Meeting the increased demands and challenges for rehabilitation nurses

        1) Increased need for services
        2) Altered practice settings
        3) Greater demand for patient and family education
        4) Increased recruitment issues and need for further education of nurses

Table 22-1. Comparison of Future Challenges in ARN's Core Curricula

Rehabilitation Nursing: Concepts and Practice (2nd ed., 1987)	*The Specialty Practice of Rehabilitation Nursing: A Core Curriculum* (3rd ed., 1993)	*The Specialty Practice of Rehabilitation Nursing: A Core Curriculum* (4th ed., 2000)
Insurance issues	Managed care	Healthcare crisis: Access, equity, reimbursement
Increased impact and influence of rehabilitation	Cost containment	
Increased knowledge and education	Increased demand for rehabilitation nursing	Changing role of rehabilitation nurses at both the basic and advanced practice levels
Increased awareness of cost-effectiveness of rehabilitation	Increased need for services	
Clearly defined and available levels of rehabilitative care	Increased recruitment and further education of nurses	Roles include case manager and expert rehabilitation clinical nurse specialist
	Increased insistence on certification	Nursing shortage and recruitment and education issues
	Greater awareness of rehabilitation and its benefit to individuals and society	Value of rehabilitation across the continuum of care
	Alteration in practice settings	Changes in practice and care settings: Hospital is more acute and rehabilitation units are changing; more clients are cared for in the home and community

5) Increased insistence on CRRN certification

6) Expansion of professional activities into consultation and research

7) Ensuring a unified voice for the specialty

b. Dealing with the implications of health-care reform as well as the need for greater awareness of rehabilitation and its benefits to individuals and society

1) Managed care

2) Cost containment

3) Legislative involvement and client activity

4) Advanced technology

5) Ethical issues

5. 1994

a. ARN updated the standards and scope of rehabilitation practice

b. ARN published *Basic Competencies for Rehabilitation Nursing Practice*

6. 1995: ARN published *21 Rehabilitation Nursing Diagnoses: A Guide to Interventions and Outcomes*

7. 1996: ARN published the scope and standards of advanced clinical practice in rehabilitation nursing

8. 1997

a. ARN published *Advanced Practice Nursing in Rehabilitation: A Core Curriculum*

b. The Certified Rehabilitation Registered Nurse-Advanced (CRRN-A) credential was introduced and the first exam was held

9. 1998: ARN published *Rehabilitation Nursing in the Home Health Setting*.

10. 1999

a. ARN published *Integrating Rehabilitation and Restorative Nursing Concepts into the MDS*

b. ARN published *Restorative Nursing: A Training Manual for Nursing Assistants*

III. Future: Nurses' Perspectives on Health Care in the 21st Century

A. The Future Practice of Rehabilitation Nursing

1. Rehabilitation nursing will continue to be a prominent specialty in the new millennium.

The knowledge and expertise that rehabilitation nurses possess will continue to be recognized as valuable resources in all practice settings. The fundamentals of rehabilitation nursing will become integrated into other nursing specialties, as an even greater awareness of the unique philosophy and its positive effect on clients emerges (T. Black, personal communication, July 6, 1999)

2. The value of rehabilitation nurses will continue to increase as the healthcare system recognizes the value of rehabilitation principles across the continuum of care—from the emergency room and the intensive care unit to outpatient primary care settings (C. Jacelon, personal communication, July 1, 1999)

3. Rehabilitation nurses must differentiate and clarify their specialized role as well as adapt to the new roles that are being influenced by technical advances, genetic engineering, information technology, and new diseases and conditions (A. McCourt, personal communication, July 7, 1999)

4. Rehabilitation nurses will consult with nurses throughout the world to assist them with educational programs that focus on the prevention of disability as well as the current treatment and care for those already disabled (A. McCourt, personal communication, July 7, 1999)

5. Rehabilitation nurses must continue to define their practice, conduct and use research, ensure that rehabilitation nurses have adequate preparation, and support ARN so that it remains the strong voice for rehabilitation nurses in the healthcare community, both nationally and internationally (M. Ter Maat, personal communication, June 23, 1999)

6. Rehabilitation nurses will continue to possess a unique and diverse skill set that will support clients' movement through the continuum of care and will have an impact on the delivery of healthcare services (T. Black, personal communication, July 6, 1999)

7. Rehabilitation nurses with advanced degrees, including doctoral, will be needed to act in many capacities:

a. As experts in research-based practice

b. As advocates and managers for large populations requiring restorative care

c. As promoters of public policy for people with disabilities at the local and national levels (A. McCourt, personal communication, July 7, 1999)

8. The advanced practice rehabilitation nursing role will combine the knowledge and skills of both the nurse practitioner (NP) and the clinical nurse specialist (CNS)

9. Nurses will become even more instrumental in decision making and providing efficient and effective rehabilitation care (T. Black, personal communication, July 6, 1999)

10. Nurses will have a greater role in measuring and monitoring client outcomes (T. Black, personal communication, July 6, 1999)

B. The Effect of Changing Demographics on the Demand for Rehabilitation Nurses and Practice Settings

1. As the population continues to age, the need for professional nurses who have the skills to treat chronic illnesses and their effects on function, quality of life, and access to care will grow significantly (C. Tracey, personal communication, June 10, 1999)

2. Nurses will have countless opportunities to be involved in the health care of the aging population (K. Johnson, personal communication, July 12, 1999)

3. Rehabilitation nurses will see a shift of the distribution of illness from acute to chronic and a shift in the kinds of injuries clients will have. Traumatic brain and spinal cord injuries from accidents will decrease, but violence-related injuries and disabilities related to multiple medical problems will increase (C. Jacelon, personal communication, July 1, 1999)

4. The average age and age range of clients will continue to increase as the percentage of the general population that is elderly increases (C. Jacelon, personal communication, July 1, 1999)

5. There will be an increase in the demand for skilled pediatric rehabilitation nurses as the success rate increases in saving the lives of premature infants and infants with congenital disabilities (C. Jacelon, personal communication, July 1, 1999)

6. The sequelae resulting from spinal cord injury, traumatic brain injury, and strokes will reverse, creating the need for a very different continuum of care (A. McCourt, personal communication, July 7, 1999)

7. Rehabilitation nurses must market their unique skill set with less focus on the word *rehabilitation* and more focus on the uniqueness of the approach and philosophy (C. Tracey, personal communication, June 10, 1999)

8. Professional rehabilitation nurses will work in settings across the continuum and possess knowledge of physical functioning, chronic illness, adjustment and adaptation, and tertiary prevention (T. Thompson, personal communication, June 22, 1999)

9. Rehabilitation nurses will continue to be autonomous and viewed as experts in promoting functional activities of daily living, quality of life, and the overall well-being of clients (T. Black, personal communication, July 6, 1999)

10. Rehabilitation nurses, who are particularly suited to the role of case manager, need to market their approach and philosophy to a variety of employers, insurance companies, inpatient settings, physicians, and other community-based services (C. Tracey, personal communication, June 10, 1999)

11. The hospital will be more acute, and the rehabilitation unit that presently exists will change as more patients are cared for in their homes, retirement centers, and other living arrangements in the community (B. Warner, personal communication, July 7, 1999)

12. The shift in care from inpatient settings to community settings will continue. The use of acute rehabilitation settings will decrease due to changes in reimbursement, and the acuity and complexity of care in all settings will continue to increase. Also, the application of rehabilitation concepts in long-term care settings will increase (C. Jacelon, personal communication, July 1, 1999)

13. Rehabilitation nurses will continue to work in long-term inpatient care and home care and will move into more community-based areas such as adult day care, assisted living, and other programs that promote living in

the least restrictive environment (C. Tracey, personal communication, June 10, 1999)

C. The Impending Nursing Shortage and Recruitment Issues

1. A large number of the nursing workforce will reach retirement age in the years 2000 to 2010. This decrease in the workforce will come at a time when there is also declining enrollment in nursing schools and declining interest in young people in the nursing profession (K. Johnson, personal communication, July 12, 1999)

2. Recruitment and education issues will arise because of the nursing shortage (M. Ter Maat, personal communication, June 23, 1999)

3. Rehabilitation nurses must find ways to entice people into the profession and pay them equitably for what they do (K. Johnson, personal communication, July 12, 1999)

4. The demand for rehabilitation clinical nurse specialists will increase as the nursing workforce decreases

5. With an overabundance of therapy practitioners and a shortage of nursing healthcare practitioners, the challenge for rehabilitation nurses will be to identify the value of what they do, clarify that it takes a registered nurse to do it, and help recruit the younger generation into the field (K. Johnson, personal communication, July 12, 1999)

D. The Healthcare Crisis: Access, Equity, and Reimbursement Issues

1. As managed care continues to cut back on or tighten reimbursement, cost and access to care will continue to be big issues (C. Tracey, personal communication, June 10, 1999)

2. Access and equity of care for all will be big issues, as well as who will be allowed to provide rehabilitation services: Access will be an issue because of changes in Medicaid eligibility and managed care programs, and equity will be an issue for those who may be denied benefits (T. Thompson, personal communication, June 22, 1999)

3. Health care will continue to be at a crisis level, and the lack of funding and other

resources will severely change the landscape of the delivery system (K. Johnson, personal communication, July 12, 1999)

4. Problems with environmental, financial, and geographic access to services and the availability of practitioners who understand the needs of patients who are elderly, chronically ill, and disabled will be important issues (K. Johnson, personal communication, July 12, 1999)

E. Primary Care for Individuals with Disabilities

1. Individuals with disabilities and chronic diseases will need primary care and preventive care (B. Warner, personal communication, July 7, 1999)

2. AAPMR formed a special interest group for primary care for people with disabilities to look at the issues of service delivery models, especially collaborative models with other specialties (B. Warner, personal communication, July 7, 1999)

F. Ethical Issues and Dilemmas

1. Nurses will increasingly face the challenge of working with individuals choosing to end their own life (B. Warner, personal communication, July 7, 1999)

2. Nurses will have to consider their position on laws dealing with patients' rights and choices

3. Nurses will need to consider how to appropriately involve patients in issues relating to quality and end-of-life decision making (M. Ter Maat, personal communication, August 29, 1999)

4. Nurses will need to assess their own feelings and attitudes related to ethical issues and dilemmas such as cloning, organ transplantation, and assisted suicide

G. Decision Making

1. Nurses will have an even more instrumental role in decision making and providing efficient and effective rehabilitation care (T. Black, personal communication, July 6, 1999)

2. Nurses will have a greater role in measuring and monitoring client outcomes (T. Black, personal communication, July 6, 1999)

Reference

McCourt, A.E. (Ed.). (1993). *The specialty practice of rehabilitation nursing: A core curriculum* (3rd ed.). Skokie, IL: The Rehabilitation Nursing Foundation of the Association of Rehabilitation Nurses.

Suggested resources

Allan, W. (1958). *Rehabilitation: A community challenge*. New York: John Wiley.

Association of Rehabilitation Nurses (ARN) 20th Anniversary Task Force. (1994). *Celebrating 20 years of magic*. Skokie, IL: ARN.

Bitter, J. (1979). *Introduction to rehabilitation*. St. Louis: Mosby.

Edwards, P.A. (1992). The evolution of rehabilitation facilities for children. *Rehabilitation Nursing, 17*, 191-192.

Mumma, C. (Ed.). (1987). *Rehabilitation nursing: Concepts and practice* (2nd ed.). Evanston, IL: Rehabilitation Nursing Foundation.

Novak, S., & McCourt, A. (1994, September). *History in the making*. Session presented at the ARN 20th Anniversary Educational Conference, Orlando, FL.

Acknowledgments

Thanks go to Terrie Black, Cynthia Jacelon, Kelly Johnson, Ann McCourt, Marilyn Ter Maat, Teresa Thompson, Cathy Tracey, and Barbara Warner for sharing their insights on the future of rehabilitation nursing.

Appendix A: Case Studies

These case studies represent individuals at five different developmental stages with various problems and rehabilitation needs. The cases can be used in classroom teaching, review sessions for certification, and as an individual learning activity. As you read the cases and answer the questions, refer to related sections of the core curriculum for specific content.

Case Study 1

Linda L. Pierce, PhD RNC CNS CRRN
Associate Professor, Medical College of Ohio, School of Nursing, Toledo, OH

Joe was 80 years old, had Type II Diabetes Mellitus, and had recently suffered a left cerebrovascular accident that left him with right hemiplegia and mild aphasia. Joe never married. Until he retired, Joe was a high school reading teacher and active in various social programs in his community. After retirement, he continued working for the Association of Teachers, serving as an adviser on literacy issues. He lived in a small apartment on the second floor of a large building. When his brother Jim's wife died a year earlier, Jim moved in with Joe because the two brothers had always been very close.

As Joe recovered from his stroke, he participated in an intensive rehabilitation program in an inpatient hospital and then continued his therapy in a skilled nursing facility. He was an active participant in physical, occupational, speech, and recreational therapies. Joe worked with determination to learn to walk with a cane and gain back his ability to speak fluently. The staff gave Joe much encouragement, which made him feel proud of his accomplishments. He learned to stand up and sit down, put on most of his clothes, shower independently, and walk from one end of the hall to the other. Speech therapy helped him to substitute certain words and make himself understood. When the time came to be discharged from the facility, Jim was willing to help Joe with daily activities. Jim learned to give medications and manage the treatment regimen for diabetes care. Jim's daughter, who lived in the same apartment building, took over the heavy household chores for the two men.

On returning to his apartment, Joe was elated to be back in his own home. However, he soon realized that he was a burden to the others, having to ask for help to complete even simple tasks. Joe was increasingly bothered by his niece, who lovingly attended to his needs before he even had a chance to ask for help. At times, Joe responded gruffly and noticed that he hurt his niece's feelings. Joe then felt guilty, although he kept quiet about it. Nonetheless, he was unable to shake off his anger about his helpless situation. When home alone, Joe fully perceived the losses he had never dealt with before, and he realized how unrealistic it was to expect a return to his old lifestyle. Rather than being active and going places, Joe felt trapped in his apartment without being able to independently master the stairs to his front door. For Joe, reading was the most difficult problem. When he tried to write a note, he noticed that the words did not look right.

Joe's anger grew day by day and was directed at his condition. Jim and his daughter suffered from Joe's moods, his many complaints, demands, nagging about little things, and his lack of gratitude for their help. Then Joe refused to bathe, dress, walk, or even eat. One day, his niece, unable to tolerate the tension, exploded with anger. She shouted that she could not stand Joe's behavior and that Joe should shape up or she would leave. That night Joe swallowed a handful of sleeping pills. Jim discovered the empty pill bottle and called an ambulance just in time to save Joe.

After spending a few days in the acute care hospital, Joe found himself in another nursing home. A psychiatric evaluation diagnosed Joe with reactive depression. Jim informed the nurse of earlier events and Joe added some information from his perspective. In order to gain a fuller understanding of the extent of Joe's losses, the nurse contacted Joe's rehabilitation nurse case manager. Together, the nurses examined Joe's life processes before and after his stroke and connected this information with Joe's potential of regaining certain functions.

Questions for Thought

1. Discuss Joe's circumstances from a developmental theory/framework approach. Describe his situational and maturational state of affairs.
2. Choose a family theory and complete an assessment of Joe's family.
3. Identify at least one priority physical, psychological, and social nursing diagnosis. State several interventions for each nursing diagnosis and how these interventions can be evaluated.
4. Give examples of how the rehabilitation team can deal with these complex problems within a developmental framework.
5. Describe strategies that the nurse can use to guide the team toward a successful outcome for Joe's family.

Case Study 2

Bonnie J. Parker, MSN RN CRRN
Rehabilitation Nurse Consultant, Private Practice,
Waterford, VA

Mike was a 21-year-old college sophomore going to school on a football scholarship at a campus approximately 4 hours from his home. During a pickup game, he jumped for a ball, had his feet taken out from under him, and landed flat on his back. He sustained a C3-C4 spinal cord injury and was insensate with no motor function from the C4 level down.

He went through an acute spinal cord injury program at a freestanding rehabilitation facility. His parents were very supportive and his mother worked diligently to be a caregiver, advocate, and case manager for her son. His father was the primary financial support for the family. Mike's rehabilitative care was funded through his father's insurance and a catastrophic insurance policy held by the school. Upon discharge, Mike returned to his parents' home. The catastrophic policy paid to have his parents' home and a home near his college modified for accessibility. A van was purchased with a lift, which allowed him to be out in the community. He had 24-hour nursing care to meet his self-care and home maintenance needs. The catastrophic policy had a cap of $100,000 per year for home healthcare services. This amount was not adequate to meet his yearly needs; however, his father's policy provided the supplemental insurance necessary to meet Mike's healthcare needs and maintain his living arrangements in his home environment. Although he was not ventilator dependent, Mike required assistance for all activities of daily living. He required intermittent catheterization every 4 hours and was on an every-other-day bowel program.

Mike decided to return to school. At this time his father changed jobs and, unfortunately, Mike's condition was now considered preexisting and the insurance company would not provide for Mike's care. Although the catastrophic policy insurance company had a telephonic nurse case manager, she was not an active participant in Mike's care. Mike was dependent for meeting his self-care needs. However, he could direct his care and was motivated to maintain control of his life. He received a letter from the catastrophic policy insurance company stating that his home care benefits would expire before the end of the year. His mother petitioned the insurance company. After many letters and telephone calls, Mike and his mother were successful in getting the insurance company to agree to "go out of policy" and continue his benefits for the year.

Despite this concession, Mike was told by the insurance company this benefit would not be granted for the following year. They added that his coverage would be dropped at age 22, because he no longer qualified as a dependent. This decision led to a great deal of frustration for both Mike and his mother. The insurance company would not pay for care unless it was delivered through a licensed home-health agency. Mike could have gotten his care much less expensively by hiring his own personal care attendants. Additionally, because of the level of service that Mike required (intermittent catheterization and a bowel program) this care could be provided only by licensed staff as directed by the nurse practice act in his state of residence.

Out of frustration and a desperate attempt to maintain control over his own life, Mike sought the assistance of an attorney to defend his right to remain in his home and ultimately control his own life. Mike was granted a temporary injunction that provided him with home healthcare benefits until his case could go to trial.

Questions for Thought

1. If you were the case manager how would you have managed this case differently?
2. Are there other resources available for a client like Mike?
3. What ongoing educational needs should be addressed related to prevention of complications requiring rehospitalization?
4. What changes in policy with third-party payers should be considered to better maximize independence and control for the client?

Case Study 3

Lyn R. Sapp, BSN RN CRRN
Rehabilitation Department, Children's Hospital and
Regional Medical Center, Seattle, WA

Six-year-old Tommy was visiting a horse, well known to him and his family. His father looked over and saw Tommy on the ground. It was presumed the horse had kicked him. No one could have predicted the roller coaster of events that followed. Tommy sustained a left fronto-temporal depressed skull fracture. After emergency aid and services, Tommy was in a coma, his family waiting for Tommy to "wake up." He went from intensive care to a long-term care facility at Rancho level II. The family hoped this would be short-term placement. After a 6-week "asleep" coma, Tommy began to have more awakening response. Three months after his original injury, Tommy transferred to the inpatient rehabilitation unit at Rancho level III.

For the next 8 months, Tommy learned to eat, talk, dress, walk, toilet, curb behaviors, and work through frustrations of word finding, medication side effects, equipment use, and reintegration back into community life. Feeding remained a critical issue, as Tommy had a silent aspiration confirmed by a videofluroscopic swallowing study. A gastrostomy tube had been placed early in his recovery for nutritional support. The nursing staff monitored Tommy's progress with the speech therapist, as oral feeds were slowly introduced. The rehabilitation nurses also began teaching the family gastrostomy tube management and feeding/water supplementation, as it was going to be a slow process. Because of the postinjury hydrocephalus, a craniectomy left a large area of no bone protection for his brain. A bike helmet was required for 6 months. Tommy had difficulty with compliance, so the nursing team collaborated with the therapy team and developed a sticker reward program. This provided Tommy with a positive outcome for helmet-wearing compliance.

When Tommy was on the rehabilitation unit, it was evident that he was a survivor. His strong will came through, especially at times when he did not want to participate in therapies, get ready for the day, or settle in for the night's sleep. It took creative strategies by the nursing team, family, and therapy team to help him want to participate, and overcome some of the obstinance that the head injury exacerbated. He struggled with disinhibition, acting before thinking of consequences, and there were times of rage and anger followed by sweetness and remorse.

During acute rehabilitation, Tommy worked with a hospital-based school teacher. Reintegration to school was part of his rehabilitation plan. Communication was crucial to the school system for the school nurse, teacher, school psychologist, and therapist. The transition from acute rehabilitation to outpatient follow-up incorporated inpatient and outpatient nurse care management. Care issues included toileting, access, feeding, safety, and supervision by an adult at all times with the "two feet on the ground" rule. The hospital-based teacher worked with Tommy's school district, and helped develop an individualized education plan. Tommy was discharged to a program he could best participate in, a self-contained classroom.

The primary nurse worked with the family and rehabilitation team to identify educational issues preparatory to discharge. The following topics were addressed: general acquired brain injury (ABI) information and resources, medications, supervision, elimination control strategies, functional mobility in the home and community environments, acceptable behavior, and strategies for modifying challenging behaviors. Goals were defined and a discharge teaching plan was developed. The rehabilitation nurses, therapists, and physicians worked together with the family to implement the plan, track progress, and make modifications as needed.

Questions for Thought

1. What nursing interventions are indicated when behavior goes out of control, including combativeness, refusal of care, and verbal and physical anger, in the pediatric rehabilitation hospitalized setting?
2. List ongoing strategies that Tommy will need for successful transition to an independent lifestyle?
3. What community resources are available to Tommy and his family?
4. How are family members, especially siblings, affected in such cases, and how can they be supported and incorporated into care?

Case Study 4

Marjorie J. Culbertson, MSE MSN RN CS
Instructor of Nursing, Medical College of Ohio,
School of Nursing, Toledo, OH

Karen was a 50-year-old single woman. She had repeated hospitalizations for pain management, an exacerbation of asthma, and depression, resulting in 10 weeks of hospital stay over 5 months. Her medical problems consist of degenerative disc disease, asthma, obesity, a cerebral vascular accident and bipolar disorder. Karen received a BA degree in education and pursued graduate studies in special education. She taught elementary school for several years before she became ill. She had been without long-term employment for 5 years because of her physical and mental problems. She was on disability. While out of the hospital, she lived with her two cats on the second floor of a low-income apartment building with an elevator. She had a tub chair and a raised toilet seat in the bathroom.

Her weight was 173 pounds; she was 5 feet tall. She gained 50 pounds within a year. She attributed the weight gain to the prednisone she took for asthma and to medications for depression. Her eating pattern was sporadic. She relied on microwave dinners, crackers and peanut butter, and fast food restaurants. She had no food allergies.

Her degenerative disk disease advanced over the years and she used a walker for ambulating. She wore a back brace for stability and pain reduction. Lack of pain management kept Karen from physical exercises that might help with her weight management. In addition, her extra weight aggravated the back pain. She took Nuprin q4 h for pain. Because of her inactivity, she was rarely sleepy at bedtime, and took medication to help her sleep. She slept about 10 hours at night and denied taking naps during the day. She went to physical therapy three times a week to help her regain her balance and strength. The right cerebral vascular accident resulted in left-sided weakness and, consequently, her gait was unsteady. In addition, she had a vision deficit. The combination of weakness and her vision deficit contributed to four falls at home in 3 months.

Karen viewed the health system as supportive of her needs. A visiting nurse saw Karen once a week to check her blood pressure, to see if she was taking her medications correctly, and to assess her physical and mental condition. Karen saw her psychologist once a week and her psychiatrist twice a month. Her psychiatrist prescribed an MAO inhibitor, so she coped with learning to eat foods that are not contraindicated with this medication. She admitted to experiencing some relief of depression since taking the new medication. She eventually experienced some urinary incontinence and constipation. The constipation and extra weight may have contributed to the incontinence. Incontinence did not keep her from socializing, since she protected herself. She was knowledgeable about Kegel exercises, but would not follow a Kegel program. She admitted that she did not drink water and only three glasses of liquid per day.

Even though she enjoyed socializing, her social contacts were few. She did not keep in close contact with family. Her best friend, Betty, was elderly but quite healthy. Another of Karen's friends, Judy, who also suffered with depression, was a supportive, caring friend for many years. But one day Judy took her own life when Karen was out of town. Judy's death affected Karen deeply, but she stated that she resolved the loss through her belief in a merciful God. Karen admitted to having had suicidal thoughts in the past, but she never had a plan. Financially, Karen had a hard time making ends meet. Her disability check paid for rent, cable television, car maintenance, medications, clothing, and food. She also rented a hospital bed at $60 per month. Medications were a major expense, and sometimes she went without them when she needed food or incurred other bills.

Questions for Thought

1. What are Karen's self-care capabilities and limitations? What specific problems can you identify?
2. What community resources are there to help with the identified problems?
3. Who might you contact to discuss her financial needs?
4. What nursing interventions might help keep Karen from having an exacerbation of asthma?
5. What realistic outcomes might you propose for Karen?

Case Study 5

Jenecia Fairfax, MSN RN
Instructor, Community Health Nursing, Medical
College of Ohio, School of Nursing, Toledo, OH

Gloria was a 65-year-old African-American who worked as a nurse in a youth home until she retired on disability at age 50. Her husband lived in another city during the week because of his job as a nurse in a psychiatric hospital, and they divorced last year. Her daughter and granddaughter lived in the same city as Gloria, but the relationship with them was always problematic. She lived in a townhouse cooperative with bedrooms and a full bath on the second floor and a laundry in the basement.

Fifteen years ago, she experienced pain in her right hip after a fall. She was told that she had a pulled muscle in the groin. The pain continued for several months. Consultation with an orthopedist revealed a fracture of the right hip with displacement and nonunion. She was also diagnosed with osteoporosis. A total hip replacement was performed. Her recovery was uneventful. She continued to live independently, attend church, and participate in committees and youth programs at her church, but she retired from her job.

Ten years later, Gloria fell in a supermarket and damaged her right hip. A second hip replacement was performed. After surgery she spent 2 weeks at a rehabilitation hospital where she received physical therapy, including stair climbing. After discharge she continued physical therapy at home for a month. She was able to go up and down stairs independently and prepare her own meals. Her husband did the grocery shopping on the weekends and friends would take her to the bank and do other errands. The relationship with her daughter and granddaughter was somewhat improved and Gloria received a substantial settlement from the supermarket where her injury occurred.

Last winter, Gloria fell in the parking lot of her cooperative and experienced pain in the right hip. She did not visit a doctor. In the spring she saw an orthopedist at the urging of a friend, a nurse, who noted that she was not only walking with a limp but that there was visible displacement of the right hip. X rays showed that the prosthesis was damaged and would need to be replaced. She was admitted for a total hip replacement; however, a large pocket of infection was discovered. Two Jackson Pratt drains were inserted. She remained in the hospital for a week, receiving intravenous antibiotics, and was discharged home on oral antibiotics for a month with daily dressing changes. She refused home care and a friend did daily dressing changes. During a visit the nurse friend noticed a large amount of beer in the second upstairs bedroom. On several occasions the friend noted that Gloria's speech was slurred and it was hard to follow her conversations during telephone calls. During this time Gloria continued to live alone. Friends did her shopping, cleaning, cooking, and banking. At the time of admission Gloria decided to stop smoking. She had smoked a pack of cigarettes a day for the past 30 years.

In the fall, Gloria returned to the hospital. The infection had not cleared up. The orthopedist did extensive debridement and again inserted two Jackson Pratt drains. Intravenous antibiotics were started. She remained in intensive care for a week, then transferred to the orthopedic unit to a private room, to minimize the chance of her becoming infected with any opportunistic organisms. The need for IV antibiotics every 4 hours prevented Gloria from being discharged to her home. She was transferred to an extended care facility for 6 weeks. It was determined that, when she was free of infection, a total hip replacement would be done.

Nowadays, Gloria continues to be optimistic about her future. She feels that the infection will clear up and surgery will be successful. She has made plans to go to a rehabilitation facility after surgery. She spends her time reading romance novels and watching television. She plans to continue to live in her current home. She feels that her friends will continue to be of assistance and that she will be able to navigate the stairs once a day. The relationship with her daughter has become strained. She recently obtained a restraining order against the daughter after she "stole" $200 from her.

Questions for Thought

1. Discuss Gloria's ability to remain independent, including the role of social supports (family, friends, church members, and neighbors).
2. Discuss the impact of her present illness on Gloria's developmental stage.
3. What are Gloria's self-care deficits?

Note. These case studies are composites based on many sources: clients, families, and readings; thus, they do not represent any one particular individual.

Appendix B: Community and Health-Related Resources

··

This appendix contains a list of resources on many health-related topics. The list includes names, addresses, and telephone numbers as well as Web sites that can be used to obtain further information. Information was confirmed at press time but is subject to change. This is not a complete listing; rather, it is meant to serve as a starting point.

Acquired Immune Deficiency Syndrome
CDC National AIDS Hotline (NAH)
Centers for Disease Control and Prevention
National Center for HIV, STD and TB Prevention
Divisions of HIV/AIDS Prevention
800-342-2437
www.cdc.gov/nchstp/hiv_aids/hivinfo/nah.htm

Alzheimer's
Alzheimer's Association
919 North Michigan Avenue, Suite 1000
Chicago, IL 60611-1676
312-335-8700/800-272-3900
www.alz.org

Alzheimer's Disease Education and Referral Center (ADEAR)
PO Box 8250
Silver Spring, MD 20907-8250
800-438-4380
www.alzheimers.org

Amputation
American Amputee Foundation
Box 250218, Hillcrest Station
Little Rock, AR 72225
501-666-2523

National Amputation Foundation
38–40 Church Street
Malverne, NY 11565
516-887-3600
www.va.gov/vso/naf.htm

Architectural and Transportation Barriers
Accessibility Concepts, Inc.
6408 Woodbeach Drive
Fort Worth, TX 76133
817-263-5153
www.accessibilityconcepts.com

Architectural and Transportation Barriers Compliance Board (U.S. Access Board)
1331 F St. NW
Washington, DC 20004
800-872-2253/202-272-5434
www.access-board.gov

Overcoming Mobility Barriers International (OMBI)
1022 S. 41st St.
Omaha, NE 68105
402-342-5731
www.arcat.com/arcatcos.cos08/arc08659.cfm

The Center for Universal Design
North Carolina State University School of Design
Box 8613, 219 Oberlin Road
Raleigh, NC 27695-8613
919-515-3082/800-647-6777
www.design.ncsu.edu/cud/center/contacts/contactus.htm

Arthritis
Arthritis Foundation
1330 West Peachtree St.
Atlanta, GA 30309
404-872-7100/800-283-7800
www.arthritis.org
(Includes information for the American Juvenile Arthritis Organization.)

Assistive Technology
ABLEDATA
8401 Colesville Road, Suite 200
Silver Spring, MD 20910
800-227-0216
www.abledata.com/sire_2/default.htm

Assistive Technology Industry Association
526 Davis St., Suite 217
Evanston, IL 60201-4686
877-687-2842/847-869-1282
www.atia.org

Massachusetts Assistive Technology Partnership (MATP)
Children's Hospital
1295 Boylston St., Suite 310
Boston, MA 02215
617-355-7820
www.matp.org

Asthma and Allergy
American College of Allergy, Asthma and
Immunology
85 West Algonquin Road, Suite 550
Arlington Heights, IL 60005
http://allergy.mcg.edu

American Lung Association
1740 Broadway
New York, NY 10019
212-315-8700/800-586-4872
www.lungusa.org

Asthma and Allergy Foundation of America
1233 20th St. NW Suite 402
Washington, DC 20036
202-466-7643
www.aafa.org

The Allergy and Asthma Network
2751 Prosperity Ave., Suite 150
Fairfax, VA 22031
800-878-4403/703-641-9595
www.aanma.org

Blindness
American Council of the Blind
1155 15th St. NW, Suite 1004
Washington, DC 20005
202-467-5081/800-424-8666
www.acb.org

American Foundation for the Blind
11 Penn Plaza, Suite 300
New York, NY 10001
212-502-7600/800-232-5463
www.afb.org

National Federation of the Blind
1800 Johnson St.
Baltimore, MD 21230
410-659-9314
www.nfb.org

Cancer
Cancer Information Service
454 Brookline Ave.
Boston, MA 02115
800-422-6237
http://cis.nci.nih.gov/contact

National Cancer Institute
Public Inquiries Office
Building 31, Room 10A02
31 Center Drive, MSC 2580
Bethesda, MD 20892-2580
301-435-3848/800-4-Cancer
www.nci.nih.gov

American Cancer Society
800-ACS-2345
www.cancer.org

Children and Families
Children's Defense Fund
25 E. Street NW
Washington, DC 20001
202-628-8787
www.childrensdefense.org

Family Caregiver Alliance
690 Market Street, Suite 600
San Francisco, CA 94104
415-434-3388
www.caregiver.org

Family Village
Waisman Center
University of Wisconsin–Madison
1500 Highland Avenue
Madison, WI 53705-2280
www.familyvillage.wisc.edu

Family Voices
PO Box 769
Algodones, NM 87001
505-867-2368/888-835-5669
www.familyvoices.org

National Information Center for Children and Youth
with Disabilities
PO Box 1492
Washington, DC 20013-1492
800-695-0285/202-884-8200
www.nichcy.org

Diabetes

American Diabetes Association
1701 North Beauregard Street
Alexandria, VA 22311
800-372-2383
www.diabetes.org

Joslin Diabetes Center
One Joslin Place
Boston, MA 02215
617-732-2400
www.joslin.harvard.edu

Juvenile Diabetes Foundation
120 Wall Street
New York, NY 10005
212-785-9500/800-JDF-CURE
www.df.org

National Diabetes Information Clearinghouse
One Information Way
Bethesda, MD 20892-3560
www.niddk.nih.gov/health/diabetes

Disability Services

American Heart Association National Center
7272 Greenville Ave.
Dallas, TX 75231
800-AHA-USA1
www.americanheart.org

Canine Companions for Independence
PO Box 446
Santa Rosa, CA 95402-0446
800-572-2275
www.caninecompanions.org

Clearinghouse on Disability Information
U.S. Department of Education, Switzer Building,
Room 3132
Washington, DC 20202-2524
202-205-8241

Council for Disability Rights
205 West Randolph, Suite 1650
Chicago, IL 60606
312-444-9484
www.disabilityrights.org

Disability Rights Center
2500 Q St. NW, Suite 121
Washington, DC 20007
202-337-4119

March of Dimes
1275 Mamaroneck Ave.
White Plains, NY 10605
888-663-4637
www.modimes.org

Leukemia Society of America
600 Third Ave.
New ork, NY 10016
800-955-4LSA/212-573-8484
www.leukemia.org

National Easter Seals Society
230 West Monroe Street, Suite 1800
Chicago, IL 60606
312-726-6200
www.easter-seals.org

National Rehabilitation Information Center
1010 Wayne Ave., Suite 800
Silver Spring, MD 20910
301-562-2400/800-346-2742
www.naric.com

Elderly

National Institute on Aging
Public Information Office
Building 31, Room 5C27
31 Center Drive, MSC 2292
Bethesda, MD 20892
301-496-1752
www.nih.gov/nia

Head Injury

The Brain Injury Association, Inc.
105 N. Alfred Street
Alexandria, VA 22314
703-236-6000
www.biausa.org

National Head Injury Foundation
1776 Massachusetts Avenue, NW, Suite 100
Washington, DC 20036
202-296-6443/800-444-6443
www.healthy.net/pan/cso/cioi.NHIF.htm

Healthcare Facilities and Programs

American Health Care Association
1201 L Street, NW
Washington, DC 20005
202-842-4444
www.ahca.org

American Hospital Association Headquarters
One North Franklin
Chicago, IL 60606
312-422-3000
www.aha.org

CARF...The Rehabilitation Accreditation
    Commission
4891 E. Grant Road
Tucson, AZ 85712
520-325-1044
www.carf.org

Joint Commission on Accreditation of Healthcare
    Organizations
One Renaissance Boulevard
Oakbrook Terrace, IL 60181
630-792-5000
www.jcaho.org

Healthcare-Related Federal Agencies
Agency for Healthcare Research and Quality
2101 East Jefferson Street
Rockville, MD 20852
800-358-9295
www.ahcpr.gov

Department of Health and Human Services
www.hhs.gov

Medicaid
www.hcfa.gov/medicaid

Medicare
800-633-4227
www.medicare.gov

Children's Health Insurance Program (CHIP)
877-543-7669
www.hcfa.gov/init/children.htm

National Institute on Disability and Rehabilitation
    Research
www.ed.gov/offices/OSERS/NIDRR

Rehabilitation Services Administration
www.ed.gov/offices/OSERS/RSA

Hearing and Speech
Better Hearing Institute
5021-B Backlick Road
Annandale, VA 22003
800-EAR-WELL
www.betterhearing.org

Hearing, Speech and Deafness Center
1620 18th Ave.
Seattle, WA 98122-2798
888-328-2974/206-323-5770
www.hsdc.org

Incontinence
Simon Foundation for Incontinence
PO Box 835
Wilmette, IL 60091
800-23-SIMON
http://urologychannel.com/education/ed_
incontinence.html

Neurologic and Muscular Disorders
ALS Association National Office
27001 Agoura Road, Suite 150
Calabassas Hills, CA 91301-5104
800-782-4747/818-880-9007
www.alsa.org

Epilepsy Foundation of America
4351 Garden City Drive
Landover, MD 20785
800-EFA-1000/301-459-3700
www.efa.org

Guillain-Barré Syndrome Foundation International
PO Box 262
Wynnewood, PA 19096
610-667-0131
http://terri.adsnet.com/jsteinhi/html/gbs/gbsfi

Myasthenia Gravis Foundation of America
123 W. Madison St., Suite 800
Chicago, IL 60602
800-541-5454/312-853-0522
www.myasthenia.org

Multiple Sclerosis Foundation
6350 N. Andrews Avenue
Fort Lauderdale, FL 33309
954-776-6805/800-441-7055
www.msfacts.org

Muscular Dystrophy Association National
Headquarters
3300 E. Sunrise Drive
Tucson, AZ 85718
800-572-1777
www.mdausa.org

National Center for Neurogenic Communication
Disorders
The University of Arizona PO Box 210071
Tucson, AZ 85721
www.shs.arizona.edu

Osteogenesis Imperfecta Foundation, Inc.
804 W. Diamond Ave., Suite 210
Gaithersburg, MD 20878
800-981-2663/301-947-0083
www.oif.org

Parkinson's Disease Foundation, Inc.
710 W. 168th Street
New York, NY 10032-9982
800-457-6676
www.pdf.org

Spina Bifida Association of America
4590 MacArthur Blvd. NW, Suite 250
Washington, DC 20007-4226
800-621-3141/202-944-3285
www.sbaa.org

United Cerebral Palsy
1660 L Street NW, Suite 700
Washington, DC 20036
800-872-5827
www.ucpa.org

Nursing Organizations

American Association of Neuroscience Nurses
4700 W. Lake Ave.
Glenview, IL 60025-1485
888-557-2266/847-375-4733
www.aann.org

American Association of Spinal Cord Injury Nurses
(AASCIN)
75-20 Astoria Blvd.
Jackson Heights, NY 11370-1177
718-803-3782
www.aascin.org

American Holistic Nurses Association
PO Box 2130
Flagstaff, AZ 86003-2130
800-278-AHNA
http://ahna.org

American Nurses Association
600 Maryland Avenue SW, Suite 100 West
Washington, DC 20024
800-274-4ANA/202-651-7000
www.ana.org

American Society of Pain Management Nurses
7794 Grow Drive
Pensacola, FL 32514-7072
850-473-0233

Association of Nurses in AIDS Care
11250 Roger Bacon Dr., Suite 8
Reston, VA 20190-5202
800-260-6780/703-925-0081
www.anacnet.org

Association of Rehabilitation Nurses
4700 W. Lake Ave.
Glenview, IL 60025-1485
800-229-7530/847-375-4710
www.rehabnurse.org

Nursing Ethics Network
Boston College SON, Cushing Hall
140 Commonwealth Ave.
Chestnut Hill, MA 02467
616-552-2230
www.bc.edu/bc_org/avp/son/ethics/nen.html

Society of Pediatric Nurses
2170 S. Parker Road, #350
Denver, CO 80231
800-723-2902
www.pednurse.org

Society of Urologic Nurses and Associates
East Holly Ave., Box 56
Pitman, NJ 08071-0056
856-256-2351

Pain

American Pain Society
4700 W. Lake Ave.
Glenview, IL 60025
847-375-4715
www.ampainsoc.org

Rehabilitation Professionals

American Academy for Cerebral Palsy and
Developmental Medicine
6300 North River Road, Suite 727
Rosemont, IL 60018-4226
847-698-1635
http://aacpdm.org

American Academy of Physical Medicine and
   Rehabilitation
One IBM Plaza, Suite 2500
Chicago, IL 60611-3604
312-464-9700
www.aapmr.org

American Occupational Therapy Association
4720 Montgomery Lane, PO Box 31220
Bethesda, MD 20824-1220
301-652-2682
www.aota.org

American Physical Therapy Association
1111 North Fairfax St.
Alexandria, VA 22314-1488
888-386-7200
www.apta.org

American Speech-Language-Hearing Association
10801 Rockville Pike
Rockville, MD 20852
888-321-ASHA
www.asha.org

National Rehabilitation Association
633 S. Washington St.
Alexandria, VA 22314
703-836-0850
www.nationalrehab.org

National Therapeutic Recreation Society
22377 Belmont Ridge Road
Ashburn, VA 20148
703-858-0748
www.nrpa.org

Sexuality
Sexual Health Network
3 Mayflower Lane
Huntington, CT 06484
203-924-4623
www.sexualhealth.com

Sexuality Information and Education Council of the
U.S. (SIECUS)
130 West 42nd St., Suite 350
New York, NY 10036-7802
212-819-9770
www.siecus.org

Spinal Cord Injury
Christopher Reeve Paralysis Foundation
500 Morris Ave.
Springfield, NJ 07081
800-225-0292
http://paralysis.apacure.org

The Miami Project to Cure Paralysis
www.miamiproject.miami.edu

Paralyzed Veterans of America
801 18th St. NW
Washington, DC 20006-3517
800-424-8200
www.pva.org

Sports and Recreation
Disabled Sports USA
451 Hungerford Dr., Suite 100
Rockville, MD 20850
301-217-0960
www.dsusa.org

Special Olympics, Inc.
1325 G St. NW, Suite 500
Washington, DC 20005
202-628-3630
www.specialolympics.org

Wheelchair Sports USA
3595 E. Fountain Blvd., Suite L-1
Colorado Springs, CO 80910
719-574-1150
www.wsusa.org

Stroke
National Institute for Neurologic Disorders and Stroke
National Institutes of Health
PO Box 5801
Bethesda, MD 20824
www.ninds.nih.gov

National Stroke Association
9707 East Easter Lane
Englewood, CO 80112-3747
800-787-6537/303-649-9299
www.stroke.org

Index